MW01133908

Sarcoma

Robert M. Henshaw

Editor

Sarcoma

A Multidisciplinary Approach
to Treatment

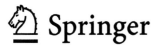 Springer

Editor
Robert M. Henshaw
Medstar Orthopedic Oncology
Washington Cancer Institute
Washington, District of Columbia, USA

ISBN 978-3-319-43119-2   ISBN 978-3-319-43121-5   (eBook)
DOI 10.1007/978-3-319-43121-5

Library of Congress Control Number: 2017941711

Printed on acid-free paper

This Springer imprint is published by Springer Nature
The registered company is Springer International Publishing AG
The registered company address is: Gewerbestrasse 11, 6330 Cham, Switzerland

Contents

List of Contributors

Albert J. Aboulafia, M.D., M.B.A. Cancer Institute, National Center for Bone and Soft Tissue Tumors, MedStar Franklin Square Medical Center, Baltimore, MD, USA

Sanjeev Agarwal, M.D. Department of Orthopaedic Surgery and Rehabilitation Medicine, SUNY Downstate Medical Center, Brooklyn, NY, USA

Osman Ali, M.D. Hematology and Oncology, Brooklyn Cancer Care, Medical PC, Brooklyn, NY, USA

Francesca Beaman, M.D. Division of Musculoskeletal Radiology, Radiology and Orthopedic Surgery, University of Kentucky College of Medicine, Lexington, KY, USA

Peter J. Brown, M.B.A. Mattie Miracle Cancer Foundation, Washington, DC, USA

Caitlin Cicone, D.O. Department of Orthopaedic Surgery and Rehabilitation Medicine, SUNY Downstate Medical Center, Brooklyn, NY, USA

Tanya DiFrancesco, M.D. Hematology and Oncology, Brooklyn Cancer Care, Medical PC, Brooklyn, NY, USA

Jeffrey S. Dome, M.D., Ph.D. Divisions of Hematology and Oncology, Children's National Health System, George Washington University School of Medicine and Health Sciences, Washington, DC, USA

Helen Findlay, M.Sc. Orthopaedic Surgical Oncology, Glasgow Royal Infirmary, Glasgow, Scotland, UK

Wei Guo, M.D., Ph.D. Department of Orthopedic Oncology, Bone Tumor Research Laboratory, Musculoskeletal Tumor Center, Peking University People's Hospital, Beijing, China

Marie Kate Gurka, M.D. Radiation Oncology, University of Louisville, Louisville, KY, USA

Mansur Halai, B.Sc. (Hons), M.B.Ch.B. Glasgow Royal Infirmary, Glasgow, Scotland, UK

K. William Harter, M.D. Clinical Radiation Medicine, Department of Radiation Medicine, Georgetown University, Washington, DC, USA

Kimberly Haynes, D.N.P., A.P.R.N. Sarcoma Center, The University of Kansas Cancer Center, Overland Park, KS, USA

Robert M. Henshaw, M.D. Georgetown University School of Medicine, Washington, DC, USA

Department of Orthopedics, MedStar Washington Hospital Center, Washington, DC, USA

Division of Orthopedic Oncology, MedStar Georgetown Orthopedic Institute, Washington, DC, USA

MedStar Washington Cancer Institute, Washington, DC, USA

Orthopedic Oncology, Children's National Medical Center, Washington, DC, USA

Surgical Branch, National Cancer Institute, Bethesda, MD, USA

Jonathan Hwang, M.D. Urology, Georgetown University School of Medicine, Washington, DC, USA

Julio Jauregui, M.D. Department of Orthopaedic Surgery and Rehabilitation Medicine, SUNY Downstate Medical Center, Brooklyn, NY, USA

James S. Jelinek, M.D., F.A.C.R. Department of Radiology, Musculoskeletal Radiology, MedStar Washington Hospital Center, Washington, DC, USA

Shah Alam Khan, M.D. Department of Orthopaedics, All India Institute of Medical Sciences, Ansari Nagar, New Delhi, India

Ratesh Khillan, M.D. Department of Orthopaedic Surgery and Rehabilitation Medicine, SUNY Downstate Medical Center, Brooklyn, NY, USA

AeRang Kim, M.D., Ph.D. George Washington University School of Medicine and Health Sciences, Washington, DC, USA

Children's National Health System, Washington, DC, USA

Dhruv Kumar, M.D. Anatomic Pathology, MedStar Washington Hospital Center, Washington, DC, USA

Venkatesan S. Kumar, M.D. All India Institute of Medical Sciences, Ansari Nagar, New Delhi, India

Mary Jo Kupst, Ph.D. Medical College of Wisconsin, Milwaukee, WI, USA

Ashish Mahendra, B.M.Sc. (Hons), M.B.Ch.B. Scottish Sarcoma Managed Clinical Network, Glasgow Royal Infirmary, Glasgow, Scotland, UK

Aditya V. Maheshwari, M.D. Orthopaedic Oncology Service, Department of Orthopaedic Surgery and Rehabilitation Medicine, SUNY Downstate Medical Center, Brooklyn, NY, USA

Eish Maheshwari Department of Orthopaedic Surgery and Rehabilitation Medicine, SUNY Downstate Medical Center, Brooklyn, NY, USA

Holly J. Meany, M.D. George Washington University School of Medicine and Health Sciences, Washington, DC, USA

Solid Tumor Program, Pediatric Hematology Oncology, Children's National Health System, Washington, DC, USA

Neil Mulchandani, M.D. Department of Orthopaedic Surgery and Rehabilitation Medicine, SUNY Downstate Medical Center, Brooklyn, NY, USA

Susan J. Neuhaus, M.B.B.S., Ph.D., F.R.A.C.S. Department of Surgery, University of Adelaide, Adelaide, SA, Australia

Xiaohui Niu, M.D. Department of Orthopedic Oncology Surgery, Beijing Ji Shui Tan Hospital, Beijing, China

Kelly E. O'Mara, D.P.T., P.C.S. Children's National Health System, Washington, DC, USA

Neel Pancholi, M.D. Department of Orthopaedic Surgery and Rehabilitation Medicine, SUNY Downstate Medical Center, Brooklyn, NY, USA

Paul A. Pipia, M.D. Department of Orthopaedic Surgery and Rehabilitation Medicine, SUNY Downstate Medical Center, Brooklyn, NY, USA

Rishi Ram Poudel, M.D. All India Institute of Medical Sciences, Ansari Nagar, New Delhi, India

Mohan Preet, M.D. Department of Orthopaedic Surgery and Rehabilitation Medicine, SUNY Downstate Medical Center, Brooklyn, NY, USA

Dennis A. Priebat, M.D. George Washington University School of Medicine, Washington, DC, USA

Medical Oncology, MedStar Washington Hospital Center, Washington, DC, USA

Lee Ann Rhodes, M.D. Pain Management, Department of Anesthesia, MedStar Washington Hospital Center, Washington, DC, USA

Howard G. Rosenthal, M.D. Orthopedic Surgery, Sarcoma Center, University of Kansas Cancer Center, Overland Park, KS, USA

Victoria A. Sardi-Brown, Ph.D., L.P.C. Mattie Miracle Cancer Foundation, Washington, DC, USA

Aziza T. Shad, M.D. Pediatric Hematology/Oncology, The Herman & Walter Samuelson Children's Hospital at Sinai, Baltimore, MD, USA

Pediatrics & Oncology, Georgetown University School of Medicine, Baltimore, MD, USA

Allison B. Spitzer, M.D. Department of Orthopaedic Surgery and Rehabilitation Medicine, SUNY Downstate Medical Center, Brooklyn, NY, USA

Mark A. Steves, M.D. Department of Surgical Oncology, MedStar Washington Hospital Center, Washington, DC, USA

Luca Szalontay, M.D. Division of Hematology, Oncology and Stem Cell Transplantation, Department of Pediatrics, Morgan Stanley Children's Hospital of New York, Columbia University Medical Center, New York, NY, USA

Nicholas Tedesco, D.O. Orthopedic Oncology and Complex Reconstruction, Oregon Medical Group, Eugene, OR, USA

David M. Thomas, F.R.A.C.P., Ph.D. Faculty of Medicine, St. Vincent's Clinical School, East Melbourne, VIC, Australia

The Kinghorn Cancer Centre, Cancer Division, Garvan Institute of Medical Research, East Melbourne, VIC, Australia

Keith R. Unger, M.D. Clinical Radiation Medicine, Georgetown University, Washington, DC, USA

Uchechi Uzoegwu, M.D. Hematology and Oncology, Brooklyn Cancer Care, Medical PC, Brooklyn, NY, USA

Mohan Verghese, M.D., F.A.C.S., F.I.C.S. Section of Urologic Oncology, Department of Urology, MedStar Washington Hospital Center, Washington, DC, USA

David T. Wallace, B.M.Sc (Hons), M.B.Ch.B. Golden Jubilee National Hospital, Glasgow, Scotland, UK

Glasgow Royal Infirmary, Glasgow, Scotland, UK

Matthew T. Wallace, M.D., M.B.A. National Center for Bone and Soft Tissue Tumors, MedStar Franklin Square Medical Center, Baltimore, MD, USA

Lori Wiener, Ph.D., D.C.S.W. Psychosocial Support and Research Program, Behavioral Science Core, National Cancer Institute, Bethesda, MD, USA

Lu Xie, M.D. Musculoskeletal Tumor Center, Peking University People's Hospital, Beijing, China

Jie Xu, M.D. Musculoskeletal Tumor Center, Peking University People's Hospital, Beijing, China

Andrew Yang, M.D. Department of Orthopaedic Surgery and Rehabilitation Medicine, SUNY Downstate Medical Center, Brooklyn, NY, USA

Peter S. Young, B.Med.Sci., B.M.B.S. University of Glasgow, Glasgow, Scotland, UK

Scottish Sarcoma Research Group, Glasgow, Scotland, UK

Glasgow Royal Infirmary, Glasgow, Scotland, UK

Chunlin Zhang, M.D. Division of Orthopaedic Oncology, Department of Orthopaedic Surgery, Shanghai Tenth People's Hospital, Tongji University, Shanghai, China

Haitao Zhao, M.D. Department of Orthopedic Oncology Surgery, Beijing Ji Shui Tan Hospital, Beijing, China

Zhongsheng Zhu, M.D. Department of Orthopaedic Surgery, Central Hospital of Fengxian District, Shanghai Sixth People's Hospital, Shanghai Jiaotong University, Shanghai, China

Kun Peng Zhu, M.D. Department of Orthopaedic Surgery, Central Hospital of Fengxian District, Shanghai Sixth People's Hospital, Shanghai Jiaotong University, Shanghai, China

Part I

Multidisciplinary Approaches to the Care of Sarcoma Patients in the United States

Robert M. Henshaw

It is widely accepted that a multidisciplinary approach is necessary to ensure the optimal care of patients with cancer, a complex disease that frequently requires a combination of treatments (e.g., surgery, chemotherapy, radiation therapy) to offer patients a chance at long-term survival. However, little has been written on how such multidisciplinary care should best be organized and/or delivered to patients suffering from sarcoma, a rare family of bone and soft tissue cancers. The purpose of this book is to explore the rationale and specific methods for providing multidisciplinary care for these challenging patients. As with most complex issues, there is no single solution that will fit into every community or organization dealing with this disease. Therefore, we have invited a variety of authors from sarcoma centers and practices in the United States and from around the world, emphasizing best practices that can be translated into local and regional groups seeking to improve access and care delivery for these patients.

At its core, a multidisciplinary approach is simply the application and coordination of individuals and/or teams representing different specialties working together and applying their knowledge and skills in their respective fields in order to solve or overcome a challenging problem. The term multidisciplinary is often interchangeably used with the terms interdisciplinary and transdisciplinary, particularly

R.M. Henshaw, M.D.
Professor, Clinical Orthopedic Surgery (Orthopedic Oncology), Georgetown University School of Medicine, Washington, DC, USA

Vice Chair, Department of Orthopedics, MedStar Washington Hospital Center, Washington, DC, USA

Director, Division of Orthopedic Oncology, MedStar Georgetown Orthopedic Institute, Washington, DC, USA

Director, Orthopedic Oncology, MedStar Washington Cancer Institute and Children's National Medical Center, Washington, DC, USA

Consultant, Surgical Branch, National Cancer Institute, Washington, DC, USA
e-mail: robert.m.henshaw@medstar.net

© Springer International Publishing Switzerland 2017
R.M. Henshaw (ed.), *Sarcoma*, DOI 10.1007/978-3-319-43121-5_1

within the medical literature. Each of these terms has its own unique definition and represents, in order: additive care from each specialty, interactive care among specialties, and an overall holistic integration of all specialties [1]. However, for simplicity and clarity, we will use the term multidisciplinary to represent each of these related concepts.

Recognition that the increasing complexity of scientific knowledge extends beyond the purview of a given specialty and that better understanding of a scientific field requires a synthesis of multiple viewpoints dates back to the 1920s [2]. In prior decades, the primary scientific paradigm was based on simple causality, with efforts focused on identifying the underlying cause for an observed outcome. While this simplistic view allowed for significant progress in areas of research, scientists began to realize that many problems in nature could not be reduced to a simple cause and effect model. The concept of complexity within a system, where interrelated and interdependent causes would lead to a specific outcome, required a fresh approach. Specialists in any given field began to find that progress could only be made by integrating their knowledge with colleagues from different specialties. The introduction and development of such multidisciplinary teams became widely accepted during the Second World, as exemplified by the rise of what became known as the military industrial complex, which grew to support efforts during the war. Perhaps the ultimate example of the success of the multidisciplinary model was the Manhattan Project; the physical creation of a new community, Los Alamos, placed scientists from a wide variety of esoteric fields into a massive cooperative group dedicated to the development of the atomic bomb [3]. This highly successful project, along with the subsequent Apollo lunar program under NASA, heralded the success of "Big Science" as an effective way of approaching and solving complex problems beyond the ken of any individual person or specialty.

1.1   Multidisciplinary Approach in Medicine

Medicine has undergone a renaissance similar to that seen in high technology fields, with increasing detailed knowledge of biologic processes and systems as well as the development of entirely new areas of specialization including the ever-expanding scope of genomics and proteonomics. As with other fields, this change was driven by a move beyond simple causality (a single cause leading to a defined effect) to a complex systems approach [4]. The rapid expansion of knowledge within medicine has effectively led to the demise of the traditional general physician single handedly providing comprehensive care for to patients [5]. Multidisciplinary approaches began in hospitals and large healthcare systems, first, to deal with complex medical issues and then, with increasing recognition of the value of such approaches, to ensure proper patient care. Most recently, multidisciplinary approaches have been widely adopted to promote efficiency within the healthcare arena, maximizing cost savings while emphasizing patient safety.

Beginning in the late 1990s, team approaches were successfully instituted for a variety of complex, often chronic, illnesses. These ran the gamut of medical conditions, including such conditions as geriatric medicine [6], chronic back pain [7], diabetes [8], renal failure [9], and heart disease [10]. The first big campaign to conquer cancer, the National Cancer Act of 1971, was signed into law by President Richard Nixon, leading to the creation of the National Cancer Institute. Researchers, supported by this national effort, quickly realized the complexity of cancer, best thought of as a multitude of separate diseases requiring a multitude of different treatments. This recognition led physicians to adopt various forms of multidisciplinary approaches to deal with this complexity.

1.2 The Multidisciplinary Tumor Board

One of the earliest forms of multidisciplinary cancer care was the institutional tumor board, where frank discussions among specialists helped to guide patient care. Comprised of a team of oncologist specialists, including representatives of medical and surgical as well as diagnostic specialties, the tumor board would review individual cases and make treatment recommendations for further workup and/or treatment. This model was instrumental in helping move care of individual patients out of highly specialized research centers and into community facilities, greatly increasing access to quality care for the majority of patients with cancer [11]. The acceptance of the tumor board model as a successful method of administering multidisciplinary care is evident as disease-specific tumor boards/cancer conferences became requirements for program certification under the American College of Surgeons Commission on Cancer [12]. Using the tumor board model, the National Comprehensive Cancer Network (NCCN) has produced a monthly series of Internet broadcast disease-specific conferences (webinars) featuring a multidisciplinary analysis and discussion of care [13]. However, despite this widespread acceptance, a large multi-institutional study has questioned the actual benefit of tumor boards relative to individual patients and their outcomes [14]. Advocates for the tumor board model of care note that they remain valid methods for applying practice guidelines, identifying patients for clinical trials, and they suggest that better training of the multidisciplinary team members may lead to better patient outcomes [15].

1.3 Multidisciplinary Care Teams

As a natural extension of the multidisciplinary tumor boards, multidisciplinary care teams, organized by tumor subtype, formed to provide optimal and coordinated care for patients. While this was certainly beneficial for patients with common cancers such as breast cancer, perhaps the most important application was for patients with rare diseases such as sarcoma. Sarcomas, of which there are more than 70 subtypes commonly recognized, arise from mesenchymal tissue and can be found in any region of the body. Different subtypes have predilections for occuring in particular regions of the body as well as at specific age ranges. This broad assortment of tumor subtypes, each having different biologic potential and response to chemotherapy and/or radiation, makes it extremely difficult to compile information on a large number of patients with similar clinical characteristics. As a result, there are no consensus guidelines supported by level I evidence clinical trials to recommend specific treatments for an individual patient. Accordingly, a multidisciplinary care team comprised of surgical oncologists, medical oncologists, radiation oncologists, diagnostic radiology, musculoskeletal pathology, and other related fields with specific interest and expertise in sarcoma is needed to help ensure that each individual patient receives a personalized recommendation based upon input from all points of view.

A variety of clinical care models have been introduced in support of a multidisciplinary care approach. A simple and common model is that of a "Cancer Institute", where patients can be seen by a variety of oncologic specialists within a single building. A more integrated approach is the concept of a disease-specific clinic, where multiple specialists come together as a team, to see patients and discuss care, often sequentially or simultaneously in a single exam room. An example of such an approach is the multidisciplinary sarcoma clinic held at Children's National Medical Center in Washington DC. Sarcoma patients are seen every other week by a team staffed by pediatric medical oncology, orthopedic oncology, physical therapy, and diagnostic radiology. All patients are discussed in a team meeting after which patients are physically seen simultaneously by representatives of each specialty. This will be discussed further in the chapter on pediatric oncology. The rationale and benefits of a multidisciplinary clinic specifically for bone and soft tissue sarcomas have been recently outlined [16] in the Journal of Multidisciplinary Healthcare, an open access journal dedicated to publishing research in healthcare areas delivered by practitioners of different disciplines on a yearly basis.

The rarity of sarcomas has led to the development of some innovative models of care in an effort to improve efficiency and to further gain experience in patient care. An interesting example of an innovative approach to this rare disease is the virtual tumor clinic developed in Scotland and discussed later in this book. The virtual clinic enables a dedicated care team to review potential patients and to coordinate ongoing care over a wide geographic area. Perhaps one of the most unique care models is the pediatric and wild-type GIST tumor clinic at the National Cancer Institute. This highly specialized clinic was developed in recognition that the pediatric form of this already rare disease is strikingly different from adults GIST both in clinical presentation tumor response and molecular mutations. The National Institute of Health, starting in 2008, has held biannual clinics in which researchers and clinicians are brought together at the NIH campus with patients with this rare disease to gather clinical information, facilitate communication, discuss and implement experimental agents, and assess patients for clinical trials [17]. The success of this clinic has enabled researchers to gather clinical data on 50 patients and collect tissue samples on 20 of these patients in 2 years.

The introduction of Internet-based technologies has also played a role in the development of multidisciplinary care for sarcomas. One example is the use of a videoconferencing bridge enabling remote sites to participate in a multidisciplinary sarcoma tumor board. Hosted by the Mayo Clinic, a total of eight sarcoma programs remotely participated in a weekly conference reviewing 342 cases in 2012; a survey of participants demonstrated agreement that HIPAA rules were followed, the conference was educational, recommendations were evidence-based or reasonable, and that 86% of participants felt that input from other sites change their management of patients [18].

1.4 Surgical Care Teams

Historically, the mainstay of treatment for sarcomas has been surgical resection whenever possible. Due to the mesenchymal origin of sarcomas, these tumors typically will involve multiple anatomic regions and structures, particularly when they occur around the pelvis or shoulder girdles. These regions with complex regional anatomy offer significant challenges, and optimal surgical resection may require the expertise of a variety of different surgical subspecialties. The concept of a multidisciplinary care team can be expanded to include surgical oncologists trained in a variety of differing fields such as orthopedics, thoracic surgery, general surgery, vascular surgery, neurosurgery, urology, and gynecology, as well as reconstructive plastic surgery. Again, from a historical perspective, the surgeon was originally trained and expected to act as the one and only person required to provide any procedure for their patient. Today, however, the explosion of knowledge in surgical techniques and disease processes has led to the formation of multiple surgical subspecialties. Of note is that the majority of the basic surgical training that physicians in each of these fields undergo is typically in isolation from other specialties and is depended upon their own skill sets and training to perform specific procedures. It is only after surgeons become involved in the care of complex diseases such as sarcoma that they may begin to work in coordinated teams where the "captain of the ship" may change multiple times or maybe shared by two or more surgeons in order to achieve an optimal outcome for patient.

1.5 Barriers to Multidisciplinary Care

There are many barriers to providing multidisciplinary care, in part arising from the rarity of sarcoma, as well as inherent limitations in the current United States healthcare system. The rarity of this disease and the limited number of dedicated centers specializing in sarcoma may mean that patients often have to travel substantial distances to recieve optimal care. Many times patients will have limited understanding of their disease and may not appreciate the value in seeking out such centers. As with all types of cancer, patient fears and anxieties may lead to neglect and denial of their disease, particularly in the early stages. This may be a significant factor in poor urban areas, where a general distrust of the medical system can lead to delays in presentation, leading to poor outcomes [19] that only serve to reinforce the community distrust of medicine in general. Certain urban myths, such as a biopsy or surgery will expose a tumor to air and cause it to spread [20], can lead to further delays and patient choices that negatively impact their health. A reluctance to seek medical attention may be compounded with further delays when patients and/or families are asked to travel to distant academic centers where they may be asked to participate in a clinical trial, raising signficant fears including that of receiving experimental treatment and being treated like a guinea pig by the healthcare system. Similar barriers and concerns can also be seen in the rural population, where lack of resources and access to specialized care can lead to delays and suboptimal care [21].

Financial barriers can further hinder patient care, particularly when insurance plans limit access to specialty consultations outside of their network and when access to specialists is artificially restricted by the need for preapproved referrals. Seeing multiple specialists on the same day, either in a multidisciplinary clinic or through multiple appointments in a cancer center, raises problems with coding and billing, particularly for patients in managed care programs. There are no easy solutions that address all of the barriers to optimal care; we as clinicians must continue to strive to educate not only patients and families but the healthcare system around us in order to improve and grow our efforts in patient care.

The chapters that follow will attempt to highlight many of the problems patients and their families encounter in dealing with a sarcoma dignosis, with specific examples given by authors how they (and their institution) strive to overcome barriers to providing optimal multidisciplinary care for these patients.

References

1. Choi BC, Pak AW. Multidisciplinarity, interdisciplinarity and transdisciplinarity in health research, services, education and policy: 1. Definitions, objectives, and evidence of effectiveness. Clin Invest Med. 2006;29(6):351–64, 451–64.
2. Smuts JC. Holism and evolution. London: Macmillan and Company Limited; 1927.
3. Hughs J. The Manhattan project: big science and the atom bomb. Cambridge: Icon Books; 2002.
4. Wilson T. Complexity and clinical care. BMJ. 2001;323(7314):685–8.
5. Plsek P. The challenge of complexity in health care. BMJ. 2001;323:625.
6. Tanaka M. Multidisciplinary team approach for elderly patients. Geriatrics & Gerontology International. 2003;3(2):69–72.
7. Shirado O, Ito T, Kikumoto T, Takeda N, Minami A, Strax E. A novel back school using a multidisciplinary team approach featuring quantitative functional evaluation and therapeutic exercises for patients with chronic low back pain: the Japanese experience in the general setting. Spine. 2005;30(10):1219–25.
8. Larsson J, Stenström A, Apelqvist J, Agardh C-D. Decreasing incidence of major amputation in diabetic patients: a consequence of a multidisciplinary foot care team approach? Diabet Med. 1995;12(9):770–6.
9. Ravani P, Marinangeli G, Tancredi M, Malberti F. Multidisciplinary chronic kidney disease management improves survival on dialysis. J Nephrol. 2003;16(6):870–7.
10. Peterson E, Albert N, Amin A, Patterson J, Fonarow G. Implementing critical pathways and a multidisciplinary team approach to cardiovascular disease management. Am J Cardiol. 2008;102(5A):47G–56G.
11. Gross G. The role of the tumor board in a community hospital. CA Cancer J Clin. 1987;37(2):88–92.
12. Green F. Cancer program standards 2012: ensuring patient-centered care. Chicago: Am College of Surgeons; 2012.
13. Monthly Oncology Tumor Board Series. NCCN. 2015. https://education.nccn.org/tumor-boards. Accessed 14 Aug 2015.

14. Keating N, Landrum M, Lamont E, Bozeman S, Shulman L, McNeil B. Tumor boards and the quality of cancer care. J Natl Cancer Inst. 2013;105(2):113–21.
15. El Saghir N, Keating N, Carlson R, Khoury K, Fallowfield L. Tumor boards: optimizing the structure and improving efficiency of multidisciplinary management of patients with cancer worldwide. In: Dizon D, editor. American Society of Clinical Oncology educational book. Alexandria: American Society of Clinical Oncology; 2014.
16. Siegel G, Biermann J, Chugh R, et al. The multidisciplinary management of bone and soft tissue sarcoma: an essential organizational framework. J Multidiscip Healthc. 2015;8:109–15.
17. Kim SY, Janeway K, Pappo A. Pediatric and wildtype gastrointestinal stromal tumour (GIST): new therapeutic approaches. Curr Opin Oncol. 2010;22(4):347–50. doi:10.1097/CCO.0b013e32833aaae7.
18. Attia S, Maki R, Trent J, et al. A model for multi-institutional, multidisciplinary sarcoma videoconferencing. J Clin Oncol. 2013; (suppl; abst 10521).
19. Lai Y, Wang C, Civan JM, et al. Effects of cancer stage and treatment differences on racial disparities in survival from colon cancer: a United States population-based study. Gastroenterology. 2016;150(5):1135–46. doi:10.1053/j.gastro.2016.01.030.
20. American Cancer Society. A guide to cancer surgery: does surgery cause cancer? http://www.cancer.org/treatment/treatmentsandsideeffects/treatmenttypes/surgery/surgery-surgery-and-cancer-spread. Last Revised 24 Sep 2014. Accessed 5 Mar 2016.
21. Charlton M, Schlichting J, Chioreso C, Ward M, Vikas P. Challenges of rural cancer care in the United States. Oncology (Williston Park). 2015;29(9):633–40.

The Role of Tumor Boards and Referral Centers

Neil Mulchandani, Eish Maheshwari, Sanjeev Agarwal, and Aditya V. Maheshwari

Tumor Boards, often referred to as Multidisciplinary Team Meetings in recent literature, are an integral element of cancer care around the world today [1]. Most generally, they involve regularly conducted meetings of healthcare providers who specialize in all aspects of cancer-related care, from diagnosis to treatment and subsequent follow-up. The attendees include, but are not limited to, oncologic surgeons, medical oncologists, radiologists, pathologists, radiation oncologists, pertinent medical specialists, research coordinators, fellows, resident staff, medical students, social workers, and case managers [1]. They all participate in a collaborative effort not only to learn from prior patient cases and outcomes but also to provide insight on many cases prospectively. This can manifest in confirmation of a diagnosis and establishment of an encompassing treatment plan [2]. The significance of such teamwork among medical professionals must not be understated and plays a crucial role in the present and future of cancer care.

2.1 Objectives of the Tumor Board

The goals of the tumor board are multifocal; however, they are all based on the underlying objective to improve the care of cancer patients. First and foremost, this is accomplished by establishing a forum for exchange of information and ideas among healthcare professionals of varying disciplines [3]. Collectively reviewing a

N. Mulchandani, M.D. • S. Agarwal, M.D. • A.V. Maheshwari, M.D. (✉)
Department of Orthopaedic Surgery and Rehabilitation Medicine,
SUNY Downstate Medical Center, Brooklyn, NY, USA
e-mail: aditya.maheshwari@downstate.edu

E. Maheshwari
Department of Orthopaedic Surgery and Rehabilitation Medicine,
SUNY Downstate Medical Center, Brooklyn, NY, USA

patient's signs and symptoms, imaging and pathology shortly after their initial presentation can help the patient's oncologist and surgeon arrive at a more accurate diagnosis. This should then allow for a discussion on the ideal treatment plan for that patient. With attendance of many of the healthcare providers involved in the potential treatment plan, this will not only improve continuity of care but also encourage more efficient, multidisciplinary, disease-specific implementation [2]. Second, with expanded participation, especially from research coordinators, knowledge of ongoing clinical trials that may be suitable for specific patients should improve, resulting in increased enrollment and potential establishment of new treatment options [1]. Third, the case conferences may also include a review of past cases and patient outcomes to provide a critical educational experience for physicians in practice as well as physicians in training [1].

Beyond educating current and future healthcare professionals, tumor boards serve as an avenue for quality improvement [3]. Although anecdotes of the effectiveness of certain treatment modalities will be commonly discussed in any physician-run forum, the conference allows a venue for a more structured database when evaluating care of cancer patients. Retrospectively analyzing the outcomes of patients presented at conferences of patients with similar conditions may allow us to determine areas of improvement, both within the institution and within the community [2]. Ongoing studies are continuously being performed to evaluate the difference in healthcare outcomes in those patients whose cases are presented or whose physicians are involved in regular tumor board meetings [4]. Keating et al. assessed the effects that tumor boards had within the United States Veterans Affairs Health System on patient's provided treatment plan [4]. They found minimal agreement among the treatment recommendations given by each tumor board in patients with the same diagnosis. This suggests that although a tumor board may have the potential to positively change the management of cancer, implementing a new standard of care or novel treatment algorithm may be difficult. Others have found the contrary and have shown that having a formal tumor board allowed reassessment of treatment plans in 17% of patients and guided 89% of patients to receive the treatment recommended by the board [5]. The resounding thought process is that this disparity is mostly due to organizational and implementation pitfalls and that tumor boards are fundamentally sound and logical; however, there will undoubtedly always be room for improvement [6].

The current shift in healthcare toward quality improvement is one that not only has pushed the requirement of tumor boards in certain institutions but also forces the boards into a dynamic role. The American College of Surgeon's Commission on Cancer Program accreditation requires an institution to hold multidisciplinary cancer conferences to prospectively discuss patient cases and treatment options [4, 7]. For physicians who practice in non-cancer centers, the tumor board at a cancer center can serve as a second opinion for physicians on the management of their patients [3]. In addition, tumor boards allow for better implementation of clinical practice guidelines and adjustment of those guidelines based on available resources [1].

2.2   The Role of Tumor Boards in Sarcoma

As alluded to earlier, most of the current literature surrounding the efficacy of tumor boards surrounds breast, colorectal, lung, prostate, and hematologic cancers. While the outcome data is currently mixed on the efficacy of tumor boards, as a majority relates to those more heavily researched and institutionally supported cancers, the tumor board has the potential to play an extremely critical and very unique role in sarcoma, especially with regard to musculoskeletal pathology.

Compared to the aforementioned cancers, bone sarcomas are rare with a national annual incidence of approximately 3000, and soft tissue sarcomas are only slightly more common with an annual incidence of approximately 12,000 [8]. They comprise approximately only 0.2 and 0.8% of all cancer cases, respectively [8]. This not only makes it more difficult for physicians to recognize these tumor in their offices and hospitals but also makes it a challenge to direct appropriate treatment. Sarcomas, as with other malignancies, also benefit from a true multidisciplinary approach to formulate an effective treatment plan [9]. Unlike many other cancers with long-standing and increasingly clear treatment algorithms, widely accepted clinical practice guidelines are only just beginning to surface for sarcomas [10]. This has become more important in recent years with advances in imaging, adjuvant chemotherapy, radiation oncology, surgical care, and implant/prosthetic design driving modern limb-salvage treatment approaches for more of these formerly amputation-destined candidates.

The ideal treatment of sarcomas can vary significantly depending upon the correct diagnosis and classification of the tumor. Although it has often been the case that the orthopedic oncology surgeon has to significantly advocate for their patient to find specialists to assist him or her to successfully treat the patient, a sarcoma tumor board or sarcoma conference can assist in this inefficient and wearisome endeavor. Rather than seeking out a musculoskeletal radiologist who could assist with reviewing images and performing a CT-guided biopsy or a musculoskeletal pathologist who could more accurately distinguish between the malignant and benign nature of the tumor, the tumor board serves as an easier and indispensable alternative [2, 3]. Expertise levels of physicians in the field vary tremendously, as is to be expected, but by uniting multiple specialists with different perspectives, we can guide patients toward their best chance at cure or at least find a way to improve their lifespan and/or quality of life. In addition, having imaging and diagnostic reports all in one place with a case presented in an organized manner can streamline care by minimizing delay of diagnosis and treatment [1]. This should ultimately ease the stressors on the physician and improve healthcare delivery.

Sarcomas are uncommon and therefore the amount of exposure that most physicians have to them is minimal; this underlying truth is what arguably makes tumor boards more useful in sarcoma than any other cancer. For the community physician, tumor boards serve as an excellent resource to turn to when faced with these diagnostic dilemmas [3]. Some argue that all community hospitals should have active tumor boards as many have had significant success in guiding the primary physician through the decision-making process and, more importantly, helping them decide which patients to refer to specialists [1]. Others suggest that tumor boards should only be held at major academic centers that are more up-to-date on the literature and have the specialized staff and resources to carry out the necessary testing and therapy [2]. Modernists advocate for tumor boards to be held regionally among smaller community hospitals and health centers through video conferencing with larger academic centers [7]. They support this notion with the fact that technology has progressed to the point where diagnostic data and visuals can be shared with minimal effort, allowing much to gain. Virtual Tumor Boards (VTBs) have been tested between referral and referring centers within the VA Health Care System and have been received with a high overall acceptance rate and effectiveness reported by the participating physicians [11]. In such situations, community physicians can engage in discussion, learn, and gain feedback and confidence in their overall assessment and treatment plan.

2.3 Referral Centers

As increasing specialization and improving efficiency in healthcare delivery continue to be the driving forces of change as we enter the next era of medicine, it is possible that referral centers may become the future of cancer care. This may ultimately cause community tumor boards to serve more of a triage role in making that critical decision of when to refer a patient to a dedicated cancer center, where the case can be discussed on a more intricate level. Although the MD Anderson Cancer Center has been around for quite some time, the initiation of its Sarcoma Center is a prime example of how effective cancer-specific healthcare delivery systems can work [9]. From the moment a patient is referred to the center, they are assigned a primary physician and nurse practitioner who will perform an intake evaluation and present their case in front of a team of pathologists, radiologists, oncologists, and surgeons. Following the initial discussion, further diagnostic testing as needed will be conducted. Once a consensus diagnosis is achieved, the clinicians collectively meet with the patient to formulate an appropriate management plan. If this requires surgery, a second conference is held with an in-depth look at the imaging studies and a discussion had among surgeons, radiologists, and the primary physician to establish a detailed preoperative plan [9].

The Tumor Board continues to demonstrate various implementation models and will continue to adapt to the ever-changing healthcare landscape; whether that be community hospitals engaging in virtual tumor boards or specialized referral centers becoming more widespread, one thing is for certain; a multidisciplinary team approach is essential to enhance the care of the sarcoma patient.

2.4 Summary

The effectiveness of Tumor Boards and Referral Centers in the multidisciplinary treatment of sarcoma demonstrates the importance of these entities as we embark on the next chapter in cancer care. While they undoubtedly help enhance the treatment of sarcoma, the management of sarcoma is a dynamic process that should be assessed and reviewed on an ongoing basis as medical technology continues to improve and advances in sarcoma research are accomplished.

References

1. El Saghir NS, Keating NL, Carlson RW, Khoury KE, Fallowfield L. Tumor boards: optimizing the structure and improving efficiency of multidisciplinary management of patients with cancer worldwide. Am Soc Clin Oncol Educ Book. 2014:e461–6.
2. Jazieh AR. Tumor boards: Beyond the patient care conference. J Cancer Educ. 2011;26(3):405–8.
3. Gross GE. The role of the tumor board in a community hospital. CA Cancer J Clin. 1987;37(2):88–92.
4. Keating NL, Landrum MB, Lamont EB, Bozeman SR, Shulman LN, McNeil BJ. Tumor boards and the quality of cancer care. J Natl Cancer Inst. 2013;105(2):113–21.
5. Nemoto K, Murakami M, Ichikawa M, Ohta I, Nomiya T, Yamakawa M, et al. Influence of a multidisciplinary cancer board on treatment decisions. Int J Clin Oncol. 2013;18(4):574–7.
6. Lamb BW, Sevdalis N, Benn J, Vincent C, Green JS. Multidisciplinary cancer team meeting structure and treatment decisions: A prospective correlational study. Ann Surg Oncol. 2013;20(3):715–22.
7. Scher KS, Tisnado DM, Rose DE, Adams JL, Ko CY, Malin JL, et al. Physician and practice characteristics influencing tumor board attendance: results from the provider survey of the Los Angeles women's health study. J Oncol Pract. 2011;7(2):103–10.
8. SEER cancer statistics factsheets: bone and joint cancer. Bethesda: National Cancer Institute. http://seer.cancer.gov/statfacts/html/bones.html. Accessed 20 Nov 2015.
9. Moon BS. The MD Anderson cancer care series. In: Lin PP, Patel S, editors. Bone sarcoma. New York: Springer; 2013. p. 270.
10. Group ESESNW. Bone sarcomas: ESMO clinical practice guidelines for diagnosis, treatment and follow-up. Ann Oncol. 2014;25(Suppl 3):iii113–23.
11. Marshall CL, Petersen NJ, Naik AD, Vander Velde N, Artinyan A, Albo D, et al. Implementation of a regional virtual tumor board: a prospective study evaluating feasibility and provider acceptance. Telemed J E Health. 2014;20(8):705–11.

Academic and Community Collaboration

3

Andrew Yang and Aditya V. Maheshwari

The treatment of patients with cancer and more specifically sarcomas is often fragmented and isolated, leading to inconsistent results. Even in thoroughly studied acute and chronic conditions with availability of proven clinical therapy, healthcare outcomes in the community have been lower than anticipated [1]. Due to the rarity and complexity of sarcoma treatment, management of these patients also relies heavily on a multidisciplinary approach with support from a large number of stakeholders. Among the team involved in the management of such patients, both the academic and community hospitals play a pivotal role. Community-based institutions are primarily accessible to the general population and focus on cost-effective treatment and preventive medicine. Community in this sense includes primary care physicians, community hospitals, and community programs. Academic-based institutions are often closely affiliated with a university and have a heavy emphasis on research and improving current standards of practice [2]. Due to these two distinct branches of healthcare with the same goals, there is a continuous need for academic and community collaboration for improved outcomes.

3.1 Need for Academic-Based Collaboration in Cancer Treatment

Most cancer diagnosis and management happens in community hospitals [3]. It is therefore imperative that communication and collaboration between community and academic institutions exist. Outreach of cancer centers to community physicians regarding advances in treatment and interventions has been shown to substantially reduce cancer morbidity and mortality [4]. For example, it has been

A. Yang, M.D. • A.V. Maheshwari, M.D. (✉)
Department of Orthopedic Surgery and Rehabilitation Medicine,
SUNY Downstate Medical Center, Brooklyn, NY, USA
e-mail: adityavikramm@gmail.com

© Springer International Publishing Switzerland 2017
R.M. Henshaw (ed.), *Sarcoma*, DOI 10.1007/978-3-319-43121-5_3

demonstrated that community physicians that were involved in virtual tumor boards with academic partners reported increased familiarity with available clinical trials and were more likely to enroll patients in clinical trials [4].

3.2   Need for Academic-Community Collaboration in Sarcoma Treatment

The complex algorithm involved in treatment of bone and soft tissue sarcomas, and the relatively low incidence of sarcomas, makes the need for academic-community communication and collaboration critical. Alterations and inconsistencies in treatment guidelines can have a large impact on outcomes [5, 6]. Two landmark studies by Mankin et al. [5, 6] demonstrated significant risks of sarcoma management in inexperienced institutions. Problems related to poor biopsy technique occurred three to five times more frequently when performed at a referring institution compared with a specialized treatment center [5]. Poor biopsy technique led to 18.2% of patients requiring alteration from optimum treatment plan, 4.5% required unnecessary amputation, and 8.5% had prognosis and outcome adversely affected. In a follow-up study 14 years later, he again demonstrated that complications and changes in outcome were still 2–12 times greater ($p < 0.001$) when biopsies were performed at institutions inexperienced with sarcoma treatment, pointing out the persisting gap between the two setups [6]. Due to the obvious complexity of sarcoma treatment and documented evidence of complications associated with inappropriate management, collaboration between academic and community institutions is vital to treatment success.

3.3   Community-Based Research of Sarcomas

Data collection and research in the community have several distinct advantages as demonstrated by the success of academic-community collaboration of the National Cancer Institute (NCI) Community Oncology Research Program. Community-based research allows access to a larger more diverse population allowing for generalizability of study findings, feasible testing of new interventions, and accelerated accrual to clinical trials [7].

The relatively low incidence of sarcomas in the general population necessitates the importance of thorough and complete data collection. Through collaboration with community hospitals and physicians, the academic institutions experienced in sarcoma treatment and management have access to a larger data pool to guide clinical practice. Voluntary participation of data collection by community-based hospitals and physicians ensures appropriate data collection and close follow-up.

Community-based research decreases healthcare disparities and gaps between evidence-based medicine and community practice. Issues of external validity, practicality, stakeholder view of relevance, and sustainability can be taken into consideration when creating guidelines for standards of care [8].

3.4   Community-Academic Collaboration to Reduce Health Disparities

Wells et al. [8] described an example of multi-organizational academic-community collaboration, the Community Health Improvement Collaboration (CHIC) (Fig. 3.1). CHIC was an initiative created to address health disparities in local populations of Los Angeles, CA. The main purpose of the CHIC initiative was to create a sustainable academic-community partnership that supported healthcare research in both the local community and academic setting. Utilizing four tracer conditions (depression, violence, diabetes, obesity), authors identified four important priorities and six challenges for sustainable academic-community partnership. The partnership priorities included:

1. Equal partnership
2. Sharing of expertise and resources
3. Focus on capacity development
4. Community involvement in evaluation and research

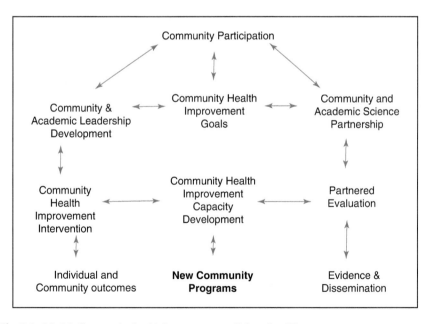

Fig. 3.1 Model: Community health improvement collaborative [8]

The six challenges identified were:

1. Obtaining adequate funding
2. Required modifications of evidence-based programs in underserved communities
3. Incorporation of diverse community priorities to be relevant in communities
4. Achieving the scale and data sets for evaluation of impact
5. Competing needs of partners
6. Learning effective communication and understanding differences between academia and community practice

The authors concluded that the challenges go beyond the significant methodologic and operational issues and include building a sustainable capacity for research, community programs, and partnership across diverse communities and stakeholder organizations even when funding sources are not fully aligned with these goals. Their model work with the CHIC initiative gives insight to important considerations and challenges that may be extrapolated to community-academic collaboration to sarcoma treatment.

3.5 A Practical Method of Academic-Community Collaboration in Sarcoma Treatment

Fung-Kee-Fung et al. described a "community of practice" infrastructure developed to address difficulties of providing cancer treatment [9]. The authors identified the key elements in implementing regional collaboration as:

1. A deliberate community of practice platform supported by the involved institutions
2. Coordinating oversight committee
3. Hub-and-spoke supporting infrastructure

A deliberate community of practice platform requires the cooperation and support from the multidisciplinary team and multi-organizations involved in sarcoma treatment. All members involved in the treatment of sarcomas, including orthopedic surgeons, radiologists, oncologists, and primary care physicians, need to establish a trusting relationship to facilitate diagnosis and treatment, with access to specialist consultation via single point of contact ensuring timely access.

Administrative coordination is facilitated via an oversight committee comprised of leaders from each respective institution for organization of care, data collection and distribution, and resource allocation.

A tertiary center experienced in the management and treatment of sarcomas acts as the regional hub, providing access to specialist consultation, diagnostic and treatment measures, and guidelines. Community-based organizations and primary care physicians act as the spokes of the infrastructure, providing standardized care in the scope of their capacity, each contributing to the multi-organizational research database. Implementing quality standards of care developed by experienced academic institution into community-based organizations ensures appropriate and timely management of bone and soft tissue sarcomas.

3.6   Evaluation of Academic-Community Collaboration

Over the years, studies have identified important components and conflicts of successful academic-community collaboration. Teal et al. [10] found that a history of positive interaction between academic and community partners and authentic commitment to academic-community collaboration by leadership facilitated successful relationships. In 2002, a study was initiated called the Latinos in a Network for Cancer Control (LINCC) [11]. The purpose of this study was to evaluate the synergistic and antagonistic factors in a long-standing community-academic collaboration. By utilizing a standardized systems model, Corbin et al. [11] were able to analyze multiple aspects of partnership functioning as well as enabled comparison with other community-academic partnerships. In addition to various new insights, authors confirmed that sustained partner interactions and positive view of leadership were essential for successful academic-community collaboration, whereas overreliance on a single leader leads to limitations. Following the study, authors concluded that:

1. Long-lasting, informal, inclusive networks provided an optimal environment for academic-community collaboration.
2. These types of interactions provide meaningful connections that lead to opportunities for future projects and funding.
3. These types of networks are valuable and should have available funding accordingly.
4. It is important to recognize that there are trade-offs in partnerships and these must be taken into account before decisions are made.

3.7   Outcomes of Community-Academic Collaboration

The utilization of community-academic collaboration has shown very promising results. Fung-Kee-Fung et al. [9] report a significant increase in regional collaboration of community and academic institutions not only in delivery of care but also in data collection and patient education. Compliance with evidence-based guidelines also saw significant improvement. The authors reported that regional clinical pathway utilization improved remarkably by 76%, with 20% improvement in colon cancer retrieval of ≥ 12 lymph nodes and 10% reduction in positive surgical margins in prostate cancer.

Partridge et al. [12] also described significant improvements in their study that utilized community-academic collaboration to eliminate cancer healthcare disparities in the African-American population in the Deep South. The authors described a mean increase in mammography utilization by 6.8% in the interventional counties versus 3% in the control population.

Conclusion

The successful treatment of sarcoma patients relies heavily on a multidisciplinary approach with support from a large number of stakeholders. The academic and community hospitals and overall healthcare systems should coordinate to provide the best possible care for these patients. This multidisciplinary model may not only aid in diagnosing and treating sarcomas, but it may also increase the quality and volume of the current research performed, which will later improve outcomes and decrease morbidity and mortality in these patients.

References

1. Lenfant C. Shattuck lecture--clinical research to clinical practice--lost in translation? N Engl J Med. 2003;349(9):868–74.
2. Chiu CG, Hari DM, Leung AM, Yoon JL, Sim MS, Bilchik AJ. Are community hospitals meeting the same standards as academic hospitals for the multimodal management of rectal cancer? Am Surg. 2012;78(10):1172–7.
3. Gross GE. The role of the tumor board in a community hospital. CA Cancer J Clin. 1987;37(2):88–92.
4. El Saghir NS, Keating NL, Carlson RW, Khoury KE, Fallowfield L. Tumor boards: optimizing the structure and improving efficiency of multidisciplinary management of patients with cancer worldwide. Am Soc Clin Oncol Educ Book. 2014;34:e461–6.
5. Mankin HJ, Lange TA, Spanier SS. The hazards of biopsy in patients with malignant primary bone and soft-tissue tumors. J Bone Joint Surg Am. 1982;64(8):1121–7.
6. Mankin HJ, Mankin CJ, Simon MA. The hazards of the biopsy, revisited. Members of the Musculoskeletal Tumor Society. J Bone Joint Surg Am. 1996;78(5):656–63.
7. Jones L, Wells K. Strategies for academic and clinician engagement in community-participatory partnered research. JAMA. 2007;297(4):407–10.
8. Wells KB, Staunton A, Norris KC, Bluthenthal R, Chung B, Gelberg L, et al. Building an academic-community partnered network for clinical services research: the Community Health Improvement Collaborative (CHIC). Ethn Dis. 2006;16(1 Suppl 1):S3–17.
9. Fung-Kee-Fung M, Boushey RP, Watters J, Morash R, Smylie J, Morash C, et al. Piloting a regional collaborative in cancer surgery using a "community of practice" model. Curr Oncol. 2014;21(1):27–34.
10. Teal R, Moore AA, Long DG, Vines AI, Leeman J. A community-academic partnership to plan and implement an evidence-based lay health advisor program for promoting breast cancer screening. J Health Care Poor Underserved. 2012;23(2 Suppl):109–20.
11. Corbin JH, Fernandez ME, Mullen PD. Evaluation of a community-academic partnership: lessons from Latinos in a network for cancer control. Health Promot Pract. 2015;16(3):345–53.
12. Partridge EE, Fouad MN, Hinton AW, Hardy CM, Liscovicz N, White-Johnson F, et al. The deep South network for cancer control: eliminating cancer disparities through community-academic collaboration. Fam Community Health. 2005;28(1):6–19.

Pathology of Bone and Soft Tissue Sarcomas

4

Dhruv Kumar

Sarcomas are malignant tumors of connective or other non-epithelial tissue. The term sarcoma comes from a Greek word meaning fleshy growth. Normal connective tissues include fat, blood vessels, nerves, muscles, fibrous tissue, bones, and cartilage. Sarcomas are divided into two main groups, bone sarcomas and soft tissue sarcomas. They are further subclassified based on the type of presumed cell of origin found in the tumor. The majority of the sarcomas arise in the extremities, and they all share certain microscopic characteristics and have similar symptoms. This is in contrast to malignant tumors originating from epithelial cells, which are termed carcinoma. Human sarcomas are quite rare. Common malignancies, such as breast, colon, and lung cancer, are almost always carcinoma.

4.1 Soft Tissue Tumors

4.1.1 Epidemiology and Etiology of Soft Tissue Tumors

The majority of soft tissue tumors are benign, superficial, and less than 5 cm in diameter. At least 30% of the benign soft tissue tumors are lipomas, 30% are fibro-histiocytic and fibrous tumors, 10% are vascular tumors, and 5% are nerve sheath tumors. The annual incidence of soft tissue sarcomas (STS) is less than 1% of all malignant tumors. The majority of soft tissue sarcomas are located in the extremities (most common in the thigh) and are deep. About 10% of patients have detectable metastases (most commonly in the lungs) at time of diagnosis of the primary tumor. Soft tissue sarcomas become more common with increasing age, but can occur at any age [1].

D. Kumar, M.D.
MedStar Washington Hospital Center, Washington, DC, USA
e-mail: Dhruv.kumar@gunet.georgetown.edu

© Springer International Publishing Switzerland 2017
R.M. Henshaw (ed.), *Sarcoma*, DOI 10.1007/978-3-319-43121-5_4

The etiology of most benign and malignant soft tissue tumors is unknown. In rare cases, the following factors may cause sarcomas: (1) Chemical carcinogens (phenoxyacetic herbicides, chlorophenols, and their contaminants (dioxin) in agricultural or forestry work). (2) Radiation (the risk increases with dose, and the median time between exposure and tumor diagnosis is about 10 years). (3) Viral infection and immunodeficiency (HHV8 plays a role in the development of Kaposi sarcoma, and EBV is associated with smooth muscle tumors in patients with immunodeficiency). (4) Genetic susceptibility (neurofibromatosis is associated with multiple benign nerve sheath tumors and malignant peripheral nerve sheath tumor). (5) Li–Fraumeni syndrome predisposes to development of sarcomas, as does germline mutation of the retinoblastoma gene. There are isolated reports of sarcomas arising in scar tissue, at fracture sites, and close to surgical implants. Some angiosarcomas arise in regions of chronic lymphedema, particularly after radiation (Stewart–Treves syndrome).

4.1.2 Techniques for diagnosis of Soft Tissue Tumors

4.1.2.1 Biopsy
Biopsy is performed in bone and soft tissue tumors to (a) identify malignancy, (b) establish the exact diagnosis (grade and subtype), and (c) guide the appropriate treatment [2]. Biopsy tissue can be obtained through a fine needle aspiration (FNA), through a wider coring needle (CNB), or through an open surgical incision (incisional biopsy). Studies show that in sarcoma diagnosis, CNB is more accurate than FNA on all accounts, and open biopsy is more accurate than both. Incisional biopsy is rarely performed because of the high accuracy rate of CNB, expense involved, and high complication rate, including hematoma, tumor spread, and wound problems that may interfere with adjuvant treatments. CNB is the preferred method for diagnosis because a block of tissue allows the pathologist to examine tumor architecture and cellular interrelation, improving the diagnosis of histologic subtype and grade compared to FNA. In one study FNA was found to be 64% accurate and core 83% accurate in establishing a specific diagnosis in soft tissue masses [3].

4.1.2.2 Intraoperative Consultation
Intraoperative consultations for soft tissue tumors are obtained mainly for determination of margins of resection [4]. Large deep soft tissue tumors undergo core needle biopsy routinely, and a diagnosis of sarcoma has usually been made prior to surgery. In smaller tumors (less than 5 cm) or superficial tumors, where a biopsy has not been performed, intraoperative consultation is sometimes obtained for diagnosis. In such cases, a designation of benign versus malignant is sufficient. This helps the surgeon to excise the tumor adequately. In some cases, distinction between a cellular benign lesion and a low-grade sarcoma can be difficult.

Evaluation of margins is of paramount importance intraoperatively. Resected soft tissue tumors are oriented with sutures by the surgeon. In our institution, the entire external surface of the specimen is colored with six different colored inks indicating the various margins, e.g., red ink for anterior/superficial margin, blue for lateral margin, orange for superior margin, green for inferior margin, yellow for medial margin, and black for posterior/deep margin. The specimen is then serially sectioned along the short axis. The relationship of the tumor to the ink is evaluated grossly and one or more sections obtained for frozen section. The section(s) are taken as perpendicular margins and not en face margins. In case of positive or close margin(s), additional tissue may be taken by the surgeon if possible.

Other tasks that can be performed during operating room consultation are: (a) Fresh tissue for cytogenetic studies. The tumor submitted must be viable and sterile. Approximately 1.0 cm^3 (if possible) should be placed in a transport medium. Tissue may be obtained for research studies in a similar manner. (b) Small sections of the tumor can be saved frozen in small vials for molecular diagnostic studies, if required. Many such studies can now be performed on formalin-fixed paraffin-embedded tissue. (c) If lymphoma is suspected, fresh tissue should be saved in normal saline and submitted for flow cytometry as soon as possible. (d) In rare cases a small portion of tumor can be cut into small cubes (less than 0.1 cm) and fixed in glutraldehyde for possible electron microscopy.

4.1.3 Grossing of Soft Tissue Tumors

Soft tissue tumors are often difficult to diagnose, and special studies (immunohistochemistry, cytogenetics, and in rare cases electron microscopy) are often requested for appropriate classification and their separation for carcinomas, melanomas, and lymphomas.

4.1.3.1 Soft Tissue Tumor Biopsy

In case of needle biopsy, obtaining multiple cores is important to sample different areas of a heterogeneous tumor. Biopsies performed under CT guidance undergo on-site cytologic preparation and evaluation to check for adequacy and narrow the differential diagnosis. Many different cores can be obtained, while specific quadrants of the tumor can be selectively biopsied. The areas which are necrotic can be avoided, and the areas with higher grade components can be resampled, significantly enhancing the ability to accurately diagnose and grade tumors more accurately. Sufficient representative samples are fixed in formalin for histopathology. Additional tissue may be saved for cytogenetics, freezing at −70 °C for molecular analysis, and electron microscopy. A separate container with fresh tissue for flow cytometry is submitted if lymphoma is suspected. Gross description of a soft tissue mass biopsy should include specimen type (needle, incisional), number of fragments, size, color, consistency, and presence of necrosis or hemorrhage.

4.1.3.2 Soft Tissue Tumor Resections

Grossing of tumor resections begins with orienting the specimen according to the labeling sutures and identifying the anatomic landmarks [5]. The outer surface of the specimen should be evaluated for structures present (muscle, bone, nerve, vessels, organs). The specimen is then measured in three dimensions and inked as previously described. The specimen is serially sectioned leaving the sections attached at one side. The exposed tumor is then described under the following headings: size in three dimensions, color, borders (infiltrating, pushing), consistency (soft, myxoid, firm, hard, rock hard) or hemorrhage or cyst formation, variation in appearance in different areas of the tumor, and involvement of, or origin from, adjacent structures, e.g., nerves, vessels, skin, subcutaneous tissue, fascia, or muscle. Any satellite nodules should be identified and described. The closest gross distance from all margins should be documented.

After proper fixation in formalin (at least 10–12 h), perpendicular sections are taken from the margins, the interface between normal and tumor tissue, and different areas of the tumor. One to two sections are taken from the margin depending on the distance between the tumor edge and the margin. At least one section per cm of the tumor's largest dimension is submitted for histologic examination.

4.1.4   Histopathologic Diagnosis of Soft Tissue Tumors

Minimum requirements for diagnosis of a soft tissue tumor are some clinical information (age, location of tumor, and growth characteristics) and adequate, well-processed tissue. Age is important because in general there is little overlap between soft tissue tumors occurring in children and those seen in adults. Location helps in developing a differential diagnosis because sarcomas, in general, develop as deeply located masses. Some superficially occurring sarcomas include dermatofibrosarcoma protuberans, epithelioid sarcoma, angiomatoid fibrous histiocytoma, plexiform fibrohistiocytic tumor, myxofibrosarcoma, angiosarcoma, Kaposi sarcoma, and atypical fibroxanthoma.

Growth characteristics are less helpful because there is a great deal of overlap between manner of presentation of benign and malignant soft tissue tumors. A neoplastic soft tissue mass could be (a) a mesenchymal neoplasm, (b) metastatic carcinoma (lung and renal carcinomas are the most common tumors to metastasize to soft tissues), (c) melanoma, or (d) a hematopoietic tumor. In majority of cases, this distinction can be made using morphology and immunohistochemistry. In case of a mesenchymal tumor, the most important priority is to determine if the lesion is a sarcoma or not. If a diagnosis of sarcoma can be made confidently, an attempt should be made to classify and grade the lesion. It is difficult to distinguish grade 2 from grade 3 sarcomas, and it is usually sufficient to grade them "low grade" or "high grade," with high-grade tumors encompassing both grade 2 and grade 3 tumors.

4.1.4.1 Grading of Soft Tissue Sarcomas
The most widely used system for grading soft tissue sarcomas is the FNCLCC system. Three factors are used for defining the grade: degree of differentiation of the tumor, mitotic activity, and necrosis. A score is assigned to each parameter, and the grade is obtained by adding these attributed scores (Tables 4.1 and 4.2).

Table 4.1 FNCLCC Grading system for Soft Tissue Sarcomas

Histological parameter	Definition
Tumor differentiation (see Table 4.2)	Score 1: sarcomas closely resembling normal adult mesenchymal tissue and potentially difficult to distinguish from the counterpart benign tumor
	Score 2: sarcomas for which histological typing is certain (e.g., myxoid liposarcoma, myxofibrosarcoma)
	Score 3: embryonal and undifferentiated sarcomas, synovial sarcomas, sarcomas of doubtful type
Mitotic count (HPF, high-power field)	Score 1: 0–9 mitoses per 10HPF
	Score 2: 10–19 mitoses per 10 HPF
	Score 3: >19 mitoses per 10 HPF
Tumor necrosis	Score 0: no necrosis
	Score 1: <50% tumor necrosis
	Score2: ≥50% tumor necrosis
Histological grade	Grade 1: total score 2, 3
	Grade 2: total score 4, 5
	Grade 3: total score 6, 7, 8

Table 4.2 FNCLCC system for histological grading of Soft Tissue Sarcomas

Histological type	Differentiation score
Well-differentiated liposarcoma	1
Well-differentiated leiomyosarcoma	1
Malignant neurofibroma	1
Well-differentiated fibrosarcoma	1
Myxoid liposarcoma	2
Conventional leiomyosarcoma	2
Conventional MPNST	2
Conventional fibrosarcoma	2
Myxofibrosarcoma	2
Myxoid chondrosarcoma	2
Conventional angiosarcoma	2
High-grade myxoid (round cell) liposarcoma	3
Pleomorphic liposarcoma	3
Dedifferentiated liposarcoma	3
Rhabdomyosarcoma	3
Poorly differentiated/pleomorphic leiomyosarcoma	3
Poorly differentiated/epithelioid angiosarcoma	3
Poorly differentiated MPNST	3
Malignant Triton tumor	3
Synovial sarcoma	3
Extraskeletal osteosarcoma	3

(continued)

Table 4.2 (continued)

Histological type	Differentiation score
Extraskeletal Ewing sarcoma	3
Mesenchymal chondrosarcoma	3
Clear cell sarcoma	3
Epithelioid sarcoma	3
Alveolar soft part sarcoma	3
Malignant rhabdoid tumor	3
Undifferentiated (spindle cell and pleomorphic) sarcoma	3

Grading remains one of the most powerful ways of assessing prognosis, and consequently a grade should be provided by the pathologist whenever possible. Grading is usually based on the least differentiated areas of the tumor unless it comprises a very minor component of the overall tumor.

4.1.4.2 Classification of Soft Tissue Tumors

Classification of soft tissue keeps evolving due to identification of new cytogenetic and molecular genetic information. The purpose of the following review is to clarify how the new terminology relates to the old and also to clarify some of the confusing closely related terms in soft tissue tumors, particularly in myxoid neoplasms. Detailed descriptions of classification are available in many textbooks. Below is a discussion of changes in some common sarcoma terminology. Soft tissue tumors are classified according to the tissue of origin, i.e., adipose tissue tumors, fibroblastic/myofibroblastic tumors, smooth muscle tumors, cartilage, bone, etc. Among each of these categories, tumors are subclassified into benign, intermediate (locally aggressive or rarely metastasizing), and malignant categories [6, 7].

1. Adipocytic tumors: Atypical lipomatous tumor is synonymous with well-differentiated liposarcoma. It is an intermediate (locally aggressive) malignant tumor with no potential for metastasis unless it undergoes dedifferentiation. The use of the term well-differentiated liposarcoma is justified in the retroperitoneum and mediastinum.
2. Recent WHO classification [8] has deleted the term "round cell liposarcoma." Round cell liposarcoma has been used to identify a subset of myxoid liposarcomas that show histologic progression to hypercellular or round cell morphology, which is associated with a poorer prognosis. Myxoid liposarcoma should be graded using a three-tier system as low, intermediate, or high grade based on the degree of cellularity.
3. The term hemangiopericytoma has been deleted. It is used only to describe a histological pattern shared by many different entities. Hemangiopericytoma is now termed extrapleural solitary fibrous tumor.
4. The category of malignant fibrous histiocytoma (MFH) has been deleted. MFH and some of its subtypes have been renamed "undifferentiated sarcoma" and reclassified under the undifferentiated/unclassified sarcomas. These account

for up to 20% of all sarcomas and are the most common radiation-associated soft tissue sarcomas.

5. Rhabdomyosarcomas were previously classified into embryonal (spindle cell, botryoid, and anaplastic variants), alveolar, and pleomorphic types. The category of "spindle cell/sclerosing rhabdomyosarcoma" has been separated from embryonal type because these tumors are well recognized and lack genetic changes observed in embryonal rhabdomyosarcoma.

4.1.4.3 Microscopic Examination of Soft Tissue Tumors

Microscopically soft tissue neoplasm can be broadly classified into (a) spindle cell tumors, (b) myxoid tumors, (c) epithelioid tumors, (d) round cell tumors, and (e) pleomorphic tumors.

1. Spindle cell tumors: These tumors comprised a large group of tumors, both benign and malignant. Common benign spindle cell tumors include schwannoma and fibromatosis. Common spindle cell sarcomas include undifferentiated spindle cell sarcoma, synovial sarcoma, MPNST, leiomyosarcoma, spindle cell rhabdomyosarcoma, and fibrosarcoma.

2. Myxoid tumors: Many soft tissue tumors can have focal myxoid areas, but tumors that consistently display a predominately myxoid morphology are included in this category. Common benign myxoid tumors include intramuscular myxoma, myxoid lipoma, and myxoid neurofibroma. Common sarcomas in this category include myxoid liposarcoma, myxofibrosarcoma, and extraskeletal myxoid chondrosarcoma. The terminology of malignant myxoid tumors can be confusing. A brief description of these tumors follows:

    (a) Myxoid liposarcoma: Myxoid liposarcoma is a malignant tumor classified under adipocytic tumors. It is composed of round- to oval-shaped cells admixed with a variable number of univacuolar lipoblasts in a prominent myxoid stroma with a delicate arborizing vascular pattern. It has a predilection for deep soft tissues of the extremities in young adults.

    (b) Myxoinflammatory fibroblastic sarcoma/atypical myxoinflammatory fibroblastic tumor (old name, inflammatory myxohyaline tumor of the distal extremities with virocyte or Reed–Sternberg-like cell): This is a rare intermediate (rarely metastasizing) tumor which has a predilection for the hands and feet and occurs in young adults. It has a myxoid stroma, inflammatory infiltrate, and virocyte-like cells.

    (c) Myxofibrosarcoma (old name, myxoid MFH): Myxofibrosarcoma is one of the most common sarcomas in elderly patients. About two thirds of these tumors develop in the dermal/subcutaneous tissues. Histologically, they are malignant fibroblastic lesions with a variable myxoid stroma, pleomorphism, and a distinctive curvilinear vascular pattern.

    (d) Low-grade fibromyxoid sarcoma (Evans tumor): Low-grade fibromyxoid sarcoma (Evans tumor) is a variant of fibrosarcoma characterized by an admixture of collagenized and myxoid zones, with bland spindle cells, a whorling pattern, and arcades of blood vessels. It is a rare sarcoma that typically affects young adults. It typically involves proximal extremities or trunk, and majority occur in subfascial location.

(e) Ossifying fibromyxoid tumor: Ossifying fibromyxoid tumor is a rare inter-mediate (rarely metastasizing) tumor of uncertain differentiation, with cords and trabeculae of ovoid cells embedded in a fibromyxoid matrix, often sur-rounded by a partial shell of the lamellar bone.

(f) Extraskeletal myxoid chondrosarcoma: Extraskeletal myxoid chondrosar-coma is a rare malignant soft tissue tumor characterized by a multinodular architecture, abundant myxoid matrix, and malignant chondroblast-like cells arranged in cords, clusters, or delicate networks.

3. Epithelioid tumors: When a tumor with an epithelioid morphology is identified, it is important to exclude metastatic carcinoma, melanoma, and anaplastic large cell lymphoma. Common sarcomas with an epithelioid morphology include epithelioid sarcoma, alveolar soft part sarcoma, predominately epithelioid monophase synovial sarcoma, and vascular tumors with epithelioid histology (epithelioid hemangioendothelioma and epithelioid angiosarcoma).

4. Round cell tumors: Similar to epithelioid tumors, when a round cell tumor is encoun-tered, metastasis (lymphoma, carcinoma, melanoma) should be excluded. In round cell tumors, in general, age of the patient helps to narrow the differential diagno-sis, e.g., in children these lesions include Ewing sarcoma, rhabdomyosarcoma, and neuroblastoma. In adults round cell liposarcoma, mesenchymal chondrosarcoma, and undifferentiated round cell sarcoma are in the differential diagnosis.

5. Pleomorphic sarcomas: Undifferentiated pleomorphic sarcoma is the most common pleomorphic sarcoma. Other tumors that can sometimes have a pleo-morphic morphology include pleomorphic liposarcoma, pleomorphic rhabdo-myosarcoma, pleomorphic leiomyosarcoma, and dedifferentiated liposarcoma. Immunohistochemistry can greatly help in distinguishing these tumors.

EORTC-STBSG [9] has recently published criteria for standardization of the macroscopic and microscopic pathological examination and reporting of STS resec-tion specimens after neoadjuvant radio- and/or chemotherapy. The surgeon should suture mark the specimen topographically to facilitate three-dimensional orienta-tion. Total weight and size in three dimensions are mandatory. The surface must be marked with permanent ink according to the surgical markings (up to five colors can be used depending on the number of margins). The specimen should be processed into 1 cm thick slabs from proximal to distal in the transversal axis. The area of total macroscopic necrosis should be approximated for the entire tumor, in order to have an initial impression of treatment effect. A representative complete central slab of the specimen should be embedded entirely in a grid manner. The position of each respective sample of the embedded slab should be marked on a photograph or diagram. Therapy response is expressed as a percentage of total tumor area that is viable. All margins should be sampled perpendicular to the margin, with at least two sections being taken from the closest margin and one to two sections from all other margins.

The data suggest that in STS, patients with clear margins have a better prognosis [10]. However, to preserve functionality, surgery may result in a close (considered to be <1 cm after formalin fixation) or even microscopically positive margin. In this circumstance, the use of preoperative or postoperative radiation should be considered. The combination of RT with surgery allows for limb salvage by using radiation to biologically "sterilize" microscopic extensions of disease and to spare neurovascular and osseous structure. Local recurrences have been observed even when negative margins are achieved with surgery and with the combination of surgery and RT, suggesting that tumor characteristics other than margin status are important. At this time, there is no evidence to support the use of postoperative chemotherapy in STS that have been treated with intralesional or marginal excisions. Clearly, other factors—tumor type, grade, and biology or even the type of tissue at the margin (e.g., fascia)—affect the rate of both local and systemic recurrence.

The management of soft tissue sarcoma requires integrated care. Unfortunately, a large proportion of patients with soft tissue sarcoma may be subject to an initial suboptimal surgery, more often when the multidisciplinary team is not utilized, which may result in the need for more extensive surgery and radiation than the original tumor may dictate.

4.2 Bone Tumors

4.2.1 Epidemiology and Etiology of Bone Tumors

Bone sarcomas are rare and account for 0.2% of all neoplasms. The incidence rates of specific bone sarcomas are age-related and, as a group, have a bimodal distribution. The first well-defined peak occurs during the second decade of life, while the second occurs in people aged >60 years.

Majority of primary bone tumors arise de novo. Predisposing lesions that lead to the development of bone sarcomas are Paget disease, radiation injury, bone infarction, chronic osteomyelitis, certain preexisting benign tumors, implanted metallic hardware, joint prostheses, and bone grafts. Genetic predisposition has been seen in osteosarcoma, the most frequent primary malignancy of the bone. It can develop in patients with retinoblastoma, Li–Fraumeni syndrome, and Rothmund–Thomson syndrome. Patients with Ollier disease, Maffucci syndrome, and multiple osteochondromatosis have an increased incidence of developing chondrosarcoma.

4.2.2 Techniques for diagnosis of Bone Tumors

4.2.2.1 Biopsy
Principles and techniques for needle biopsies in bone tumors are similar to those in soft tissue tumors.

4.2.2.2 Intraoperative Consultation

In bone tumors, intraoperative consultation is needed for various reasons. It may be needed to determine if sufficient lesional tissue is present for eventual diagnosis on permanent sections and special studies. It is sometimes obtained to confirm lesional tissue, e.g., nidus of an osteoid osteoma. In rare cases, a diagnosis of benign versus malignant is requested, and this distinction may not always be possible. Most frequently, the reason for frozen section in bone tumors is to evaluate the bone resection margin in resections for osteosarcoma and other malignant bone tumors. The specimen is obtained as bone marrow curettings. The specimen usually contains bone debris which should not be mistaken for osteoid. Another reason for an open biopsy and intraoperative consultation is apportionment of tissue for special studies, e.g., flow cytometry for lymphomas and cytogenetic studies for Ewing sarcoma.

4.2.3   Grossing of Bone Tumors

4.2.3.1 Bone Biopsy and Bone Curettings

Grossly examine for presence of bone and soft tissue. Pure soft tissue fragments should not be decalcified. Small non-necrotic soft tissue can be taken for special studies, if required, as described under soft tissue above. However, in the majority of cases, the entire specimen should be fixed in formalin for routine sections. The specimen should be fixed overnight and then gently decalcified. Overnight decalcification is usually sufficient for core biopsies and small curettings. Larger bone fragments can be checked periodically to see if the bone is soft. Decalcification solution should be changed frequently for adequate and faster decalcification.

4.2.3.2 Bone Tumor Resections

Resection for bone tumors can be in the form of resection of a portion of the bone or a major limb amputation or disarticulation. The specimens should be measured in three dimensions, and each separate structure present within the specimen should be measured. In disarticulations and amputation specimens, the bone involved with the tumor should be identified and dissected out carefully making sure that the tumor remains intact. Relationship to the vessels should be noted. The resection margins, as applicable, should be inked and sections taken.

Soft tissue over the tumor should be incised in a plane that will demonstrate the greatest extent of the tumor. A band saw is used to bisect the specimen along the long axis. Gently brush away the bone dust under running water. For large bones (femur, tibia, humerus, etc.), additional 0.5 cm parallel cuts are made to produce multiple-cut sections of the tumor. Description of the tumor should include size in three dimensions, color, evidence of bone or cartilage formation, necrosis, areas of bone involved (epiphysis, metaphysis, diaphysis, intramedullary, periosteal), whether the tumor destroys the cortex or not, extent of soft tissue involvement, relationship to surrounding structures (vessels, muscle), extension into joint space, vascular involvement, skip metastasis, and distance from each margin. Partial resection of long bones (the most common type of bone resection) should be inked similar to what is described under soft tissue resections in six colors. Soft tissue and bone margins should be taken perpendicular to the tumor and distance from the tumor noted.

The entire specimen is fixed in formalin overnight. The sections ("slabs") of bone are then decalcified. The specimen is checked every few hours to prevent over-decalcification. Over-decalcification can damage cellular morphology and cause problems with staining, particularly nuclear staining. This can cause difficulties in distinguishing necrotic and viable areas of the tumor and falsely negative immuno-histochemical staining. Sections are taken from various areas of the tumor demon-strating the relationship of the tumor to the adjacent structures (cortex, joint space, soft tissues). In cases of treated osteosarcomas and Ewing sarcoma, it is important to determine the percentage of necrosis. A whole section (slab) with the largest amount of tumor is mapped out (drawing, photocopy, photograph) and submitted for histological examination.

4.2.4 Histopathologic Diagnosis of Bone Tumors

Correlation of the core biopsy especially for bone tumors can be improved by care-ful review of the radiographic, CT, and MR appearance of the bone lesion with a musculoskeletal tumor radiologist. A core biopsy may have a sampling error, whereas the radiograph, CT, or MR may visualize the entire tumor revealing a much more aggressive appearance especially for chondrosarcomas. Radiologic-pathologic correlation is extremely important for bone tumors, as demonstrated by the follow-ing examples.

Case 1. 61-year-old woman presented with a 3-month history of progressive pain around the left shoulder girdle. Examination of the left shoulder did not show any masses. Plain X-rays and MRI showed a poorly defined permeative lytic lesion with significant loss of cortex in the humeral neck and a second area lower down in the proximal humerus. The shoulder joint itself was well preserved. Chest X-ray was negative for tumor. Given her age and radiographic appearance, possibility of metastasis was a strong consideration although a primary bone tumor could not be excluded. Arrangements were made for her to undergo a CT-guided core needle biopsy. Core biopsy showed a malignant cartilage tumor with two distinct histolo-gies. One area shows a low-grade cartilage tumor and the other a high-grade pleo-morphic sarcoma. A diagnosis of a dedifferentiated chondrosarcoma was made in conjunction with the radiographic appearance of the lesion. Resection of the tumor confirmed the biopsy diagnosis (Figs. 4.1).

Case 2. This active 37-year-old female presented with pain in the left leg around the knee. On physical examination she had tenderness in the metadiaphyseal por-tion of the distal femur circumferentially. There was no appreciable mass. Plain X-rays and MRI showed a large intramedullary lesion completely filling the canal

Fig. 4.1 Core needle biopsy of a tumor in the proximal humerus. Atypical cartilage tumor (low-grade chondrosarcoma) with adjacent high-grade sarcoma. Histology is that of a dedifferentiated chondrosarcoma

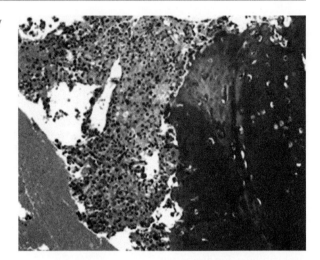

Fig. 4.2 Needle biopsy of a painful lesion in the distal femur. The histology is that of a low-grade cartilage tumor which could either be an enchondroma or an atypical cartilage tumor (low-grade chondrosarcoma). The clinical history of pain and the radiological findings of a large cartilage tumor filling the medullary canal and causing endosteal scalloping confirmed the diagnosis of an atypical cartilage tumor

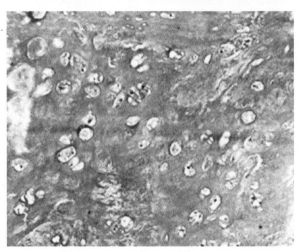

with evidence of endosteal scalloping, but no evidence of cortical breakthrough. A CT-guided biopsy showed a bland-cartilage tumor. The patient underwent extensive curettage of the lesion followed by cryosurgery. Both the biopsy and curettage specimen showed similar histopathology of a low-grade cartilage tumor with mild atypia. These tumors are labeled as atypical cartilaginous tumor/chondrosarcoma grade 1, and their cytology is indistinguishable from that of an enchondroma. Diagnosis is based on the clinical findings and the radiographic appearance of the lesion (Fig. 4.2).

4.2.4.1 Grading of Bone Sarcomas

In bone tumours, cellularity and nuclear features of the tumor cells are the most important criteria used for grading. The more cellular the tumor, the higher the grade. Irregularity of the nuclear contors, enlargement and hyperchromasia of the nuclei are correlated with grade. Mitotic figures and delete necrosis are additional features useful in grading. Many studies have shown that histological grading correlates with prognosis in chondrosarcoma and malignant vascular tumours. Tumors which are monomorphic, such as small cell malignancies (Ewing sarcoma, malignant lymphoma and myeloma), do not lend themselves to histological grading. Mesenchymal chondrosarcomas and dedifferentiated chondrosarcomas are always high grade, whereas clear cell chondrosarcomas are low grade.

4.2.4.2 Classification of bone tumors
Recent changes in the terminology are as follows:

1. Cartilage tumors are now classified into benign, intermediate (locally aggressive), and malignant types. Grade 1 chondrosarcoma is now reclassified as an intermediate (locally aggressive) tumor and termed "atypical cartilaginous tumor." These tumors are locally aggressive and metastasize only extremely rarely.
2. Fibrohistiocytic tumors: Malignant fibrous histiocytoma of the bone has been removed from the classification. High-grade pleomorphic malignant tumors that lack a specific line of differentiation are classified as "undifferentiated high-grade pleomorphic sarcoma."
3. The term primitive neuroectodermal tumor (PNET) has been removed as a synonym for Ewing sarcoma.
4. Hemangioma is now separated from epithelioid hemangioma, a recently characterized locally aggressive tumor composed of small vessels lined by epithelioid endothelial cells. Epithelioid hemangioma should be distinguished from epithelioid hemangioendothelioma which is a malignant neoplasm.

4.2.4.3 Microscopic Examination of Bone Tumors
A diagnosis of bone tumor should not be made without integrating clinical, radiological, and histologic appearances. Biologically different types of tumors may have overlapping histologic appearance. Histologic features to consider include pattern of growth (eg., sheets of cells seen in sarcomas such as Ewing's Sarcoma and Osteosarcomas vs. lobular architecture seen in most Chondrosarcomas). Cytologic characteristics of the cells can help distinguish benign and malignant bone tumors. Malignant tumors often have pleomorphic and hyperchromatic nuclei, although many low grade malignant tumors can have bland appearing nuclei. Presence of necrosis is usually seen in malignant tumors but can be seen in Giant cell tumors of the bone. A diagnosis of Osteosarcoma cannot be made without demonstrating osteoid matrix production by the tumor cells. Multiple sections may be needed to identify such matrix production. Chondrosarcomas usually have abundant cartilaginous matrix.

4.3 Immunohistochemistry in Sarcoma Diagnosis

Immunohistochemistry is a technique where antibodies are used to detect antigens in tissue sections. Antibodies are tagged to reagents which generate a colored reaction product which is commonly brown or red. Immunohistochemistry is used only in conjunction with routine H&E staining for diagnosis. There are no immunohisto-chemical markers that will distinguish benign from malignant tumors. The following is a brief discussion of commonly used antibodies:

1. Cytokeratins are sensitive markers for identifying carcinomas and distinguishing them from lymphomas, melanomas, and sarcomas. Among the sarcomas, synovial sarcoma and epithelioid sarcoma manifest true epithelial differentiation and express cytokeratins. Anomalous cytokeratin expression is seen in smooth muscle tumors, melanomas, endothelial cell tumors, and some small round cell tumors (Ewing sarcoma, rhabdomyosarcoma, desmoplastic small round cell tumor, Merkel cell carcinoma).
2. Desmin is a very sensitive marker of smooth muscle and skeletal muscle differentiation. It is positive in rhabdomyosarcoma and leiomyosarcomas. It is not 100% specific, and desmin expression can be seen in Ewing sarcoma, desmoplastic small round cell tumor, and giant cell tumor of tendon sheath.
3. Smooth muscle actin: Monoclonal antibody is expressed in smooth muscle and myofibroblasts. It can be used to distinguish smooth muscle tumors from skeletal muscle tumors.
4. S-100 protein: In soft tissue tumors, S-100 is most useful in the diagnosis of MPNST and melanomas. S-100 is diffusely and strongly positive in schwannomas, whereas in MPNST positivity is focal and weak. This staining pattern can be helpful in distinguishing cellular schwannomas from MPNST. S-100 protein staining is, however, not specific, and its expression may be seen in synovial sarcoma, rhabdomyosarcoma, and leiomyosarcoma.
5. CD99: The most important use of CD99 antibodies is for diagnosis of Ewing sarcoma, but its expression is not specific, and many small round cell tumors (lymphoblastic lymphoma, rhabdomyosarcomas) and other tumors (synovial sarcoma, undifferentiated round cell sarcoma, mesenchymal chondrosarcoma, and desmoplastic round cell tumor) are positive.
6. CD34 is expressed in the majority of vascular tumors and is a sensitive marker for Kaposi sarcoma. It is also expressed in DFSP, solitary fibrous tumors, MPNST, GIST, and epithelioid sarcoma. Its expression is helpful in distinguishing epithelioid angiosarcoma (which are cytokeratin positive) and epithelioid sarcoma, from carcinoma.
7. CD31 is the most sensitive and specific endothelial marker, and its expression is not seen in any non-endothelial tumor. It is expressed in more than 90% of angiosarcomas, hemangioendotheliomas, hemangiomas, and Kaposi sarcoma.
8. Vimentin: Vimentin is expressed in all mesenchymal cells. It is also expressed in sarcomatoid carcinomas, lymphomas, and melanomas. Vimentin expression is preserved in which all other immunoreactivity has been lost. Therefore, vimentin immunoreactivity is a good marker of tissue preservation.

Table 4.3 summarizes the utility of immunohistochemistry in the differential diagnosis of soft tissue and bone tumors.

Table 4.3 Commonly used immunohistochemical stains in the diagnosis of Soft Tissue Sarcomas

	Cytokeratin	S 100	ASMA	Desmin	CD 45	CD 99	CD34	CD 31	Other markers
Spindle cell tumors:									
Synovial sarcoma	Positive	Variable	Negative	Negative	Negative	Variable	Negative	Negative	EMA
MPNST	Negative	Positive	Negative	Negative	Negative	Negative	Variable	Negative	CD 57
Fibrosarcoma	Negative	Negative	Variable	Negative	Negative	Negative	Negative	Negative	
Leiomyosarcoma	Rare	Rare	Positive	Positive	Negative	Negative	Rare	Negative	
Solitary fibrous tumor	Rare	Negative	Negative	Negative	Negative	Variable	Positive	Negative	
Angiosarcoma	Variable	Negative	Negative	Negative	Negative	Negative	Positive	Positive	
Round cell tumors:									
Small cell carcinoma	Positive	Negative	Negative	Negative	Negative	Negative	Negative	Negative	Chromogranin, synaptophysin
Lymphoma	Negative	Negative	Negative	Negative	Positive	Variable	Negative	Negative	B- and T-cell markers
Ewing sarcoma	Variable	Variable	Negative	Rare	Negative	Positive	Negative	Negative	FLI-1
Rhabdomyosarcoma	Rare	Rare	Negative	Positive	Negative	Variable	Negative	Negative	Myogenin, myo D1
Epithelioid tumors:									
Carcinoma	Positive	Negative	Negative	Negative	Negative	Negative	Negative	Negative	
Melanoma	Variable	Positive	Negative	Negative	Negative	Negative	Negative	Negative	Melan A, HMB 45, tyrosinase
Epithelioid sarcoma	Positive	Negative	Negative	Negative	Negative	Negative	Variable	Negative	Loss of INI-1

4.4 Molecular Genetics Pathology of Sarcoma

Sarcomas can be divided into two groups for the discussion of genetic alterations in these tumors, (a) sarcomas that have a specific translocations and (b) those with complex karyotypes.

(a) Genetics of some major sarcomas with specific translocation:
  1. Synovial sarcoma is characterized by the t (x; 18) (p11; q11) translocation, which is found exclusively in this tumor. This translocation or variants thereof are present in >95% of all cases, often as a sole abnormality. Fluorescence in situ hybridization (FISH) and RT-PCR techniques are commonly used to detect this translocation.
  2. Ewing sarcoma: Approximately 85% of Ewing sarcomas have a reciprocal chromosomal translocation, t (11; 22) (q24; q12), that fuses EWSR1 to FLI1 to generate EWSR1-FLI1 oncoprotein. In other cases, alternate translocations fuse EWSR1 to other ETS family members. In rare cases, FUS-ERG or FUS-FEV fusions are present instead. The diagnosis of Ewing sarcoma may be made by the presence of a positive RT-PCR result or supported by a split EWSR1 FISH signal, while still considering the diagnoses of other EWSR1-rearranged tumors, such as desmoplastic round cell tumor, extraskeletal myxoid chondrosarcoma, myxoid liposarcoma, or clear cell sarcoma, among others. Additional chromosomal abnormalities, e.g., trisomies, and additional unbalanced chromosomal translocation are often present in Ewing sarcoma. Although absence of molecular confirmation should prompt a review of the clinical, histological, and immunohistochemical features, it should not rule out the diagnosis of Ewing sarcoma by itself.
  3. Alveolar rhabdomyosarcoma: Approximately 60–70% of ARMS involve a t (2; 13) (q35; q14) leading to PAX3-FKHR gene fusion, and 10–20% have a t (1; 13) (p36; q14) representing the variant PAX7-FKHR gene fusion. However, 10–30% of ARMS fail to exhibit any of these translocations. Furthermore, PAX3-FKHR-positive tumors appear to be significantly more aggressive than those containing PAX7-FKHR, although the tumors expressing these two translocations appear morphologically identical.
  4. Myxoid/round cell liposarcoma: MLS is characterized by the recurrent translocation t (12; 16) (q13; p11) that results in FUS-DDIT3 gene fusion, present in >95% of cases. In the remaining cases, a variant t (12; 22) (q13; q12) is present in which DDIT3 fuses with EWSR1, a gene which is related to FUS. The presence of FUS-DDIT3 fusion is highly sensitive and specific for MLS and is absent in other morphologic mimics, including myxoid well-differentiated liposarcoma, dedifferentiated liposarcoma, and myxofibrosarcoma.
  5. Extraskeletal myxoid chondrosarcoma: Approximately 75–80% of EMC contain a characteristic t (9; 22) (q22; q12) in which the EWS gene becomes fused to a gene located at 9q22 encoding an orphan nuclear receptor belonging to the steroid/thyroid receptor gene superfamily, NR4A3. In another 15–20% of EMC, a gene at 17q11 highly related to EWS, TAF15, fuses with NR4A3 instead. In addition, two additional variant fusions involving NR4A3

have been reported. The NR4A3 fusions have not been found in any other sarcoma and may therefore be considered as a hallmark of this disease.

6. Alveolar soft part sarcoma: Cytogenetically ASPS is defined by a specific alteration, der (17) t (x; 17) (p11; q25). This translocation results in the fusion of TFE3 transcription factor gene (from x p11) with ASPSCR1 at 17q25. ASPSCR1-TFE3 RT-PCR and FISH for TFE3 rearrangement are both good methods for molecular diagnosis. Although the presence of the ASPSCR1-TFE3 fusion appears to be highly specific and sensitive for ASPS among sarcomas, the same gene fusion is also found in a small subset of renal cell carcinomas, often affecting young patients.

7. Low-grade fibromyxoid sarcoma: The cytogenetic hallmark of these tumors is the t (7; 16) (q33; p11), which is present, often as a sole change, in approximately two thirds of cases. Another 25% of cases show a supernumerary ring chromosome. Both aberrations result in fusion of the FUS gene and the CREB3L2 gene. A rare variant t (11; 16) (p11; p11) results in a FUS-CREB3L1 fusion. FUS-CREB3L2 and FUS-CREB3L1 fusion genes occur in 76–96% and 4–6% of cases, respectively. Low-grade fibromyxoid sarcomas arising in atypical locations and those with giant rosettes or foci resembling sclerosing epithelioid fibrosarcoma also display t (7; 16)/FUS CREB3L2.

8. Clear cell sarcoma of soft tissue: The genetic hallmark of CCS is the presence of reciprocal translocation t (12; 22) (q13; q12), resulting in the fusion of EWSR1 with ATF1 in >90% of cases. A related variant translocation, t (2; 22) (q32.3; q12), resulting in an EWSR1-CREB1 fusion has been described in 6% of CCS. In CCS, EWSR1-ATF1 fusion protein targets the melanocyte-specific MITF promoter, required for cell proliferation as well as triggering ectopic melanocytic differentiation.

9. Desmoplastic small round cell tumor (DSRCT) is characterized by a recurrent chromosomal translocation t (11; 22) (p13; q12), resulting in the fusion of the EWSR1 gene in 22q 12 and Wilms tumor gene, WT1, in 11 p13. Rare variants including additional exon of EWSR1 can also occur. Detection of the EWSR1-WT1 gene fusion can be especially useful in cases with unusual clinical or histological features. EWSR1-WT1 is expressed in tissues derived from the intermediate mesoderm, primarily those undergoing transition from mesenchyme to epithelium. This recapitulates the epithelial differentiation noted in DSRCT.

(b) Sarcomas with complex karyotypes:

Soft tissue sarcoma with complex unbalanced karyotypes lacking specific translocations includes pleomorphic and dedifferentiated liposarcomas, angiosarcoma, leiomyosarcoma, neuroblastoma, mesothelioma, adult fibrosarcoma, and undifferentiated pleomorphic sarcoma. Inactivation of the p53 pathway appears to be a key differentiating factor between sarcomas with simple genetic alterations and those with karyotypic complexity. In sarcomas with nonspecific genetic alteration, p53 pathway inactivation may be a common early event, needed to overcome checkpoints triggered by senescence telomere erosion or double-strand breaks in the progression of these sarcomas.

4.5   Summary

The rarity of bone and soft tissue sarcomas requires a systematic multidisciplinary team approach for management of patients with these diseases [11]. These rare tumors require sophisticated pathologic diagnosis and imaging interpretation. Incorrect biopsy technique may compromise surgical options and resectability. Treatment of bone and soft tissue sarcomas routinely includes surgery, medical management (routinely used for high-grade sarcomas), and radiation therapy given for select tumors either in lieu of surgery or as an adjunct. Together, these issues mandate close cooperation and multidisciplinary care to optimize outcome. In other types of cancers, pathologic interpretation may be performed based solely on the examination of the retrieved specimen. In soft tissue and bone tumors, however, interpretation frequently necessitates understanding of the clinical presentation, along with symptom quality, duration, intensity, and radiographic interpretation of aggressiveness and site. In low-grade cartilage tumors of bone, the specimen cannot be interpreted in a vacuum, excluding clinical and radiographic factors. A multidisciplinary team is well equipped to discuss image interpretation and clinical presentation with the diagnosing pathologist. Similarly, in the interpretation of biopsy specimens, multidisciplinary exchange is essential to determine if a seemingly non-diagnostic biopsy can be interpreted in the clinical and imaging context; if not, future diagnostic maneuvers can be discussed and optimized, leading to fewer unproductive interventions and tests. A core group of dedicated and experienced physicians can accomplish this goal.

References

1. Weiss SW, Goldblum JR. Enzinger and Weiss's soft tissue tumors. 5th ed. St. Louis: Mosby Elsevier; 2008.
2. Kasraeian S, Allison DC, Ahlmann ER, Fedenko AN, Menendez LR. Comparison of fine-needle aspiration, core biopsy, and surgical biopsy in the diagnosis of extremity soft tissue masses. Clin Orthop Relat Res. 2010;468(11):2992–3002.
3. Yang YJ, Damron TA. Comparison of needle core biopsy and fine-needle aspiration for diagnostic accuracy in musculoskeletal lesions. Arch Pathol Lab Med. 2004;128:759–64.
4. Lester SC. Manual of surgical pathology. 3rd ed. Philadelphia: Elsevier Saunders; 2010.
5. Westra WH, Hruban RH, Phelps TH, Isacson C. Surgical pathology dissection: an illustrated guide. 2nd ed. New York: Springer; 2003.
6. Doyle LA. Sarcoma classification: an update based on the 2013 World Health Organization Classification of Tumors of Soft Tissue and Bone. Cancer. 2014;120(12):1763–74.
7. Saanna GA, Bovée J, Hornick J, Lazar A. A review of the WHO classification of tumours of soft tissue and bone. ESUN. 2013;10:3.
8. Fletcher CDM, Gronchi A. WHO classification of tumors of soft tissue and bone. 4rth ed. Lyon: IARC; 2013.
9. Wardelmann E, Haas RL, Bovée JV, Terrier P, Lazar A, Messiou C, LePechoux C, Hartmann W, Collin F, Fisher C, Mechtersheimer G, DeiTos AP, Stacchiotti S, Jones RL, Gronchi A, Bonvalot S. Evaluation of response after neoadjuvant treatment in soft tissue sarcomas; the European Organization for Research and Treatment of Cancer–Soft Tissue and Bone Sarcoma Group (EORTC–STBSG) recommendations for pathological examination and reporting. Eur J Cancer. 2016;53:84–95.

10. Kandel R, Coakley N, Werier J, Engel J, Ghert M, Verma S. Sarcoma Disease Site Group of Cancer Care Ontario's Program in Evidence-Based Care. Surgical margins and handling of soft-tissue sarcoma in extremities: a clinical practice guideline. Curr Oncol. 2013;20(3):247–54.
11. Geoffrey W, Siegel J, Biermann S, Chugh R, Jacobson JA, Lucas D, Feng M, Chang AC, Smith SR, Wong SL, Hasen J. The multidisciplinary management of bone and soft tissue sarcoma: an essential organizational framework. Multidiscip Healthc. 2015;8:109–15.

Musculoskeletal and Interventional Radiology in the Management of Sarcoma Patients

5

James Jelinek and Francesca Beaman

This chapter is designed for the primary physician, orthopedic oncologist, surgical oncologist, medical oncologist, radiation oncologist, and other health-care providers to understand modern imaging techniques in the diagnosis, percutaneous biopsy, and follow-up of bone and soft tissue sarcomas. There are many excellent textbooks describing the imaging appearance and differential diagnosis of both bone and soft tissue sarcomas [1–3]. The goal of this chapter is more focused on the newest approaches to sarcoma diagnosis, staging biopsy, and follow-up. Compared to a decade ago, there is more reliance on MRI in the initial staging and increasing usage of image-guided percutaneous needle biopsy for initial diagnosis and proof of recurrence as well as an increasing utilization of PET-CT in the staging and surveillance of sarcomas [4]. The value and limitations of these strategies are discussed.

5.1 Initial Diagnosis

The initial diagnosis of a bone or soft tissue mass is sometimes incidental as identified by a routine joint pain MRI (such as a shoulder or knee MRI) or may be made based on clinical symptoms. The presence of clinical symptoms related to the "incidental" findings is often different in significance for bone versus soft tissue masses. Painful bone masses warrant much closer attention. Chondroid lesions of the bone which are malignant (chondrosarcoma) are painful, whereas benign enchondromas are typically painless. The opposite is often the case for soft tissue masses. Unless they have achieved a large size or are compressing a nerve, most soft tissue

J. Jelinek, M.D., F.A.C.R. (✉)
MedStar Washington Hospital Center, Washington, DC, USA
e-mail: James.s.jelinek@medstar.net

F. Beaman, M.D.
University of Kentucky College of Medicine, Lexington, KY, USA

© Springer International Publishing Switzerland 2017
R.M. Henshaw (ed.), *Sarcoma*, DOI 10.1007/978-3-319-43121-5_5

sarcomas are not painful. Most painful soft tissue masses are benign lesions such as myositis ossificans, thrombosed hemangiomas/angiolipomas, posttraumatic hematomas, nerve sheath tumors, glomus tumors, or myositis.

The best imaging practice for bone and soft tissue tumors is outlined in the American College of Radiology (ACR) Appropriateness Criteria [5]. This lists in detail the best (and least appropriate) tests for the diagnosis of primary sarcomas of bone and soft tissue. There are also online references of the American College of Radiology (ACR), Society of Pediatric Radiology, and the Society of Skeletal Radiology on consensus recommendations as outlined in the ACR Practice Guidelines for the Performance and Interpretation of Computed Tomography and Magnetic Resonance Imaging of Bone and Soft Tissue Tumors. Just because a patient has a sarcoma does not mean they must have every single exam including CT, MRI, X-rays, bone scan, and PET-CTs. For example, many soft tissue sarcomas of the extremity do not need an extremity CT or bone scan. We need to image wisely. A skilled musculoskeletal radiologist can be helpful in delineating which exams are useful and which would likely add little benefit to the patient. Excess radiation, whenever possible, should be avoided in young patients likely to have many follow-up exams.

5.1.1 Plain Film Radiographs

The initial evaluation of both bone and soft tissue sarcoma typically begins with plain film radiographs [3]. There is increasing usage of MRI in the evaluation of the extremities and joints without use of a plain film radiograph. For many sports injury of the shoulder and knees, this may be appropriate; however, evaluating tumors of bone and soft tissue without plain film radiographs can result in the misdiagnosis of benign lesions as malignant and malignant lesions misdiagnosed as benign. X-rays may define the presence of margins and matrix in soft tissue masses. A soft tissue mass with a sharply defined calcific rim seen on X-ray may not be seen on MRI; the presence of the calcification may be diagnostic of a myositis ossificans as opposed to a soft tissue sarcoma. Radiographs are also helpful to identify whether the tumor is truly arising from bone or soft tissue (Fig. 5.1). The evaluation of bone tumors should always start with plain film radiographs.

Sarcomas of the bone: The correct diagnosis of bone tumors begins with an appreciation of the patient age and specific location of the bone tumor. The X-ray appearance in terms of the margins is critically important in establishing the degree of aggressivity of the bone tumor. Sharply defined lesions with sclerotic borders are rarely malignant, and the diagnosis of a bone sarcoma can be excluded. A skilled bone radiologist can provide additional confidence to the treating oncologist/surgeon that follow-up studies or biopsy of a benign bone lesion may not be warranted. On an increasing level of aggressiveness, bone lesions which demonstrate a less well-defined to ragged margin without a sclerotic border represent more aggressive processes. Age is important. Many benign childhood lesions such as histiocytosis X

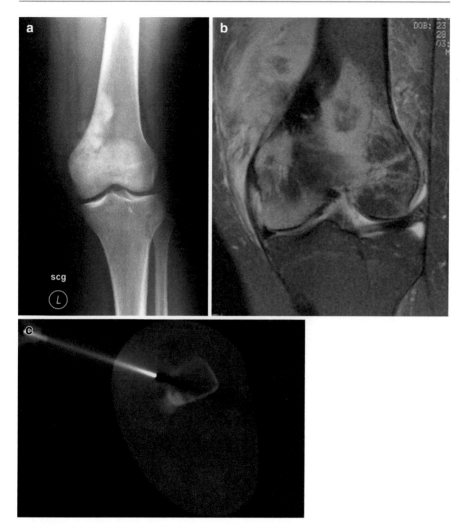

Fig. 5.1 A 24-year-old pregnant female with 4-month history of painful leg. X-rays of the leg were previously deferred because of the pregnancy. Biopsy and surgically proven osteoblastic osteosarcoma. (**a**) AP X-ray of the knee shows osteoid matrix in the distal medial femoral metaphysis. More importantly there is poorly mineralized osteoid extending medially into the soft tissues. (**b**) Coronal T2-weighted MRI shows the soft tissue component, but dense osteoid matrix of an osteoblastic osteosarcoma is not identifiable. (**c**) Axial CT scan during large core needle biopsy of the tumor

(Langerhans cell histiocytosis), bone cysts, and enchondroma do not necessarily have a prominent well-defined sclerotic rim but usually have sharply defined margins. On the other hand, in adults, especially over the age of 40 years, it is not uncommon for such tumors as multiple myeloma and metastatic disease to present with sharply defined punched-out ("cookie cutter") lesions. The presence of a lytic lesion with poorly defined margins signifies a bone tumor as an aggressive process and likely malignant. While the vast majority of lytic lesions of the bone over the age of 40 years are likely due to metastatic disease or multiple myeloma, the possibility of a primary bone sarcoma should still be considered. For example, a patient in their fourth or fifth decade with a bone tumor with poor margins and subtle calcifications with arcs and swirls signifies that this represents a chondroid tumor such as a chondrosarcoma or a chondroblastic osteosarcoma. Dense cloud-like osteoid matrix within a bone lesion usually suggests this represents an osteoblastic tumor (Fig. 5.1). Small lesions with a minimally spiculated borders might simply signify a benign bone island in particular if the patient is asymptomatic, and the finding is incidental. A blastic lesion, especially if multiple, in a patient over the age of 40 could represent metastatic disease. A history of breast cancer would make a sclerotic lesion more worrisome for metastatic disease. A sclerotic bone lesion in a male should suggest the potential for metastatic prostate cancer, and the next appropriate step is to evaluate with a serum prostate-specific antigen (PSA). A male patient with incidental bone islands or enostosis will likely have a normal or high normal PSA level. Metastatic prostate cancer to the bone almost invariably is associated with a PSA level greater than 10 at initial presentation.

Soft tissue sarcoma: The role of plain film radiographs is less appreciated for soft tissue sarcomas. MRI clearly has the major role in the assessment of the imaging appearance of the soft tissue sarcoma. Furthermore, MRI is very accurate in establishing the local extension of tumor and its relationship to important neurovascular structures [6]. However, MRI is likely to miss internal calcification or ossification within a soft tissue tumor (Fig. 5.2). The presence of internal soft tissue calcification may be an important clue that the lesion may represent a synovial sarcoma which often presents with findings of sand-like calcifications [1]. The matrix of an extraskeletal osteosarcoma or extraskeletal chondrosarcoma will be missed by MRI. The extension of the soft tissue tumor to the bone can be better depicted by plain film radiographs. Long-standing benign tumors such as juxtacortical chondromas often have a sharply defined margin with thick cortical reaction suggesting a long-term lesion that would not be obvious by MRI. Sarcomas of soft tissue can erode the bony cortex without a sclerotic reaction and often have no bone reaction (just lytic) or a feathery pattern. Expert evaluation of the periosteal reaction of a soft tissue tumor on radiographs can predict an aggressive versus long-term process.

The use of plain film and the adjunctive use of CT are particularly essential when assessing a large osteoblastic or osteoid producing lesion. In general, benign lesions such as myositis ossificans or heterotopic ossification typically have a well-defined sharply corticated margin without evidence of an adjacent soft tissue mass. Malignant processes, which include parosteal osteosarcoma, periosteal osteosarcoma, extraskeletal chondrosarcoma, or extraskeletal osteosarcoma, will have dense osteoid matrix [3, 7] (Fig. 5.2). A careful evaluation of the margins of these malignant tumors will show that the peripheral edge (paint brush margins) are less well

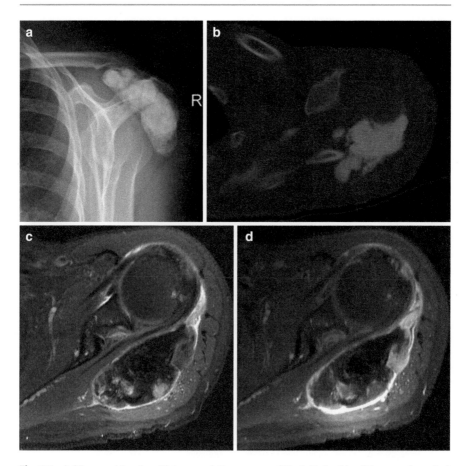

Fig. 5.2 A 37-year-old male with bony soft tissue mass of the left shoulder. Biopsy and surgical proven osteosarcoma. (**a**) AP X-ray of the scapula demonstrates a large osteoid mass. Mistakenly called myositis ossificans or bony exostosis. Experience with these entities would suggest this would not be typical for this diagnosis. CT is strongly recommended on multiple occasions despite initial reluctance of general orthopedic surgeon. (**b**) CT shows "paint brush" borders on the outside and other soft tissue components of poor mineralization, worrisome features for malignancy. The peripheral margins are not sharply defined. (**c**) Axial T2-weighted MRI shows peripheral areas of high signal intensity not consistent with mature bone. (**d**) Axial post-contrast-enhanced T1-weighted MRI shows both lateral and posterior nodular areas of enhancement

defined and are often associated with soft tissue masses (Fig. 5.2). The internal component of these tumors typically may have either no internal matrix or a solid homogeneous osteoid pattern. It is the presence or absence of a sharp-defined margin of the cortex that indicates whether an otherwise large dense osteoid mass is benign or represents a soft tissue sarcoma. Defined margins of myositis ossificans have a very distinct sharply marginated cortex without a peripheral soft tissue mass.

5.1.2   CT Evaluation

CT is a major diagnostic tool in the assessment of bone and soft tissue tumors. Plain film radiographs have limitations in the assessment of tumor especially those that are superimposed over complex bony structures such as tumor present within the pelvis or scapula. In some cases, the radiograph findings are extremely subtle as to the presence or absence of matrix. Matrix can be missed on X-rays. CT is valuable in the assessment of the presence and type of matrix especially in the shoulder and pelvis. Chondroid matrix signifying a chondroid tumor is often subtle on plain film and better defined on CT (Fig. 5.3).

CT can be invaluable in the assessment of the soft tissue tumors when the presence or absence of matrix is being assessed or when the extent of cortical erosion may be present. In the absence of matrix, as might be seen on plain film X-ray, and the absence of bone erosion, CT may not be warranted. Many of our soft tissue sarcoma patients never get an extremity CT.

The presence of calcification or ossification within a soft tissue mass is not in itself diagnostic of a malignant or benign process. For example, long-standing lipomas and liposarcomas can both contain calcification. The interaction between the musculoskeletal radiologist and the clinician is very important in the proper evaluation of such small lesions. A small chondroid tumor with minimal scalloping of the cortex can be either an enchondroma or a chondrosarcoma. If the patient has significant pain referable to that area, then strong clinical suspicion and more careful assessment of chondrosarcoma is advised.

The soft tissue sarcomas with the highest incidence of calcifications include synovial sarcoma [8], malignant fibrous histiocytoma (today most malignant fibrous histiocytomas have been reclassified as undifferentiated pleomorphic sarcomas (UPS)), and the rarer extraskeletal osteosarcoma and extraskeletal chondrosarcoma.

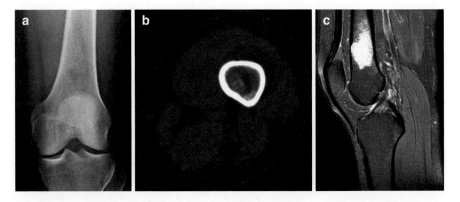

Fig. 5.3 A 37-year-old female with bone pain left distal femur. Surgically proven low-grade chondrosarcoma. (**a**) X-ray shows subtle matrix in the distal left femur. (**b**) CT scan shows definite chondroid matrix without involvement of the cortex. (**c**) Sagittal T2-weighted MRI shows the lesion of distal femur with anterior endosteal scalloping

5.1.3 Ultrasound Examination

Initial evaluation of a sarcoma typically does not include the use of ultrasound. Ultrasound provides poor discrimination of the type of bone tumor present. Ultrasound is valuable in the assessment of soft tissue masses when a lesion is suspected to be "cystic" such as a simple cyst or ganglion or pseudoaneurysm. The major role for ultrasound is to show that a lesion is purely a cystic lesion and using color flow Doppler to show that the lesion is avascular either and a cyst or a cystic tumor. Ultrasound examination can show communication between the central portion of a soft tissue mass, and extension to the joint capsule with characteristic imaging appearance diagnostic of a synovial ganglion. Ultrasound readily demonstrates large soft tissue hematomas. The assessment of a soft tissue hematoma, however, should be performed with caution. The addition of color flow Doppler ultrasound may be helpful in the assessment for neovascularity or nodules within the cystic mass. A cystic mass with internal nodules with hypervascularity should suggest that the soft tissue mass represents a soft tissue sarcoma rather than a hematoma. Any hematoma diagnosed by ultrasound should be assessed for the lack of internal vascularity and should be correlated with clinical history as to whether the patient has an appropriate recent injury to cause a hematoma. Typical hematomas related to trauma or muscle tears are less well defined, track down the entire compartment of the injured muscle, and have an overall length which greatly exceeds the cross-sectional diameter of the lesion (hot dog shaped). On the other hand, soft tissue sarcomas typically are round or elliptical (ball or football shaped). It is unusual for a soft tissue sarcoma to have a length which exceeds more than three times the maximal cross-sectional diameter of the lesion. Follow-up of any hematoma is always warranted as change over time may be diagnostically significant. Unfortunately, many of the tumors which are diagnosed by CT, MRI, or ultrasound are initially described as hematomas. The referring physician often takes the phrase "hematoma" as a diagnosis rather than a pure description that the mass in fact represents blood products of uncertain etiology. Hematomas which turn out to represent a soft tissue sarcoma are typically very high-grade. There is a controversial theory that high grade sarcomas with underlying hemorrhage have a worse prognosis than those soft tissue tumors which do not have evidence of internal hemorrhage [9]. In our experience the presence of hemorrhage within a tumor suggests the tumor is not a low-grade lesion but high-grade. The one exception is that some ancient schwannomas may have internal hemorrhage.

5.1.4 MRI Examination

MRI should be the imaging modality of choice for the local staging of soft tissue and bone sarcomas. MRI is not used as the test to make a correct diagnosis of a bone tumor but is the essential imaging tool in the assessment of the full staging of the lesion. MRI is very accurate in the assessment of the extent of the tumor within the bone (i.e., medullary canal), as well as identifying cortical erosion and the presence of extraosseous extension, and is clearly superior to both CT and plain film radiograph in this regard [9].

Many benign soft tissue masses can be correctly identified and diagnosed with MRI. Many of the more common benign "tumors" for which MRI is diagnostic include meniscal cysts, ganglion, hemangiomas, lipomas, intramuscular myxoma, fibromatosis, and benign peripheral nerve sheath tumor such as schwannomas and neurofibromas [1]. In many cases, based on the MR appearance, patient age, and tumor location, the lesion can be simply followed over time, particularly when the lesion is not easily amendable to percutaneous biopsy. Furthermore, the imaging appearance of some soft tissue sarcomas is also diagnostic based on the MR appearance [1]. For example, many liposarcomas, including the myxoid liposarcoma and the well-differentiated liposarcoma (atypical lipomatous tumor), and synovial sarcomas have a characteristic appearance on MR. The MR imaging appearance however should never preclude a biopsy of a suspected sarcoma, and the more important role is to correctly define the extent of tumor and to assess the invasion of adjacent neurovascular structures. No other modality comes close to MRI in the assessment of local invasion of nerves, arteries, veins, bony cortex, and other adjacent organs (Fig. 5.4).

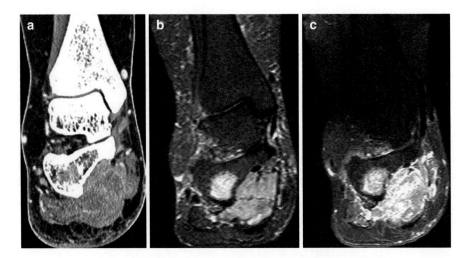

Fig. 5.4 A 58-year-old female with slightly painful growing soft tissue mass of the medial foot. Biopsy and surgically proven extraosseous sarcoma with cortical invasion and bony involvement. (**a**) Coronal contrast-enhanced reformatted CT with soft tissue window shows a soft tissue mass with probable cortical erosion of the medial cortex of the calcaneus. Cystic appearing areas present. (**b**) Coronal T2-weighted MRI shows large soft tissue mass with obvious invasion of the body of the calcaneus. (**c**) Coronal T1-weighted post-contrast-enhanced image shows no significant cystic or hemorrhagic areas present

5.1.4.1 MRI Technique

There are many different MR scanners and sequences. The strength of the MR magnet (Tesla (T) units) has limited importance compared to other uses of MRI within the brain and body. Most MRI scanners used today are 1.5 T. The problem with low-field 0.5 T is poor spatial resolution and blurring. If a patient can tolerate a 1.5 T MR, then they should have a 1.5 T MR. The use of high-field MRI at 3 T is increasing; 3 T MRI has a more prominent role in neuroimaging of stroke, MR tractography, and MR angiograms. Increasing use of 3 T MRI with joints shows improved conspicuity of articular cartilage. There is no significant literature to support that 3 T MR improves diagnosis or staging of sarcomas compared with traditional 1.5 T MRI.

Sequences: With regard to musculoskeletal imaging, the type of MRI sequences utilized can effect whether soft tissue and/or bone sarcomas are correctly diagnosed. There are myriad of MRI sequences: T1, T2, proton density, FLASH, GRE, FLAIR, STIR, SPIR, HASTE, diffusion with ADC mapping, etc. The imaging sequences used for general abdominal MRI, in particular assessment of the liver, kidneys, and pelvic organs, differ significantly from those used for musculoskeletal imaging. Even within the musculoskeletal MRI protocols, there are significant differences in the type of sequences utilized to assess pathology. For example, most MR sequences to evaluate the sports injuries of the knees, hips, shoulders, and wrists are optimized to improve the appearance of both hyaline and fibrocartilage. Typically, these studies use fast sequences and proton-weighted or balance sequences to help in the detection of cartilage lesion of the labrum and condyles. The proton-weighted sequences are of significantly less benefit in the evaluation of tumor as a balance, or proton-weighted sequence minimizes the signal of pathologic processes relative to that of bone or soft tissue. We have specific and differing musculoskeletal sequences that are defined as either sports injury/joint protocols or tumor protocols. Optimal MRI sequences for the assessment of bone and soft tissue tumors should include simple T1-weighted and water-sensitive sequences with fat suppression. The most commonly used water-sensitive sequences included T2-weighted with fat saturation and STIR sequences. T2-weighted sequences without fat saturation make it difficult to differentiate a tumor from the adjacent subcutaneous fat or from the adjacent intramedullary fat (within bone marrow). Other optional sequences such as gradient echo sequences are more sensitive to the presence of internal hemorrhage. Gradient echo images are not as commonly used in ordinary follow-up of tumors but may be used when internal hemorrhage is suspected.

MR contrast: The use of contrast agent for MRI can be valuable in many cases [10]. All of the commonly used agents for MR contrast are based on gadolinium which is one of the basic elements of the periodic table. Gadolinium is frequently chelated with other molecules to provide different biochemical properties. MR contrast agents are significantly safer than the iodinated contrast agents used for CT scans. There is little to no crossover of reactivity with regard to allergic reactions to iodinated contrast agent for CT and the gadolinium contrast agents used for MRI. The frequency of the minor contrast reactions is significantly less for MRI than for contrast agent used for CT. Typically, the incidence of MRI contrast agent reactions is less than 1%, with most of these representing headaches and rashes. The incidence of reactions to CT iodinated contrast agents is two to four times higher. Likewise, the incidence of severe anaphylactic reactions to MR gadolinium contrast agents is also extremely rare and much less likely than the severe allergic reactions to CT iodinated contrast agents [11]. Note that the new iso-osmolar CT iodinated contrast agents have a significantly safer biochemical profile than those iodinated contrast agents used a decade ago. The incidence of both minor and major allergic reactions to both the CT and MR contrast agents has significantly declined of the last two decades. Shellfish allergy is not a contraindication to either CT or MRI contrast agents. Rather, allergic individuals who have several allergic reactions to such products as seafood, nuts, cheeses, and pollens with atopy have an increased likelihood compared to the general population of having an acute anaphylactic reaction to either iodinated CT or gadolinium-based MR contrast agents [12].

The value of MR contrast is somewhat controversial if used in all cases. Many tumors can be well seen on the typical T1-weighted and water-sensitive sequences. The addition of contrast often does improve the conspicuity of the margins of the tumor. Where MR with contrast is more helpful is in the assessment of the internal content of the lesion. For example, a cystic lesion such as a synovial ganglion or meniscal cyst should not show internal enhancement on early post-contrast sequences. In some cases, contrast may leach into a ganglion or meniscal cyst on delayed post-contrast sequences. A large tumor which is very "cystic" in appearance based on the T1-weighted and the T2-weighted images may in fact represent a myxoid tumor. Myxoid tumors whether benign intramuscular myxoma or malignant myxoid liposarcoma or myxoid MFH will show significant internal enhancement on post-contrast sequences. The best way to accurately characterize tumor as a cyst versus a cystic tumor is based on the use of contrast. Furthermore, large bone and soft tissue sarcomas may have large areas of internal hemorrhage or necrosis. Preoperative biopsy planning of a suspected malignancy may be affected if the area to be sampled contains a large area of central necrosis or hemorrhage. The value of a contrast MRI (or contrast CT) is that the area of greatest contrast enhancement will typically represent the area of greatest tumor viability and is the most optimal site of biopsy whether the biopsy is performed as a CT-guided core needle biopsy or performed as an open surgical biopsy. For a large tumor with central areas suggesting "cystic" changes, careful review of the enhancement pattern is invaluable to optimizing the biopsy procedure. Central areas showing no enhancement should be carefully avoided. In addition, the value of contrast with MRI is extremely important when biopsying vascular lesions of a high-grade sarcoma containing large feeder vessels and extensive neovascularity. These large vessels can be easily identified on the earlier arterial phase sequences. It is important to carefully avoid the large vessels to minimize the risk of post-biopsy hemorrhage. Avoidance of vascular structures can be more easily done with CT/MR guidance than with an open biopsy because they can be directly visualized. This is also discussed in the following biopsy section. Invasion of important adjacent structures can deem a tumor unresectable or at least has a major impact on long-term survival [13].

Direct osseous invasion is sometimes obvious from MR or CT. Other times invasion is less obvious. Some useful rules of thumb include the extent of contiguous contact with adjacent structures. Typically, when more than 5 cm of contiguous contact is present then invasion of the associated osseous, chest wall, or vascular structures is likely even if no obvious penetration is visible. Similarly, if tumor encases a structure by more than 180° such as a bone or neurovascular bundle, then the likelihood of invasion is also high [14].

The limitations of an MRI are becoming less of an issue with modern MRI scanners. Newer MRI scanners can hold patients up to 600 pounds. The new generation MRI scanner is shorter in overall length (length of the tube), and the bore or the internal cross-sectional diameter has greatly increased. This results in decreased claustrophobia. Nonetheless, the MR examination takes significantly longer than a CT scan. New CT scan protocols typically can be completed in less than 5 minutes, whereas the average tumor protocol for MRI is typically 45 minutes, especially if contrast is given. A patient felt to be minimally claustrophobic should have an appropriate discussion of whether premedication with an antianxiety medication such as benzodiazepine medication Valium (diazepam) or Ambien (zolpidem) may be beneficial in decreasing the patient's anxiety. Even minimal movement of the patient significantly degrades the overall quality of the MR imaging study. Almost all patients with a joint replacing prosthesis can be safely imaged by MRI. Patient with various other implants can often be easily imaged. A useful reference for whether an implant or prosthesis is MR compatible can be assessed by the excellent website called "MRI Safety.com" (MRISafety.com). Almost all patients who have had recent cardiac or peripheral vascular stents can be safely imaged. These usually do not represent contraindications after the first week of insertion. Most of the modern intracranial aneurysm clips are also MR compatible. Only the older intracranial aneurysm clips used more than two decades ago were not MRI compatible. Today, the single most common contraindication for an MRI is an actively used implanted pacemaker or defibrillator. There are an increasing number of hospitals which can image patients with pacemakers. The newest pacemakers such as the Revo pacing system by Medtronic are considered MR compatible, and in the future more widespread MR compatible pacemakers will become available. Nonetheless, the patients do require careful assessment for the mode of the pacemaker settings. A cardiologist or pacemaker technician should be around to access the pacemaker and, in some cases, turn off the pacemaker and then reset it post MR imaging. Other active implanted stimulators include bone stimulators, and spinal cord stimulators that are functioning are typically contraindicated.

Newer technologies in MRI include the use of MR spectroscopy which may allow better differentiation between benign and malignant primary soft tissue masses. The assessment is based on differences in choline peaks, but the results have been mixed [6, 15]. Diffusion MR is another sequence that is being widely applied to oncology imaging and is widely used in the assessment of prostate, liver, colorectal, and brain tumors. Its application to primary sarcomas has not been defined [16, 17].

5.2   Staging of Primary Tumors

The staging of primary tumors can be separated into the assessment of the local tumor site and then the assessment for metastatic disease. As described above, MRI is the chief modality to assess both bone and soft tissue sarcoma for local extent as well as the tumor's relationship to the nerves, arteries, veins, destruction of bony cortex, and local invasion of the other organs. MRI is clearly superior to CT (Fig. 5.4); however, for those patients who cannot have an MRI, CT staging is also quite accurate. The multiplanar capability of MRI is more useful for surgical planning. Contrast improves the visibility of tumor necrosis and vessels within a sarcoma.

The vast majority of sarcomas of bone and soft tissue typically metastasize to the lungs. As such, the assessment of lung metastasis is performed using multidetector CT. While most pulmonary nodules are easily seen without contrast, the addition of the CT contrast agents is helpful in assessing tumors adjacent to vascular structures as well as for the assessment of adenopathy in the chest. There are some sarcomas which have unusual metastatic pathways to lymph nodes such as epithelioid sarcoma and synovial sarcoma. Additionally, leiomyosarcomas and myxoid liposarcomas can metastatize to the intrapelvic or abdominal lymph nodes, bone, liver, and peritoneum [18–20].

The second most common site of metastatic disease of sarcomas is to the bone, especially for the most common sarcomas of the bone. Nuclear medicine bone scan has been the typical imaging modality for the assessment of bone metastasis. After lung metastasis, spread to bone is common for osteosarcoma and Ewing's and other aggressive soft tissue sarcomas such as leiomyosarcomas and rhabdomyosarcomas. While MRI is considered most sensitive and specific for the local assessment of a bone sarcoma, it is nearly impossible to adequately image the entire appendicular and central axial skeleton with MR imaging. The time would be extensive and most patients could not tolerate the long MR scanning time. Shortened MR protocols to two sequence whole-body scanning have been employed primarily for research assessment but are not commonly the modality of choice for whole-body screening for bone metastasis. The sensitivity and accuracy of total body nuclear bone scanning is effective from both a clinically tolerated perspective and practical cost and time perspective.

Recent total body nuclear bone scanning technique for metastatic disease has been improved by the replacement of the most commonly used bone scan agent methylene diphosphonate (MDP). In years past the typical bone scan agent used was technetium MDP. In many imaging centers, the technetium MDP agent is being replaced by sodium fluoride. The advantage of these sodium fluoride bone scanning agents is that in addition to the whole-body scanning, low-dose combined CT can be performed to improve the spatial resolution of the location of the lesion as well as improve specificity by differentiating increased activity related to arthritis adjacent to the joint versus a tumor adjacent to a joint. There is some concern the sodium fluoride SPECT-CT may be too sensitive with false-positive studies as compared to technetium MDP.

The other evolving technology which may replace nuclear medicine bone scan and basic CT scanning of the body is the use of a combined high-resolution diagnostic CT with PET-CT. The study is performed using fluorodeoxyglucose (FDG) as the most commonly used agent. There are other agents which been utilized, including radioactive carbon-11, nitrogen-13, oxygen-15, or rubidium-82. However, in clinical practice, these other agents are rarely utilized. PET-CT with high-resolution diagnostic CT allows the areas of greatest activity to be visualized on a high-resolution CT scan as well. The combination of detecting the areas of greatest uptake with the multidetector CT scanner allows precise localization of uptake within specific structures detected on CT. For example, a small or normal-sized lymph node seen on CT with a very high degree of specific uptake value (SUV) is likely pathologic. Most normal organs and lymph nodes have a low degree of activity (SUV < 3), whereas high-grade tumors typically have an uptake (SUV > 5). But this is a gross simplification because acute inflammation can have a high degree of uptake, whereas a low-grade sarcoma can have a low degree of uptake; this is a source of confusion for referring clinicians, nuclear medicine physicians, and radiologists. Knowing type and grade of a sarcoma can be very helpful in assessing what the value of a low degree of uptake in a specific location means. There are papers that would suggest that the SUV max of a primary sarcoma is an independent prognostic factor for long-term survival [21]. While the high-resolution CT and the PET-CT are performed in one setting, the two components, including the PET and the CT images, are fused and co-registered together. It is also possible for a PET study to be co-registered or fused with an outside-referring facility CT or MRI study performed shortly before or after the MR study. However, to improve the accuracy of the fusion or co-registration, it is best performed at the same setting so as to not have other factors such as exact body positioning come into play.

PET-CT, in some cases, may replace the need to perform a bone scan. For example, in the staging of Ewing's sarcoma, lytic bone lesions are better depicted by PET-CT [22, 23]. On the other hand, blastic bone lesions are better detected with traditional Tc-MDP bone scan [23].

In the past, PET-CT has had limited coverage by payers including Medicare and Medicaid and other large third-party payers. Fortunately, new guidelines for the coverage of oncology FDG PET-CT now provide more widespread coverage of most malignancies, including bone and soft tissue sarcomas. Exceptions to the initial staging and diagnosis use of PET-CT exclude staging for prostate, breast, cervix, and melanoma (Centers for Medicare & Medicaid Services (CAG-00181R4)). There is increasing literature to support PET-CT for high-grade tumors such as Ewing's sarcoma as the more appropriate test to stage these tumors [23]. PET-CTs for other common tumors, such as early-stage colorectal and renal cancers, are not usually approved. Furthermore, inpatient PET-CTs in many hospitals are not covered because of the DRG-related cost issues; therefore, hospitals are typically not willing to absorb the cost related to an inpatient stay. Furthermore, most PET-CT scans are limited in frequency of usually not more often than one every 6 months. For a fast changing tumor, this is a significant restriction on tumor assessment. Undoubtedly new proven evidence-based medicine supporting the valuable role of PET-CT will increase the type of tumors that are covered for this study.

5.3   Image-Guided Biopsy

Over the last decade, there has been an increasing role in image-guided biopsy for accurate tissue diagnosis [24]. Routine use of open surgical biopsy in many cases is neither cost-effective nor safer [25]. In the past, the most common reason for open surgical biopsies was that radiologists were untrained in sarcoma biopsies, had performed few of them, and universally failed to obtain enough tissue. In large cancer centers where musculoskeletal radiologists work closer with their surgical oncologists, the biopsies can be performed by very experienced interventional musculoskeletal radiologists who understand and respect the importance of surgical planes of resection. When performed with appropriate CT or ultrasound guidance and with identification of important neurovascular structures and large tumor vessels, multiple (6–10) large cores can safely be obtained [26]. CT may be more useful for deep bone biopsies. Ultrasound is faster and easily identifies vascular structures and may be preferable for more superficial soft tissue masses.

Fine needle aspirates are usually not satisfactory for demonstrating sarcoma micro-architecture, which can be critical to proper classification of the tumor. In our institution we have highly trained cytopathologists who can accurately evaluate the viability versus necrosis/hemorrhage of core biopsy samples. Areas showing hemorrhage or necrotic tumor can be avoided and the biopsy directed to other regions of tumor without utilizing a different puncture site. Using CT guidance, the more aggressive area of bone sarcoma can be identified and selectively biopsied. For example, areas of parosteal osteosarcoma that have a more lytic appearance should be biopsied rather than areas of bland osteosclerosis [7]. With dedifferentiated chondrosarcomas, the more aggressive areas are more likely to have soft tissue breakthrough and less bland appearing enchondroma chondroid appearance [3].

In addition, CT or ultrasound-guided biopsy can be scheduled same day or within a day or so of initial discovery. CT or ultrasound-guided needle biopsy does not require general anesthesia or operating room time; CT or ultrasound core biopsies are often done with moderate sedation with IV midazolam and fentanyl. After a needle core biopsy, there are no problems with wound healing and neoadjuvant chemotherapy, or radiation can be started immediately. The likelihood of procedural complication such as hematoma or infection from a needle biopsy in experienced hands should be much less than an open biopsy [6].

The technique of a CT or ultrasound-guided core needle biopsy of a potential sarcoma is different from a CT or ultrasound fine needle biopsy of a primary or metastatic lung or liver cancer [24–26]. First, the biopsy of a possible sarcoma should be set up to obtain maximal core samples (6–10). The most common tumor biopsies of lesions from metastatic lung, breast, colon, or head and neck cancer are usually performed with a 22G needles. The route chosen for the biopsy is usually the "safest." For example, a lung biopsy is performed with the biopsy pathway closest to the pleural surface of the lesion, minimizing the risk of pneumothorax or hemorrhage. The performing interventional radiologist will identify his/her chosen approach at the time of the biopsy. In some cases as few as two or three passes may be diagnostic. Because only a few passes are made with 22G needle, sedation may not be required. The tissue diagnosis of a primary sarcoma is optimized by maximal core sample size and number. For soft tissue sarcomas, multiple 14 or 16G cores are obtained with a biopsy gun. For lesions near the skin surface that are easily palpable, this can be accomplished in the clinic setting; deeper soft tissue tumors require image CT guidance. Dense or sclerotic bone sarcomas may require a larger 8 or 11G bone needle to penetrate the cortex and penetrate through the sclerotic tumor (Fig. 5.5). Again, multiple large core samples are obtained. Because of the greater size of the needles and the number of needle passes required (four to six versus two or three passes), moderate sedation is required for patient comfort. Additionally, because large needle sizes are being used (8–16G versus 22G needle), the risk of tumor seeding of the tract is increased. Oncologic surgeons typically remove any previous incomplete surgical excision or biopsy tract of a proven sarcoma at the time of definitive surgery. If the core needle biopsy is not performed in the plane of resection, this might result in the need to perform a second incision at the time of resection. While most interventional experts recommend direct consultation with the treating oncologic surgeons and strict adherence to compartmental anatomy, there is a recent article suggesting not all biopsies must be done with strict adherence to compartmental anatomy. This study, however, was performed by a highly skilled large musculoskeletal radiology group with excellent rapport with their surgical oncologists [27]. We recommend all sarcoma biopsies be reviewed with a surgical oncologist before the procedure. For cases of potential sarcoma referred by a general physician, we consult with our surgical oncologists on a potential approach even if the patient is not known to them. According to Mankin, even today an inappropriate initial biopsy or partial excision of a sarcoma by a general surgeon, orthopedic surgeon, or radiologist is still a common cause of complications resulting in additional surgery or even amputation [28, 29]. This study showed no improvement in mismanagement by initial biopsy or surgical approach over 14 years, and 19 patients required amputation because of improper initial biopsy and surgery. It is still common that orthopedic oncologists are required to make a second incision at the time of definitive surgery because the initial open surgical or needle biopsy was not done near the expected surgical plane of resection.

Newer needles have dramatically improved the quality of core specimens obtained both for bone and soft tissue sarcomas. New bone needles have hand drill bits which allow much easier control and penetration of an intact cortex or sclerotic bone lesions. Many of these needles have just become available in the last several years. In general, for larger sclerotic bone tumors, we use bone core needles between

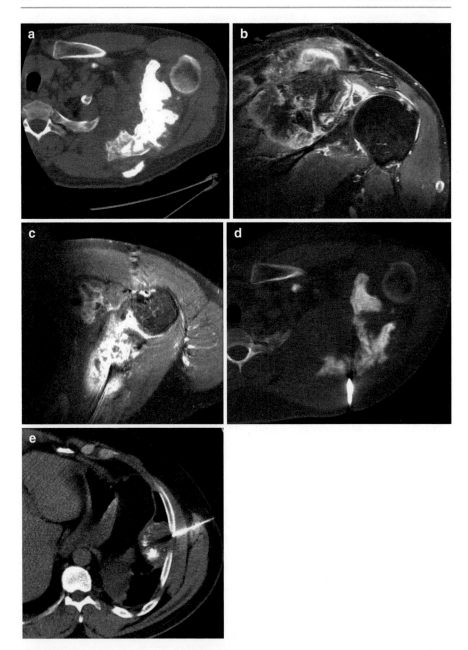

Fig. 5.5 A 54-year-old male with history of progressively enlarging mass of the right scapula. Previous limited open biopsy by general surgeon and core needle biopsy at outside hospital showed only benign fibro-osseous cells. CT biopsy showed low-grade osteosarcoma. But follow-up showed pulmonary metastases and repeated biopsy showed high-grade tumor. (**a**) CT shows large osteoid producing tumor in the body of the left scapula. Initial biopsies were benign. (**b**) Coronal MRI T1 post-contrast shows enhancing mass. (**c**) Axial MRI T1 post-contrast image shows central enhancement in the scapula at the level of the glenoid. (**d**) Repeat CT biopsy acquiring multiple 8 gauge cores through the areas of enhancement and less dense osteoid matrix. (**e**) CT biopsy of the left lung for metastatic disease

8 and 14 gauge. Newer soft tissue biopsy guns allow better quality and quantity of soft tissue cores and range from 14 to 18 gauge needles. Image-guided control and the ability to limit the 2.5 cm "throw" of the core sample allow improved safety.

The result today is that image-guided biopsies are equally accurate and safer and cost-effective than open biopsies [30].

We are often asked to perform a repeat biopsy on tumor cases where there has been a nondiagnostic limited partial resection or prior needle biopsy (Fig. 5.5). This is by no means a contraindication and often valuable if the previous biopsy went into hemorrhagic or necrotic areas, or large core samples were not obtained. The two most common scenarios include tumors with significant internal hemorrhage/necrosis or lymphomas. Either scenario is common and does not mean that a large open biopsy must be performed. Lymphomas often require more tissue for flow cytometry and larger cores. Since lymphomas are on many occasions hypovascular, it is not unsafe to obtain several 14 or 16 gauge cores. Previous tumors that have been diagnosed as necrotic, hemorrhagic, or too scant viable cells for diagnosis require a different approach. Utilization of contrast-enhanced MRI or CT examinations is very helpful. Studies are first done without contrast and then in the early arterial phase, venous phase, and, finally, delayed sequences. Areas showing the maximal amount of enhancement are the tumor areas most likely to contain viable tumor cells, and repeat biopsy should be specifically targeted to these regions. We often perform this type of contrast-enhanced CT exam immediately before the biopsy, as this significantly increases the yield of tumor diagnosis.

Another asset that is not used often enough is to have pathologists or specifically trained cytology technologists present at the time of the biopsy to review the material during the biopsy (similar to a frozen section). Assessing viable tumor cells will then guide the radiologist performing more targeted CT-guided biopsy to those regions. While the availability of a skilled pathologist may not be practical in some places, it is extremely valuable and reasonably done at major centers with multidisciplinary teams.

Asking the pathologists help in advance might enable the pathology department to provide support of the biopsy when they would not ordinarily be able to. For sarcomas in particular, the clinical and radiologic evaluations of these tumors can affect accurate tumor diagnosis and grading of the tumor. Pathologists must be given as much detailed information as possible. In cancer centers of excellence, radiologists and pathologists frequently confer on the imaging appearance of sarcomas, especially for osseous tumors. Having a pathologist routinely diagnose primary tumors of bone without benefit of the radiologic findings is unacceptable and can lead to errors in the primary tumor diagnosis and grade.

For optimal and consistent tumor biopsies, a dedicated team starting with an orthopedic oncologist is optimal. The musculoskeletal interventional radiologists must have a strong rapport with the oncologic surgeons. There must be give-and-take. Occasionally, there are cases where the radiologists may feel a biopsy is not necessary due to the benign appearance of the lesion. However, the radiologist is not the one seeing the patient, who may have come from a far distance, with the expectation that a definitive diagnosis requires a biopsy. This is frequently the only reason the patient was sent to the orthopedic oncologist to begin with. There are other cases where the radiologists may push to have additional imaging studies performed before biopsy, many times trying to identify areas where there is maximal tumor enhancement and better assess tumor vascularity. A healthy respect for each physician with expertise in their specialty leads to better outcomes.

A general interventional radiologist may not have a strong experience in bone and soft tissue tumors. We have had brisk hemorrhages when atypical hemangiomas were aggressively core biopsied where a confidant musculoskeletal radiologist could have convinced the oncologist that a biopsy was not necessary. Most general interventional radiologists know little about orthopedic surgical planning and appropriate planes of biopsy approach, leading to potentially significant errors in management.

Other members of the orthopedic oncology biopsy service should include a dedicated technologist who is familiar with the various bone needles ranging in gauge from 7 to 22G. There are many different bone needles with different advantages. For soft tissue sarcomas, we employ biopsy guns that range from 14 to 18 gauge. These needles each have different types of introducers, and since progressively large needles may be used during a biopsy if the tumor is not highly vascular, it is important to know what needles will fit through what introducers. The technologist should make sure various needles are available for each biopsy. In some cases of blastic lesions, a mallet may be used to get purchase and advance a needle. There are several battery-powered drills that are useful to the bone radiologists, and the biopsy technologist should make sure they are charged and available. An interventional radiology nurse is also essential. Since many of these biopsies require core samples with large needles, moderate sedation is usually required for sarcoma biopsies. Frequently, patients with pathologic fractures may have extreme pain. The consent and "pause for the cause" is best done before these patients are moved. Moderate sedation and analgesia can be started before moving the patient onto a CT or ultrasound table. Most of our patients are far more comfortable leaving the CT or ultrasound suite than when they come in. An unsedated patient in pain will not tolerate 8–10 cores, especially when pushing on a pathologic fracture site.

Lastly a biopsy coordinator is helpful for a busy biopsy service. Many patients may need to be scheduled urgently, and others may be traveling a long distance. Switches in the schedule may need to be made. For some musculoskeletal biopsies, particularly in older patients, anticoagulant medication such as Plavix (clopidogrel), Coumadin (warfarin), Lovenox (enoxaparin), and aspirin should be stopped. In some cases, the risk of stopping the medication may outweigh the risk of intraprocedural bleeding. The scheduling coordinator can work with the nurse navigators of the orthopedic oncology service to address these issues as well as to answer patient questions. Another major role of the biopsy coordinator and the orthopedic oncology nurse navigators and nurse practitioners is to help surmount the ever difficult insurance approval for the biopsy service. There are still payer plans that will not pay for a CT biopsy but ironically will pay for an open surgical procedure to the detriment of the patient. Working with the third-party payers to understand the benefit (and cost savings) of CT or ultrasound-guided biopsy takes time and patience.

5.4   Ablation of Unresectable or Recurrent Sarcoma

Various ablative technologies exist, including radiofrequency ablation (RFA), cryo-ablation, microwave, laser interstitial thermal therapy, and focused ultrasound therapy. Ablative therapies are becoming widely used in the treatment of recurrent sarcomas or for those sarcomas that are not resectable. Tumors may not be resectable because of tumor invasion of vital neurovascular structures or because the patient is frail and unable to tolerate definitive surgery. In addition, patients with repeated multiple recurrences may be best treated with ablative techniques (Fig. 5.6).

The most common musculoskeletal ablative application is for the treatment of osteoid osteomas. RFA is the gold standard with high success rates (often >90%) and requiring shortened convalescence in comparison to surgery [31]. Osteoid osteoma is a benign but painful bone tumor occurring primarily in young adults. The tumor nidus is targeted, and tissue necrosis is achieved through the application of high-frequency, alternating current producing lethal heat causing cellular death. RFA may also be used to ablate small tumors. This procedure is performed with CT guidance and will be briefly described. As the procedure is often painful, general or spinal anesthesia is required. Grounding pads must first be placed on the patient.

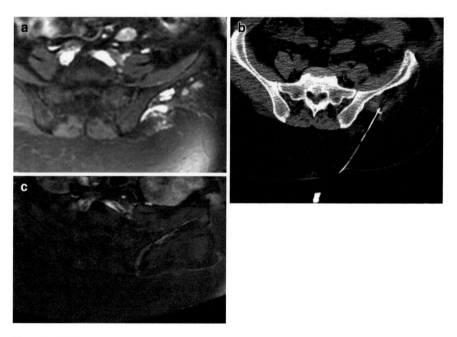

Fig. 5.6 A 54-year-old female with locally recurrent leiomyosarcoma despite multiple resections. Cryoablation performed for local control. (**a**) Axial T1-weighted MRI post-contrast shows enhancing tumor of the left gluteus muscles. (**b**) Cryoablation of the soft time mass performed. (**c**) Axial T1-weighted MRI 6 weeks post-cryoablation shows no residual enhancing tumor

Then, under CT guidance, a bone biopsy needle is used for drilling into the bone. Once the lesion is entered, an insulating cannula is inserted through the guide needle. The insulating cannula must be placed within the center of the lesion. The metal bone biopsy needle is then withdrawn to avoid unwanted heating of the metal which could lead to potential soft tissue damage. The radiofrequency electrode is inserted through the insulating cannula and ablation performed. Pain management is required following ablation, with some institutions hospitalizing patients for one night to allow for adequate pain control.

Other applications of RFA include the treatment of osseous and soft tissue metastatic lesions for disease control and pain relief. In patients with metastatic disease, complete surgical resection affords the best long-term survival, and long-term, intermittent treatment may be required. However, some patients may not be surgical candidates or may decline surgery. Various investigators have shown that percutaneous ablation offers a minimally invasive therapeutic option for controlling metastatic disease and increasing disease-free survival. Nakamura et al. evaluated 20 patients with pulmonary metastasis secondary to musculoskeletal sarcomas [32]. In patients with complete tumor ablation, one and three-year survival rates increased.

Cancer-related pain is a pervasive challenge for oncologists, often uncontrolled or poorly controlled by conventional therapies including external beam radiation, surgery, systemic therapies, and analgesics. Following ablation, cancer pain management improves. Nair et al. showed significant reduction in patient's baseline pain immediately following treatment and at six-week follow-up [33].

Cryoablation achieves cellular death through the application of extreme cold (Fig. 5.6). This system delivers argon gas through a closed-loop insulated probe placed into a lesion. The gas rapidly expands across an internal nozzle, causing a precipitous drop in temperature. Consequently, targeted tissues undergo a swift freeze with the formation of an ice ball. Following a determined length of freezing, thawing is accomplished by infusion of helium gas into the probe. It is emerging as a therapeutic option in the treatment of metastatic disease to bone and soft tissues [34].

5.5   Follow-Up Strategies of Sarcomas

Sarcoma patients, after initial treatment, require meticulous follow-up to ensure they remain disease-free; this process requires details of the tumor location, the type of tumor, and likelihood of unusual metastatic sites. As a general rule, bone and soft tissue sarcomas are followed by MRI of the primary site and CT of the chest without contrast for detection of pulmonary metastasis [35]. As alluded to earlier, there are some tumors such as myxoid liposarcoma, leiomyosarcoma, Ewing's sarcoma, and clear cell sarcoma which will spread to unusual sites including lymph nodes, peritoneum, and liver [18–20]. In general, high-grade tumors are more likely to recur earlier (at 6 months to a year), and lower-grade tumors may occur at a much later time. Early diagnosis of local recurrence and/or metastatic disease may improve long-term disease-free survival. Even pulmonary metastasis can be resected with long-term survival especially if few in number. Newer chemotherapy options may delay the onset of recurrent tumor.

Ultrasound: Ultrasound imaging can be useful in the local assessment of recurrent tumor but is not often performed as the study is operator dependent and not as reliably consistent in terms of localization to the surgeon for resection. Indeterminate palpable lesions can be assessed and checked for vascularity and differentiated from a postoperative seroma or hematoma.

Computed tomography: CT, typically without contrast, is used for surveillance of pulmonary metastasis. In general, contrast does not help in the detection of pulmonary nodules, and most sarcomas do not cause mediastinal or hilar adenopathy. A comment should be made about the increasing awareness of CT safety, especially when young patients are likely to receive many follow-up CTs of the chest. No CT should be performed unnecessarily particularly in children where the concern and potential risk is greatest. We should "Image wisely and gently." The lowest possible diagnostic CT doses should be used. Pediatric CT doses should be much lower than adults. Although no study has demonstrated a proven case of cancer caused by diagnostic imaging, statistical studies show an increasing likelihood of potential carcinogenesis. Risks and benefits should be discussed with the patients and parents. The sarcomas of the pediatric population, including rhabdomyosarcoma, Ewing's, and osteosarcoma, do have a very high likelihood of metastasizing to the lung. Early detection and treatment may be lifesaving. Modern CT scanners with new reconstruction and software techniques can be used with a much lower radiation dose. Annual whole-body radiation dose from background radiation to a person living in the mid-Atlantic region of the United States is about 3 mSieverts. Those living in Denver or Santa Fe typically have an annual radiation dose of 6 mSieverts. CT scans of the chest should be performed in that dose range (3–6 mSieverts) or effectively the same as dose as living for a year. Pediatric CT doses should be even less. In addition to the risk of the pediatric population, not all parts of the body are equally sensitive to the carcinogenic risks of radiation. The breast and thyroid are among the most sensitive regions. Increasing usage of thyroid and breast shields is recommended in the younger population. Finally, CT scans should not be repeated in the same setting. There is usually no reason to perform a CT scan for sarcoma follow-up without and with contrast or multiple-phased dynamic contrast-enhanced CTs. This has a low diagnostic yield and doubles the radiation dose. The Center for Medicine Services (CMS) tracks hospital utilization for the frequency of performance of CT scans performed without and with contrast as opposed to a study just done once. Radiologists should be able to confidently discuss with patients, parents, physicians, and other health-care providers how they are keeping radiation doses as low as possible. CT is lifesaving but must be, respectively, utilized with the lowest possible radiation dose.

Magnetic Resonance Imaging: MRI is the modality of choice for assessing local recurrence of bone and soft tissue tumors. MRI does not expose the patient to radiation and provides both superior contrast and spatial resolution compared with CT or PET-CT. A small field of view as possible should be used to increase spatial resolution. The use of contrast is debatable but is commonly used in most places. Contrast improves the confidence in a true negative or positive study and differentiates from post-operative findings of seromas and hematomas [36]. Not all seromas and hematomas resolve in 6 months. Typically, MRIs are performed initially every 3 months after a surgery for high-grade lesions and every 6 months for lower-grade tumors. Immediate postradiation or post-operative MRIs should not be performed as residual edema and swelling lead to determinant results and worry both the patient and treating physician. Local recurrence is also unlikely in the immediate posttreatment period. Obviously if there is a compelling clinical finding, then imaging may be warranted. For those patients who cannot undergo MRI because of an active pacemaker or implanted spinal cord stimulator, then CT with contrast may serve as an acceptable alternative.

Positron emission tomography: PET is now universally available combined with computed tomography (PET-CT) performed with the CT done at low resolution/low radiation dose for localization in most cases. In selected patients, the PET can be performed with high-quality contrast CT with excellent resolution [37]. The types of tumors that are approved by third-party payers for follow-up imaging are rapidly changing. Nonetheless, the frequency of follow-up imaging is usually limited to every 6 months to a year. For typical sarcomas such as osteosarcoma and malignant fibrous histiocytoma (undifferentiated pleomorphic sarcoma) where the follow-up assessment has been straightforward, e.g., an MRI of the local site and CT scan of the chest for pulmonary metastases, PET-CT may not have a role. However, patients with complicated advanced sarcomas such Ewing's sarcoma or leiomyosarcoma, which can spread to the regional nodes, lung, liver, and/or bone, would likely benefit from follow-up PET-CT [23]. Of interest, some tumors may increase in size during treatment while paradoxically responding to therapy; this can be established by decreased SUV value on follow-up imaging [38].

The follow-up of patients with known metastatic disease should not be simply a description of findings. Radiographic assessment should include specific measurements of the largest masses. Lymph nodes typically are measured by their short-axis dimension. Most research protocols follow a more systematic approach. The most widely used assessment follows Response Evaluation Criteria of Solid Tumors (RECIST) 1.1 criteria. These criteria include identifying the size and number of target lesions. Target lesions are most typically pulmonary nodules, liver masses, brain metastases, and lymph nodes. All but the lymph nodes are measured by their single greatest diameter. In the new RECIST 1.1 criteria, only two target lesions (decreased from five in the prior version) per organ are counted. A minimum size of 1 cm is required (otherwise it is considered a nontarget lesion). Only a total of five target lesions are counted. Lymph nodes are measured by their short axis and must be a minimum of 1.5 cm; lymph nodes measuring between 1.0 and 1.5 cm are considered nontarget lesions. Without the use of PET-CT, lymph nodes less than 1 cm short axis are not considered pathologic. Other sites of metastatic disease that are recorded as nontarget metastatic disease include sclerotic bone metastases, malignant pleural effusions, and malignant ascites. The total tumor burden is scored by a summation of the measurements of the target organ greatest length and sum of the short-axis dimension of pathologic lymph nodes (>1.5 cm). It is useful for follow-up studies to be interpreted in a similar fashion to avoid confusion to accurately confirm tumor response or progression. Radiologists should be familiar with these criteria and dictate them in their reports. Likewise, specific formula-based percent increase or decrease in size of target lesions and lymph nodes is used to consistently classify tumor response as: complete response, partial response, stable disease, and progressive disease. In general terms, a complete response means that the target lesions have disappeared, and lymph nodes measure under 1.0 cm short axis. Stable disease is defined as less than a 20% change in total lesion sum has occurred. Progressive disease is present when the sum of lesions' length has a greater than 20% increase and an absolute increase of at least 5 mm.

More recently, because of the new technology, newer classification schemes have been employed to formally assess tumor response. Newer classifications and modifications include the use of PET-CT response. The appearance of a new lymph node, even if less than 1 cm in size, might be considered progressive disease if it is a new lymph node with a significant PET activity (SUV). In addition, many molecular-targeted therapies discussed elsewhere in the book can cause significant internal hemorrhage, myxoid degeneration, and necrosis but without decreasing (or para-doxically increasing) the overall tumor size. Classic examples of this response are seen in tyrosine kinase inhibitors such as imatinib (Gleevec) used for gastrointestinal stromal tumors (GIST) or melanoma. Tumors undergoing internal necrosis or myxoid degeneration may paradoxically increase in size [39]. The Choi criteria therefore states that a greater than 15% decrease in lesion internal CT attenuation (density) may be included in a partial response to therapy even if the lesion increases in size. Whether newer MR characteristics such a diffusion imaging will be useful to assess response to therapy remains to be seen.

5.6 Multidisciplinary Approach with Advanced Musculoskeletal Radiologists and Interventional Radiologists

A multidisciplinary approach to cancer treatment affords the best long-term patient outcomes [40]. This approach also holds true in the diagnosis and treatment of bone and soft tissue sarcomas. While the members of a multidisciplinary sarcoma team may vary, a standard group may include orthopedic oncology, surgical/medical oncology, radiation therapy, radiology, pathology, and patient care coordinators.

Collaboration between radiology and pathology is critical in challenging and rare cases. Radiologic/pathologic concordance should be established in all cases. Conversely, discordance should require further evaluation prior to instituting definitive therapy. While many musculoskeletal tumors have diagnostic pathologic appearances, pathologists also encounter nonspecific lesions which require description of cellular composition, mitotic rate, and stroma. Thus, radiologic features suggesting an indolent versus aggressive lesion will aid in guiding the orthopedic oncologist with the surgical decision. The converse may also hold true with a non-specific radiologic appearance but bland versus highly mitotic pathologic appearance guiding the initial treatment plan.

In a national survey of oncology, radiation, and surgical clinicians, Wasif et al. confirmed that physician specialty is an important factor in shaping treatment recommendations [41]. Each subspecialist brings varying expertise, and thus, by combining knowledge, the patient is afforded the best overall care in initial treatment, continued disease surveillance, and in cases of disease recurrence. Open discussion mitigates treatment bias. While individual physicians may offer differing options regarding the exact course of patient therapy, collaborative knowledge affords patients the best treatment pathway through consideration of different regimens including the eligibility of promising clinical trials [40–42]. As a specific example, we had a patient with an aggressive looking soft tissue tumor which on CT and MRI showed destruction of the femoral cortex. The patient had had a prior open biopsy that was read as benign. We repeated a CT-guided biopsy with multiple cores, and this also came back with similar pathology. Despite the fact that we had done the biopsy and the patient had had an open biopsy, we expressed strongly that the tumor was very likely malignant and that, if malignant, needed more aggressive management of the femur erosion. An open deep biopsy with an available musculoskeletal pathologist on hand to review the frozen section was carefully planned. A more extensive surgery was also designed in case the tumor was malignant on frozen. The deep portion of the tumor was found to be a high-grade sarcoma, and a partial femoral resection was formed with a femoral prosthesis available for the planned resection.

There is no absolute formula for the creation of a multidisciplinary team; rather the key concept is providing best practice patient care through subspecialty expertise. Teams usually meet in a conference setting, which may occur weekly, biweekly, or monthly. Frequency is determined by case volume. At our institutions, the orthopedic oncologist serves as team leader by creating a list of patients for discussion and functioning as conference director. Any team member may present relevant cases. Patient care coordinators record recommendations and functions as patient liaisons navigating patients through various appointments and stages of their care.

The multidisciplinary approach is an effective tool to reach treatment consensus and mitigate subspecialty bias, thus affording the best disease-free outcomes [41, 42].

References

1. Kransdorf M, Murphey M. Imaging of soft tissue tumors. 2nd ed. Philadelphia, PA: Lippincott Williams & Wilkins; 2006.
2. Miettinen M. Modern soft tissue pathology: tumors and non-neoplastic conditions. Cambridge: Cambridge University Press; 2010.
3. Resnick D, Kransdorf M. Bone and joint imaging. 3rd ed. Philadelphia, PA: Elsevier Saunders; 2005.

4. Tateishi U, Yamaguchi U, Seki K, Terauchi T, Arai Y, Kim E. Bone and soft-tissue sarcoma: preoperative staging with fluorine 18 fluorodeoxyglucose PET/CT and conventional imaging. Radiology. 2007;245(3):839–47.
5. American College of Radiology. (n.d.). 2013. Retrieved 2014 from http://www.acr.org/Quality-Safety/Appropriateness-Criteria
6. Beaman F, Jelinek J, Priebat D. Bone and soft-tissue sarcoma: current imaging and therapy of malignant soft tissue tumors and tumor-like lesions. Semin Musculoskelet Radiol. 2013;17(02):168–76.
7. Jelinek J, Murphey M, Kransdorf M, Shmookler B, Malawer M, Hur R. Parosteal osteosarcoma: value of MR imaging and CT in the prediction of histologic grade. Radiology. 1996;201(3):837–42.
8. Murphey M, Gibson M, Jennings B, Crespo-Rodriguez A, Fanburg-Smith J, Gajewski D. From the archives of the AFIP: imaging of synovial sarcoma with radiologic-pathologic correlation. Radiographics. 2006;26(5):1543–65.
9. Malawer M, Sugarbaker P. Musculoskeletal cancer surgery treatment of sarcomas and allied diseases. Dordrecht: Kluwer Academic; 2001.
10. Barile A, Caulo M, Zugaro L, Di Cesare E, GAllucci M, Masciocchi C. Staging and re-staging of soft tissue sarcoma using. Usefulness of contrast. Radiol Med. 2001;101(6):444–55.
11. Widmark J. Imaging-related mediations: a class overview. Proc Baylor Univ Med Cent. 2007;20(4):408–17.
12. Dozo G, Serra MT, Menso E, Herrera R, Alesso E. Allergy-immune profile of high risk patients for low osmolality contrast media (LOCM) adverse drug reactions (ADRs): a basis for prevention. Drug Saf. 2008;31(10):885–960.
13. Panicek DM, Go SD, Healey JH, Leung DH, Brennan MF, Lewis JJ. Soft-tissue sarcoma involving bone or neurovascular structures: MR imaging prognostic factors. Radiology. 1997;205(3):871–5.
14. Jungmann PM. 21st Annual Scientific Meeting of the European Society of Musculoskeletal Radiology (ESSR), Riga, Latvia, June 26–28, 2014. Skelet Radiol. 2014;43(6):849–74.
15. Fayad L, Barker P, Bluemke D. Molecular characterization of musculoskeletal tumors by proton MR spectroscopy. Semin Musculoskeletal Radiol. 2007;11(3):240–5.
16. Subhawong TK, Jacobs MA, Fayad LM. Insights Into quantitative diffusion-weighted MRI for musculoskeletal tumor imaging. Am J Roentgenol. 2014;203(3):560–72.
17. Kwee TC, Takahara T, Ochiai R, Nievelstein RA, Luijten PR. Diffusion-weighted whole-body imaging with background body signal suppression (DWIBS): features and potential applications in oncology. Eur Radiol. 2008;18(9):1937–52.
18. Noble J, Moskovic E, Fisher C, Judson I. Imaging of skeletal metastases in myxoid liposarcoma. Sarcoma. 2010;2010:1–6.
19. Schwab J, Boland P, Guo T, Brennan M, Singer S, Healey J, Antonescu C. Skeletal metastases in myxoid liposarcoma: an unusual pattern of distant spread. Ann Surg Oncol. 2007;14(4):1507–14.
20. Brewer P, Abudu A, Carter S, Grimer R, Sumathi V, Jeys L, Tillman R. Primary leiomyosarcoma of bone: analysis of prognosis. Sarcoma. 2012;2012:1–4.
21. Hong S, Lee S, Choi Y, Seo S, Sung K, Koo H, Choi J. Prognostic value of 18F-FDG PET/CT in patients with soft tissue sarcoma: Comparisons between metabolic parameters. Skelet Radiol. 2014;43(5):641–8.
22. Ulaner G, Magnan H, Healey J, Weber W, Meyers P. Is methylene diphosphonate bone scan necessary for initial staging of Ewing sarcoma if FDG PET/CT is performed? Am J Roentgenol. 2014;202(4):859–67.
23. Meyer J, Schomberg P, Marina N, Nadel H, Kailo M, Lessnick S, Womer R. Imaging guidelines for children with Ewing sarcoma and osteosarcoma: a report from the Children's Oncology Group Bone Tumor Committee. Pediatr Blood Cancer. 2008;51(2):163–70.
24. Jelinek J, Murphey M, Welker J, Henshaw R, Kransdorf M, Shmookler B, Malawer M. Diagnosis of primary bone tumors with image-guided percutaneous biopsy: experience with 110 tumors. Radiology. 2002;223(3):731–7.

25. Nouh M, Shady H. Initial CT-guided needle biopsy of extremity skeletal lesions: diagnostic performance and experience of a tertiary musculoskeletal center. Eur J Radiol. 2014;83(2):360–5.
26. Le H, Lee S, Munk P. Image-guided musculoskeletal biopsies. Semin Intervent Radiol. 2010;27(02):191–8.
27. Omura M, Motamedi K, Uybico S, Nelson S, Seeger L. Revisiting CT-guided percutaneous core needle biopsy of musculoskeletal lesions: contributors to biopsy success. Am J Roentgenol. 2011;197(2):457–61.
28. Mankin H, Mankin C, Simon M. The hazards of eh biopsy, revisited. Members of the Musculoskeletal Tumor Society. J Bone Joint Surg Am. 1996;78(5):656–63.
29. Mankin H, Lange T, Spanier S. The hazards of biopsy in patients with malignant primary bone and soft-tissue tumors. J Bone Joint Surg Am. 1982;64(8):1121–7.
30. Pohlig F, Kirchhoff C, Lenze U, Schauwecker J, Burgkart R, Rechl H, et al. Percutaneous core needle biopsy versus open biopsy in diagnostics of bone and soft tissue sarcoma: a retrospective study. Eur J Med Res. 2012;17(1):29.
31. Obyrne J, Eustace S, Cantwell C. Current trends in treatment of osteoid osteoma with an emphasis on radiofrequency ablation. Eur Radiol. 2004;14(4):607–17.
32. Nakamura T, Shimizu T, Abo D, Takeda K, Nakatsuka A, Takaki H, Uchida A. Lung radiofrequency ablation in patients with pulmonary metastases from musculoskeletal sarcomas. Cancer. 2009;115(16):3774–81.
33. Nair R, Vansonnenberg E, Shankar S, Morrison P, Gill R, Tuncali K, Silverman S. Visceral and soft-tissue tumors: radiofrequency and alcohol ablation for pain relief--initial experience. Radiology. 2008;248(3):1067–76.
34. Callstrom M, Wong G, Atwell T, Brown K, Maus T, Welch T, Charboneau J. Painful metastases involving bone: percutaneous image-guided cryoablation--prospective trial interim analysis. Radiology. 2006;241(2):572–80.
35. Watts A, Teoh K, Evans T, Beggs I, Robb J, Porter D. MRI surveillance after resection for primary musculoskeletal sarcoma. J Bone Joint Surg. 2008;90-B(4):484–7.
36. Grande FD, Subhawong T, Weber K, Aro M, Mugera C, Fayad LM. Detection of soft-tissue sarcoma recurrence: added value of functional MR imaging techniques at 3.0 T. Radiology. 2014;271(2):499–511.
37. Tewfik J, Greene G. Fluorine-18-deoxyglucose–positron emission tomography imaging with magnetic resonance and computed tomographic correlation in the evaluation of bone and soft-tissue sarcomas: a pictorial essay. Curr Probl Diagn Radiol. 2008;37(4):178–88.
38. Sanford Z, Israelsen S, Sehgal R, Cheung FH. Atypical growth on MRI in a case of Ewing's sarcoma despite lower SUV on PET. Skelet Radiol. 2013;43(6):819–25.
39. Stacchiotti S, Collini P, Messina A, Morosi C, Barisella M, Bertulli R, Casali PG. High-grade soft-tissue sarcomas: tumor response assessment—pilot study to assess the correlation between radiologic and pathologic response by using RECIST and Choi criteria 1. Radiology. 2009;251(2):447–56.
40. Zhang J, Mayros M, Cosgrove D, Hirose K, Herman JM, Smallwood-Massey S, Kamel I, Gurakar A, Anders R, Cameron A, Geschwind JF, Pawlik TM. Impact of a single-day multidisciplinary clinic on the management of patients with liver tumors. Curr Oncol. 2013;20(2):123–31.
41. Wasif N, Tamurian R, Christensen S, Do L, Martinez S, Chen S, Canter R. Influence of specialty and clinical experience on treatment sequencing in the multimodal management of soft tissue extremity sarcoma. Ann Surg Oncol. 2012;19(2):504–10.
42. Castell P. Multidisciplinary and medical decision, impact for patients with cancer: sociological assessment of two tumor committees' organization. Bull Cancer. 2012;99(4):34–42.

The Role of Surgery in the Multidisciplinary Care of Sarcoma

6

Robert M. Henshaw

6.1 Introduction

Primary malignant neoplasms of the musculoskeletal system, defined as sarcomas, arise from mesenchymal tissue and can occur at any age and in any location of the body. These tumors rank among the most uncommon neoplasms seen by physicians and are frequently mistaken for other conditions due to the fact that many physicians remain unfamiliar with the presenting signs and symptoms of these rare tumors. Despite this, it is interesting to note that these rare tumors have historically garnered great interest in the medical profession due to their ability to reach extraordinary size with resulting massive deformities and disabilities when left untreated (Fig. 6.1). The natural history of a sarcoma is characterized by unrelenting circumferential growth and metastatic spread via hematologic pathways. In extremity locations, unchecked growth of the tumor can lead to disabling pain (from compression and secondary involvement of peripheral nerves) and expansion of the tumor through the skin (tumor fungation), resulting in persistent bleeding and subsequent secondary infection of the exposed tumor (Fig. 6.2). Prior to the introduction of effective adjuvant treatments, sarcoma patients would often turn toward surgeons in

R.M. Henshaw, M.D.
Professor, Clinical Orthopedic Surgery (Orthopedic Oncology), Georgetown University School of Medicine, Washington, DC, USA

Vice Chair, Department of Orthopedics, MedStar Washington Hospital Center, Washington, DC, USA

Director, Division of Orthopedic Oncology, MedStar Georgetown Orthopedic Institute, Washington, DC, USA

Director, Orthopedic Oncology, MedStar Washington Cancer Institute and Children's National Medical Center, Washington, DC, USA

Consultant, Surgical Branch, National Cancer Institute, Bethesda, MD, USA

MedStar Washington Cancer Institute, Washington, DC, USA
e-mail: Robert.m.henshaw@medstar.net

© Springer International Publishing Switzerland 2017
R.M. Henshaw (ed.), *Sarcoma*, DOI 10.1007/978-3-319-43121-5_6

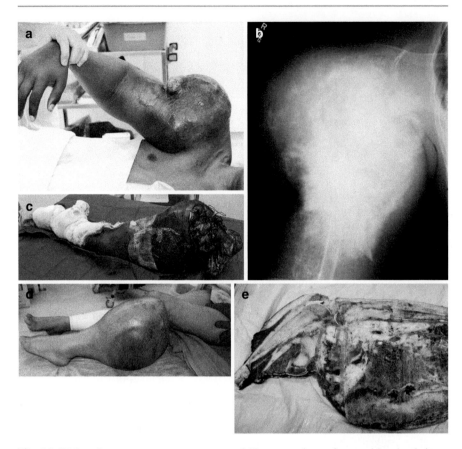

Fig. 6.1 Neglected osteosarcoma can grow to astonishing proportions, often requiring drastic intervention. (**a**) Young male with untreated osteosarcoma unable to walk as his arm was bigger than his chest. (**b**) X-ray demonstrating massive bone formation. (**c**) Palliative forequarter amputation was performed, allowing him to independently ambulate and leave the hospital. He eventually succumbed to metastatic disease. (**d**) Young woman unable to ambulate or lay down due to massive osteosarcoma of the leg. (**e**) Resection specimen after palliative amputation demonstrating massive tumor dwarfing of her knee joint, femur, and tibia. Amputation allowed her to ambulate and leave the hospital

Fig. 6.2 Fungating undifferentiated soft tissue sarcoma destroying the hand and axilla in a 6-month-old, progressing on chemotherapy. Parents were unable to hold him due to the size and weight of his hand; palliative forequarter amputation permitted him to be held and to leave the hospital

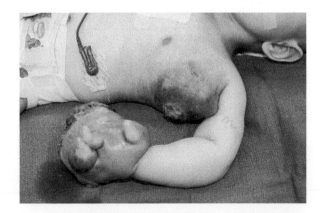

the hope of having the tumor removed. Experienced surgeons recognized the futility of incomplete resections (debulking procedures), which often hastened fungation of the tumor as it recurred through the surgical site (Fig. 6.3). Accordingly, surgeons were forced to perform major amputations, such as hemipelvectomy (hindquarter amputation) (Fig. 6.4) or scapulothoracic disarticulation (forequarter amputation)

Fig. 6.3 Tumor fungation seen on referral after an unplanned intralesional excision of a mass involving the index fingertip. Treated with an amputation through the middle phalanx

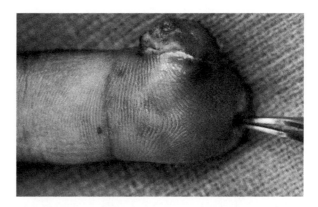

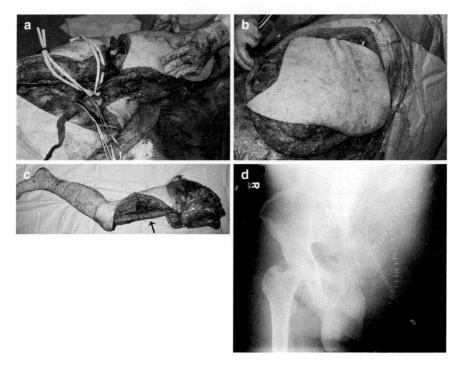

Fig. 6.4 Anterior flap hemipelvectomy. (**a**) A full-thickness pedicle flap consisting of the quadriceps muscles and anterior skin is raised with the superficial femoral vessels (looped with Penrose drains). (**b**) The flap is positioned over the pelvic defect, taking care to avoid kinking the vessels. (**c**) Resection specimen showing the hemipelvis and lower extremity with the anterior defect from the flap (*arrow*). (**d**) Postoperative x-ray showing the flap outlined by skin staples

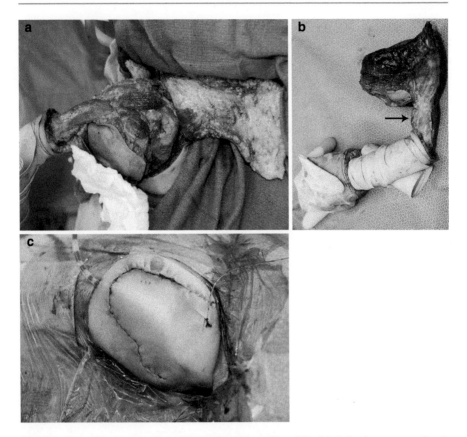

Fig. 6.5 Forequarter amputation of 6-month-old boy (Fig. 6.2). (**a**) A fasciocutaneous flap is raised from the posterior arm prior to the amputation. (**b**) Resection specimen demonstrating shoulder girdle and upper extremity with a defect from raising the flap (*arrow*). (**c**) Coverage of the chest wall with the posterior flap

(Fig. 6.5), for any and all patients presenting with such masses in the hopes of controlling disease and improving (palliating) patient's quality of life. Frequently, patients treated with such aggressive surgical techniques would succumb to the cancer due to metastatic spread beyond the area removed by the surgeon. However, a small but measurable number of patients would survive beyond 5 years, helping to justify the role of surgery in these diseases; data for patients with primary sarcoma of the bone, defined as osteosarcoma, showed an expected survival after radical amputation around 20% at 2 years [1].

The advent of radiographic imaging along with the introduction of histologic analysis by pathologists started a slow but progressive revolution in the management of these malignancies. A key step was taken by James Ewing, a pathologist at General Memorial Hospital (the forerunner to the Memorial Sloan Kettering Cancer Center), who in 1921 published a case series on "diffuse endothelioma of the bone" [2], (later named as Ewing's sarcoma of the bone by Dr. Ernest Codman), where he differentiated this aggressive round cell tumor from other musculoskeletal tumors that featured a spindle cell appearance. He demonstrated that patients with this specific tumor would clinically respond to exposure to radiation from the newly available radioactive element radium, differentiating it from osteosarcoma, laying the foundation for radiotherapy as a form of adjuvant treatment for sarcomas [3]. Of interest, Ewing established one of the first funds for cancer research and founded the American Association for Cancer Research in 1907, now known as the American Cancer Society.

Despite poor survival with amputation, surgeons of that era had already begun investigating the role of conservative "limb-sparing" surgery for low-grade tumors. Building on the early pioneering work of Dallas Phemister who introduced key concepts in limb-sparing surgery in the 1940s [4, 5], Frank Parrish reported the use of large bone grafts to reconstruct defects following the local resection of bone tumors [6], while Ralph Marcove reported the use of liquid nitrogen (cryosurgery) in the treatment of primary and metastatic bone tumors [7]. Surgical advances were also reported in the treatment of sarcoma metastases; Judson McNamara demonstrated that pulmonary resection for isolated metastatic osteosarcoma to the lungs was potentially curative [8]. The discovery of effective chemotherapy agents, such as Adriamycin and methotrexate, offered new hope to patients with osteosarcoma [9]. Advances in imaging included the use of angiography to evaluate tumor vasculature [10], the development of computerized axial tomography (CT scan) by Hounsfield [11] and Ambrose [12], and the introduction of the technetium (Tc^{99m})-labeled polyphosphate bone scan by Subramanian [13]. All of these imaging modalities provided surgeons with new methods of visualizing the anatomy of a given tumor and its relationship to the surrounding anatomic structures within the surgical field.

These advances led to increased interest in limb-sparing surgery, driven by improved understanding of anatomy and a new confidence in techniques for limb reconstruction. William Enneking introduced the resection-arthrodesis technique of limb salvage, using local bone grafts combined with intramedullary rods to replace and fuse the knee following limb-sparing tumor resections [14] (Fig. 6.6). Henry Mankin demonstrated that large defects could be reconstructed with massive homologous bone grafts (allografts) [15] (Fig. 6.7). Ralph Marcove reported that massive metallic implants (endoprostheses) could be used to replace the entire femur and the knee [16]. Gerald Rosen, working with Ralph Marcove, introduced the concept of preoperative (induction) chemotherapy, which enabled treatment while patients were waiting for the manufacturing of a custom limb salvage implant [17]. Donald Morton and Frederick Eilber reported on successful limb-sparing resection for soft tissue sarcomas when combined with chemotherapy and radiation [18] and began asking if amputation was always necessary for sarcomas [19]. The same advances in imaging and chemotherapy driving limb-sparing surgery also led to further interest in surgery for metastatic disease involving the lungs [20, 21].

This brief historical overview illustrates the cascading and synergistic effects of different subspecialties upon each other. The interrelationship between surgeons, medical oncologists, radiation oncologists, pathologists, and radiologists becomes

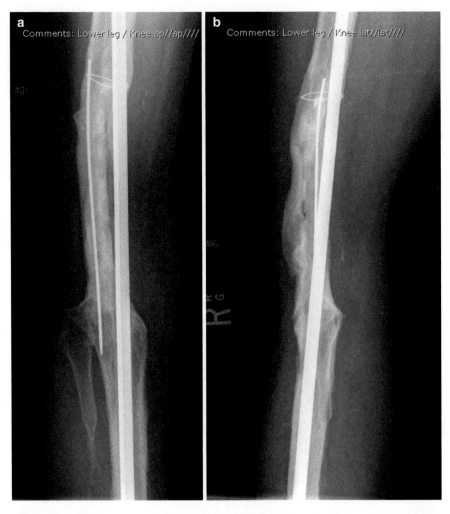

Fig. 6.6 (**a**) AP radiograph and (**b**) lateral radiograph of a long-term survivor of osteosarcoma treated with a resection arthrodesis performed by Enneking 45 years ago with a full-length Sampson rod and ipsilateral fibular autograft bridging the skeletal defect

increasingly critical as advances in each individual specialty impact and drive innovation in the other specialties. This was the impetus behind the development of multidisciplinary treatment teams for sarcoma. The surgical specialist has become the de facto gatekeeper of the treatment team by virtue of the fact that patients with masses are often first referred to a surgical specialist for initial evaluation. The introduction of cancer centers on a regional and now community basis has helped further the central role of the surgeon in the care of these patients. Today, the orthopedic or surgical oncologist must be prepared to diagnose patients and help them (and their

Fig. 6.7 Massive osteoarticular allograft reconstruction of the proximal tibia in a 7-year-old boy after resection of an osteosarcoma. The graft eventually fractured and he was successfully converted to a proximal tibial endoprosthesis

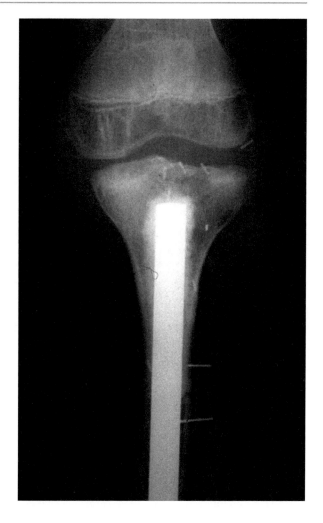

families) understand and navigate multiple specialties (not to mention the current healthcare system) to ensure appropriate and timely treatment for their disease.

As members of the MedStar Orthopedic Institute and the MedStar Georgetown Oncology Network, our service provides patient care in a comprehensive cancer center featuring a fully implemented multidisciplinary team approach at the MedStar Washington Cancer Institute and at Children's National Medical Center. Per our departmental surgical database (as of January 2016), our group has operated on 5813 patients with musculoskeletal tumors, including 3450 patients with cancer (1896 bone and 1554 soft tissue); the majority of these cases have been performed by the author. Of the cancer patients, only 8% required an amputation, for an overall limb salvage rate of 92%. This large clinical experience provides the basis for much of the information included in this chapter.

6.2   Surgical Evaluation of Sarcoma Patients

The typical sarcoma patient seeks medical attention after becoming aware of a mass or after experiencing a new onset of pain or discomfort. In the case of soft tissue sarcomas, which frequently present without pain (at least until tumor growth results in nerve irritation or compression), patients may ignore a mass for weeks or months due to the lack of any other symptoms. A primary care (or urgent care) physician is frequently the first medical practitioner the patient sees, although alternatively some patients may be seen by chiropractors, podiatrists, physical therapists, massage therapists, or physical trainers who discover a mass while laying hands on the patient. Delays in referral may be due to lack of patient concern, denial of a physical problem, or lack of recognition that a painless mass may be more than a simple lipoma. Once a patient has been referred to a surgical specialist, it is incumbent upon the surgeon to perform a detailed physical exam and obtain pertinent clinical history in order to identify a potential sarcoma. During the initial evaluation, plain radiographs of the affected site can often provide significant clues as to the nature of the problem, particularly when the tumor arises from or involves the bone. General surgeons and orthopedists must be prepared to recognize a potential sarcoma and be willing to make an appropriate referral to an oncologic subspecialist prior to performing invasive testing or biopsy. Studies have shown that inappropriate procedures and/or biopsies remain a leading cause of amputation in cases otherwise suited to limb-sparing surgery due to unplanned contamination of multiple surgical compartments [22]. It is the position of the Musculoskeletal Tumor Society (MSTS) that the physician arranging for or performing a biopsy of a suspected sarcoma be prepared to perform the definitive surgical resection in the advent of a musculoskeletal malignancy.

Physical examination of the patient by the surgical specialist requires a detailed knowledge of anatomy and surgical compartments. Tumor characteristics including size, shape, texture, and mobility are often readily apparent with careful palpation of the mass. Assessment of vascular and neurologic status is important, particularly in planning a biopsy and subsequent surgery. Detailed history and physical examination of the entire body is important to rule out multifocal conditions, such as lipomatosis or neurofibromatosis, skip lesions/metastases, and other medical conditions that have potential bearing not only on the diagnosis but also on patient suitability for surgical resection. This assessment serves to confirm the suspicion of a musculoskeletal neoplasm and provides a rational basis for appropriate advanced imaging and biopsy techniques as discussed in more detail in Chap. 5. Imaging should include the entire mass as well as its anatomically relevant compartment; for plain radiographs, this should include the joint above and below the tumor, while for MRI and CT scans, the field of view should include the entire muscular compartment in which the tumor resides. Additional imaging for the purposes of staging routinely includes a high-resolution chest CT (in preference to chest x-ray) as well as bone scan or PET/CT in selected cases. Preliminary planning for surgical intervention can be discussed with the patient, who often can be reassured that treatment options exist and that they are not alone in having such a problem. Patients often relate that uncertainty in diagnosis and delays in being referred to a qualified specialist are some of the most stressful portions of their interaction with the health-care system. The role of the surgeon includes addressing the anxiety, fear, and concern of patients and their families with regard to their potential treatment. Mid-level practitioners working with the surgeon can be instrumental in providing such support, as detailed in Chap. 17.

Following the initial encounter, a diagnostic biopsy to confirm the presence of a sarcoma as well as its grade needs to be performed. For some patients, the biopsy can easily be performed at the same time as the initial evaluation in the clinic. Patient selection is critical in deciding who can undergo a successful office-based procedure. The goal is to obtain diagnostic tissue with minimal contamination of adjacent compartments that might interfere with definitive surgical resection. In general, tumors that can easily be palpated in the extremities and that are not involving neurovascular structures can easily be sampled with a core needle without radiographic imaging [23]. This technique requires proper sterilization/prepping of the skin, the use of a local anesthetic such as 1% lidocaine, and a large gauge core biopsy needle that can be inserted several times into the mass in order to harvest adequate tissue for pathology (Fig. 6.8). Occasionally, tumors that involve or extend

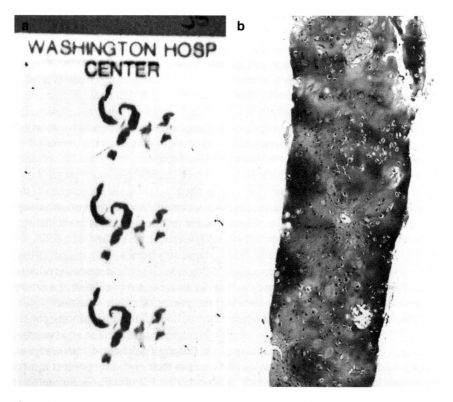

Fig. 6.8 (**a**) Glass slide showing multiple sections of a core needle biopsy. (**b**) Low-power microscopic view of the slide demonstrating the preserved architecture of the tumor. The relationship between neoplastic cells, stromal cells, and extracellular matrix is critical to the proper diagnosis of musculoskeletal tumors

included the use of angiography to evaluate tumor vasculature [10], the development of computerized axial tomography (CT scan) by Hounsfield [11] and Ambrose [12], and the introduction of the technetium (Tc^{99m})-labeled polyphosphate bone scan by Subramanian [13]. All of these imaging modalities provided surgeons with new methods of visualizing the anatomy of a given tumor and its relationship to the surrounding anatomic structures within the surgical field. These advances laid the groundwork for a new understanding of the biologic behavior and growth patterns of sarcoma and permitted surgeons to prepare and plan for procedures that previously were deemed too risky.

With these advances in place, William Enneking introduced several concepts that placed surgical management of sarcomas on a scientifically sound basis. One of the key elements he introduced was the concept of a surgical compartment, ranging from a single entire bone or muscle to entire muscle groups confined by strong fascial boundaries [28]. The recognition that sarcoma growth was frequently limited by fascial boundaries and the ability to demonstrate compartmental involvement using the newly introduced imaging techniques allowed surgeons to plan for precise resections. Enneking created a framework for classifying and defining the type of resection performed using the concept of the tumor pseudocapsule (reactive zone) as a delineation between the tumor and the surrounding tissue. For the first time, surgeons could easily understand how an amputation, if it violated the tumor pseudocapsule, could easily fail to control the disease with local recurrence occurring within the amputation stump. This classification of surgical margins allowed surgeons to understand and convey information in a reproducible fashion, further advancing efforts to perform limb-sparing surgery. Enneking also showed that the risk of local recurrence following removal of the tumor varies not only on the grade of the tumor but also on the type of resection that was performed [28]. This data help to validate the scientific underpinnings of his classification scheme, leading to its widespread adoption by surgeons performing limb-sparing resections (limb salvage surgery) for patients with malignant tumors. Enneking introduced a surgical staging system for musculoskeletal tumors with individual stages dependent upon the tumor grade and whether it was confined to a single compartment [30]. He subsequently used the staging system to analyze his clinical experience and showed that a patient's surgical stage was prognostically significant with regard to their oncologic outcome [31]. These tools formed the basis by which surgeons could select appropriate patients for limb-sparing surgery.

In addition to this fundamental framework, Enneking introduced a method of reconstructing skeletal defects around the knee following tumor resection which he termed as resection arthrodesis, consisting of local bone grafts combined with intramedullary rods to replace and fuse the knee following limb-sparing tumor resections [14]. Around the same time, Henry Mankin demonstrated that large defects could be reconstructed with massive homologous bone grafts (allografts) [15], and Ralph Marcove reported that massive metallic implants (endoprostheses) could be used to replace the entire femur and the knee [16]. While many traditional surgeons criticized these efforts at putting patients' lives at risk, careful analysis of patient outcomes showed otherwise. Results from the first International Society of Limb Salvage (ISOLS) meeting in 1981 were later summarized by Enneking as such:

"532 resections were reported with a local recurrence rate of 18% and a surgical failure rate in reconstruction of 15% for an overall failure rate of 1 in 3 attempts" [32]. After the 1989 ISOLS meeting, he noted: "more than 2,500 resections were reported with a combined local recurrence and surgical failure rates of 1 in 10 attempts—a remarkable decrease in the short span of one decade" [32].

In addition to his work with bone sarcomas, Enneking also showed that his concepts of resection margin and compartmental status were valuable in the treatment of soft tissue sarcomas [33]. Donald Morton and Frederick Eilber reported on successful limb-sparing resection for soft tissue sarcomas when combined with chemotherapy and radiation and began asking if amputation was always necessary for sarcomas [19]. The introduction of magnetic resonance imaging (MRI), based on the Nobel prize-winning work of Lauterbur and Mansfield [34] and approved by the FDA in 1984, gave surgeons an unprecedented and noninvasive look into patient and tumor anatomy. Multiaxial imaging with the ability to distinguish abnormal from normal tissue allowed surgeons to plan limb-sparing oncologic resections in areas of significant anatomic complexity such as the shoulder girdle and the pelvis. Similar progress was seen in efforts to resect retroperitoneal sarcomas, where complete resection was associated with significant improvements in survival [35]. Anatomic imaging also allowed surgeons to plan and perform effective oncologic resections based upon sound anatomic principles for tumors of the spine.

6.4   Endoprosthetic Reconstruction

A significant advance in the medical treatment of sarcomas was the use of preoperative (induction) chemotherapy, introduced by Gerald Rosen while working with Ralph Marcove, which enabled treatment of the tumor while patients were waiting for the manufacturing of a custom limb salvage implant [17]. This helped to spur the acceptance of endoprosthetic reconstruction as a means of limb-sparing surgery for patients with large skeletal defects. Interest in endoprosthetic reconstruction attracted the attention of engineers and implant manufacturers, leading to an evolution from unique custom implants requiring weeks of manufacturing lead time to modular implants featuring off the shelf flexibility in matching patient anatomy with improved manufacturing quality controls [36, 37]. The introduction of modular implants led to a significant change in reconstructive trends away from allograft reconstruction, which was prevalent in the 1980s, toward endoprosthetic reconstruction in the 1990s [32]. Data presented at the 2007 ISOLS meeting showed that the majority of sarcoma patients were candidates for limb-sparing surgery, with satisfactory functional outcomes doubled than that of amputation [32].

Early adopters of modular implants demonstrated that this form of reconstruction offered significant advantages, including improved patient outcomes and early return to function [38]. Subsequent studies have reported the long-term outcomes of these implants, demonstrating excellent survival compared to custom implants while noting that mechanical failures, now rare, have been replaced by aseptic loosening and infection as the most common forms of implant failure [39]. Recent work has focused on solving these specific issues, particularly aseptic loosening [40]. Rapid implementation of changes has been facilitated by the modularity of implant systems as improved design concepts can be incorporated into existing proven implant systems by creating a new component(s) that joins with the existing system, leading to improved implant survival [41, 42]. Wide variations in the rate of aseptic loosening of cemented stems have been reported by various centers; mechanical factors and cement technique may account for these differences, with best results seen when stem sizes are matched to patient anatomy [40]. Porous-coated uncemented stems have been introduced to avoid aseptic loosening, paralleling trends seen in total joint arthroplasty [43, 44]. A new method of biologic fixation, compressive osteointegration, was introduced to address stress shielding seen in total joints with mechanically rigid stems by creating significant mechanical loads directly at the implant/cortical bone junction through a novel loading mechanism [45]. This device has subsequently been incorporated into a modular endoprosthetic system for limb salvage after tumor resection [46] and may reduce the risk of aseptic loosening [47] (Fig. 6.9).

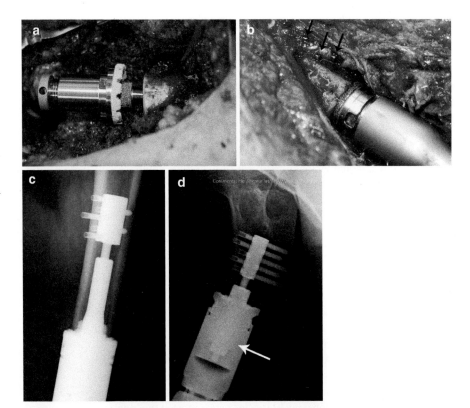

Fig. 6.9 Compressive osteointegration demonstrated using a Biomet (Warsaw, IN) Compress limb salvage system. (**a**) Porous-coated spindle that matches the machined end of the bone, designed to permit bone ingrowth between the cortical bone and the implant. (**b**) The spindle is secured to the bone by an anchor plug fixed intramedullary with transfixion pins (*arrows*). (**c**) X-ray showing a standard anchor plug with bi-cortical transfixion pins. (**d**) The spindle is loaded (compressed) against the bone using a Belleville washer spring mechanism located in the spindle (*arrow*)

Significant advances have occurred in implants designed to address unique challenges encountered in anatomically complex locations as well as in skeletally immature patients. While allograft reconstructions may still be considered by some, the introduction of mechanically reliable implants continues to drive the increasing acceptance of endoprosthetic reconstruction. Improvement in designs, surgical techniques, methods of fixation, and new joint articulations continue to be introduced, often as modifications to more conventional total joint arthroplasty. For example, shoulder stability following proximal humeral resection can now be significantly improved with the adoption of a reverse total shoulder replacement articulation, originally introduced for patients with massive rotator cuff tears [48] (Fig. 6.10). Successful endoprosthetic reconstruction has been performed for segmental replacements of complex joints such as the scapula (shoulder) [49], elbow [50], acetabulum (hip) [51] and ankle [52], and even smaller bones such as the ulna (Figs. 6.11, 6.12, 6.13, and 6.14).

Similarly, expandable implants for skeletally immature patients where loss of growth plates would result in a significant limb length discrepancy have also undergone significant advances. Originally described by Lewis in 1986 [53],

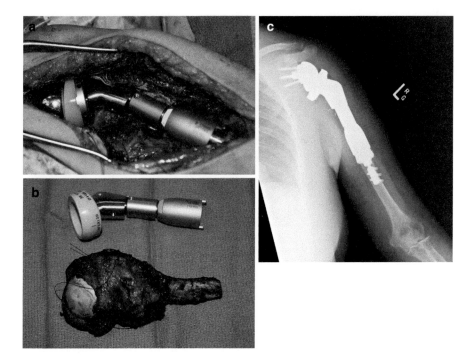

Fig. 6.10 Proximal humeral replacements have suffered from instability/dislocation as well as poor active function of the shoulder; their primary benefit is to stabilize the upper arm so that patients can perform useful activities with their hand. (**a**) The reverse total shoulder arthroplasty, originally designed for shoulder replacement in the rotator cuff-deficient patient, can be used in conjunction with a proximal humeral replacement as seen with this Biomet (Warsaw, IN) Compress endoprosthesis. It offers superior stability and improved function following repair of the deltoid insertion by providing a stable fulcrum for the arm to actively abduct against. (**b**) Resection specimen from this patient with a high-grade chondrosarcoma arising from the proximal humerus. (**c**) Postoperative xray showing relationship of the scapula and glenoid hemisphere to the proximal humeral implant

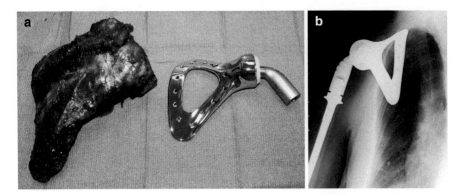

Fig. 6.11 Total scapula replacement with a constrained shoulder joint, Stryker/Howmedica (Mahwah, NJ) GMRS system, for reconstruction following resection of the scapula. (**a**) Resection specimen and implant. (**b**) X-ray demonstrating relationship of the scapular implant to the chest wall and lateralization of the shoulder arthroplasty

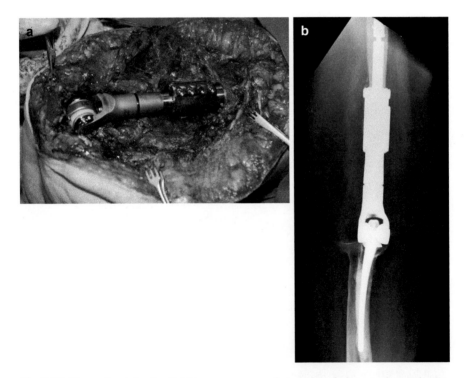

Fig. 6.12 Tumors involving the distal humerus are rare, but can benefit from modern endoprosthetic reconstruction. (**a**) Distal humeral replacement following resection of the distal humerus and (**b**) follow-up x-ray showing a Biomet (Warsaw, IN) Discovery elbow combined with a Compress limb-sparing system

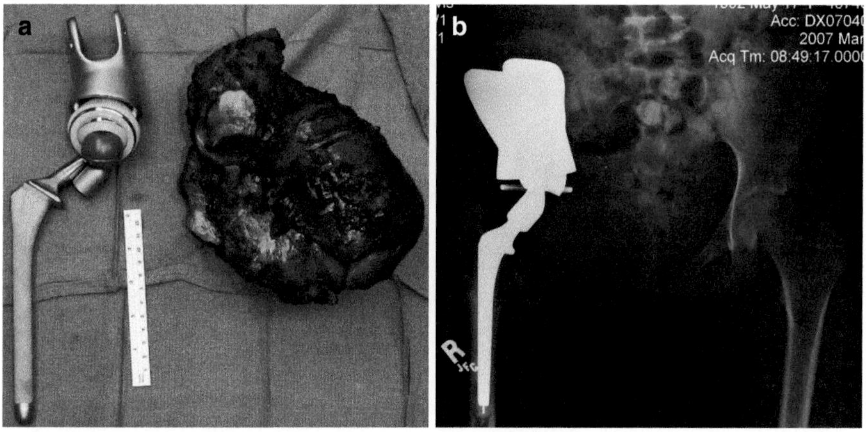

Fig. 6.13 Reconstruction of the acetabulum following tumor resection poses multiple challenges due to the complex anatomy and the risk of infection. (**a**) Combined type II/III pelvic resection specimen for a pelvic chondrosarcoma with a trial periacetabular replacement (PAR, Stryker/Howmedica (Mahwah, NJ)) and (**b**) follow-up x-ray showing positioning of the pelvic component on the residual ilium with restoration of the hip position and center of rotation. Depending on the amount of tissue saved, patients with a PAR reconstruction can achieve function similar to a total hip replacement

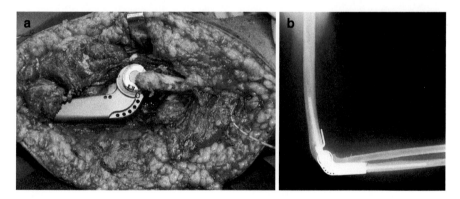

Fig. 6.14 Custom endoprosthetic reconstruction can be utilized in a number of unusual locations, as determined by the oncologic needs of the patient. A 16-year-old girl with a soft tissue sarcoma secondarily destroying the proximal ulna underwent wide resection, which necessitated sacrifice of the ulnar nerve. (**a**) Custom proximal ulnar replacement with a Biomet (Warsaw, IN) Discovery elbow for reconstruction of the skeletal defect. (**b**) Follow-up x-ray at 5 years showing positioning of the implant

expandable implants have traditionally required multiple operative procedures to physically access the expansion mechanism and frequently suffered mechanical failure [54]. Modern versions of this expansion system utilize an internal screw mechanism adjusted by a percutaneously inserted screwdriver (Fig. 6.15). Recent designs have incorporated noninvasive mechanisms utilizing external electromagnetic fields which transcutaneously activate internal mechanisms

Fig. 6.15 Custom mechanically expandable proximal femoral replacement, Biomet (Warsaw, IN), for replacement of the proximal femur in a 4-year-old with Ewing's sarcoma. This implant can be lengthened using a percutaneously inserted screwdriver to turn a worm gear along the lateral surface of the implant (*arrow*)

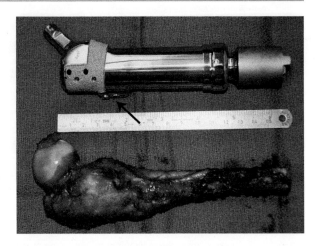

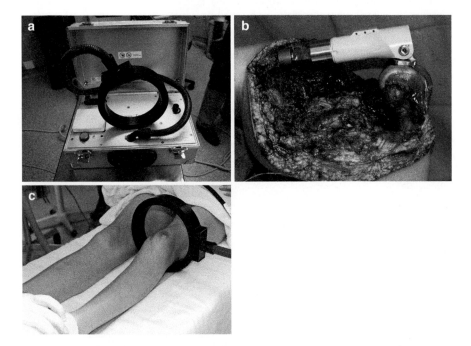

Fig. 6.16 Noninvasive expandable implants are activated by an externally applied power source. The FDA approved Repiphysis implant from Wright Medical (Memphis, TN) features an internal spring mechanism held in compression until released by an externally applied radio-frequency coil. (**a**) Radio-frequency coil. (**b**) Repiphysis distal femoral replacement, demonstrating its unique plastic housing that surrounds the internal mechanism. (**c**) Patient undergoing lengthening of the distal femur. Older children can often be treated without sedation, with an average of 4 mm length achieved per session

within the implant to incrementally lengthen the implant in a controlled fashion. Examples include the use of a radio-frequency coil to release a compressed internal spring mechanism [55] (Fig. 6.16) and a magnetic field generator to power an internal motor coupled by gears to the expansion mechanism [56] (Fig. 6.17). Engineering challenges such as the durability of the internal expansion mechanism [57] (Fig. 6.18) and compatibility issues with MR imaging remain for these implants [58].

Today, significant emphasis has been placed on the development of techniques and strategies designed to lower the risk of surgical site infections. The incidence of infection following massive endoprosthetic reconstruction in an oncology population is approximately ten times of that seen following routine total joint arthroplasty [39]. Host factors such as relative immunosuppression due to chemotherapy, effects of radiation on local tissue, and indwelling long-term central catheters as well as surgical factors including extensive surgical approaches, blood loss requiring immunosuppressive allogenic blood transfusions, and the

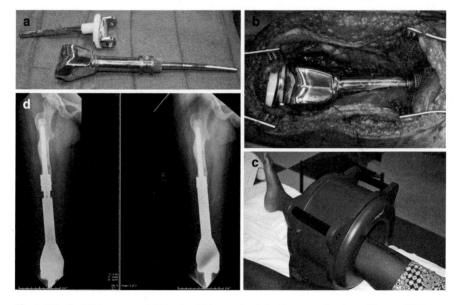

Fig. 6.17 The FDA-approved JTS extendible prosthesis by Stanmore Implants (Elstree, UK) uses an internal motor induced by an external magnetic field to power the expansion mechanism. (**a**) Distal femoral replacement featuring a semiconstrained rotating hinge knee mechanism. (**b**) Intraoperative view of JTS reconstruction following resection of an osteosarcoma of the distal femur. (**c**) Limb lengthening performed in a clinic without sedation showing the affected limb placed into the external magnetic unit. (**d**) Pre- (*right*) and post (*left*) images showing 16 mm expansion of implant after two lengthening sessions. In the event of a problem, the implant can be shortened by reversing the polarity of the magnetic field

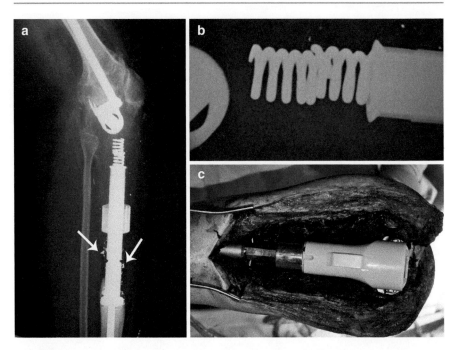

Fig. 6.18 Expandable implants still suffer from a much higher mechanical failure rate than adult modular endoprosthetic systems. (**a**) Failure of a Repiphysis (Wright Medical (Memphis, TN)) proximal tibial replacement which occurred as the patient achieved skeletal maturity. One of the signs of implant failure is the presence of metallic debris along the implant body (*arrows*). The patient presented with pain and acute shortening of the limb. (**b**) Closeup view demonstrating fractured internal spring mechanism. (**c**) Intraoperative view of failed implant showing marked metallic staining of the prosthetic pseudocapsule. The patient was salvaged using an adult modular proximal tibial replacement after extraction of the failed implant and resection of the pseudocapsule

size of the implants required for reconstruction likely account for this elevated risk [39, 59]. Methods of sterile skin preparation, such as DuraPrep (3M Health Care, St Paul, MN) and ChloraPrep (BD, Vernon Hills, IL) that create a film barrier locking skin bacteria into place have been shown to significantly reduce the risk of surgical site infections [60]. Preoperative testing and treatment of patients colonized by *Staphylococcus aureus* effectively reduce infections following orthopedic surgery [61]. Heat-stable antibiotics, such as tobramycin, when added to bone cement have been shown to reduce the risk of infection following joint arthroplasty [62]. The addition of an antimicrobial silver coating to a prosthetic stem has also shown a reduction in periprosthetic infection [63]. The use of a dilute betadine soak of the prosthesis after implantation can significantly reduce the risk of periprosthetic infection [64] (Fig. 6.19). These

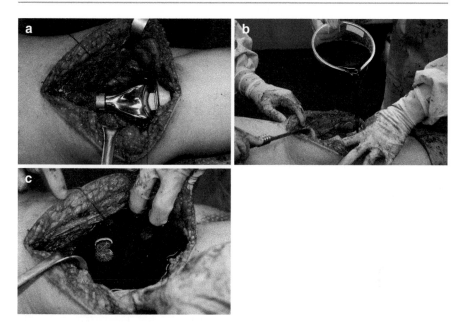

Fig. 6.19 Infection remains a significant concern following endoprosthetic reconstruction. (**a**) Cemented Stryker/Howmedica (Mahwah, NJ) GMRS distal femoral replacement for reconstruction after resection of an osteosarcoma. (**b**) A dilute betadine solution is poured into the open wound, covering the implant. This has been shown to reduce periprosthetic infections after total joint arthroplasty. (**c**) The solution is allowed to soak for 5 min prior to a final washout with a pulsatile lavage. Wound closure is then performed

and other innovative techniques hold promise of minimizing the incidence of surgical site infections and sparing patients the devastating consequences of a periprosthetic infection following limb-sparing surgery [39].

6.5   Surgical Planning

Proper evaluation of a patient presenting with a sarcoma requires an understanding of the biologic behavior of the tumor and detailed knowledge and familiarity with the local anatomy in the vicinity of the tumor. Advanced imaging, particularly MRI and high-resolution CT scans, can greatly aid the surgeon in identifying the relationship between the tumor and surrounding critical anatomy, including neurovascular structures, adjacent muscle groups, and skeletal structures. These relationships must be evaluated in order to determine if a limb-sparing resection can be performed safely. As a general rule of thumb, any single muscular compartment

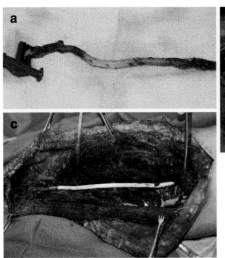
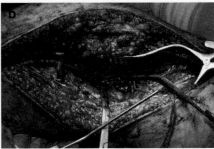

Fig. 6.20 (**a**) Harvested saphenous vein graft, filled with heparin solution. (**b**) The reversed graft undergoing an end-to-end anastomosis for reconstruction of a segmental defect of the superficial femoral artery following resection of a soft tissue sarcoma. 6-0 Prolene, Ethicon (Somerville, NJ), visible under magnification, is used to repair the anastomosis (*arrow*). (**c**) PTFE (Gore-Tex) vascular graft replacing the superficial femoral artery resected en bloc with a soft tissue sarcoma in a patient expected to undergo postoperative radiation. Artificial grafts are frequently used for long segments and when high-dose radiation is anticipated

can be removed with minimal functional loss due to the redundancy within the muscular system. Loss of an entire functional compartment may require adaptive bracing (lower extremity) or tendon transfers (upper extremity) in order to achieve an adequate functional outcome. Loss of a major nerve is often surprisingly well tolerated, although adaptive bracing may be necessary if there is significant loss of muscular function (e.g., an ankle-foot orthosis to support the ankle after resection of the sciatic nerve [65]). In selected cases, a major artery may be resected en bloc with the tumor safely provided that an appropriate vascular reconstruction (graft) is performed to restore sufficient blood flow to the affected extremity (Fig. 6.20).

The decision to sacrifice important structures is dictated by the type of resection chosen by the surgeon for a given tumor in its specific location. This is a direct application of Enneking's classification of resection margin; high-grade tumors require, at a minimum, a wide resection to ensure complete removal of the tumor pseudocapsule [28]. When a sarcoma arises from or engulfs a nerve or an artery, attempts to preserve those structures inevitably result in violation of the pseudocapsule, converting the attempted wide resection into an intralesional procedure with the result of greatly increasing the risk of local recurrence. In cases where crucial and/or multiple anatomic structures are involved, the surgeon is often faced with either performing a primary amputation (a wide resection through a limb outside of the tumor pseudocapsule) or, in selected cases, using chemotherapy and/or radiation therapy in a preoperative or neoadjuvant setting in the hope of downsizing the tumor

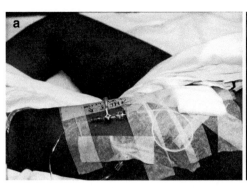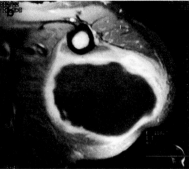

Fig. 6.21 (**a**) Intra-arterial catheterization for administration of cisplatin as part of a neoadjuvant chemotherapy regimen for soft tissue sarcoma. (**b**) Posttreatment MRI image showing extensive central necrosis of the tumor. This patient underwent successful limb-sparing surgery and remains alive 15 years later

and potentially converting the patient to a limb-sparing candidate. Neoadjuvant treatment (Fig. 6.21) can facilitate surgical resection through reduction of the size of the tumor and through sterilization of the tumor pseudocapsule (by killing tumor cells within the reactive zone) allowing for a plane of dissection much closer to the tumor than one would normally choose [25, 66].

A necessary component of the surgical planning is of course evaluating a patient's overall health and their ability to withstand a complex procedure that can be very long and entail significant blood loss. Even young patients, who typically are ideal surgical candidates, can develop significant comorbidities such as heart failure or renal failure from induction chemotherapy. The surgeon must be familiar with the potential complications from induction and adjuvant therapies, as detailed in Chap. 19, and make appropriate decisions keeping the patient's best interest in mind at all times.

A unique challenge that occurs far too often is the patient who has undergone a previous, unplanned, intralesional, or marginal biopsy or excision. Surgical planning must take into account not only the volume of the original and possibly residual tumor but also the tissue potentially contaminated during the original procedure. In addition to increasing the volume of tissue that needs to be resected, the risk of recurrence is also increased, potentially leading to poor outcomes and even legal action, as explained in Chap. 9.

6.6   Surgical Resection of Sarcomas

Significant advances in the surgical management of sarcomas have occurred over the past 50 years [67]. Once a plan of action has been determined by the surgeon for the safe oncologic resection of the tumor, the surgery itself consists of three separate but interrelated steps. First is the actual resection of the tumor with identification and preservation or sacrifice of key anatomic structures as determined by the surgical plan. A number of well-written references [68, 69] detail the surgical approaches and exposures when performing limb-sparing surgical resections and will not be duplicated here. Second, following the oncologic resection, reconstruction of the surgical defect is performed with the purpose of improving functional outcome. This can include the use of muscle transfers for functional reconstruction or, when bone has been removed, the use of endoprosthetic implants, bone grafts, internal fixation, or combination of these techniques in order to restore skeletal stability. Finally, reconstruction of the soft tissues and skin is performed, covering exposed vessels and nerves and any skeletal reconstruction that has been performed, in order to ensure proper healing of the surgical wound. This can include the use of flaps or muscle transfers or skin grafts depending upon the size and location of the surgical defect, particularly after preoperative radiation [70, 71].

Orthopedic oncology has traditionally focused upon methods of reconstructing significant skeletal defects as the key step in limb-sparing surgery. This was partly driven by the inherent limitations of radiographic imaging in the early days of the field, x-rays and bone scan which were the primary imaging tools available at that time and the lack of effective neoadjuvant treatments. This led to surgeons selecting very wide margins relative to the tumor in order to be certain of achieving a proper oncologic resection, often creating significant skeletal defects in the extremities, even for resection of primary soft tissue sarcomas. The reconstruction performed in these cases often varied upon the institutional experience and surgical training of the specific orthopedic oncologist. Well-accepted forms of skeletal reconstruction included Enneking's resection arthrodesis [14], massive osteoarticular allograft reconstructions as popularized by Mankin [15], endoprosthetic reconstruction (as discussed above), and hybrid reconstruction combining implant and bone graft as an allograft-prosthesis composite (APC) [72]. However, soft tissue reconstruction plays a significant role in determining the potential function following a limb-sparing resection due to the effect of the resection on the functional muscle groups which power the affected limb and adjacent joints. Additionally, proper soft tissue coverage helps to facilitate wound healing and minimizes the risk of potentially devastating infection following major resections and reconstructions [70].

High-resolution imaging has greatly improved the ability of the surgeon to visualize where the pseudocapsule boundary is, allowing for a planned resection that minimizes the amount of normal tissue removed with the tumor. Smaller resection volumes permit the preservation of more functional tissue which translates into improved functional outcomes. An additional benefit of smaller resections is the associated reduction in insensate fluid and blood loss as well as shorter operative times. Reduction of resection volume is especially applicable when preoperative or neoadjuvant therapies have shrunk the tumor with sterilization of the pseudocapsule [25]. This ongoing trend toward more precise surgery and preservation of otherwise normal tissue has led to additional downstream advances, including reduced length of stay, need for postoperative drains, and major reconstructive procedures, and has helped facilitate earlier mobilization and rehabilitation of limb-sparing patients. Smaller resections may also reduce the risk of postoperative complications,

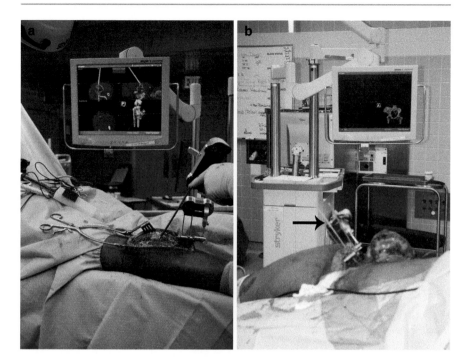

Fig. 6.22 (**a**) Computerized navigation used during hemi-cortical surgical resection of a posterior tibial chondrosarcoma (Fig. 6.27), demonstrating real-time positioning of instruments relative to a multiplaner view of the patient's anatomy seen on the computer monitor. (**b**) The NAV system, Stryker (Kalamazoo, MI), can be used in a variety of locations, as seen in this intraoperative view for resection of a pelvic chondrosarcoma. The system is registered and keyed to a system tracker that is secured to the bone by the surgeon (*arrow*)

particularly in distal sites [73, 74]. The use of computerized navigation systems with three-dimensional and multiplanar modeling of tumors based on preoperative imaging and the use of real-time feedback systems showing anatomic location relative to the tumor can greatly facilitate complex resections, permitting closer margins and preservation of a more normal tissue (Fig. 6.22).

Despite efforts to improve early diagnosis and techniques to reduce tumor volume prior to surgery, there are still patients with massive tumors that require extensive surgery, particularly in complex anatomic regions such as the pelvis, spine, and shoulder girdles. As with other locations, these cases benefit from advanced imaging for planning of surgical resections. Many times, such cases are best performed by teams of experienced surgeons representing different subspecialties, including diverse fields such as orthopedic oncology, surgical oncology, thoracic oncology, vascular surgery, plastic surgery, urology, and neurosurgery (Fig. 6.23). This multidisciplinary approach combined with surgery can benefit not only the patient but also the individual surgeon, by leveraging the respective experiences of each surgeon and sharing the physical labor and risks involved in each step of a

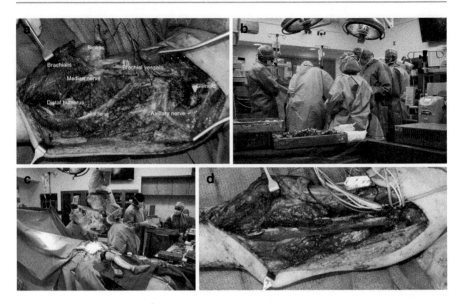

Fig. 6.23 Complex cases often require teams of surgical specialists to ensure optimal outcomes. (**a**) Resection of the majority of the humerus in a 5-year-old with Ewing's sarcoma. (**b**) Intraoperative photo of surgical teams representing orthopedic oncology, plastic surgery, and microvascular surgery. The team approach permitted simultaneous resection of the tumor with harvesting of the contralateral fibula as a microvascular free flap. (**c**) Following insertion of the fibula, the microvascular team performed the anastomosis. (**d**) Intraoperative view of the secured free flap prior to wound closure. The patient had a successful limb salvage and had intact peroneal nerve function in the harvested leg

complex procedure. This is particularly true when there is a respectful and collegial environment among the surgical team. Oncologic surgery presents unique stresses and challenges to any surgeon, and their response to stress may either facilitate or inhibit their ability to work as part of a team. In order to work effectively together, surgeons must be prepared to take a subordinate assistant role at times when another surgeon's skill sets dictate they should be in the lead. The author's personal experience is that surgeons who actively train residents and fellows often have the necessary skills to be effective members of a multidisciplinary surgical team. This is likely due to their frequent interaction and guidance of surgeons in training at varying skill levels in whom they are trying to instill the ability to operate independently upon graduation.

6.7   The Surgical Management of Bone Sarcomas

There are a limited number of sarcomas that arise from the bone, and these are generally classified based upon the type of matrix produced by the tumor, namely, osteoid-forming tumors (osteosarcomas), chondroid-forming tumors (chondrosarcomas), fibrous tumors (MFH and fibrosarcomas), and the round cell sarcomas

(Ewing's family of tumors). These tumors are extremely rare and account for less than 1% of all malignancies that occur on a yearly basis. Osteosarcoma, which is the most common of the primary bone sarcomas, is often used as the archetype for discussing treatment. Surgical management consists of complete removal of the entire tumor with negative margins, i.e., a wide resection as defined by Enneking [28]. Since osteosarcoma, and the other bone sarcomas, arise from and primarily involve the bone, this inevitably entails resection of the involved portion of the bone. Typically, these rapidly growing tumors have extended into the surrounding soft tissues by the time of initial presentation; this complicates surgical resection in the sense that the soft tissue component must be removed en bloc with the rest of the tumor. Osteosarcoma has a predilection for occurring in the metaphyseal portions of the long bones although they may arise anywhere within the axial or appendicular skeleton. When wide resection of the metaphyseal segment is necessary, the adjacent epiphysis and therefore joint are typically affected. Planning of the surgical resection as outlined above requires careful evaluation of the tumor and its relationship to the surrounding structures. As detailed in Chaps. 11 and 12 on chemotherapy, there is good evidence for the use of induction (neoadjuvant) chemotherapy specifically for osteosarcoma [75]; the evidence for chemotherapy in the treatment of fibrosarcoma/MFH of the bone is very weak; and there is no evidence to support the use of induction treatment for chondrosarcoma of the bone. Ewing's sarcoma is widely recognized to respond significantly to both induction chemotherapy and radiation; the role of surgery for Ewing's sarcoma has become much more accepted as it has been shown to be as effective as radiation for achieving local control while eliminating the potential long-term risks of radiation, particularly in extremity locations [76, 78].

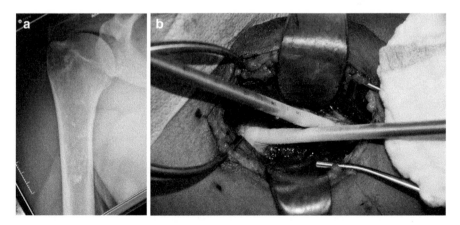

Fig. 6.24 (**a**) Low-grade enchondrosarcoma of the proximal humerus characterized by new onset of night pain, tumor length greater than 5 cm, entire canal filled by tumor, and endosteal scalloping of the bone. (**b**) Following curettage and high-speed burring (curettage/resection) of the lesion, cryosurgery was performed as a physical adjuvant using two 8 mm Endocare (Healthtronics (Austin, TX)) cryoprobes placed into the open defect

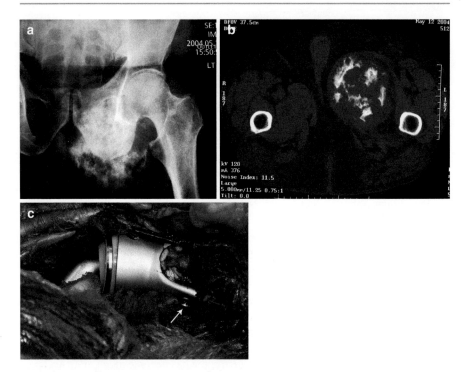

Fig. 6.25 (a) Radiograph of a primary pelvic chondrosarcoma arising from the pelvic floor, involving the acetabulum. (b) Axial CT scan showing classic chondroid matrix within a predominately unmineralized mass worrisome for a high-grade tumor. (c) Following type II/III resection, reconstruction was performed using a periacetabular replacement (PAR, Stryker/Howmedica (Mahwah, NJ)). Intraoperative view demonstrates cement filling of the iliac component with additional transfixation screws (*arrow*) securing implant to the bone. The iliac vessels are visible to the left of the constrained hip socket

Chondrosarcomas are relatively resistant to the effects of both chemotherapy and radiation; therefore, surgical resection remains the primary treatment option. Low-grade chondrosarcomas, often arising as secondary lesions from underlying enchondromas, are amenable to intralesional curettage and a physical adjuvant such as cryosurgery (Fig. 6.24). Primary chondrosarcomas have a propensity for proximal and central locations, often necessitating complex surgical approaches to the spine or pelvis (Fig. 6.25). Likewise, chordoma, a rare malignancy arising from notochordal remnants, often occurs in the sacrum and coccyx. They also are resistant to induction therapy and often require significant surgical resections of the sacrum (Fig. 6.26). Due to the lack of effective adjuvant treatment, patients with these tumors are especially at risk of local relapse and often benefit from close follow-up for extended periods of time compared to other sarcomas.

When induction treatment is used, it is important to completely restage the tumor with appropriate imaging prior to the surgical resection; changes in the tumor size, favorably or unfavorably, can affect the surgical plan, and adjustments must be made accordingly. As with all surgical resections, an extensile surgical approach is ideally performed, as it offers the most flexibility to the surgeon. Many of the extensile

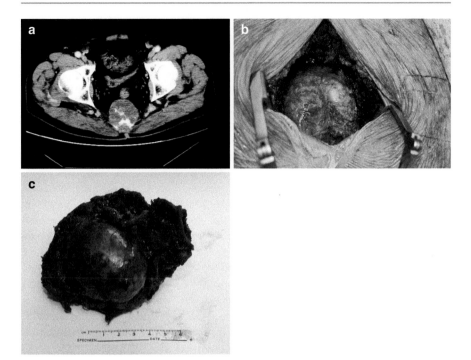

Fig. 6.26 (**a**) Axial CT scan showing a midline destructive tumor arising from the sacrum, typical for a sacral chordoma, confirmed after needle biopsy. Chordomas are typically resistant to chemotherapy and radiation. (**b**) Intraoperative view showing a posterior approach to the sacral mass during sacrectomy. (**c**) Resection specimen showing the anterior (presacral) surface of the mass that was lying on the rectum

approaches in use today were first described in detail by Henry [78]. These approaches dictate the placement of the surgical incision, which can be modified as needed for the particular features of a specific tumor and its anatomic location. The surgeon, with the help of preoperative imaging, must identify the involved compartments and surrounding structures in order to be able to safely remove the entire tumor. Traditional orthopedic approaches to the bone, such as those described by Hoppenfeld [79], typically recommend the use of intra-nervous planes and approaches that avoid major vascular structures. While this is perfectly appropriate for general orthopedic cases, oncologic cases require identification and preservation of these same structures; once the surgeon has identified and protected all of the key structures to be saved, the entire tumor and surrounding tissue can safely be removed.

Following surgical resection of the tumor, skeletal reconstruction is then performed in order to restore limb stability as well as overall function. The use of endoprosthetic reconstruction offers the advantage of immediate stability and rapid functional rehabilitation of the patient following treatment [41]. A variety of manufacturers offer modular systems that feature a variety of stem sizes and implant lengths permitting the creation of a customized implant sized to the patient using off-the-shelf components [38]. Methods of fixation include traditional cemented stems, porous-coated press-fit stems, and compression-loaded osteointegration stems (Fig. 6.10). Implants are available for replacing virtually any portion of the large appendicular bones in the body; custom implants are also available for those rare cases involving other bony sites such as the scapula (Fig. 6.11) and pelvis (Fig. 6.13) [49, 51]. Multiple series have shown the viability of endoprosthetic reconstruction in the oncologic setting; complications, which are typically manageable, include infection, implant loosening, mechanical breakage, and occasionally joint dislocation [39, 80].

Proper sizing of the implant is important for multiple reasons including restoration of the functional length of the surrounding musculature to optimize postoperative strength, stability of the affected joint to reduce the risk of dislocation or instability, and for prevention of vascular spasm and difficulty closing the soft tissue due to over lengthening of the limb. The use of trial components and trial reduction as well as careful measurement of the resection specimen can facilitate selection of the proper implant size. In addition to the implant length, selection of an appropriate stem diameter may be important in reducing the risk of aseptic loosening; a large stem diameter relative to the canal size appears to be important in both cemented and cementless systems [40, 81]. However, the body diameter, i.e., the portion of the implant between the bone stem interface and the adjacent joint, is not critical other than to provide strength for the implant and smaller body diameters do facilitate soft tissue closure particularly in cases where a relatively small amount of soft tissue has been removed.

In rare cases, the tumor to be resected may be relatively small, permitting the surgeon to remove a portion of the bone that is not segmental; this form of resection is referred to as a hemi-cortical resection given that a portion of the cortex is left intact along with the entire length of the resection (Figs. 6.27 and 6.28). This form of resection has the benefit of maintaining cortical continuity, preserving limb length and anatomic alignment in all planes. While more commonly applicable to benign tumors, examples of sarcomas that may be amenable to this form of resection include parosteal osteosarcomas (which are unique due to their low grade and relatively latent biology), relatively small periosteal osteosarcomas, and secondary chondrosarcomas arising from osteochondromas. Reconstruction of these hemicortical defects must be focused upon prevention of pathologic fracture, while biologic reconstruction of the missing cortex must be performed to restore the cortical circumference and bone stability. A combination of locking plate fixation and autogenous bone graft can often be performed in these cases. Purely diaphyseal tumors (such as a classic Ewing's sarcoma) are amenable to segmental resection with preservation of the adjacent joints and, in skeletally immature patients, even the adjacent growth plates (Fig. 6.29). A variety of segmental intercalary implants are available for reconstruction following a diaphyseal resection [28], while intercalary allografts with internal fixation (Fig. 6.30) can also be used effectively [82, 83].

Following restoration of skeletal length and adjacent joint stability, soft tissue reconstruction is performed in order to power the mechanical joint and to provide coverage of the metallic implant; these goals are not mutually exclusive and are often interrelated. As a rule of thumb, functional outcome following limb-sparing surgery is often related to the amount of soft tissue that is resected, i.e., preservation of more

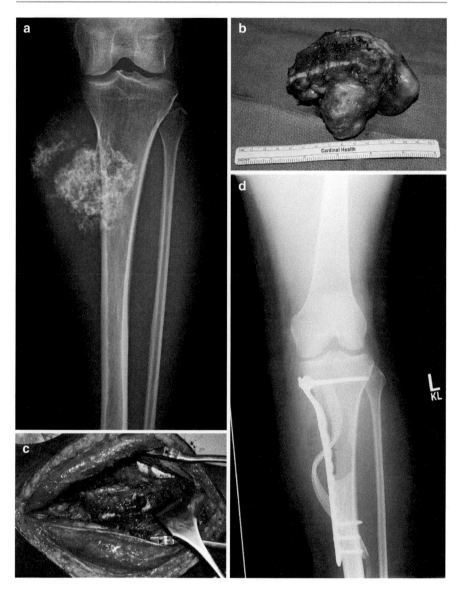

Fig. 6.27 (**a**) Rapidly enlarging secondary chondrosarcoma arising from a posterior tibial osteochondroma. Radiograph demonstrates calcified matrix with radiolucent regions concerning for chondrosarcoma. (**b**) Hemi-cortical resection specimen demonstrating the normal tibial cortices following a multiplaner complex osteotomy of the posterior tibia using a high-speed router (Midas Rex, Medtronic (Washington DC)) attached to a computerized navigation tracker for real-time guidance of the cut (Fig. 6.22a). (**c**) Intraoperative view of the resulting bony defect. Note that the anterior cortex of the tibia remained intact. (**d**) Postoperative radiograph demonstrating prophylactic fixation of the tibia using an AxSOS 3 Periarticular Locking Plate, Stryker (Kalamazoo, MI). The defect was filled with a bone graft substitute, DBX demineralized bone matrix, Synthes (West Chester, PA)

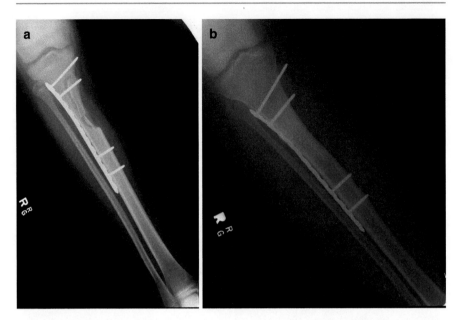

Fig. 6.28 (a) Physeal-sparing hemi-cortical resection for a periosteal osteosarcoma in a skeletally girl with Li-Fraumeni syndrome (p53 mutation). Reconstruction was performed using a tri-cortical iliac crest autograft and a Synthes (West Chester, PA) locking plate inserted submuscularly from the lateral side in a minimally invasive fashion. (b) Radiograph 7 years postsurgery demonstrating complete incorporation of the bone graft, interval growth, closure of the physis, and metaphyseal remodeling resulting in the proximal screw tips becoming prominent. The patient just recently undergone resection of a new osteosarcoma involving her entire humerus

functional muscle groups and compartments lead to increased strength and function of the limb following rehabilitation. In cases of significant soft tissue resection, particularly when major peripheral nerves are sacrificed, significant loss of strength must be anticipated, even to the point of requiring long-term bracing to support weight-bearing joints such as the knee or ankle. Frequently, this can be anticipated preoperatively based upon radiographic imaging and surgical planning and should be discussed with the patient to ensure appropriate expectations following surgery.

Fig. 6.29 (a) Surgical plan for a physeal-sparing intercalary resection of the femur after induction chemotherapy for Ewing's sarcoma. (b) Resection specimen with a customized intercalary double Compress, Biomet (Warsaw, IN) implant. (c) Intraoperative view of the inserted implant prior to coverage with the vastus lateralis muscle. (d) Postoperative radiograph demonstrating short Compress anchor plugs and intact physeal plates. (e) Follow-up radiograph demonstrating continued normal growth of both physeal plates

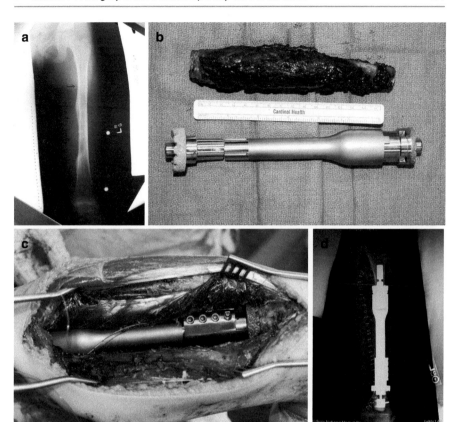

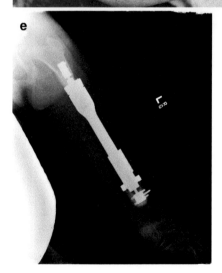

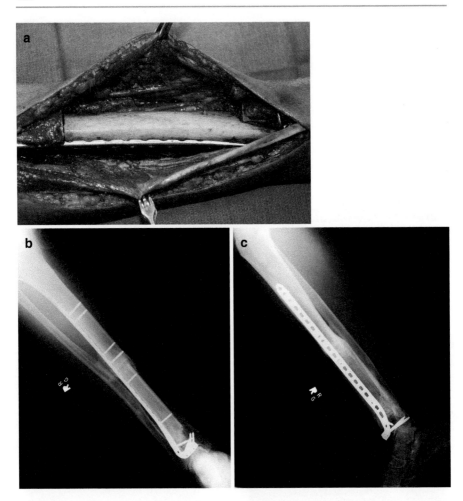

Fig. 6.30 (**a**) Intraoperative view of a femoral allograft inserted following resection of a cystic adamantinoma of the distal tibia, preserving 1.5 cm of the tibia above the ankle joint. Bridging fixation was accomplished using a Synthes (West Chester, PA) periarticular locking plate to secure the allograft, with a step cut at the distal junction to increase the contact surface area. Both host and allograft junctions were also grafted with iliac crest autograft to facilitate healing. (**b**) AP radiograph and (**c**) lateral view of the tibia 5 years post-op showing a stable allograft with incorporation at the host junctions. Patient has a normal gait with full ROM of the ankle joint

Loss of a complete functional compartment due to soft tissue resection or sacrifice of a major peripheral nerve (such as the femoral or sciatic nerve) can result in a permanent disability, but one that often remains far more functional than an amputation performed at the same level. Advances in bracing, physical therapy and

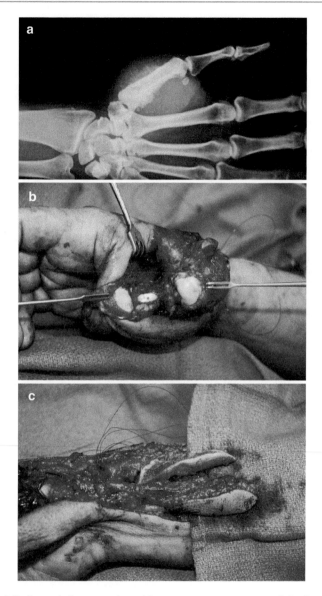

Fig. 6.31 (a) Radiograph demonstrating a biopsy-proven osteosarcoma of the dominant thumb metacarpal. (b) Intraoperative view following resection of the tumor, disarticulating the CMC and MCP joints. (c) Osteocutaneous pedicle flap from the distal radius fed by the radial artery was raised by plastic surgery. (d) Placement of the flap into the surgical defect. (e) View of the hand after closure of the wound. The cutaneous portion of the flap filled the defect from the tumor resection. (f) Follow-up x-ray showing stable reconstruction of the thumb metacarpal

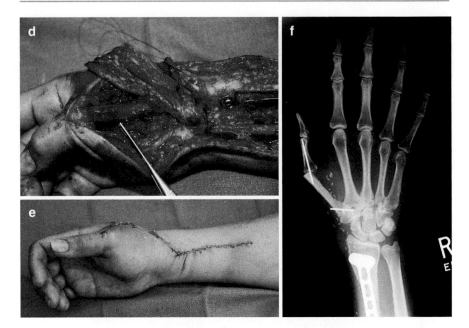

Fig. 6.31 (continued)

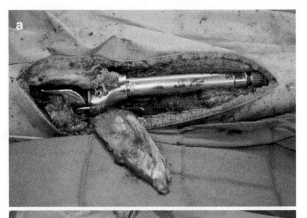

Fig. 6.32 (**a**) Medical gastrocnemius flap is routinely performed after proximal tibial replacement, as in this skeletally immature osteosarcoma patient reconstructed with an expandable JTS implant (Stanmore, Elstree, UK). The extensor mechanism (patellar tendon remnant) is directly attached to the implant over a porous-coated surface with 3 mm Dacron tapes. (**b**) The flap covers the proximal implant and the extensor reconstruction, helping to reinforce it. Patients are kept in full extension for 6 weeks prior to starting ROM; many patients have full active extension without extensor lag

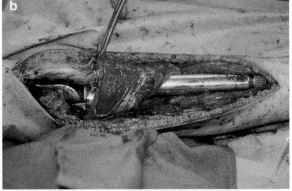

rehabilitation, and in selected cases appropriate tendon transfers or free flaps, can help patients achieve satisfactory to excellent outcomes [84–86] (Fig. 6.31).

Coverage of the implant following reconstruction may necessitate significant rotational or advancement flaps of surrounding muscles; common examples include the use of the medial gastrocnemius flap following resection of the proximal tibia (Fig. 6.32) and hamstring transfer to the patella following resections of the distal femur and quadriceps [84]. It is important to ensure complete muscular coverage of the skeletal reconstruction in order to minimize the risk of infection particularly as soft tissue complications including delayed wound healing and marginal skin necrosis can occur in up to 10% of cases. The use of full-thickness fasciocutaneous flaps, whenever possible, can help prevent superficial wound issues; however, this may not be possible after resection of large tumors affecting the skin or in cases of improperly positioned biopsy tracks that require significant skin resection en bloc with the underlying tumor. A recent advance in the management of soft tissue wounds involves the use of incisional vacuum dressings, which help to reduce swelling and can prevent fluid collections from jeopardizing the blood supply to the skin edges of the incision [87]. Vacuum dressings can also be applied in

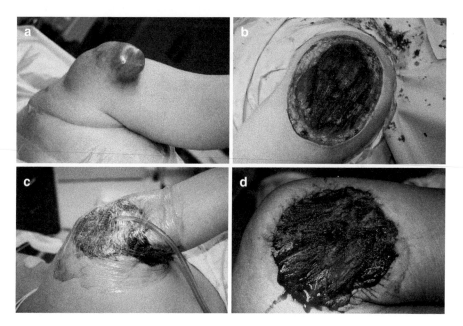

Fig. 6.33 (**a**) Large dermatofibrosarcoma protuberans (DFSP) of the lateral shoulder. (**b**) Resection of the tumor necessitated the creation of a large defect that could not be closed. (**c**) The wound was covered with a vacuum-dressing set for continuous suction, maintaining sterility of the wound and evacuation of serous fluid from the wound. (**d**) Appearance of the wound 4 days later, showing a generous granulation base highly suitable for split-thickness skin grafting. During this time, final pathology on the resection specimen confirmed that all margins were free and clear, permitting application of the final skin graft

cases where significant skin loss prevents primary closure of the wound, permitting maintenance of a sterile environment and allowing for delayed skin grafting once a granulation bed has developed (Fig. 6.33). Extremely large tumors may have the paradoxical advantage of acting like an implanted soft tissue expander such that following removal there is an excess of redundant tissue that greatly facilitates soft tissue closure.

6.8   The Surgical Management of Soft Tissue Sarcomas

Soft tissue sarcomas, which are more common than bone sarcomas, arise from any of the multiple mesenchymal-derived tissues in the body, commonly including tumors arising from fat (liposarcoma), muscle (rhabdomyosarcoma and leiomyosarcoma), nerve (malignant peripheral nerve sheath tumor), and blood vessels (angiosarcoma). For some soft tissue sarcomas, the cell of origin remains unknown (synovial cell sarcoma). As with bone sarcomas, the primary method of treatment is complete surgical resection. Unlike bone sarcomas, soft tissue sarcomas are often sensitive to radiation, which is frequently used for high-grade tumors in either a preoperative or adjuvant setting to improve local control. The role of radiation in the treatment of sarcomas is discussed in Chap. 10. The use of chemotherapy remains controversial but has been shown to be helpful for certain tumor types, as detailed in Chaps. 11 and 12.

As previously outlined for bone sarcomas, surgical management for soft tissue sarcomas begins with an accurate histologic diagnosis followed by a complete imaging of the tumor and relevant anatomy. The surgeon then selects an appropriate resection margin based upon the tumor grade and expected oncologic behavior. Enneking's concept of a surgical margin [28] applies equally well to soft tissue tumors, with each muscle representing a compartment (due to its investing fascia) and each functional group of muscles also representing a compartment. As with bone sarcomas, wide resection represents the surgical goal to ensure complete removal of the tumor with optimal local control. Frequently, deep-seated soft tissue sarcomas will be adjacent to or involve neurologic and vascular structures and may secondarily involve the bone. After a detailed review of the imaging studies, a surgical plan that addresses relevant local anatomy with respect to the oncologic need for a wide resection can be generated and discussed with the patient. If sacrifice of significant neurologic or vascular structures would be required to achieve an adequate oncologic resection, then the use of preoperative or induction therapy such as chemotherapy (Fig. 6.21) or radiation therapy (Fig. 6.34) should be considered. The choice of induction treatment often varies depending upon the age and the health of the patient [88].

Certain histologic subtypes of soft tissue sarcomas do require additional consideration during surgical planning. Although the majority of soft tissue sarcomas demonstrate hematogenous spread with metastases concentrated in the lungs, some histologic subtypes demonstrate a predilection for lymphatic spread (e.g.,

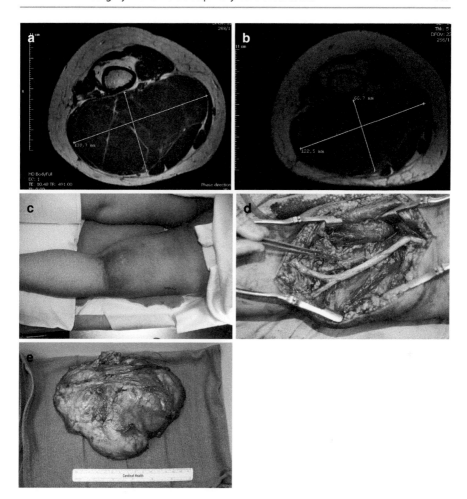

Fig. 6.34 (**a**) Biopsy-proven massive myxoid liposarcoma of the posterior thigh as seen on a T1-weighted axial MRI image. Due to the large size of the tumor, the patient was offered induction radiotherapy. (**b**) Similar cross-section MRI 2 weeks after completion of induction radiation showing shrinkage of the tumor. Clinically, the tumor continued to regress until the day of surgery. (**c**) Intraoperative view showing the posterior thigh with skin discoloration due to her radiation. (**d**) Post-resection view demonstrating the tibial and peroneal branches of the sciatic nerve which were draped over the tumor and the popliteal vessels (under the Debakey forceps) which were dissected free from the undersurface of the tumor. (**e**) Resection specimen; the patient had no wound complications and remains free of disease over 6 years post-op

rhabdomyosarcoma, epithelioid sarcoma) [89] or other unusual patterns of metastasis (e.g., myxoid liposarcoma) [90]. In such cases, consideration to additional imaging studies for accurate staging, such as PET/CT [91], and sentinel lymph node biopsy (particularly for patients with clear cell sarcoma) [92] should be included in the surgical planning. Additionally, leiomyosarcoma can arise directly from the smooth muscle adventitia of an artery or vein, necessitating removal of the involved structure. The assistance of a vascular surgeon in such cases can greatly facilitate reconstruction (Fig. 6.20).

As with bone sarcomas, functional outcomes following resection of a soft tissue sarcoma frequently depend upon the extent of the resection; preservation of

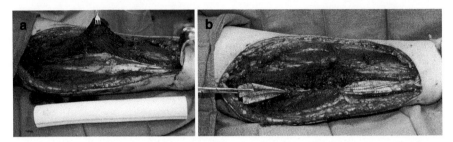

Fig. 6.35 (a) Resection of the gastro-soleus condensation into the Achilles tendon for an epithelioid sarcoma of the leg. An aortic Dacron graft is placed adjacent to the leg for sizing. (b) Reconstruction was performed by bridging the defect with the graft, attaching it with 3 mm Dacron tapes to the tendon distally and laying it between the two gastrocnemius and soleus muscles proximally. The patient was able to walk normally with active plantar flexion

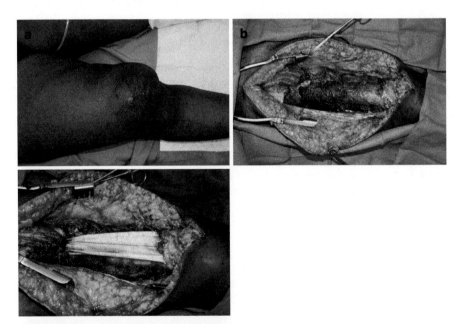

Fig. 6.36 (a) Clinical view of a massive liposarcoma of the anterior thigh extending down to the patella. (b) Intraoperative view following resection of the tumor along with the quadriceps tendon. (c) Reconstruction using an aortic Dacron graft secured to the patella distally and woven into the remaining quadriceps muscles proximally. The graft was covered subsequently with the sartorius and vastus intermedius. This elderly patient was able to ambulate without bracing with grade 4 strength in knee extension

muscle and its nervous innervation correlates with postoperative function and reha-bilitation. Loss of major tendons can occasionally be addressed with augmented reconstruction using aortic Dacron grafts, such as for the tendo-Achilles complex (Fig. 6.35) or the quadriceps tendon (Fig. 6.36). Rotation and or advancement of adjacent muscles may be necessary to reduce dead space and to provide coverage of important structures such as nerves and vessels and even bones and adjacent joints [70]. This becomes increasingly important when radiation is part of the treat-ment plan due to the risk of wound complications; vascularized flaps are relatively resistant to the effects of radiation and can reduce the size and complexity of break-downs when they occur. In cases of extensive radiation-induced necrosis, free flap reconstruction may be the best option for salvage [71].

6.9   Postoperative Considerations

Following limb-sparing surgery, the goal of the postoperative period is to ensure the overall health of the patient, proper healing of the wound, and appropriate mobiliza-tion and early functional rehabilitation. Large resection volumes and prolonged sur-gery can lead to significant fluid shifts and postoperative swelling of the limb. This can be greatly complicated by the use of anticoagulation as well as preoperative radiation particularly along with the major lymphatic channels of the limb. Meticulous attention to hemostasis in order to minimize overall blood loss and need for fluid resuscitation as well as the avoidance of extremity tourniquets can help to minimize reactive edema formation in the immediate postoperative period. The use of compression dressings (such as Ace wraps) and elevation of the limb above the heart combined with bed rest for 24 h can be helpful in cases where significant swelling is expected. The use of appropriate wound drains and, more recently, the use of incisional vacuum dressings can help reduce tension on the primary wound closure helping to protect the surrounding skin. Avoidance of chemical anticoagula-tion (i.e., low molecular weight heparins) can reduce the risk of hematoma forma-tion particularly in patients with existing coagulopathies due to chemotherapy. As a matter of standard practice, we do not use any anticoagulation in limb-sparing patients, relying instead on mechanical compressive devices or, in cases at high risk of pulmonary embolus, preoperative placement of an internal vena cava filter. In a similar fashion, we avoid routine use of tourniquets which can cause vascular inti-mal damage along with blood pooling and reperfusion injury that increase the risk of clotting, relying instead on meticulous surgical technique and direct occlusion of vessels when necessary to control bleeding. In cases where a tourniquet is neces-sary, we try to minimize the inflation pressure as well as the overall time of inflation in order to minimize damage to the underlying tissue which can result in increased pain, postoperative edema, and likely increases the risk of postoperative thrombus formation.

Maintenance of an adequate blood pressure and hematocrit is important not only to the patient's well-being but also in ensuring adequate perfusion of the limb and flaps following limb-sparing surgery. This is particularly true in the distal extremities of elderly cancer patients who may have varying amounts of preexisting atherosclerotic disease. Additionally, younger patients who have received substantial doses of chemotherapy may lack the bone marrow reserves necessary to compensate for acute intraoperative blood loss. Intraoperatively, the anesthesia team should be prepared to transfuse blood products in preference to other volume expanders, while routine monitoring of the hematocrit/hemoglobin levels during the first 24 h following limb-sparing surgery should always be performed. Nursing and blood bank personnel should be educated as to the unique needs of limb-sparing patients with regard to blood products in order to ensure adequate and timely access to the blood when needed.

Early mobilization of postoperative patients has been shown to be important in reducing hospital length of stay and helps minimize medical comorbidities related to prolonged bed rest. However, early mobilization must be distinguished from early movement of a given limb. Extensive surgical resection and reconstruction often involve tight wound closures that are adjacent to mobile joints. Immobilization of the limb using either splints or braces can protect the wound during the early critical healing phase thereby reducing the risk of wound dehiscence. This is particularly true in patients who have undergone preoperative radiation who are already at risk of wound complications. Patients may be out of bed and can even ambulate while a single limb is effectively immobilized. Early mobilization of the patient, as an integrated part of an enhanced recovery after surgery program, has been shown to reduce hospital length of stay in patients with soft tissue sarcoma [93]. Close communication with the physical therapy team is needed to ensure that proper precautions are taken to protect the surgical site. Rehabilitation for sarcoma patients is detailed in Chaps.15 and 16.

A major concern of both patients and health providers is ensuring that adequate pain control is achieved following surgery. While the use of patient-controlled analgesia (PCA) is widely accepted, intravenous narcotics often cause varying levels of sedation and/or delirium and can lead to urinary retention and constipation. In comparison, the use of regional or epidural analgesia in the postoperative period can minimize the need for systemic narcotics and can be titrated to provide excellent pain relief while still permitting sensory and motor function in the limb [94]. Patients undergoing major limb-sparing surgery may not be suited to indwelling epidural catheterization as central administration of analgesics can result in significant hypotension precluding adequate administration of medication for pain relief. A better approach is the use of peripheral nerve blocks and catheterization as peripheral administration of analgesics has a minimal effect on blood pressure. A favorable side effect of a peripheral block is the associated sympathetic block which helps improve blood flow within the limb and may help reduce the incidence of thromboembolic disease. Regional nerve sheath catheters can be introduced by the anesthesia team in either preoperative holding area or in the PACU following surgery. Direct insertion of a nerve sheath catheter by the surgeon can also be effective and is often easily performed in limb-sparing cases as many cases will require the identification and exposure of one or more major peripheral nerves within the extremity. In patients who must undergo amputation, such catheters are extremely important in minimizing postoperative pain, reducing the risk of phantom pain syndrome and allowing for early mobilization [95]. The use of an external disposable pump (e.g., On-Q pump) permits patient discharge within the indwelling peripheral nerve sheath catheter. The use of these pumps has been shown to be effective following thoracotomy [96] and is safe in children [97]. This is a powerful technique that is particularly suited to patients undergoing major amputation as these catheters can be safely maintained and utilized for days to weeks following surgery. Pain management techniques for sarcoma patients are detailed in Chap. 14.

It is important to note that the role of the surgeon in multidisciplinary management of sarcomas does not end with surgical healing of the wound. Close communication with the rest of the treatment team, particularly medical and radiation oncologists, is needed to ensure the appropriate and timely use of adjuvant treatments. A multidisciplinary sarcoma conference/tumor board can facilitate such communication and allows the surgeon to communicate the relevant details of the surgery and anatomy to the team. The surgeon can be a useful resource for the radiation oncologist in planning an appropriate treatment volume on a case-by-case basis. The surgeon should actively communicate with the physical therapist and rehab personnel to ensure that patients are both adequately protected and mobilized during the critical first 6 weeks of soft tissue healing [98]. The surgeon must also be prepared to intervene quickly; when evidence of a wound complication presents, aggressive surgical management is often required to ensure a successful and timely outcome. Unlike the routine orthopedic patient, limb-sparing patients often require close monitoring during the postoperative period. The use of experienced mid-level practitioners can significantly facilitate close monitoring and is often well received by patients, as detailed in Chap.17.

Finally, the responsibility of the surgeon does not end with the surgery alone. Sarcomas have a predilection for recurring, even in cases treated with wide resection, negative margins, and adjuvants such as radiotherapy. The time interval between treatment and recurrence can vary significantly: the time to relapse for high-grade tumors is often around the 2-year mark, while low-grade sarcomas can relapse even years later. More than anyone else in the treatment team, the surgeon is best suited to detect recurrences due to his/her intimate knowledge of the local anatomy, the precise details regarding the reconstruction that was performed, as well as having experience in performing musculoskeletal examinations. Ideally, the treating surgeon should perform routine physicals and review imaging studies along with the rest of the sarcoma follow-up team (Chaps. 19 and 20). In the event of disease relapse, complete reevaluation of the patient is a necessary step for potential salvage treatment, as seen in Chap. 13.

6.10 Summary

Patients presenting with bone and soft tissue sarcomas present many challenges to the surgeon who must work as part of a multidisciplinary team to ensure the best possible oncologic and functional outcomes for a given patient. A rational approach to diagnosing and staging patients helps to facilitate surgical planning; the concept of a surgical margin and compartment as defined by Enneking provides a framework for the surgeon to plan any oncologic resection. Functional outcomes are often determined by the amount of soft tissue that can be successfully spared during a resection, while segmental defects of bones and adjacent joints can be successfully reconstructed using a variety of techniques. Meticulous attention to soft tissue handling and postoperative care is needed to minimize the risk of wound-healing complications particularly in patients receiving radiation. Finally, the surgeon must recognize his or her role as part of a multidisciplinary team and should actively participate with the team to ensure the best possible outcomes for these challenging patients.

References

1. Link MP, Am G, Miser AW, et al. The effect of adjuvant chemotherapy on relapse-free survival in patients with osteosarcoma of the extremity. N Engl J Med. 1986;314(25):1600–6.
2. Ewing J. Diffuse endothelioma of bone. Proc NY Pathol Soc. 1921;21:17–24.
3. Cripe T. Ewing sarcoma: an eponym window to history. Sarcoma. 2011;2011: Article ID 457532, 4 pages. doi:10.1155/2011/457532
4. Phemister DB. Conservative surgery in the treatment of bone tumors. Surg Gynecol Obstet. 1940;70:355–64.
5. Phemister DB. Local resection of malignant tumors of bone. AMA Arch Surg. 1951;63:715–7.
6. Parish FF. Treatment of bone tumors by total excision and replacement with massive autologous and homologous grafts. J Bone Joint Surg Am. 1968;48A:968–90.
7. Marcove RC, Miller TR. Treatment of primary and metastatic bone tumors by cryosurgery. JAMA. 1969;207(10):1890–4.
8. McNamara J, Paulson D, Kingsley W, Urschel H. JAMA. 1968;205(7):535–6.
9. Cortes EP, Holland JF, Wang JJ, et al. Amputation and adriamycin in primary osteo-sarcoma. N Engl J Med. 1974;291:998–1000.
10. Hudson TM, Hass G, Enneking WF, Hawkins EF. Angiography in the management of musculoskeletal tumors. Surg Gynecol Obstet. 1975;141:11–21.
11. Hounsfield GN. Computerised transverse axial scanning (tomography): Part 1. Description of system. Br J Radiol. 1973;46:1016–22.
12. Ambrose J. Computerised transverse axial scanning (tomography): Part 2. Clinical application. Br J Radiol. 1973;46:1023–47.
13. Subramanian G, McAfee JG. A new complex of 99mTc for skeletal imaging. Radiology. 1971;99:192–6.
14. Enneking WF, Shirley PD. Resection-arthrodesis for malignant and potentially malignant lesions about the knee using an intramedullary rod and local bone grafts. J Bone Joint Surg Am. 1977;59(2):223–36.
15. Mankin HJ, Fogelson FJ, Thrasher DZ, et al. Massive resection and allograft transplantation in the treatment of malignant bone tumors. N Engl J Med. 1976;294:247–55.
16. Marcove RC, Lewis MM, Rosen G, Huvos AG. Total femur and total knee replacement. A preliminary report. Clin Orthop Relat Res. 1977;126:147–52.
17. Rosen G, Marcove RC, Caparros B, Nirenberg A, Kosloff C, Huvos AG. Primary osteogenic sarcoma: the rationale for preoperative chemotherapy and delayed surgery. Cancer. 1979;43(6):2163–77.
18. Morton DL, Eilber FR, Townsend Jr CM, Grant TT, Mirra J, Weisenburger TH. Limb salvage from a multidisciplinary treatment approach for skeletal and soft tissue sarcomas of the extremity. Ann Surg. 1976;184(3):268–78.
19. Eilber FR, Mirra JJ, Grant TT, Weisenburger T, Morton DL. Is amputation necessary for sarcomas? A seven-year experience with limb salvage. Ann Surg. 1980;192:431–8.

20. Martini N, Huvos AG, Miké V, et al. Multiple pulmonary resections in the treatment of osteo-genic sarcoma. Ann Thorac Surg. 1971;12:271–80.
21. Shah A, Exelby PR, Rao B, et al. Thoracotomy as adjuvant to chemotherapy in metastatic osteogenic sarcoma. J Pediatr Surg. 1977;12:983–90.
22. Mankin HJ, Mankin CJ, Simon MA. The hazards of the biopsy, revisited. Members of the Musculoskeletal Tumor Society. J Bone Joint Surg Am. 1996;78(5):656–63.
23. Welker JA, Henshaw RM, Jelinek J, et al. The percutaneous needle biopsy is safe and recom-mended in the diagnosis of musculoskeletal masses. Cancer. 2000;89(12):2677–86.
24. Zuber T. Punch biopsy of the skin. Am Fam Physician. 2002;65(6):1155–8.
25. O'Donnell PW, Manivel JC, Cheng EY, Clohisy DR. Chemotherapy influences the pseudo-capsule composition in soft tissue sarcomas. Clin Orthop Relat Res. 2014;472(3):849–55. doi:10.1007/s11999-013-3022-7.
26. Kepka L, DeLaney TF, Suit HD, Goldberg SI. Results of radiation therapy for unre-sected soft-tissue sarcomas. Int J Radiat Oncol Biol Phys. 2005;63:852–9. doi:10.1016/j.ijrobp.2005.03.004.
27. Eckert F, Matuschek C, Mueller A, et al. Definitive radiotherapy and single-agent radiosen-sitizing ifosfamide in patients with localized, irresectable soft tissue sarcoma: a retrospective analysis. Radiat Oncol. 2010;5:55. doi:10.1186/1748-717X-5-55.
28. Enneking WF, Spanier SS, Malawer MM. The effect of the anatomic setting on the results of surgical procedures for soft parts sarcoma of the thigh. Cancer. 1981;47:1005–22. doi:10.1002/1097-0142(19810301)47:5<1005::AID-CNCR2820470532>3.0.CO;2-9.
29. Eilber F, Giuliano A, Eckardt J, et al. Adjuvant chemotherapy for osteosarcoma: a randomized prospective trial. J Clin Oncol. 1987;5(1):21–6.
30. Enneking W. A system of staging musculoskeletal neoplasms. Clin Orthop. 1986;204:9–24.
31. Wolf R, Enneking WF. The staging and surgery of musculoskeletal neoplasms. Orthop Clin North Am. 1996;27(3):473–81.
32. Enneking WF. History of orthopedic oncology in the United States: progress from the past, pros-pects for the future. Cancer Treat Res. 2009;152:529–71. doi:10.1007/978-1-4419-0284-9_32.
33. Neel MD, Enneking WF. Surgical management of extremity soft tissue sarcomas. Cancer Control. 1994;1(6):586–91.
34. Pearson H. Magnetic pioneers net Nobel for putting medicine in the picture. Nature. 2003;425(6958):547.
35. Neifeld JP, Walsh JW, Lawrence Jr W. Computed tomography in the management of soft tissue tumors. Surg Gynecol Obstet. 1982;155(4):535–40.
36. Kotz R, Ritschl P, Trachtenbrodt J. A modular femur-tibia reconstruction system. Orthopedics. 1986;9(12):1639–52.
37. Malawer MM, Chou LB. Prosthetic survival and clinical results with use of large-seg-ment replacements in the treatment of high-grade bone sarcomas. J Bone Joint Surg Am. 1995;77(8):1154–65.
38. Henshaw RM, Malawer MM. Advances in modular endoprosthetic reconstruction of osseous defects. Curr Opin Orthop. 2003;14(6):429–37.
39. Shehadeh A, Noveau J, Malawer M, Henshaw R. Late complications and survival of endopros-thetic reconstruction after resection of bone tumors. Clin Orthop Relat Res. 2010;468(11):2885–95. doi:10.1007/s11999-010-1454-x.
40. Bergin PF, Noveau JB, Jelinek JS, Henshaw RM. Aseptic loosening rates in distal femo-ral endoprostheses: does stem size matter? Clin Orthop Relat Res. 2012;470(3):743–50. doi:10.1007/s11999-011-2081-x.
41. Henshaw RM, Kellar-Graney K, Malawer MM. Limb sparing endoprosthetic reconstruction following major oncologic musculoskeletal resections: improved long term results and quality of life with a modular system. Sarcoma. 2001;5(5):S1, S15.
42. Schwartz AJ, Kabo JM, Eilber FC, Eilber FR, Eckardt JJ. Cemented distal femoral endo-prostheses for musculoskeletal tumor: improved survival of modular versus custom implants. Clin Orthop Relat Res. 2010;468(8):2198–210. doi:10.1007/s11999-009-1197-8. Epub 2009 Dec 22

43. Blunn GW, Briggs TW, Cannon SR, Walker PS, et al. Cementless fixation for primary segmental bone tumor endoprostheses. Clin Orthop Relat Res. 2000;372:223–30.
44. Abraham J, Weaver M, Ready J, et al. Short-term outcomes of cementless modular endoprostheses in lower extremity reconstruction. Curr Orthop Pract. 2012;23(3):213–7.
45. Cristofolini L, Bini SA, Toni A. In vitro testing of a novel limb salvage prosthesis for the distal femur. Clin Biomech. 1998;13:608–15.
46. Avedian RS, Goldsby RE, Kramer MJ, O'Donnell RJ. Effect of chemotherapy on initial compressive osseointegration of tumor endoprostheses. Clin Orthop Relat Res. 2007;459:48–53.
47. Pedtke AC, Wustrack RL, Fang AS, Grimer RJ, O'Donnell RJ. Aseptic failure: how does the compress implant compare to cemented stems? Clin Orthop Relat Res. 2012;470(3):735–42.
48. Sirveaux F, Favard L, Oudet D, Huquet D, Walch G, Mole D. Grammont inverted total shoulder arthroplasty in the treatment of glenohumeral osteoarthritis with massive rupture of the cuff. Results of a multicenter study of 80 shoulders. J Bone Joint Surg Br. 2004;86:388–95.
49. Wittig JC, Bickels J, Wodajo F, Kellar-Graney KL, Malawer MM. Constrained total scapula reconstruction after resection of a high-grade sarcoma. Clin Orthop Relat Res. 2002;397: 143–55.
50. Kulkarni A, Fiorenza F, Grimer RJ, Carter SR, Tillman RM. The results of endoprosthetic replacement for tumours of the distal humerus. J Bone Joint Surg Br. 2003;85(2):240–3.
51. Menendez LR, Ahlmann ER, Falkinstein Y, Allison DC. Periacetabular reconstruction with a new endoprosthesis. Clin Orthop Relat Res. 2009;467(11):2831–7.
52. Shekkeris AS, Hanna SA, Sewell MD, et al. Endoprosthetic reconstruction of the distal tibia and ankle joint after resection of primary bone tumours. J Bone Joint Surg Br. 2009;91(10):1378–82.
53. Lewis MM. The use of an expandable and adjustable prosthesis in the treatment of childhood malignant bone tumors of the extremity. Cancer. 1986;57(3):499–502.
54. Eckardt JJ, Kabo JM, Kelley CM, Ward WG, et al. Expandable endoprosthesis reconstruction in skeletally immature patients with tumors. Clin Orthop Relat Res. 2000;373:51–61.
55. Gitelis S, Neel MD, Wilkins RM, Rao BN, Kelly CM, Yao TK. The use of a closed expandable prosthesis for pediatric sarcomas. Chir Organi Mov. 2003;88(4):327–33.
56. Sewell MD, Spiegelberg BG, Hanna SA, et al. Non-invasive extendible endoprostheses for limb reconstruction in skeletally-mature patients. J Bone Joint Surg Br. 2009;91(10):1360–5.
57. Maheshwari AV, Bergin PF, Henshaw RM. Modes of failure of custom expandable repiphysis prostheses: a report of three cases. J Bone Joint Surg Am. 2011;93(13):e72. doi:10.2106/JBJS.J.00841.
58. Gupta A, Meswania J, Pollock R, et al. Non-invasive distal femoral expandable endoprosthesis for limb-salvage surgery in paediatric tumours. J Bone Joint Surg Br. 2006;88(5):649–54.
59. Jeys LM, Grimer RJ, Carter SR, Tillman RM. Periprosthetic infection in patients treated for an orthopaedic oncological condition. J Bone Joint Surg Am. 2005;87(4):842–9.
60. Swenson BR, Hedrick TL, Metzger R, Bonatti H, Pruett TL, Sawyer RG. Effects of preoperative skin preparation on postoperative wound infection rates: a prospective study of 3 skin preparation protocols. Infect Control Hosp Epidemiol. 2009;30(10):964–71.
61. Rao N, Cannella B, Crossett LS, Yates Jr AJ, McGough III R. A preoperative decolonization protocol for *Staphylococcus aureus* prevents orthopaedic infections. Clin Orthop Relat Res. 2008;466(6):1343–8.
62. Parvizi J, Saleh KJ, Ragland PS, Pour AE, Mont MA. Efficacy of antibiotic-impregnated cement in total hip replacement. Acta Orthop. 2008;79(3):335–41.
63. Hardes J, von Eiff C, Streitbuerger A, et al. Reduction of periprosthetic infection with silver-coated megaprostheses in patients with bone sarcoma. J Surg Oncol. 2010;101(5):389–95.
64. Brown NM, Cipriano CA, Moric M, Sporer SM, Della Valle CJ. Dilute betadine lavage before closure for the prevention of acute postoperative deep periprosthetic joint infection. J Arthroplast. 2012;27(1):27–30.
65. Bickels J, Wittig J, Kollender Y, et al. Sciatic nerve resection. Is that truly an indication for amputation? Clin Orthop. 2002;399:201–4.
66. Xu M, Xu S, Yu X. Marginal resection for osteosarcoma with effective neoadjuvant chemotherapy: long-term outcomes. World J Surg Oncol. 2014;12:341. doi:10.1186/1477-7819-12-341.

67. Henshaw RM. Surgical advances in bone and soft tissue sarcoma: 50 years of progress. Am Soc Clin Oncol Educ Book. 2014:252–8. doi:10.14694/EdBook_AM.2014.34.252.
68. Malawer M, Sugarbaker P. Musculoskeletal cancer surgery treatment of sarcomas and allied diseases. Boston: Kluwer Academic Publishers; 2001.
69. Malawer M, Bickels J. Operative techniques in orthopedic surgical oncology. Philadelphia: Lippincott Williams & Wilkins; 2012.
70. Drake DB. Reconstruction for limb-sparing procedures in soft-tissue sarcomas of the extremities. Clin Plast Surg. 1995;22(1):123–8.
71. Barwick WJ, Goldberg JA, Scully SP, Harrelson JM. Vascularized tissue transfer for closure of irradiated wounds after soft tissue sarcoma resection. Ann Surg. 1992;216(5):591–5.
72. Gitelis S, Piasecki P. Allograft prosthetic composite arthroplasty for osteosarcoma and other aggressive bone tumors. Clin Orthop Relat Res. 1991;270:197–201.
73. Wu CC, Henshaw RM, Pritsch T, et al. Implant design and resection length affect cemented endoprosthesis survival in proximal tibial reconstruction. J Arthroplast. 2008;23(6):886–93. doi:10.1016/j.arth.2007.07.007. Epub 2008 Feb 13
74. Kawai A, Lin PP, Boland PJ, Athanasian EA, Healey JH. Relationship between magnitude of resection, complication, and prosthetic survival after prosthetic knee reconstructions for distal femoral tumors. J Surg Oncol. 1999;70(2):109–15.
75. Rosen G. Preoperative (neoadjuvant) chemotherapy for osteogenic sarcoma: a ten year experience. Orthopedics. 1985;8(5):659–64.
76. Sluga M, Windhager R, Lang S, et al. The role of surgery and resection margins in the treatment of Ewing's sarcoma. Clin Orthop Relat Res. 2001;392:394–9.
77. Bacci G, Ferrari S, Longhi A, et al. Local and systemic control in Ewing's sarcoma of the femur treated with chemotherapy, and locally by radiotherapy and/or surgery. J Bone Joint Surg Br. 2003;85(1):107–14.
78. Henry AK. Extensile exposure applied to limb surgery. Churchill Livingstone, 1945, 2nd ed. 1957, reprinted 1973.
79. Hoppenfeld S, de Boer P, Buckley R. Surgical exposures in orthopaedics: the anatomic approach. Philadelphia: Wolters Kluwer/Lippincott Williams & Wilkins; 2009.
80. Zeegen EN, Aponte-Tinao LA, Hornicek FJ, Gebhardt MC, Mankin HJ. Survivorship analysis of 141 modular metallic endoprostheses at early followup. Clin Orthop Relat Res. 2004;420:239–50.
81. Farfalli GL, Boland PJ, Morris CD, Athanasian EA, Healey JH. Early equivalence of uncemented press-fit and Compress femoral fixation. Clin Orthop Relat Res. 2009;467:2792–9. doi:10.1007/s11999-009-0912-9.
82. Benevenia J, Kirchner R, Patterson F, et al. Outcomes of a modular intercalary endoprosthesis as treatment for segmental defects of the femur, tibia, and humerus. Clin Orthop Relat Res. 2016;474(2):539–48.
83. Bus MP, Dijkstra PD, van de Sande MA, et al. Intercalary allograft reconstructions following resection of primary bone tumors: a nationwide multicenter study. J Bone Joint Surg Am. 2014;96(4):e26. doi:10.2106/JBJS.M.00655.
84. Horowitz SM, Lane JM, Healey JH. Soft-tissue management with prosthetic replacement for sarcomas around the knee. Clin Orthop Relat Res. 1992;275:226–31.
85. Muramatsu K, Ihara K, Tominaga Y, Hashimoto T, Taguchi T. Functional reconstruction of the deltoid muscle following complete resection of musculoskeletal sarcoma. J Plast Reconstr Aesthet Surg. 2014;67(7):916–20. doi:10.1016/j.bjps.2014.03.018. Epub 2014 Mar 28
86. Fischer S, Soimaru S, Hirsch T, et al. Local tendon transfer for knee extensor mechanism reconstruction after soft tissue sarcoma resection. J Plast Reconstr Aesthet Surg. 2015;68(5):729–35. doi:10.1016/j.bjps.2015.01.002. Epub 2015 Jan 24
87. Sakellariou VI, Mavrogenis AF, Papagelopoulos PJ. Negative-pressure wound therapy for musculoskeletal tumor surgery. Adv Skin Wound Care. 2011;24(1):25–30. doi:10.1097/01. ASW.0000392924.75970.b9.
88. Fairweather M, Keung E, Raut CP. Neoadjuvant therapy for soft-tissue sarcomas (review). Oncology (Williston Park). 2016;30(1):99–106.

89. Sherman KL, Kinnier CV, Farina DA, et al. Examination of national lymph node evaluation practices for adult extremity soft tissue sarcoma. J Surg Oncol. 2014;110(6):682–8. doi:10.1002/jso.23687. Epub 2014 Jun 7
90. Pearlstone DB, Pisters PW, Bold RJ, et al. Patterns of recurrence in extremity liposarcoma: implications for staging and follow-up. Cancer. 1999;85(1):85–92.
91. Becher S, Oskouei S. PET imaging in sarcoma. Orthop Clin North Am. 2015;46(3):409–15, xi. doi:10.1016/j.ocl.2015.03.001. Epub 2015 Apr 11. Review.
92. Andreou D, Boldt H, Werner M, Hamann C, Pink D, Tunn PU. Sentinel node biopsy in soft tissue sarcoma subtypes with a high propensity for regional lymphatic spread--results of a large prospective trial. Ann Oncol. 2013;24(5):1400–5. doi:10.1093/annonc/mds650. Epub 2013 Jan 31
93. Michot A, Stoeckle E, Bannel JD, et al. The introduction of early patient rehabilitation in surgery of soft tissue sarcoma and its impact on post-operative outcome. Eur J Surg Oncol. 2015;41(12):1678–84. doi:10.1016/j.ejso.2015.08.173. Epub 2015 Sep 26
94. van Boekel RL, Vissers KC, van de Vossenberg G, et al. Comparison of epidural or regional analgesia and patient controlled analgesia: a critical analysis of patient data by the Acute Pain Service in a University Hospital. Clin J Pain. 2016;32(8):681–8.
95. Morey TE, Giannoni J, Duncan E, Scarborough MT, Enneking FK. Nerve sheath catheter analgesia after amputation. Clin Orthop Relat Res. 2002;397:281–9.
96. Wheatley 3rd GH, Rosenbaum DH, Paul MC, Dine AP, et al. Improved pain management outcomes with continuous infusion of a local anesthetic after thoracotomy. J Thorac Cardiovasc Surg. 2005;130(2):464–8.
97. Pontarelli EM, Matthews JA, Goodhue CJ, Stein JE. On-Q ® pain pump versus epidural for postoperative analgesia in children. Pediatr Surg Int. 2013;29(12):1267–71. doi:10.1007/s00383-013-3342-4. Epub 2013 Jul 17
98. Shehadeh A, El Dahleh M, Salem A, Sarhan Y, Sultan I, Henshaw RM, Aboulafia AJ. Standardization of rehabilitation after limb salvage surgery for sarcomas improves patients' outcome. Hematol Oncol Stem Cell Ther. 2013;6(3–4):105–11. doi:10.1016/j.hemonc.2013.09.001. Epub 2013 Oct 24

Specific Surgical Topics: A Multidisciplinary Management of Paratesticular Sarcomas in Adults

7

Mohan Verghese and Jonathan Hwang

7.1   Introduction

Primary paratesticular sarcomas are rare, affecting primarily older men between the ages of 50 and 80 years. They are the most common tumors of the paratesticular region and usually present insidiously as an asymptomatic slow-growing mass. Because of the rarity of these tumors, there is no common consensus regarding the best management, especially in the adjuvant setting [1]. In adults, 75–80% arise from the spermatic cord and the remainder from the epididymis, tunic, or testicular appendages [2]. Among the malignant tumors, the most common histotype is liposarcoma (46.4%), followed by leiomyosarcoma (20%), malignant fibrous histiocytomas (13%), and embryonal rhabdomyosarcoma (9%) [3]. Of these, rhabdomyosarcoma, rare after the age of 40, is the most common malignant mesenchymal tumor in children and is considered the most aggressive sarcoma. It has an increased ability to spread via the lymphatic or hematogenous route [4, 5]. The main dissemination pattern of adult paratesticular sarcomas is by local invasion through the contiguous inguinal canal and less commonly via hematogenous or lymphatic channels. Surgery represents the first and the most effective therapeutic approach to most paratesticular sarcomas, and overall, the prognosis after diagnosis has been related to grading, size, depth of invasion, and surgical margin status [6].

M. Verghese, M.D., F.A.C.S., F.I.C.S. (✉)
Department of Urology, Director, Section of Urologic Oncology,
Medstar Washington Hospital Center, Washington, DC, USA
e-mail: Mohan.M.Verghese@medstar.net

J. Hwang, M.D.
Department of Urology, Robotic Surgery, Georgetown University School of Medicine,
MedStar Washington Hospital Center, Washington, DC, USA

© Springer International Publishing Switzerland 2017
R.M. Henshaw (ed.), *Sarcoma*, DOI 10.1007/978-3-319-43121-5_7

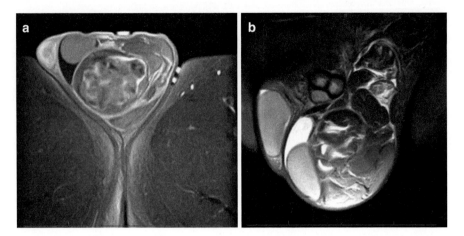

Fig. 7.1 (**a**, **b**) MRI of the inguinal-scrotal region showing an inguinal-scrotal mass with signal intensity of fat

7.2   Clinical Presentation

Paratesticular sarcomas often present as a slow-growing palpable paratesticular mass. It commonly manifests as a solid, irregular palpable mass of the inguinal canal or scrotum. Most sarcomas develop below the external inguinal ring and thus grow as a scrotal mass [2]. They may present as an inguinoscrotal mass and commonly mistaken for a hernia (Fig. 7.1). Pain and tenderness have been reported in 10–15% of patients [7]. Infrequently, the initial presentation may be acute scrotum due to necrosis or intratumoral bleeding [8]. In a minority of patients, there is a history of scrotal surgery or trauma (<6%) [9]. The rarity of these sarcomas continues to make preoperative diagnosis very challenging. More often, patients are suspected of having more common conditions in the differential diagnosis, including inguinal hernia, hydrocele, spermatocele, chronic epididymitis, or lipoma [10, 11]. The diagnosis should always be considered in patients presenting with recurrent inguinal hernia [11]. Any palpable mass of the cord structures should be evaluated with ultrasonography even though findings are often nonspecific [12]. CT/MRI can be helpful in the diagnosis and staging as the preoperative imaging modalities [1, 13] (Fig. 7.1a, b).

7.3   Surgical Management of Sarcomas of the Spermatic Cord

Sarcomas of the spermatic cord tend to spread by local extension. Simple excision alone of the spermatic cord may result in microscopic residual disease as repeat wide excision has revealed microscopic residual disease in 27% of completely excised cases [14]. Therefore, a radical inguinal orchiectomy with high ligation of

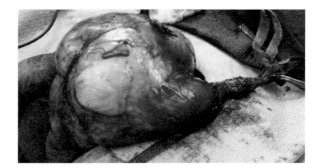

Fig. 7.2 Wide resection of a large liposarcoma with high ligation of the spermatic cord

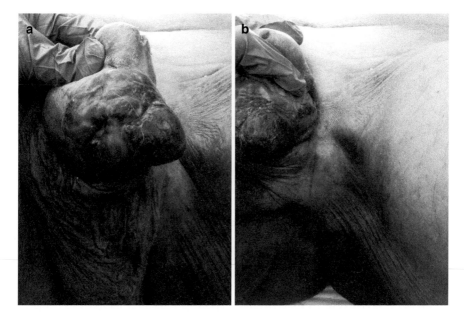

Fig. 7.3 (**a, b**) Recurrent sarcoma of the spermatic cord with invasion to the corporal bodies of the penis

the spermatic cord and wide excision of the soft tissue around the cord within the inguinal canal to achieve negative margins results in a lower rate of local recurrence (Fig. 7.2). Patients with inadequately resected disease should undergo a reoperative procedure with wide inguinal resection [15].

The long-term locoregional recurrence following radical excision has been reported to be approximately 50% [16]. Factors that increase the risk for local recurrence include large tumor size, inguinal location, narrow or positive margins, violation of the pseudocapsule, or unintentional intralesional surgery for misdiagnosed inguinal hernia [17]. Local relapse may occur in the partially resected spermatic cord, within the scrotal cavity or adjacent pelvis with or without involvement of lymph nodes [18]. Relapse in one of our cases involved invasion to the corporal bodies necessitating a total penectomy, urethrectomy, and proximal urinary diversion (Figs. 7.3a, b and 7.4). In patients presenting with local recurrence following

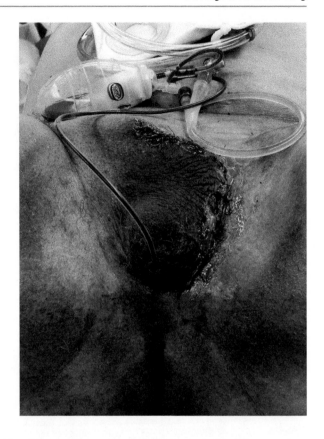

resection, reoperation with wide resection can result in decreased local recurrence [19]. If negative margins are not achieved at the time of the initial surgery, wide re-excision including the previous scar should be considered mandatory even if it involves the excision of adjacent normal structure to obtain negative margins [20]. Fiducial markers using clips can be placed to facilitate postoperative radiation to the tumor bed following resection.

Because of the anatomical constraints of the inguinal region, wide resection to achieve negative margins may not be possible without significant loss of surrounding soft tissue resulting in large defects in the inguinal region (Fig. 7.5). It is imperative to have a multidisciplinary team approach to the surgical management to cover these large defects. General anesthesia is preferable to eliminate visceral pain associated with spermatic cord manipulation in healthy males. Patient is prepared and draped to include the scrotum and the lower abdomen in the operative field. A standard inguinal incision is made overlying the spermatic cord mass from the deep inguinal to the level of the superficial inguinal ring. The skin, subcutaneous tissue, and Scarpa's layer are incised to expose the external oblique fascia which is incised in the direction of its fibers. The ilioinguinal nerve is identified and preserved. If the

Fig. 7.5 Resection of a large right paratesticular sarcoma with excision of the floor of the inguinal canal and high ligation of the cord

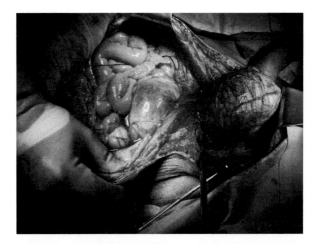

Fig. 7.6 Resected paratesticular mass with intact fascial planes

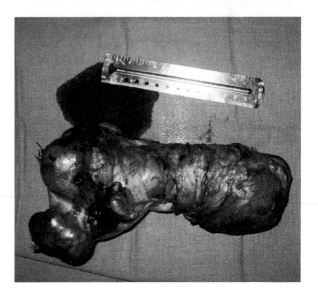

mass is large, the incision can be extended into the scrotum. In primary resection of a suspected sarcoma, it is important to preserve the integrity of the external spermatic fascia, cremasteric, and internal spermatic fascia which forms the outer tubular sheath surrounding the spermatic cord to prevent the contents of the cord spilling into the wound (Fig. 7.6). At the deep inguinal ring, the spermatic vessels are clamped, divided, and tied with permanent sutures that can be identified in the event a retroperitoneal lymphadenectomy is needed so that the remnant cord can be identified and removed. The vas deferens is tied and divided separately. The testis with its investing tunica vaginalis is delivered into the wound, and the entire specimen is removed without violating any facial layers. The wound is copiously irrigated. The external aponeurosis is closed with absorbable sutures and skin approximated with either staples or subcuticular sutures.

For patients with bulky tumor recurrences or those with radio-recurrent tumors, preoperative planning with plastic, orthopedic, and reconstructive surgeons for coverage of large defects created by wide resection should be done ahead of time (Fig. 7.5). Wide excision may include surrounding soft tissues, lower anterior abdominal wall fascia, and muscles of the thigh exposing femoral vessels and the neural bundles and exposed bone as the clinical picture dictates (Fig. 7.5). Involvement of the corporal bodies from local recurrences may require a total penectomy and urethrectomy (Fig. 7.3a, b). Patients should be counseled accordingly.

Many reconstructive options are available to repair defects in this region which include fasciocutaneous, muscle, or musculocutaneous flaps such as the tensor fascia latae, rectus abdominis, anterolateral thigh, gracilis, and the vastus lateralis flaps to cover the defects [20–23]. Overlying femoral vessel tissue loss should be covered with well-vascularized tissue to prevent or minimize local vascular complications if adjuvant RT is considered [20]. The tensor fasciae latae musculocutaneous flaps can cover a large defect including the femoral vessels [23]. The abdominal wall musculature may need to be reinforced with mesh in addition to flaps to cover larger defects. The type of flaps used will depend on the extent of resection, and with good planning, good long-term results can be achieved.

7.4   Current Adjuvant Therapy

Radiation therapy: Radiation treatment for patients with paratesticular sarcomas is most often utilized as postoperative adjuvant therapy to prevent local recurrences [24], although planned preoperative radiotherapy can be given to debulk large sarcomas. Select patients with intermediate- or high-grade pathology may benefit, though the optimum dosage is yet to be defined [25, 26]. At present, there is no consensus on the benefit of retroperitoneal lymphadenectomy or chemotherapy for paratesticular adult sarcomas [1]. The current standard of care for rhabdomyosarcoma is multimodal treatment including surgery, chemotherapy, and radiation based on disease stage, histology, and age of patient [24, 27].

Conclusion

In patients with sarcomas of the spermatic cord, wide excision via radical inguinal orchiectomy and high ligation of the cord should be the primary procedure. For local relapses, postradiation recurrences, or margin-positive initial resections, re-excision with wide margins and appropriate reconstruction with flaps should be done to provide the best outcome. Regardless of the initial therapy, the risk of local recurrence always necessitates long-term follow-up [26].

References

1. Rodriguez D, Olumi AF. Management of spermatic cord tumors: a rare urologic malignancy. Ther Adv Urol. 2012;4(6):325–34.
2. Schwartz SL, Swierzewski SJ, Sondak VK, Grossman HB. Liposarcoma of the spermatic cord: report of 6 cases and review of the literature. J Urol. 1995;153:154–7.
3. Rodriguez D, Barrisford GW, Sanchez A, Preston MA, Kreydin EI, Olumi AF. Primary spermatic cord tumors: disease characteristics, prognostic factor, and treatment options. Urol Oncol. 2014;32:52.e19–25.
4. Panagis A, Karydas G, Vasilakakis J, Chatzipaschalis E, Lambropoulou M, Papadopoulos N. Myxoid liposarcoma of the spermatic cord: a case report and review of the literature. Int Urol Nephrol. 2003;35:369–72.
5. Fisher C, Goldblum JR, Epstein JI, Montgomery E. Leiomyosarcoma of the paratesticular region: a clinicopathologic study. Am J Surg Pathol. 2001;25:1143–9.
6. Lewis JJ, Leung D, Woodruff JM, Brennan MF. Retroperitoneal soft-tissue sarcoma: analysis of 500 patients treated and followed at a single institution. Ann Surg. 1998;228:355–65.
7. Peterson JJ, Kransdorf MJ, Bancroft LW, O'Connor MI. Malignant fatty tumors: classification, clinical course, imaging appearance and treatment. Skelet Radiol. 2003;32:493–503.
8. Castineiras J, Varo C, Sanchez Bernal C, et al. Paratesticular neoplasms of mesenchymatous origin. Clinico-pathologic study (in Spanish). Actas Urol Esp. 1995;19:40–5.
9. Alyousef H, Osman EM, Gomha MA. Paratesticular liposarcoma: a case report and review of the literature. Case Rep Urol. 2013;2013:806289.
10. Fitzgerald S, MacLennan G. Paratesticular liposarcoma. J Urol. 2009;181:331–2.
11. Li F, Tian R, Yin C, et al. Liposarcoma of the spermatic cord mimicking a left inguinal hernia: a case report and literature review. World J Surg Oncol. 2013;11:18.
12. Frates MC, Benson CB, Di Salvo DN, et al. Solid extratesticular masses evaluated with sonography: pathologic correlation. Radiology. 2014;1997:43–6.
13. Guttilla A, Crestani A, Zattoni F, et al. Spermatic cord sarcoma: our experience and review of the literature. Urol Int. 2013;90:101–5.
14. Catton C, Jewett M, O'Sullivan B, Kandel R. Paratesticular sarcoma: failure patterns after definitive local therapy. J Urol. 1999;161:1844–7.
15. Rodriguez D, Olumi AF. Management of spermatic cord tumors: a rare Urologic malignancy. Ther Adv Urol. 2012;4(6):325–34.
16. Fagundes MA, Zietmman AL, Althusen AF, Coen JJ, Shipley WU. The management of spermatic cord sarcoma. Cancer. 1996;77:1873–6.
17. Folpe AL, Weiss SW. Paratesticular soft tissue neoplasms. Semin Diagn Pathol. 2000;17:307–18.
18. Merimsky O, Terrier P, Bonvalot S, Le Pechoux C, Delord JP, Le Cesne A. Spermatic cord sarcomas in adults. Acta Oncol. 1999;38:635–8.
19. Coleman J, Brennan MF, Alektiar K, Russo P. Adult spermatic cord sarcomas: management and results. Ann Surg Oncol. 2003;10:669–75.
20. Enoch S, Wharton SM, Murray DS. Management of leiomyosarcomas of the spermatic cord: the role of reconstructive surgery. World J Surg Oncol. 2005;3:23.
21. Bare RL, Assimos DG, McCullough DL, Smith DP, DeFranzo AJ, Marks MW. Inguinal lymphadenectomy and primary groin reconstruction using rectus abdominus muscle flaps in patients with penile cancer. Urology. 1994;44(4):557–61.
22. Wei F-c, Jain V, Celik N, Chen H, Chewi-chin C, Lin C. Have we found an ideal soft tissue flap? An experience with 672 anterolateral thigh flaps. Plast Reconstr Surg. 2002;109(7):2219–26.
23. Gopinath KS, Chandrashekhar M, Kumar MV, Srikant KC. Tensor fasciae latae musculocutaneous flaps to reconstruct skin defects after radical inguinal lymphadenectomy. Br J Plast Surg. 1988;41:366–8.

24. Caton CN, Cummings BJ, Fornaiser V, O'Sullivan B, Quirt I, Warr D. Adult paratesticular Sarcomas: a review of 21 cases. J Urol. 1991;146:342–5.
25. Fubiao L, Runhui T, Changju Y, Xiafan D, Hongliang W, Ning X, Kaimin G. Liposarcoma of the spermatic cord mimicking a left inguinal hernia: a case report and literature review. World J Surg Oncol. 2013;11:18.
26. May M, Seehafer M, Helke C, Gunia S, Hoschike B. Liposarcoma of the spermatic cord— report of one new case and review of the literature. Aktuelle Urol. 2014;35(2):130–3.
27. Dangle PP, Correa A, Tennyson L, Gayed B, Reyes-Mugica M, Ost M. Current management of paratesticular rhabdomyosarcoma. Urol Oncol. 2016;34(2):84–92.

Specific Surgical Topics: Surgical Management of Gastrointestinal Stromal Tumors

8

Mark Steves

Gastrointestinal stromal tumor (GIST) is the most common mesenchymal tumor of the GI tract with a new patient diagnosis of 4000–6000 per year in the USA. The pathological characterization of this tumor and the molecular basis of its treatment in the last several decades illustrate the complexity and beauty of targeted treatment for cancer.

8.1 Background

GIST typically presents as a subepithelial tumor in the GI tract with the mean presentation in the sixth decade of life. They occur primarily in the stomach and small intestine. Initial pathological classification was confusing. Early attempts to better define this group of gastrointestinal sarcomas from other types of sarcomas were difficult. Treatment decisions for patients were made with the best data at hand. At many institutions, such as the Washington Hospital Center, which is a tertiary referral center for the National Capital region, both surgeons and medical oncologists were stymied by the lack of good treatment for patients with diffuse peritoneal sarcomatosis. Systemic chemotherapy did not have any meaningful impact. In the 1990s our approach centered around surgical cytoreduction. Even with all gross diseases removed, most patients would have progressive disease, though we did have a median survival of 20 months in our group of 43 patients [1]. In retrospect the majority of these sarcomatosis patients had GIST.

M. Steves, M.D.
Department of Surgical Oncology, MedStar Washington Hospital Center,
Washington, DC, USA
e-mail: Mark.Steves@medstar.net

© Springer International Publishing Switzerland 2017
R.M. Henshaw (ed.), *Sarcoma*, DOI 10.1007/978-3-319-43121-5_8

A light began to shine in the darkness with the molecular characterization of GIST. It is thought that the majority of these tumors originate from cells in the bowel wall that are precursors to the intestinal cells of Cajal (ICC). ICC are the GI pacemaker cells that coordinate the innervation of the bowel and the smooth muscle. More importantly the majority of GIST cells express the CD117 antigen, unlike leiomyomas or leiomyosarcomas. The CD117 antigen is part of the kit tyrosine kinase receptor, which sits on the cell membrane, and is coded by the kit proto-oncogene (c-kit). This overexpression of CD117 is readily detected by immunohistochemical staining. This mutation with the resulting activation of the kit tyrosine kinase receptor induces cell proliferation.

As the importance of the tyrosine kinase receptor in the pathogenesis of GIST was emerging, inroads were being made in the pharmaceutical industry with respect to the use of agents targeted to tyrosine kinase receptors. Dr. Brian Druker and others working with Ciba-Geigy (now Novartis) found one drug, STI-571, that showed incredible promise because of its effect on the tyrosine kinases that are important in the pathogenesis of chronic myelogenous leukemia (CML). In the first clinical trials of STI-571 (imatinib), there was nearly universal response in the patients treated with appropriate dosages of drug [2]. After further studies showed similar promise, a new drug application for imatinib was submitted to the Food and Drug Administration (FDA). In rapid fashion, after 2 1/2 months, the FDA approved imatinib for the treatment of CML in May of 2001.

The extreme interest in the drug was fueled by a large grassroot movement and the drug made the cover of *TIME* magazine on the month of its approval by the FDA, touted as the "bullet against cancer." However, the historical impact of the drug on another tumor type, GIST, was yet to be felt.

The story of "patient zero" is worth repeating. A 54-year-old Finnish woman with familial ties to the pharmaceutical industry had been advised of the potential benefit of imatinib on patients with GIST because of the kit mutation commonly expressed. She started the treatment in March 2000. The remarkable effect that imatinib had on her tumor was chronicled in a *New England Journal of Medicine* (NEJM) brief report in April 2001 [3]. This effect of imatinib on GIST in the metastatic setting led to other clinical trials that showed equal promise. The FDA granted accelerated approval to imatinib in 2002 for the treatment of metastatic disease. Approval for use in the adjuvant setting had to wait until 2008 (Fig. 8.1).

8.2   Presentation

Since most GISTs are located in the stomach and the small intestine, the usual presentation to the surgeon is secondary to one or more of the following: (1) abdominal mass with or without abdominal pain, (2) gastrointestinal bleeding, (3) obstruction, (4) perforation—rare, and (5) incidental finding, which has become increasingly more common.

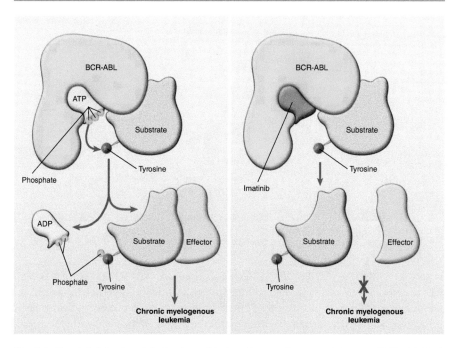

Fig. 8.1 Imatinib Mesylate: Mechanism of Action. Source: Savage and Antman. N Engl J Med. 2002;346:683.

8.3   Diagnosis/Workup

Usually by the time of surgical consultation, the diagnosis of GIST has been presumptively made by the use of a high-resolution computed tomography (CT) scan of the abdomen and pelvis with intravenous (IV) and oral contrast. It is important to maximize the amount of oral contrast to entirely fill the gastrointestinal tract. A high-quality CT scan may show early signs of metastatic peritoneal disease, namely, small nodules located between loops of small bowel (SB) and leaves of the SB mesentery. Certainly the extent of a primary small bowel GIST is easily seen with saturation of oral contrast on CT scan (Fig. 8.2). Magnetic resonance imaging (MRI) does not usually play a role in the workup but does help delineate disease in the liver and specifically in the pelvis, i.e., rectal GIST. Routinely, positron emission test (PET) scans are not obtained preoperatively on patients who are thought to be good surgical candidates. However, in patients who are not surgical candidates, PET scans can be used to monitor therapy.

Upper endoscopy and endoscopic ultrasound (EUS) play a large role in the diagnosis of gastric GIST. Upon presentation with GI bleeding, the endoscopist will usually find a submucosal mass with central ulceration. A biopsy confirming the diagnosis of GIST may be elusive since this is not a mucosal tumor. Therefore, EUS is an important modality and can reliably give the diagnosis of a gastric submucosal

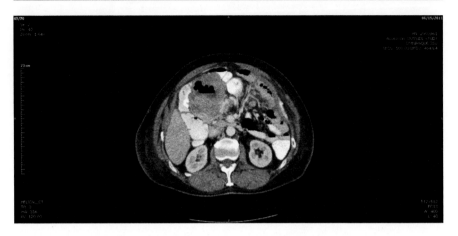

Fig. 8.2 59 year old patient with large bleeding small bowel GIST

mass based on the layer of origin of the mass. The five layers of the GI tract as seen by the conventional endoscope are (1) innermost layer is the superficial mucosa, (2) second layer is the lamina propria, (3) third layer is the submucosa, (4) fourth layer is the muscularis propria, and (5) fifth layer is the serosa. With accurate localization, which is easier with smaller lesions, a gastric lesion originating from the second layer is typically a carcinoid, and lesions arising from the fourth and fifth layers are usually lipomas. Of course there are other endoscopic and EUS features that are used to differentiate these tumors.

Though the role of EUS is key to the diagnosis and workup of GIST, the absolute need for pretreatment biopsy is only important in patients with metastatic disease at the time of presentation. The use of neoadjuvant imatinib in patients with borderline resectable tumors or definitive treatment of patients with diffuse metastatic disease will not begin without accurate pathological characterization. In operable patients with a classic clinical presentation, typical endoscopic findings of a submucosal mass with ulceration, and a CT scan showing resectability, there is not an absolute mandate for preoperative biopsy.

After preoperative workup and staging are complete, patients are categorized into three groups: (1) surgical resectable patients, (2) surgical resectable patients with potential for significant morbidity from multiorgan resection of primary tumor, and (3) unresectable patients and patients with metastatic disease. In regard to patients with resectable lesions but who face potentially morbid surgical procedures, referral should be made to a tertiary care facility for possible treatment with neoadjuvant imatinib. This will be discussed later.

8.4 Surgical Management

As with most other GI malignancies, surgery is the primary modality in resectable disease and reserved for palliation in patients with advanced disease. Occasionally, in patients who present with significant bleeding, perforation, and/or obstruction, the patient will need urgent surgical intervention, and the diagnosis is only achieved after pathological examination. However, in the face of a large epigastric palpable mass, it would behoove the surgeon to try and establish the diagnosis preoperatively with CT scan and/or endoscopy. As mentioned earlier, patients with clinical features of GIST and who are good surgical candidates may forego a preoperative biopsy.

At surgery, the basic approach should involve thorough exploration of the abdominal and pelvic cavities to rule out peritoneal disease. The right and left hemidiaphragm are inspected as well as the right and left colonic gutters; small bowel and its mesentery are also thoroughly evaluated. Pelvic structures are looked at with particular attention to the pouch of Douglas in women. Other sites of potential peritoneal disease that are worth looking at include the gastrohepatic ligament as well as the lesser sac after dividing the gastrocolic ligament. Specifically, attention should be drawn to the potential space that can exist under the pylorus and duodenal bulb. In our early work with peritoneal carcinomatosis, this was a site that was frequently not appreciated. Lastly, another area that should be inspected is the ligament of Treitz and proximal jejunum where various recesses exist and tumor cells can find a home. Once peritoneal disease is encountered, a variety of peritonectomy procedures can be used to resect small to moderate volume disease [4].

Once peritoneal disease volume has been ascertained, it is also important to quantitate any metastatic liver disease. Usually the diagnosis of metastatic liver disease can be made preoperatively with CT scan. However small lesions at the surface of the liver can be missed and should always be biopsied. Intraoperative ultrasound (IUS) of the liver may also be needed to delineate a vague mass felt in the liver as well.

Having thoroughly searched for metastatic disease, attention can then be turned to the primary site which in the majority of cases is the stomach. The overriding surgical approach is resection with negative gross margins (RO) and without spillage and/or rupture of tumor. Tumor spillage, as will be discussed later, usually portends a poor future outcome. Adequate resection of the gastric primary can be achieved without the need for an anatomic resection as is needed with gastric adenocarcinoma. Resection of nodal basis is also not needed since the spread of GIST to regional lymph nodes is rare.

Preoperatively, large GIST tumors in the stomach can look very imposing. Often these large lesions will lift out of the abdominal cavity, and resection of the primary can proceed in a more routine fashion. Adherence to adjacent tissues and organs (omentum, pancreas, and spleen) will occasionally lead to en bloc resection of these tissues.

Every attempt should be made to preserve function in the stomach, namely, preservation of the gastroesophageal (GE) junction and/or the pylorus. Since most GISTs emanate from the greater curvature, large lesions can be resected without subtotal gastrectomy using techniques similar to bariatric surgery, i.e., sleeve gastrectomy. A bougie dilator placed during surgery may minimize encroachment of the resection on the GE junction. If, however, a margin-free resection cannot be obtained without sacrifice of the GE junction, the resection of the GE junction should not lead to a total gastrectomy. A gastric reservoir can still be preserved with a proximal gastrectomy and stapled esophageal/gastric anastomosis with pyloroplasty. Though this surgical reconstruction can lead to problems with gastric reflux,

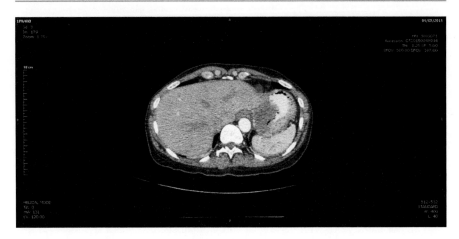

Fig. 8.3 57 year old patient with large bleeding proximal gastric GIST

the operation has been well tolerated. Anecdotally we have had minimal patient dissatisfaction over the last two decades when we have had to resort to this reconstruction (Fig. 8.3).

Surgical resection of a small bowel primary should be a more straightforward event. As mentioned nodal resection is not indicated for GIST. Macroscopically gross negative margins should be obtained.

Unfortunately, even with the most comprehensive preoperative workup, patients with localized primaries will occasionally be found to have metastatic disease in the form of peritoneal carcinomatosis or small-volume metastatic disease. The experience of the surgeon will then dictate whether the patient is closed after pathological diagnosis is confirmed or whether the surgery proceeds. It has been our practice that the primary lesion is resected if it can be done with minimal functional loss to the patient. Peritoneal disease then can be addressed in a systemic fashion much like colorectal cancer with post-op imatinib. Also if the primary site at exploration requires significant functional loss to the patient that the surgeon feels may be minimized with preoperative treatment with imatinib, the pathological diagnosis is established and the patient is then closed. Then neoadjuvant therapy (discussed later) can begin.

8.5   Staging

Once the primary tumor in the stomach or small bowel has been resected and the patient has recovered, medical oncology referral can be made. The TNM staging according to the American Joint Committee on Cancer (AJCC) for gastric and small bowel GIST is shown below (Table 8.1). Based on tumor location, tumor size, and mitotic rate, the rate of recurrent disease can be also estimated (Tables 8.2 and 8.3).

Table 8.1 TNM staging for gastrointestinal stromal tumors (GIST)

For GISTs at all sites				
Primary tumor (T)				
TX	Primary tumor cannot be assessed			
T0	No evidence for primary tumor			
T1	Tumor 2 cm or less			
T2	Tumor more than 2 cm but not more than 5 cm			
T3	Tumor more than 5 cm but not more than 10 cm			
T4	Tumor more than 10 cm in greatest dimension			
Regional lymph nodes (N)				
N0	No regional lymph node metastasis[a]			
N1	Regional lymph node metastasis			
Distant metastasis (M)				
M0	No distant metastasis			
M1	Distant metastasis			
Histologic grade (G)b				
GX	Grade cannot be assessed			
G1	Low grade; mitotic rate $\leq$5/50 HPF			
G2	High grade; mitotic rate $\geq$5/50 HPF			
Anatomic stage/prognostic groups				
Stage	*T*	*N*	*M*	*Mitotic rate*
Gastric GISTc				
IA	T1 or T2	N0	M0	Low
IB	T3	N0	M0	Low
II	T1	N0	M0	High
	T2	N0	M0	High
	T4	N0	M0	Low
IIIA	T3	N0	M0	High
IIIB	T4	N0	M0	High
IV	Any T	N1	M0	Any rate
	Any T	Any N	M1	Any rate
Small intestinal GISTd				
I	T1 or T2	N0	M0	Low
II	T3	N0	M0	Low
IIIA	T1	N0	M0	High
	T4	N0	M0	Low
IIIB	T2	N0	M0	High
	T3	N0	M0	High
	T4	N0	M0	High

(continued)

Table 8.1 (continued)

IV	Any T	N1	M0	Any rate
	Any T	Any N	M1	Any rate

Note: cTNM is the clinical classification, pTNM is the pathologic classification
[a]If regional node status is unknown, use N0 not NX
[b]Histologic grading, an ingredient in sarcoma staging, is not well suited to GISTs, because a majority of these tumors have low or relatively low mitotic rates below the thresholds used for grading of soft tissue tumors, and because GISTs often manifest aggressive features with mitotic rates below the thresholds used for soft tissue tumor grading (the lowest tier of mitotic rates for soft tissue sarcomas being 10 mitoses per 10 HPFs). In GIST staging, the grade is replaced by mitotic activity
[c]Also to be used for omentum
[d]Also to be used for esophagus, colorectal, mesentery, and peritoneum

Table 8.2 Disease progression rate for gastric gastrointestinal stromal tumors (GIST) according to tumor size and miotic rate or AFIP prognostic group

Stage	Tumor size, cm	Mitotic rate	AFIP prognostic group[a]	Observed rate of progressive disease,[a] percent
IA	≤5 (T$_{1,2}$)	Low	1, 2 (≤2–5 cm, ≤5 mit/50 hpf)	0–2
IB	>5–10 (T$_3$)	Low	3a (5–10 cm, ≤5 mit/50 hpf)	3–4
II	>5–10 (T$_3$)	High	4 (≤2 cm, >5 mit/50 hpf)	Insufficient data
	>5–10 (T$_3$)	High	5 (2–5 cm, >5 mit/50 hpf)	15
	>10 (T$_4$)	Low	3b (>10 cm, ≤5 mit/50 hpf)	12
IIIA	>5–10 (T$_3$)	High	6a (>5–10 cm, >5 mit/50 hpf)	49
IIIB	>10 (T$_4$)	High	6b (>10 cm, >5 mit/50 hpf)	86

AFIP Armed Forces Institute of Pathology, *mit* mitoses, *hpf* high-powered field
[a]Miettinen M, Sobin LH, Lasota J. Gastrointestinal stromal tumors of the stomach: a clinicopathologic, immunohistochemical, and molecular genetic studies of 1765 cases with long-term follow-up. Am J Surg Pathol. 2005; 29:52–68, with permission from Lippincott Williams & Wilkins

Table 8.3 Disease progression rate for small intestinal gastrointestinal stromal tumors (GIST) according to size and mitotic rate or AFIP prognostic group

Stage	Tumor size, cm	Mitotic rate	AFIP prognostic group[a]	Observed rate of progressive disease,[a] percent
IA	≤5 (T$_{1,2}$)	Low	1, 2 (≤2–5 cm, ≤5 mit/50 hpf)	0–2
II	>5–10 (T$_3$)	Low	3a (5–10 cm, ≤5 mit/50 hpf)	23
III A	>10 (T$_4$)	Low	3b (>10 cm, ≤5 mit/50 hpf)	49
	≤2 (T$_1$.)	High	4 (≤2 cm, >5 mit/50 hpf)	50
III B	>2–5 (T$_2$)	High	5 (2–5 cm, >5 mit/50 hpf)	73
	>5–10 (T$_3$)	High	6a (>5–10 cm, >5 mit/50 hpf)	72
	>10 (T$_4$)	High	6b (>10 cm, >5 mit/50 hpf)	89

AFIP Armed Forces Institute of Pathology, *mit* mitoses, *hpf* high-powered field
[a]Miettinen M, Makhlouf HR, Sobin LH, Lasota J. Gastrointestinal stromal tumors (GISTs) of the jejunum and ileum—a clinicopathologic, immunohistochemical and molecular genetic study of 906 cases prior to imatinib with long-term follow-up. Am J Surg Pathol. 2006; 30:477–89, with permission from Lippincott Williams & Wilkins

Of particular note in the staging system is that a T3 or T4 GIST with low mitotic activity becomes a higher stage if the primary is in the small bowel. A T3 lesion in the stomach is a stage I lesion, while in the small bowel, it is a stage II lesion. Likewise, a T4 lesion (stage II) in the stomach becomes a stage III lesion in the small bowel. Similar stage increases occur with small lesions with high mitotic activity and similarly gastric lesions being of lower stage than equal size small bowel lesions.

As shown in Tables 8.2 and 8.3, the rate of recurrent disease increases significantly with worsening stage. The biological aggressive nature of small bowel GIST is highlighted by the fact that a stage II small bowel GIST has a recurrence rate in the 20–25% range where a stage II gastric GIST has a recurrence rate in the 10–15% range despite the fact that stage II gastric GISTs include smaller lesions with high mitotic activity or large lesions (T4) with low mitotic activity.

At the heart of any staging system is the goal of stratifying the risk of recurrence. In GIST, patients with a high rate of recurrence would be started on adjuvant imatinib. Proper stratification would accurately guide the oncology team and patient. Toward that end, other classifications, such as the Joensuu stratification system, have not only included tumor site, tumor size, and mitotic rate but also tumor rupture [5]. The Joensuu system also has three categories rather than two for mitotic rate (<5, 6–10, and >10 per high-power field (HPF)). In the study that was used to validate the Joensuu risk criteria, a total of 46 (7%) out of the 640 cases in the registry database had tumor rupture. The vast majority of these ruptures happened preoperatively. Of note is that patients who were treated preoperatively with imatinib were excluded from this study. Though patients with tumor rupture did poorly, on multivariable relapse-free survival (RFS), tumor rupture did not have an independent influence. As suggested by the authors, patients with tumor rupture also have other adverse criteria, such as large size, high mitotic activity, and non-gastric tumor origin.

Along with tumor rupture, microscopic positive margin resections (R1) have also been associated with poor prognosis. McCarter et al. reviewed the 819 patient database of GIST patients that were entered in the American College of Surgeons Oncology Group (ACOSOG) Z29000 and Z29001 clinical trials [6]. ACOSOG Z29000 is a phase II trial of imatinib for resected high-risk GIST patients [7]. ACOSOG Z29001 is a phase III trial for patients with resected GIST randomized to imatinib or placebo [8]. Out of 819 patients, 72 (8.8%) had a microscopically positive resection (R1). Variables associated with R1 resection were tumor size, tumor location, and tumor rupture. Twenty-one patients of the 72 (27%) also had tumor rupture. Median follow-up was 49 months. In untreated patients the RFS was not statistically significant in patients who had R1 versus R0 resection. Similarly, in patients treated with imatinib, there was no statistical difference in patients who had R0 versus R1 resection. This data strongly calls into question the need for surgical re-resection of a "positive" margin.

8.6   Neoadjuvant Therapy

In certain clinical situations and specifically with GIST tumor in the duodenum and rectum, consideration should be given to preoperative treatment with imatinib. After pathological confirmation, neoadjuvant treatment can also start for large primary tumors in the stomach or small bowel that an experienced surgeon may feel is in need of a multivisceral organ resection (Fig. 8.4).

In the case of patients with duodenal or rectal GIST, preoperative therapy with imatinib may allow for sufficient downsizing of the primary tumor to avoid the need for a pancreaticoduodenectomy or abdominal perineal resection. Also large proximal gastric primaries may respond enough to allow the preservation of the gastro-esophageal junction.

Neoadjuvant treatment should be started and patients should be followed in a multidisciplinary fashion. Along with CT scan follow-up, PET scans may be useful

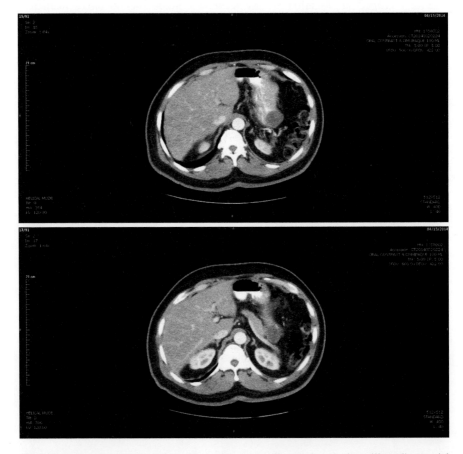

Fig. 8.4 63 year old patient with good response to neoadjuvant therapy but still needing partial gastrectomy and distal pancreatectomy

to ensure that therapy is making an impact. Evaluation of CT scan by Response Evaluation Criteria in Solid Tumors (RECIST) criteria might be difficult since large primary tumors may be responding well yet have no change in size. Effective therapy would be indicated by hypodense changes in the tumor on CT scan (even if no change in size) and minimal to no activity on PET scan. The exact length of treatment with preoperative imatinib is unknown, but stability of disease on two sequential CT scans may indicate that further preoperative treatment may not yield more effect and may put the patient at risk for potential unresectability if there is tumor growth. Continued decrease in size on sequential CT scans can be followed until maximal response. Surgery then may proceed with the expectation that a less morbid procedure will be needed.

8.7   Surgery for Small Gastric GISTs

With the more frequent use of upper GI endoscopy, a large number of small incidental lesions will be found. The natural history of small gastric GISTs (< 2 cm in size) would seem to indicate that a significant majority of these lesions will follow an indolent course [9]. Autopsy series and careful pathological examination of resected stomachs for gastric adenocarcinoma have identified small lesions frequently [10]. To address this issue, the National Comprehensive Cancer Network (NCCN) guidelines have used EUS findings to help distinguish those small GISTs that may follow a more aggressive course. Small lesions with irregular borders, cystic spaces, and tumor heterogeneity on EUS should be considered for surgical resection. Consideration of a laparoscopic resection for these small lesions by an experienced surgeon would also minimize the surgical impact to the patient.

8.8   Surgery for Metastatic or Recurrent Disease

Despite adequate surgery and appropriate postoperative therapy with imatinib, patients unfortunately may recur, usually in the peritoneal cavity and/or liver. Second-line and third-line therapy are available and will be discussed elsewhere.

The role of surgery in patients with metastatic disease is still being defined. One important point that appears to be a significant prognostic variable is the patient's response to tyrosine kinase inhibitor (TKI). When response to treatment is classified into stable disease, limited or focal progression, and generalized progression, the latter group had no benefit from reoperative surgery in a study conducted by Raut [11]. Patients with stable disease had a 1-year PFS of 80% in this study. Other studies have also borne out the futility of surgery on patients with progressive metastatic GIST while on TKI therapy [12]. As mentioned previously, the exact timing of surgery after initiation of TKI therapy is not known, but prolonged therapy will eventually give rise to secondary mutations.

8.9   Summary

The medical and surgical care of patients with GIST has dramatically changed with the advent of effective systemic therapy. Careful coordination of care between the medical oncologist and surgeon will optimize the benefit given to these patients with this fascinating disease.

References

1. Berthet B, Sugarbaker TA, Chang D, Sugarbaker PH. Quantitative methodologies for selection of patients with recurrent abdominopelvic sarcoma for treatment. Eur J Cancer. 1999;35:419–3.
2. Druker BJ, Lydon NB. Lessons learned from the development of an abl tyrosine kinase inhibitor for chronic myelogenous leukemia. J Clin Invest. 2000;105:3–7.
3. Joensuu H, Roberts PJ, et al. Effect of the tyrosine kinase inhibitor STI571 in a patient with metastatic gastrointestinal stromal tumor. N Engl J Med. 2001;344:1052–6.
4. Sugarbaker PH. Peritonectomy procedures. Ann Surg. 1995;221:29–42.
5. Rutkowski P, Bylina E, Wozniak A, et al. Validation of the Joensuu risk criteria for primary resectable gastrointestinal tumor-the impact of tumor rupture on patient outcomes. Eur J Surg Oncol. 2011;37:890–6.
6. McCarter MD, Antonescu CR, Ballman KV, Maki RG, Pisters PW, Demetri GD, et al. Microscopically positive margins for primary gastrointestinal stromal tumors: analysis of risk factors and tumor recurrence. J Am Coll Surg. 2012;215:53–9.
7. DeMatteo RP, Ballman KV, Antonescu CR, Corless C, Kolesnikova V, von Mehren M, et al. Long term results of adjuvant imatinib mesylate in localized, high risk, primary gastrointestinal stromal tumor: ACOSOG Z9000 (alliance) intergroup phase 2 trial. Ann Surg. 2013;258:422–9.
8. Corless CL, Ballman KV, Antonescu CR, Kolesnikova V, Maki RG, Pisters PW, et al. Pathologic and molecular features correlate with long term outcome after adjuvant therapy of resected primary GI stromal tumor: the ACOSOG Z9001 trial. J Clin Oncol. 2014;32:1563–70.
9. Agaimy A, Wunsch PH, Hofstaedter F, et al. Minute gastric sclerosing stromal tumors are common in adults and frequently show c-KIT mutations. Am J Surg Pathol. 2007;31:113–20.
10. Kawanowa K, Sakuma Y, Sakurai S, et al. High incidence of microscopic gastrointestinal stromal tumors in the stomach. Hum Pathol. 2006;37:1527–35.
11. Raut CP, Posner M, Desai J, Morgan JA, George S, Zahrieh D, et al. Surgical management of advanced gastrointestinal stromal tumors after treatment with targeted systemic therapy using kinase inhibitors. J Clin Oncol. 2006;24:2325–31.
12. Bamboat ZM, Dematteo RP. Metastasectomy for gastrointestinal stromal tumors. J Surg Oncol. 2014;109:23–7.

Multidisciplinary Approach to Salvage of Unplanned Sarcoma Resections

9

Nicholas S. Tedesco and Robert M. Henshaw

9.1 Introduction

Ever since the recognition of the necessity for a multidisciplinary approach to optimize care of patients afflicted with cancer, outcomes have steadily improved. This concept of "total cancer care" was first introduced by Dr. Sidney Farber in the 1950s [1]. This was further defined, expanded, explored, and promoted by Dr. Jacob Lokich in 1978 [2] paving the way for the modern multidisciplinary approach to cancer care. Dr. Mario Campanacci of the Rizzoli Institute in Balogna, Italy, noted the improvement in outcomes seen at his institution following the first formation of a sarcoma-specific multidisciplinary care group. He then championed the idea throughout the field of musculoskeletal oncology worldwide. The blossoming in improved oncologic outcomes over time seen with the multidisciplinary approach to care has paralleled developments in diagnostic techniques, surgical

N.S. Tedesco, D.O. (✉)
Orthopedic Oncology and Complex Reconstruction, Oregon Medical Group,
Eugene, OR, USA
e-mail: nicholas.tedesco@gmail.com

R.M. Henshaw, M.D.
Clinical Orthopedic Surgery (Orthopedic Oncology), Georgetown University
School of Medicine, Washington, DC, USA

Department of Orthopedics, MedStar Washington Hospital Center, Washington, DC, USA

Division of Orthopedic Oncology, MedStar Georgetown Orthopedic Institute,
Washington, DC, USA

Orthopedic Oncology, MedStar Washington Cancer Institute and Children's National
Medical Center, Washington, DC, USA

Surgical Branch, National Cancer Institute, Washington, DC, USA

MedStar Washington Cancer Institute, Washington, DC, USA

© Springer International Publishing Switzerland 2017
R.M. Henshaw (ed.), *Sarcoma*, DOI 10.1007/978-3-319-43121-5_9

protocols, additions of chemotherapy drugs and regimens, and radiation oncology technological advances. Progress in such varied fields further promotes the concept of the multidisciplinary synergy needed for optimal care of cancer patients.

The demands of sarcoma patients are no exception to the requirement of a multidisciplinary approach. When it comes specifically to patients experiencing an unplanned resection of sarcoma, these represent a nontrivial percentage of patients presenting to tertiary care institutions that provide musculoskeletal oncology care. The term "unplanned resection" was first conceived in 1985 by Giuliano and Eilber [3]. It was further defined by in 1996 by Noria et al. [4] to include patients whom have experienced attempted tumor resection without preoperative imaging or regard to the necessity for tumor resection with a margin of normal tissue. However, a more appropriate descriptor may be: "any procedural or surgical manipulation of a tumor without regard for the possibility that the tumor represents a sarcoma." This latter descriptor encompasses many aspects of unplanned resections not covered under the former definition. This proposed definition would include poorly placed or inappropriately performed biopsies (not just attempted resections), inappropriate procedures done with the presence of sarcoma missed at the time of index procedure (e.g., fixation of a missed pathologic fracture), patients not adequately locally imaged *or* systemically staged prior to treatment, patients treated without an appropriate tissue diagnosis, attempted incomplete or intralesional tumor resections, and failure of consultation with an orthopedic oncologist for expert advice in the unlikely event that the tumor does represent a sarcoma.

Unplanned resections have colloquially become known as "whoops" or "oops" surgeries among practicing community surgeons of all disciplines. These words are often the first things that come to mind when the pathology report of the manipulated, presumably benign, specimen is returned with the word "sarcoma" in the final diagnosis [5]. However, "oops" as a response far underestimates the gravity of such situations. This chapter will cover the issues associated with unplanned resection of sarcoma and the multidisciplinary considerations required for adequate care and salvage of this unique circumstance.

9.2   Epidemiology

All 69 histologic subtypes of sarcoma recognized by the WHO as of 2013 [6] collectively represent <1% of all cancers diagnosed in the United States [7]. The rarity of these cancers demand a team approach at a greater rate than their more frequently encountered carcinoma counterparts simply because of the comparative lack of general experience with these tumors. The relative paucity of knowledge, research, and experience in treating sarcoma can't be ignored when compared to carcinoma. Compare that in 2013, less than 15,000 total sarcomas were diagnosed and treated in the United States versus greater than 800,000 cases of lung, breast, prostate, and colon cancer, irrespective of the remaining numerous subtypes of carcinoma [7]. The numbers simply aren't there for appropriate study and treatment of sarcoma *without* a multidisciplinary and, possibly, multi-institutional approach.

The rarity of sarcoma almost necessitates that it take a back seat to carcinoma in an ongoing effort to cure these diseases simply based on a supply and demand model. This is no more evidenced than in federal money allotted to cancer research in the United States. In 2012, the National Cancer Institute operated on a research budget of $4.9 billion; $4.84 billion was spent on carcinoma research compared to just over $61 million on sarcoma, roughly 1.3% of the annual budget [8].

Because of the rarity of these cancers, care of a patient afflicted with sarcoma requires a multidisciplinary effort that pools together the collective knowledge and experience of many physicians and ancillary staff familiar with sarcoma care. As such, every patient is treated on an individualized, case-by-case basis; rather, there is no cookie cutter, reproducible algorithm into which sarcoma patients nicely fit. In fact, outcomes have steadily improved in the United Kingdom since government mandate of the centralization of sarcoma care and formation of a constant multidisciplinary team for care of these patients [9].

Unplanned resection of osseous and soft tissue malignancies is far more common than is typically thought among community surgeons. Several reports suggest that between 5 and 31% of osseous sarcoma referrals at major musculoskeletal oncology tertiary care centers involve patients whom have received a prior unplanned procedure [10–14]. Similarly, multiple studies have reported that anywhere from 16 to 64% of new patient referrals for soft tissue sarcoma are patients whom have received a prior unplanned resection [4, 15–33]. In pediatric patients, specifically, reports are as high as 50–81% of new patient referrals that involve unplanned resections [34, 35]. In subcutaneous sarcomas, which represent greater than 1/3 of all sarcomas, up to 91% have experienced an unplanned procedure [36].

If we look at the epidemiologic numbers of sarcomas in each studied category (osseous, soft tissue, pediatric, subcutaneous), this suggests that up to 7500 (52%) sarcomas in the United States experience inappropriate manipulation in the community before reaching an expert musculoskeletal oncology team [37]. Further, when reviewing these series over time, these numbers have not diminished [38] despite improved diagnostic techniques and intense efforts to educate the medical community at large about sarcoma (Table 9.1). In fact, the numbers are virtually identical for all types of sarcoma and anatomic regions involved, with the notable exception that osseous sarcoma seems to undergo unplanned resections at a lower rate than its soft tissue counterpart.

Table 9.1 Percentage of referred sarcoma cases that have experienced an unplanned resection in reported series over time

Year	Primary author	Sarcoma type	% of cases referred
1996	Noria [4]	Soft tissue	25
1996	Goodlad [29]	Soft tissue	40
1997	Davis [25]	Soft tissue	44
1999	Karakousis [39]	Soft tissue	85
2000	Lewis [27]	Soft tissue	37
2001	Temple [32]	Foot soft tissue	51
2002	Chui [35]	Pediatric soft tissue	81
2003	Zagars [31]	Soft tissue	54
2004	Wong [15]	Soft tissue	24
2004	Davies [28]	Soft tissue	16
2005	Manoso [24]	Soft tissue	52
2005	Rougraff [36]	Subcutaneous soft tissue	91
2006	Fiore [40]	Soft tissue	53
2006	Ayerza [13]	Osseous	7.7
2008	Chandrasekar [30]	Soft tissue	18
2008	Potter [17]	High-grade soft tissue	32
2009	Kim [10]	Osseous	5.5
2009	Rehders [18]	Soft tissue	35
2009	Puri [14]	Osseous	31
2010	Sawamura [34]	Pediatric soft tissue	50
2011	Wang [11]	Osseous	12
2011	Nishimura [33]	Foot soft tissue	36
2012	Sawamura [23]	Deep high-grade soft tissue	18
2012	Venkatesan [16]	Soft tissue	19
2012	Qureshi [22]	Soft tissue	64
2012	Alamanda [41]	Soft tissue	38
2013	Alamanda [20]	Soft tissue	34
2013	Alamanda [21]	Soft tissue	37
2013	Umer [42]	Soft tissue	38
2015	Morii [26]	Soft tissue	26

9.3   Presentation

The first issue to consider is why unplanned resection is such a frequent occurrence in sarcoma care. As discussed above, unplanned resection would appear to be more common than planned resection, likely due to the large number of subcutaneous lesions inappropriately dealt with. To determine why unplanned resections are so common, the disconnect must be explored between the presentation of a tumor and the failure to have sarcoma in the differential diagnosis by the treating physician.

One major problem is likely the educational focus on "classic" presentation of osseous and soft tissue sarcoma. However, it is the non-classic presentations of sarcoma that are more commonly unrecognized due to insufficient imaging or inaccurate interpretation [37] and receive inappropriate surgical management [3, 4, 10, 11, 13, 15–22, 24–27, 35–39, 41, 43–50]. Instead, these tumors are presumed benign and undergo attempted resection without preoperative imaging, biopsy, or proper adherence to oncological surgical principles. Up to 88% of all referred unplanned resections do not have a pretreatment MRI [51, 52] including 75% of deep tumors [51]. This latter finding begs the question that even if the lesion were indeed benign, how could the treating surgeon have any idea of the anatomic derivation, boundaries, and involvement of the tumor to have an appropriate surgical plan ready? Physical exam alone is not reliable in accurately differentiating whether or not a mass is superficial or deep to the investing muscular fascia [4, 36].

Osseous sarcomas exhibit a wide array of presentations, ranging from being virtually undetectable on plain radiographs to being very large, destructive tumors with extensive matrix formation and periosteal reaction [53]. The latter is referred to as the "classic" presentation of osseous sarcoma. However, many histologic subtypes of osseous sarcoma, particularly in older patients, may be purely lytic. This may account for the diagnostic confusion among community surgeons with other more common lytic lesions, including simple or degenerative cysts, giant cell tumor of bone, or metastatic carcinoma [46]. Many osseous sarcomas also exhibit "classic" age predilections of childhood and adolescence for both primary osteosarcoma and Ewing sarcoma [54] and middle- to older-aged adults for chondrosarcoma and secondary osteosarcoma [55].

As expected, the majority of referrals for osseous sarcoma after unplanned resection lack the classic osseous sarcoma presentation or occur in patients outside the classic age ranges for the various osseous sarcomas [10, 11]. The most common reason for referral of an inappropriately treated osseous sarcoma is failure to preoperatively consider a lesion seen as sarcoma. Frequently cited presumed diagnoses preoperatively in unplanned osseous sarcoma resections are giant cell tumor of bone, bone cyst, osteomyelitis, osteonecrosis, and metastatic carcinoma [11, 46]. Because failure to recognize a pathologic fracture is the second most common reason cited for unplanned procedures in osseous sarcoma, index of suspicion should be high for an underlying malignancy in the bone whenever there is an abnormal fracture pattern for the mechanism of injury, any osseous abnormality is seen on plain radiographs, or there is a low-energy mechanism of injury in the absence of severe osteopenia [11, 46].

The "classic" presentation of a soft tissue sarcoma (STS) is a large (>5 cm) firm, fixed, deep-seated, enlarging, painless mass or new pain in an existing painless mass [15, 16, 49]. However, STS can be any size at presentation, and more than 1/3 arise superficial to the investing muscular fascia [36]. Therefore, the vast majority of soft tissue masses lack the "classic" presentation associated with soft tissue sarcoma, contributing to the diagnostic confusion. Another large reason why sarcoma is often not considered in the differential diagnosis is that benign soft tissue tumors have been estimated to occur 300 times more often than malignant soft tissue tumors [19, 49].

Similar to osseous sarcoma, several series have reported that the majority of soft tissue sarcoma referred after an unplanned resection are more likely to have non-classic presentations, i.e., less than 5 cm, superficially located, and painless [17, 19–22, 26, 27, 35, 36, 44, 45, 56]. Likewise, rapidly growing lesions are more likely to be referred primarily, and slow-growing tumors or those found after mild trauma are more likely to be dealt with inappropriately due to their more indolent presentation [19–22, 35, 43]. The most common preoperatively presumed diagnoses in unplanned soft tissue sarcoma resections have been reported to be lipoma, cyst, hematoma, fibroma, abscess, enlarged lymph node, or other benign neoplasm [28, 43, 44, 51].

General surgeons account for 42–70% of unplanned resection referrals overall, followed by orthopedic surgeons, plastic surgeons, urologists, podiatrists, vascular surgeons, primary care providers, and dermatologists [16, 43–45]. This highlights the importance of a multidisciplinary approach not just for treatment of these patients but for education of the medical community at large with regard to appropriate extremity tumor workup and management.

9.4   Diagnosis

Accurate diagnosis and staging of the patient is crucial to determining both prognosis and treatment options [52]. There is marked heterogeneity of treatment plans offered to patients whom have experienced an unplanned resection. Each patient's treatment plan is largely dependent on histologic subtype, histologic grade, extent of previous surgical manipulation, presence of residual disease, and extent of locoregional and distant spread of the tumor.

One of the biggest challenges in the treatment of a patient with an unplanned resection is determining the presence of residual disease within the manipulated field. This knowledge is paramount to determining the necessity of additional surgery. If all a patient experienced was a percutaneous needle biopsy and they present with a continued palpable mass, the answer is obvious. However, if a patient experienced an open, marginal or intralesional resection, the clinical picture becomes less obvious.

Although management will be discussed in detail later in this chapter, most patients referred after an unplanned resection undergo re-resection of their tumor bed in an attempt to gain wide margins around the tumor [28]. Failure to attain wide margins increases local recurrence rates from 10–20% to 80–90% [33, 45]. Rates of histologically proven residual sarcoma reported in the re-resected surgical specimens are uniformly high (Table 9.2). Similar to previously discussed referral percentages for unplanned resections (Table 9.1), these numbers have not changed appreciably over time (Table 9.2). Once again, this indicates that despite educational efforts to promote recognition of soft tissue sarcoma and performance of oncologically sound procedures during any tumor resection, the medical community at large has not incorporated appropriate oncologic surgical principles into their practices. Ostensibly, it would appear that international educational efforts by the various professional organizations involved in sarcoma care have fallen well short of their goals and have not changed practice patterns over time.

In series where all patients with unplanned resections received re-excision regardless of clinical scenario, residual tumor rates in the re-resected specimen range from 24 to 72% [3, 4, 17, 19, 25–29, 36, 45, 49, 50, 57–59]. In series where

Table 9.2 Residual sarcoma found histologically in re-resected surgical beds following unplanned resection of soft tissue sarcoma as reported over time

Year	Primary author	Cases of unplanned resections reported	Cases re-resected (%)	Histologically tumor-positive re-resected specimens (%)
1985	Giuliano [3]	90	100	51
1995	Zornig [57]	67	100	45
1996	Noria [4]	65	100	35
1996	Goodlad [29]	95	100	59
1997	Davis [25]	104	100	40
1999	Karakousis [39]	63	95	63
2000	Lewis [27]	407	100	39
2000	Siebenrock [51]	16	100	63
2002	Chui [35]	94	73	48
2002	Sugiura [45]	45	100	47
2002	Kaste [52]	24	100	58
2003	Zagars [31]	666	44	46
2004	Wong [15]	18	89	56
2004	Davies [28]	111	100	57
2004	Peiper [58]	110	100	39
2005	Manoso [24]	42	91	42
2005	Rougraff [36]	75	100	65
2006	Fiore [40]	318	100	24
2008	Chandrasekar [30]	363	87	60
2008	Potter [17]	64	100	72
2008	Hoshi [44]	38	58	70
2008	Morii [59]	77	100	45
2009	Rehders [18]	143	97	31
2011	Han [50]	104	100	51
2012	Venkatesan [16]	42	95	74
2012	Qureshi [22]	134	90	48
2012	Alamanda [41]	106	100	73
2013	Kang [49]	121	100	51
2013	Morii [26]	24	100	71

strict criteria were applied (e.g., gross residual disease, positive margins, and ability to preserve functional limb) to select re-excision candidates, the rates of tumor-positive specimens are virtually identical [30, 31, 44].

Unfortunately, there appears to be no way to clinically predict residual disease in the tumor/surgical bed. Physical exam of the surgical bed is unable to detect residual gross disease when it exists in 33% of resected surgical beds with histologically proven residual disease [4]. Pathology reports from the index procedure have been shown to be incorrect after expert review regarding both diagnosis and margin status at rates of 37% [43] and 50–82% [3, 36, 43], respectively. MRI to attempt to visualize residual disease after unplanned resection has been shown to have a negative predictive value of 66–86%, a sensitivity of only 56–78%, and false-negative rates as high as 19–33% [4, 24, 28, 52]. With no accurate way to identify patients at risk, it must be presumed that all unplanned resection patients continue to have sarcoma in their surgical bed in order to avoid the pitfalls of missing the patient with active disease. Due to the poor prognosis of improperly treated sarcoma, the trend throughout the field has been to overtreat the few to avoid undertreating any.

Involving a multidisciplinary team early on is paramount to accurate diagnosis, the first step toward determining the treatment plan. Independent review of the pathologic specimen and slides from the unplanned procedure by a musculoskeletally trained pathologist is key. With greater than 1/3 of the histologic diagnoses expected to change [43] and up to 82% of the margin statuses to be reclassified [3, 36, 43], this can greatly affect the treatment options suitable to the patient.

Additionally, local MRI remains a critical portion of the workup of a patient after an unplanned resection [28, 52]. Despite the poor reliability of MRI to detect residual disease, in select patients with at least 10 mm diameter or 65 cm^3 of tumor left behind, it is sensitive enough to reveal its extent [28, 52]. Further, MRI can determine the extent of hematoma, edema, reactive inflammation, and scar tissue created by the previous procedural manipulation that is potentially contaminated with tumor spillage [28]. These latter findings greatly assist in preoperative planning for determining the anatomic boundaries required for a wide re-resection. MRI can also help denote the extent of neurovascular and cutaneous involvement [28, 52] allowing for preoperative subspecialty consultation (vascular, spinal, microsurgical, general, and/or plastic surgery), avoiding urgent intraoperative consultations.

MRI spin-echo (i.e., T1, T2, STIR) sequence with and without gadolinium of the entire involved bone or limb segment is the test of choice to evaluate the tumor and surgical bed. Tumor protocol MRI should be specified in order to avoid nondiagnostic gradient-echo (i.e., proton density, balanced weight, BLADE, FLASH) sequences often used in conventional extremity or joint MRI [5]. Involving a musculoskeletal radiologist as part of the multidisciplinary team to review both the pre- and post-unplanned resection images can greatly improve diagnostic accuracy and determine extent of anatomic involvement much more precisely. Up to 76% of unplanned resections referred with a prior MRI read by a general community radiologist do not even mention sarcoma in the differential diagnosis [43].

In only 4.3% of unplanned resections was the possibility of a malignancy considered by the primary surgeon [28]. Therefore, very few patients are adequately staged before reaching a definitively treating musculoskeletal oncology team. Staging of the tumor remains an essential part of determining a treatment plan, as the timing and types of treatments offered to each patient will vary greatly depending on stage [60]. One benefit of having an unplanned procedure is that the tissue diagnosis is often already made by the time the patient in question reaches an orthopedic oncology team for evaluation. Staging starts with local imaging of the anatomic site of tumor with MRI as outlined above and possibly a plain radiograph or CT scan if bony involvement is suspected/confirmed. Sarcomas preferentially metastasize to the lung most commonly, followed by bone, and rarely to lymphatics and other soft tissue sites [60]. Therefore, CT scan of the chest without contrast and whole-body technetium or sodium fluoride bone scan are the tests of choice to evaluate these most common metastatic sites.

Additional staging studies can be valuable depending on specific histologic subtypes of sarcoma. Myxoid liposarcoma may exhibit unusual patterns of metastasis to retroperitoneal and intrabdominal, extrahepatic sites [61], so a CT scan of the abdomen and pelvis with oral contrast is required during staging of this particular tumor. While PET imaging is still somewhat controversial, there are some histologic subtypes that can benefit from staging with a PET, including Ewing sarcoma [62], sarcomas with a predilection for lymph node metastases [63] (e.g., rhabdomyosarcoma, alveolar soft part sarcoma, clear cell sarcoma, epithelioid sarcoma, angiosarcoma, and synovial cell sarcoma [60]), and malignant peripheral nerve sheath tumors in the setting of neurofibromatosis [64]. Further, bone marrow biopsy is often required in the staging of Ewing sarcoma [62] and alveolar rhabdomyosarcoma [65] particularly in the absence of PET imaging.

9.5   Outcomes

The types of patients receiving unplanned resections have been explored to determine risk factors for referral or outcome following such instances. Insurance coverage or distance from a tertiary center with an orthopedic oncologist has not been shown to affect the types or amounts of patients being referred after an unplanned sarcoma resection [21]. Referrals based on hospital type, however, have been shown to affect outcomes. Patients referred from tertiary referral centers to a musculoskeletal oncologist have been compared to patients referred from non-tertiary centers. The tertiary center referrals have lower rates of local and distant tumor recurrence despite the patients having larger and higher-grade tumors [49]. This may be the result of more oncologically appropriate procedures being performed by surgeons with increased experience with tumor resections seen at larger centers.

When looking directly at patient outcomes following an unplanned resection, there are two broad categories that need to be addressed: oncologic and treatment-based outcomes. Oncologic outcomes are those that deal specifically with the tumor and the diseased state caused by the tumor (e.g., local recurrence, metastases, survival). Treatment-based outcomes include those directly related to the surgery, chemotherapy, and/or radiotherapy administered to the patient. This includes functional outcomes, treatment-induced morbidity and side effects, psychological outcomes, and need for further treatment.

9.5.1   Oncologic Outcomes

Oncologic outcomes have been very inconsistent among reported series on unplanned sarcoma resection. Several studies favor worse oncologic prognoses [4, 11, 13, 17, 18, 22, 25, 42, 45–47, 51] for unplanned resection patients compared to planned, while others report no difference [10, 14, 18, 19, 23, 26, 32, 33, 39, 41, 59] among the cohorts. Only one study to date reported paradoxically improved onco-logic prognosis in unplanned resections compared to planned [27].

One inherent issue as discussed previously with regard to studying sarcoma and its unplanned resection is the very low numbers available for critical review. The average number of cases reported in Table 9.2 is only 125 per study. Small study size is a frequent problem when attempting to analyze rare tumors and likely underpow-ers many of these studies [33] to detect differences in outcome. Further, with few exceptions, almost all the reported series represent a widely heterogeneous group of tumors. The prognostic implications of reaming a conventional osteosarcoma is far different than a marginal excision of a 1 cm subcutaneous, low-grade soft tissue sar-coma. However, in many series, these entities are lumped together and treated as the same circumstance of "unplanned resection" for statistical purposes. Again, the large number of small, subcutaneous sarcomas experiencing unplanned resection likely skews oncologic outcomes toward no difference from planned resections because of the better prognosis of these tumors in general [39]. Therefore, the numerous cases obviously worsened by an unplanned resection may not hold statistical weight in large series. This renders sweeping statements about the difference, or lack thereof, in outcomes in all unplanned resections very dangerous and erroneous.

A few studies have attempted to stratify the different sarcomas when determining oncologic outcomes to help elucidate the true effects of unplanned resection per prog-nostic sarcoma presentation. Most notably, worse prognosis after unplanned excision has been shown for high-grade tumors and for more advanced stage of disease when compared to similar patients with low-grade or early stage disease experiencing a planned resection [17, 22]. As predicted, one series showed no difference in metas-tases or change in disease-specific survival when the cohort of unplanned resections were compared en masse to planned resections. However, when the tumors were stratified by grade, it was found that high-grade tumors were associated with higher rates of metastases and worse disease-specific survival after an unplanned resection compared to planned [22].

Multiple studies have found increased metastatic rates and worse local recur-rence, relapse-free survival, or overall survival rates only in patients with residual disease in their re-resected specimens [17–19, 25, 26, 45]. By only reviewing sub-cutaneous sarcomas, another series demonstrated that local control cannot be as reliably obtained in this subset of patients compared to planned resections and that in tumors with their largest dimension ≥ 4 cm, disease-free survival was signifi-cantly worse than matched patients that underwent planned excision [36].

A specific outcome consideration for treatment following unplanned osseous sarcoma resection is that too little tumor is often left in the re-resected specimen to properly evaluate chemotherapy-induced tumor necrosis. This causes significant treatment dilemmas, as assessing tumor necrosis may help determine adjuvant sys-temic chemotherapy options and prognosticating outcomes [10]. Further, by com-parision, oncologic and surgical outcome alterations following an unplanned resection mimic those of a pathologic fracture through an osseous sarcoma, a poten-tial indicator of poorer prognosis [46].

One important consideration for oncologic outcomes after treatment of an unplanned resection is the manner in which re-resection is conducted. A major issue with unplanned procedures includes anatomically inappropriate positioning of a biopsy or an attempted resection surgical tract. Safe limb salvage would be precluded by use of these planes, and the decision may then be made to proceed with a standard resection approach away from the previous unplanned procedure. This can greatly increase the risk of local recurrence and secondarily worsen survival parameters if the previous tract seeded by tumor violation is not also removed in its entirety with the tumor [47, 66–68].

Only one study to date directly compared re-resected sarcoma in those whom previously experienced planned and unplanned resections. They found that overall, metastasis-free and local recurrence-free survival was no different between the two cohorts [56]. Although not specifically discussed, the re-resections in prior planned surgeries were presumably due to local recurrence, while re-resections in prior unplanned surgeries were part of the treatment standard of re-resection of any potentially contaminated tumor bed [5]. Thus, it may be inferred that overall, metastasis-free and local recurrence-free survival of unplanned resections mimic those of recurrence in planned resections, a known poor prognostic indicator [40, 47]. Interestingly, delays in definitive treatment after an unplanned resection as long as 92 days after the initial procedure have not been associated with any significant oncologic outcome alterations [19, 41, 50].

9.5.2 Treatment-Based Outcomes

Contrary to the inconsistencies seen with regard to oncologic outcomes, the literature is quite clear with regard to treatment-based outcomes: they are ubiquitously worse following an unplanned resection. Unplanned manipulation of osseous sarcoma invariably increases the risk of subsequent amputation during re-resection [10, 11, 13, 46, 47]. Due to the large amounts of anatomy now exposed to (and therefore assumed to be contaminated with) tumor, a wide (at least 2 cm cuff of normal tissue [38, 39]) margin resection for adequate oncologic treatment often obviates a postoperative functional limb. If limb salvage is still attempted at re-resection, local recurrence rates are higher [13, 46] despite tumors referred after unplanned resection being smaller than those typically referred for planned primary resection [11]. When there is a local recurrence of sarcoma, this further increases the risk of secondary amputation [12, 47].

Soft tissue sarcoma re-resections also exhibit higher amputation rates compared to planned primary resections [15–18, 22, 24, 41–45, 51, 56] for the exact same reason as osseous tumors. If major neurovascular bundles, joints, or multiple compartments have been contaminated by any previous unplanned manipulation, an oncologically sound resection often requires that the entire limb be sacrificed to obtain a tumor-free margin. Likewise, re-resection when limb salvage is possible often involves greater need for flap coverage, soft tissue reconstruction, bone grafting, nerve resection, multiple surgeries to obtain wide margins, or increased wound complications [15–18, 22, 24, 26, 41, 43–45, 51, 56, 59]. Despite these findings, functional scores and emotional acceptance appear to be equivocal between patients whom have received planned versus unplanned resections [24, 26, 45, 59]. This may be explained by many patients' willingness to accept any functional or cosmetic outcome in exchange for eradication of their cancer.

The more morbid surgery required as a result of wound contamination with tumor is nearly uniformly a result of the poor unplanned resection technique (e.g., transverse extremity incisions, wide suture closure, hematoma formation, drains placed not in-line with incision, failure to plug any bony windows, adjacent compartment violation, joint or neurovascular contamination [5, 44, 51]) and rarely due to the extent of the presenting tumor [5, 69]. It can be inferred that the vast majority of the worse surgical outcomes seen may have been avoided with an appropriately planned initial resection. Even in oncologically sound resections, inadvertent tumor spillage into the wound can worsen local control rates, which secondarily can affect distal relapse rates [68].

It has been shown that even after an unplanned resection has been performed, the treating physician often fails to realize the gravity of the situation. The recommendations and expectations conveyed to the patient after the unplanned resection have only been in concert with the final orthopedic oncologist's recommendations 45% of the time, significantly increasing patient anxiety and confusion [43]. Thus, once an unplanned resection has been identified, referral delays should be minimized and treatment recommendations should be deferred to the definitively treating musculoskeletal oncologist.

It goes without saying that adding a re-resection as a second procedure greatly increases direct medical costs for these patients. Because the re-resection is technically more demanding than a primary planned resection would be, the re-resection is often billed at a higher rate due to the increased time based upon CPT modifiers and increased procedure codes used [20]. Additionally, management of these patients often require more frequent multidisciplinary consultations due to the increased need for vascular procedures, soft tissue reconstruction, and wound complications [15–18, 22, 24, 26, 43, 44, 56]. It has been shown that professional charges increase by 33% and overall cost increases by 11% for the re-resection compared to the cost of a primary planned sarcoma resection [20]. When this cost is added to the costs already billed in the primary unplanned resection, the overall cost of treatment is more than double for these patients compared to those treated definitively with a planned resection.

Because of the worse oncologic and treatment-based outcomes, the initial physician involved in the unplanned resection often experiences medicolegal consequences. Average indemnity payments for sarcoma-related medical malpractice are several-fold higher compared to general claims within all specialties (Fig. 9.1). According to the work of Mesko et al., delay in diagnosis (81%) and unnecessary amputation (11%) account for the majority of complaints with wrongful death cited in 39% of cases. In cases decided in favor of the plaintiff, mean indemnity payments of $2.3 million (adjusted to 2012 US dollar amounts) have been awarded. The average jury verdict award amount of $3.9 million is almost triple that of the average settlement amount of $1.4 million. The greatest numbers of claims are filed against primary care specialties (34%), orthopedic surgeons (23%), and radiologists (12%) [70].

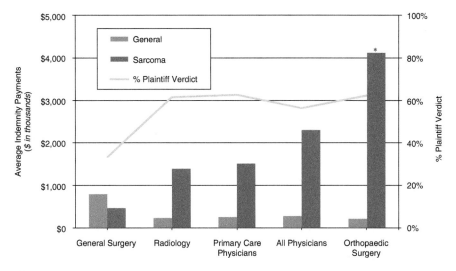

Fig. 9.1 Average indemnity payments for reported general specialty practice awards versus those specified toward sarcoma care. The blue bars represent the 2012 mean general indemnity payment within a delineated specialty. The red bars represent the mean sarcoma indemnity payment within that same specialty. The numeric values over each bar pairing represent a specialty-specific ratio of sarcoma indemnity payment to reported same-specialty general indemnity payment. (Reprinted with permission from Mesko NW, et al. J Surg Oncol 2014;110:919-929.)

9.6   Management

There have been pleas for prevention as the best treatment [5, 17, 69] to avoid unplanned resection of sarcoma ever since the problems with it were first recognized in 1985 [3]. However, these unfortunate events continue to occur at an alarmingly unchanged rate over 30 years later. The optimal management of these patients requires multidisciplinary "damage control" as a means of salvaging these difficult cases. The goal of treatment in these patients is to improve oncological prognosis while optimizing functional, cosmetic, and psychiatric outcomes.

As mentioned previously, the involvement of a multidisciplinary team should begin at initial presentation during diagnosis, workup, and staging of the patient in order to determine and administer a treatment plan in as timely a fashion as possible. Having a sarcoma tumor board or designated multidisciplinary sarcoma treatment team is the essential beginning to optimizing management and outcomes of these patients.

The core sarcoma treatment group should be composed at minimum of orthopedic (musculoskeletal) oncology, radiation oncology, medical oncology, musculoskeletal pathology, and musculoskeletal radiology [52]. Other disciplines that should serve as an ancillary team include pediatric oncology, pediatric surgery, pediatric orthopedic surgery [52], surgical oncology, vascular surgery, microsurgery, gynecologic surgical oncology, neurosurgery, urology, cardiothoracic surgery, plastic and reconstructive surgery, cosmetic surgery, otolaryngology, general practitioners, psychiatry, palliative care, and end-of-life care (e.g., Hospice), among other disciplines.

Another adjunctive team that should be involved with both the core and ancillary teams is physical medicine and rehabilitation (PM&R). This team includes a physician PM&R specialist, physiotherapists, occupational therapists, speech therapists, and vocational counselors and can include pain management specialists, prosthetists, dieticians, social workers, and case managers as well. This is the team that will be part of the care of the patient from diagnosis through treatment and follow-up that will deal with the patient's function, general well-being, and integration into the workplace with their new physical limits. These limits depend greatly on the type, anatomic area, and morbidity of the surgery received (e.g., amputation, nerve resections, muscle resections). The rehab team is optimized to obtain the greatest function possible with what the patient has left after treatment and can provide assistive devices, edema control, custom bracing, durable medical equipment, and external prosthetics when needed to improve function and provide pain relief.

9.6.1   Core Team

The core team mentioned above are the disciplines whose input should be involved in the care of all presenting sarcomas. Ideally, this team should have an established frequent "sarcoma conference" where these difficult cases can be discussed as soon as the unplanned resection patient presents to any member of the team. This disease-specific tumor board should also function to provide an environment for any other physician/discipline to present cases they believe to be unplanned resections. This can help facilitate an appropriately sequenced treatment plan, familiarize each physician to be involved in the care of the patient with the unique presentation to prevent communication errors, and eliminate treatment delays or redundancy by establishing follow-up visits and diagnostic testing plans as a group.

Optimal management for local treatment of unplanned resections includes wide re-resection of the surgical bed [28]. Orthopedic oncology is necessary for the surgical considerations of re-resection of all trunk, retroperitoneal, and extremity sarcomas. An orthopedic oncologist's experience with the behavior and natural history of the different histologic subtypes of sarcoma makes their input invaluable even if they will not be directly involved with any planned re-resection procedure (e.g., solid organ or central nervous system sarcomas, dural hemangiopericytomas, head and neck sarcomas, and gastrointestinal stromal tumors).

It has been suggested that radiotherapy as monotherapy for treatment of unplanned resections can result in high morbidity due to the field size and dosage required for adequate local control and is less effective than surgery alone or combined surgery with radiotherapy for local control [31, 48]. However, radiation oncology should still be available to offer their opinion regularly in the care of these patients precisely because of their combined role with surgery in the local control of the sarcoma [24, 68, 71]. The frequency of positive margins seen with unplanned resection [15–18, 22, 24, 26, 43, 44, 56], the number of high-grade tumors referred [23] that benefit from radiotherapy, and the fact that even some low-grade sarcomas can benefit from radiotherapy [72] are considerations that radiation oncology can add to the conversation. Further, a radiation oncologist familiar with sarcoma can help determine whether any treatment would have a greater benefit in the neoadjuvant versus the adjuvant setting with respect to the planned re-resection [37, 73].

With regard to medical oncology, ideally a sarcoma specialist or someone with a special interest in sarcoma should be included in the primary team, as there are unique dosing and chemotherapy considerations specific to sarcoma. Opinion can be obtained if there is any roll for chemotherapy in the adjuvant or neoadjuvant setting for the primary tumor. Chemotherapy is a requirement for the treatment of certain sarcomas [54, 74–77]. There is some limited data for soft tissue sarcomas to suggest outcomes are improved, the tumor can be downstaged, or resectability of a presenting tumor can be improved with neoadjuvant chemotherapy in certain circumstances [78]. The medical oncologist should be readily available to help make these determinations on a case-by-case basis. Because of the potential for increased distant relapse in unplanned resection patients [4, 11, 13, 17, 22, 25, 46, 47], the medical oncologist can be involved with long-term follow-up such that treatment can begin without delay in the event of this unfortunate circumstance.

As mentioned previously, the musculoskeletal pathologist should be involved early on to independently review the outside specimen. They should confirm the diagnosis and margin status before any treatment proceeds. Although this may require significant effort, routine review is critical given the high percentage of errors found in community pathology reports [3, 36, 43]. Further, they are paramount to care post-re-resection by determining margin status, confirming the diagnosis, determining presence of residual tumor, and denoting any areas of dedifferentiation, as all of these variables can greatly affect adjuvant treatment options and surveillance schedule [52]. The availability of prior pathology is critical to help the musculoskeletal pathologist detect and distinguish microscopic residual tumor in the re-resection specimen from the significant reactive changes that are frequently present from the prior procedure.

Likewise, the musculoskeletal radiologist should be primarily involved to review any imaging to confirm that the clinical picture matches the diagnosis and to aid in determining residual tumor and re-resection anatomic boundaries. Ideally, they should be skilled in interventional radiology for the purpose of image-guided biopsies or ablations when indicated. If not, a specific interventional radiologist should be included in the primary sarcoma team.

9.6.2 Ancillary Team

The ancillary team should be available for the unique, case-by-case needs of the unplanned resection patients due to the heterogeneity of their presentation. Any member of this team can and should be part of the core team if they have a special interest or are routinely involved in the care of sarcoma patients, which varies from institution to institution. Physicians often involved in the care of these patients that should be included in the ancillary team when needed include primary care specialties and any additional surgical or medical subspecialty that may be indicated depending on patient comorbidities or specific anatomic considerations of the tumor and its spread.

The members of this team are those involved when special circumstances dictate. If complex reconstruction following resection is being considered (e.g., soft tissue flaps, vascular-pedicled bone autografts), plastic surgery, vascular surgery, or microsurgery should be considered. If specific anatomic involvement is present (e.g., spinal canal, head/neck, thorax, abdominopelvic organs), then the surgical subspecialty specific to that area should be involved with the definitive resection. Further, because there can be benefit from oligometastatic disease resection or ablation [79, 80], the specific subspecialist or interventionalist should be consulted depending on the location of metastatic involvement when the clinical situation dictates.

Finally, the clinical management of the patient as a whole must be comprehensive for optimal management of sarcoma patients. Particularly, the complex situation of increased anxiety after a cancer diagnosis has been determined, and the poorer outcomes seen following unplanned resection often require the need for psychiatric, clerical, palliative, or end-of-life care. Dealing with cancer can be very difficult for the individual patient as well as friends and family, from the standpoint of grief, disbelief, monetary issues from medical costs, and often anger toward the initial physician involved in the unplanned resection [81]. Palliative care alone has been shown in several randomized trials to improve outcomes, decrease anxiety, and actually prolong life in the care of terminal cancer patients [82, 83]. The benefit and importance of these ancillary disciplines can't be overstated.

9.7   Case Examples

As shown above, there is a litany of outcomes that can come as a result of an unplanned resection. These can range from no change in surgical or oncological outcome as a result of the tumor manipulation, to rapidly fatal progression of disease in extreme cases. As alluded to earlier, statistical measures often fall short of truly describing the issues associated with unplanned resections. Because not all studied tumors exist in a homogeneous patient population, carry the same anatomic boundaries, or possess identical intrinsic biology and aggressiveness, it is difficult to truly study these small numbers without lumping them all together.

Below are case examples of the most common outcome categories seen in unplanned resections and the multidisciplinary considerations that were applied to each patient in an effort to minimize the morbidity and mortality that can follow from an unplanned resection. The heterogeneity of the cases highlights the way certain aspects can be easily overlooked if all of these cases were to be combined into one series of "unplanned resections." All cases discussed below presented and were treated in 2014 at the authors' institutions and serve to highlight ongoing contemporaneous issues associated with unplanned resection of sarcoma.

Fig. 9.2 Axial fat-satured T1-weighted MRI with gadolinium contrast enhancement of a massive thoracic superficial back sarcoma with large necrotic/hemorrhagic central contrast void

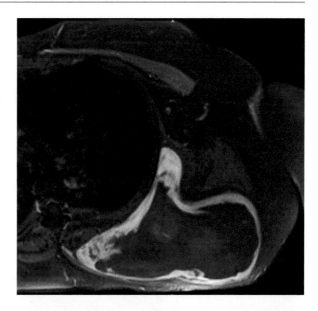

Fig. 9.3 Transverse incision with wide mattress closure following community-based open biopsy of a massive back sarcoma

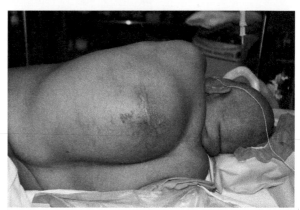

Case 1: *No alteration of outcome*

As discussed previously, small, subcutaneous lesions often undergo unplanned resection with very little consequence [36, 51]. However, even large, deep, high-grade tumors can experience an unplanned resection with little effect on outcome when treated appropriately. To reiterate, the major oncologic goal of treatment during salvage of an unplanned resection is to restore prognosis to identical that of a planned resection.

An example of such a case involves a 61-year-old female referred to a community general surgeon with a massive upper back tumor (Fig. 9.2). The surgeon performed an open intralesional biopsy via a large transverse incision with very wide suture closure (Fig. 9.3). The subsequent pathology report revealed a histologic diagnosis of high-grade undifferentiated pleomorphic sarcoma, and thus the patient

Fig. 9.4 (**a**) Axial CT denoting a plural-based pulmonary nodule (*arrow*) suspicious for metastatic disease at initial patient presentation. Of note, the left-sided massive soft tissue mass can be seen in the dorsal soft tissues. (**b**) Six-month postoperative axial CT demonstrating no interval growth of the pulmonary nodule (*arrow*). Of note, the left-sided massive soft tissue mass has been resected from the dorsal soft tissues

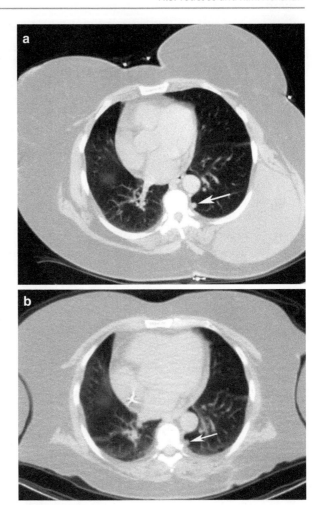

was then referred to orthopedic oncology. However, this referral came 3 months after her initial referral to the general surgeon.

She was immediately discussed in a multidisciplinary sarcoma conference with confirmation of the diagnosis by a musculoskeletal pathologist. Because of the massive size of the tumor, the lack of patient comorbidities, and a subcentimeter pulmonary nodule suspicious for metastatic disease (Fig. 9.4a), the general consensus reached at the conference was that she was an ideal candidate for induction adriamycin/ifosfamide chemotherapy. The patient tolerated the chemotherapy well and had an excellent clinical response to the chemotherapy with softening of the mass and stabilization of the pulmonary nodules.

She subsequently underwent wide re-resection taking the large surgical tract en bloc with the tumor (Fig. 9.5). Because of the unique location on the back, excision of the 10 cm wide tract of skin was able to be easily apposed with a tension-free closure (Fig. 9.6). The patient healed uneventfully and returned to daily swimming at 3 months postoperatively. The pulmonary nodule has remained stable at the latest

Fig. 9.5 (a) Intraoperative photograph during re-resection of a massive back soft tissue sarcoma following unplanned inappropriate biopsy procedure. (b) Wound closure with trapezius advancement to gain appropriate coverage, post-operative function, and tension-free closure

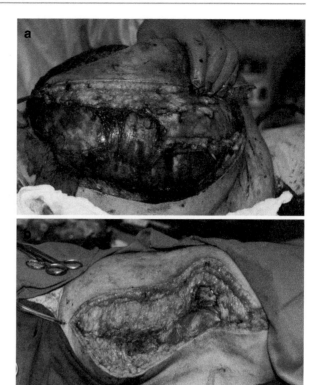

Fig. 9.6 Six-month follow-up evaluation showing a well-healed longitudinal incision and excellent functional outcome with symmetric overhead shoulder range of motion despite partial resection of periscapular musculature to obtain wide surgical margins at the time of tumor re-resection

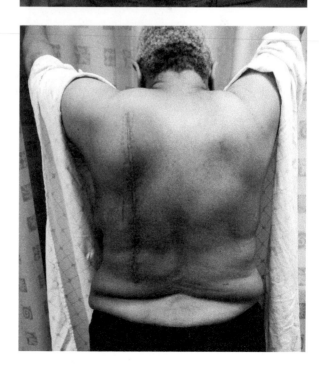

follow-up 6 months postoperatively (Fig. 9.4b) with no evidence of recurrent disease at the surgical site. It would appear her risk for local and distant relapse at this point is identical that of a planned primary resection in the same clinical setting. However, because of the time gap in referral, she may have been spared the chemotherapy had she been primarily referred to orthopedic oncology sooner.

Case 2: *Increased morbidity of surgery without additional reconstruction needed*
Often an unplanned resection can be salvaged with a more morbid re-resection that doesn't necessarily need to involve amputation or complex reconstruction. Such a case involves a 31-year-old male who had a "bump" on his back for several years before rapid growth of it commenced approximately 1 year prior to his presentation to a musculoskeletal oncology team.

Unfortunately, he presented to three outside surgeons first who all attempted an incision and drainage for presumed refractory abscess. The last two surgeons sent a portion of the evacuated tissue to a community pathologist that returned the diagnosis of a benign fibrous tumor. By the time he was referred to a musculoskeletal oncology team, he had experienced three separate unplanned procedures through three separate widely spaced incisions, had no local advanced imaging or systemic staging, and experienced continued rapid growth of his tumor throughout his pre-referral course (Fig. 9.7).

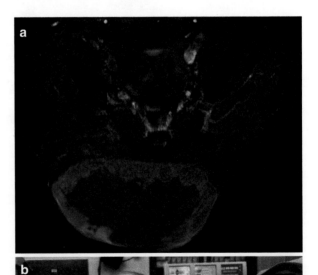

Fig. 9.7 (**a**) Axial fat-satured T1-weighted MRI with gadolinium contrast enhancement of a massive superficial lower back sarcoma with fungation and large necrotic/hemorrhagic central contrast void.
(**b**) Clinical photograph of the patient's tumor with central malignant ulceration noted by extensive eschar formation

Following consultation with a multidisciplinary sarcoma treatment group, the outside pathology slides were reviewed resulting in a diagnosis of dermatofibrosarcoma protuberans (DFSP). The patient underwent wide re-resection of the tumor and surrounding skin from the region of fungation and prior procedures. This left a massive defect over his lower back (Fig. 9.8), but because of the amount and mobility of truncal skin, he was able to be closed via multiple V-Y advancement flaps by the plastic and reconstructive surgery team (Fig. 9.9). He did not require free flaps, tissue transfers, or skin grafting, but a significant portion of the skin could have been saved obviating the morbid closure had he not had multiple scattered incisions into the tumor across the lower back or had he been referred sooner when his tumor was much smaller. He did go on to heal his wounds and secondarily granulate the open confluence by 2 months postoperatively.

His resected tumor (Fig. 9.10) was meticulously evaluated for signs of fibrosarcomatous degeneration, given its massive size [84], but no such histopathologic change was not found. Because DFSPs are characteristically indolent with a tendency to locally recur, but with a low propensity to metastasize [85], it is likely that his oncologic outcome is and will be similar to a planned DFSP resection. However, the massive scarring and months-long healing process may have been avoided with appropriate workup and primary planned resection at the time of his initial presentation to an outside facility 1 year prior, while the lesion was most certainly smaller and no additional incisions had been made in the skin. Correct initial pathologic analysis by a musculoskeletally trained pathologist may have facilitated earlier referral as well.

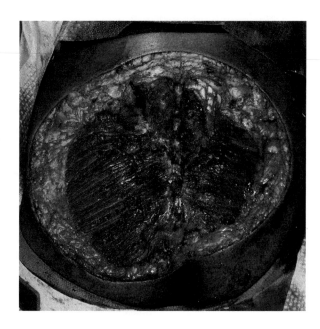

Fig. 9.8 Intraoperative photograph demonstrating massive skin loss with uncoverage of nearly the entire dorsal sacral and buttock region at the expense of an oncologically-sound re-resection of the sarcoma

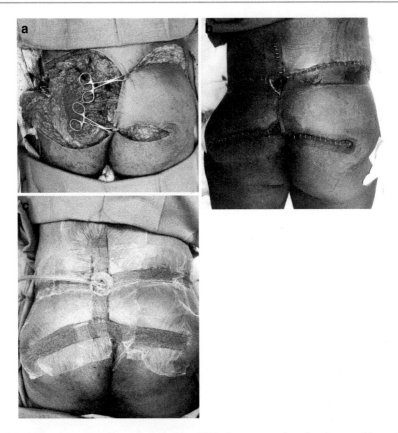

Fig. 9.9 (**a**) Intraoperative photograph showing V-Y advancement flaps for closure without tissue transfer. (**b**) Final wound closure with (**c**) open central confluences treated with vacuum-assisted closure for healing by secondary intention

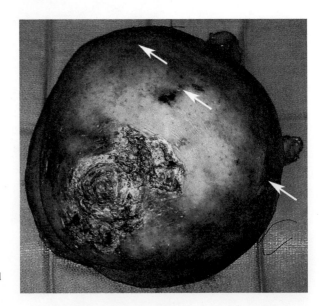

Fig. 9.10 Clinical photograph of the re-resected fungating sarcoma and adjacent skin with multiple, wide-spread unplanned procedure healed incisions (*arrows*)

Case 3: *Increased morbidity of surgery with additional reconstruction needed*
Many post-procedural contaminated tumor fields require very large segments of tissue removal in order to attain a wide, tumor-free margin at re-resection. As a result, adjacent bone, skin, muscle, and/or neurovascular bundles have to be sacrificed that otherwise were not involved with the primary tumor in situ. Quite often this additional resection in the setting of limb salvage requires some form of reconstruction to maintain a functional limb: bone grafting or endo-prosthetics for bony defects, neurovascular grafting or bipass for vital neuro-vascular bundle resections, and flaps, skin grafting, or free tissue transfers for soft tissue defects.

This predicament was seen in a 75-year-old male who required soft tissue recon-struction for limb salvage after unplanned resection without overt alteration of his oncologic outcome. He initially presented to a community institution with signs, symptoms, and plain radiographs consistent with end-stage degenerative gonarthro-sis. He was taken to the operating room for a total knee arthroplasty, but upon skin incision, a juxta-articular mass was encountered. This was presumed to be a menis-cal cyst and was removed piecemeal with a rongeur. However, the surgeon recog-nized upon the intralesional procedure that the mass was not cystic at all and astutely abandoned proceeding further until pathology was known on the resected specimen.

Unfortunately, the pathology report came back consistent with a pleomorphic rhabdomyosarcoma, a highly aggressive tumor that carries with it a very poor oncologic prognosis in older adults [74, 75]. The patient was promptly referred to orthopedic oncology and discussed at the biweekly sarcoma conference. Given the rarity of this pathology in adults, the first step was confirmation of the diagno-sis by a musculoskeletal pathologist and MRI review by a musculoskeletal radi-ologist (Fig. 9.11). Once the diagnosis and anatomic boundaries were confirmed, the patient was staged with PET-CT that was negative for metastatic disease (Fig. 9.12a). Because of the anticipation of a large soft tissue defect upon review of MRI, plastic surgery was consulted, and a combined surgical resection and staged reconstruction plan was developed between them and orthopedic oncology. Because of the well-coordinated multidisciplinary effort, the patient was able to undergo re-resection within 2 weeks of presentation to the orthopedic oncologist.

The re-resection required burring of the adjacent tibia and removal of a very large region of skin overlying the knee joint (Fig. 9.13a). Once final margins were determined to be negative, plastic surgery performed a local gastrocnemius flap reconstruction with split thickness skin graft several days later (Fig. 9.13b). The wound did heal by 6 weeks postoperatively (Fig. 9.13c), but the patient's function was limited secondary to pain, leg weakness, and edema. However, con-sistent with the aggressivity of the patient's disease [74, 75], he subsequently developed locoregional lymph node metastases 3 months postoperatively. He was immediately evaluated by the medical oncologist in the core sarcoma treatment team who already had familiarity with the patient from the sarcoma conference

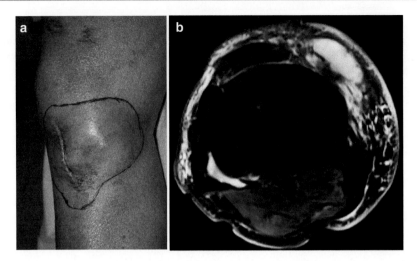

Fig. 9.11 A 75-year-old male with confirmed pleomorphic rhabdomyosarcoma following unplanned resection. (**a**) Clinical photograph of the patient's incision and palpable tumor/postoperative hematoma outlined with the methylene blue pen. (**b**) Axial fat-saturated T2-weighted MRI following the unplanned resection. Note the large anteromedial residual tumor focus with extensive perilesional post-surgical edema and hematoma formation

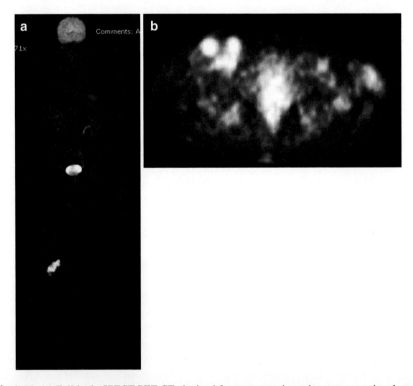

Fig. 9.12 (**a**) Full-body SPECT PET CT obtained for tumor staging prior to re-resection demonstrating isolated increased metabolic activity about the right knee. (**b**) Axial PET CT obtained for tumor restaging 3 months postoperatively demonstrating marked avidity of the ipsilateral inguinal lymph nodes that contained confirmed metastatic disease by biopsy

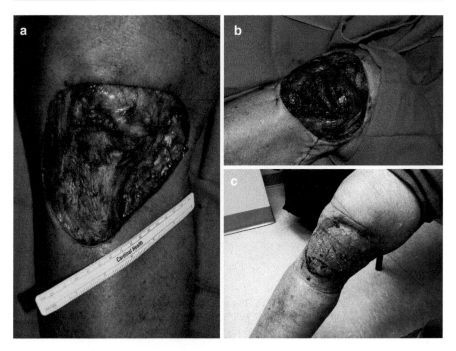

Fig. 9.13 (**a**) Intraoperative photograph following wide re-resection of a pleomorphic rhabdomyosarcoma demonstrating exposed tibia and adjacent knee joint capsule with no remaining soft tissue coverage. (**b**) Pedicled local gastrocnemius flap used for soft tissue coverage of the surgical defect performed 5 days after re-resection once permanent specimen margins were confirmed negative. (**c**) Complete healing of the gastrocnemius flap covered by split-thickness skin graft 6 weeks post-operatively

meetings. However, the patient progressed rapidly with widespread metastases (Fig. 9.12b) and succumbed to his disease 4 months postoperatively, not ever able to begin chemotherapy.

Because of the intrinsic biology of his presenting tumor, it is likely that his oncologic outcome and death were not related to the intralesional procedure; although, there is no way to definitively conclude this. However, the requirement of the large soft tissue reconstruction and bone burring could have been prevented with an appropriate planned resection. Although the patient died of metastatic spread of the disease, he may have had a better functional outcome with better pain control for his remaining life with an oncologically sound initial resection.

Case 4: *Unnecessary amputation*
A 69-year-old female with a history of uncontrolled atrial fibrillation and severe dilated cardiomyopathy presented with a massive dominant arm antecubital soft tissue tumor with impending fungation (Fig. 9.14). She had experienced 3 prior unplanned, intralesional debulkings and irrigation/debridements over a 5-year period prior to referral. She was immediately discussed at the biweekly multidisciplinary sarcoma conference. She was offered a percutaneous biopsy, which revealed

Fig. 9.14 Clinical photograph of a massive antecubital soft tissue sarcoma with impending fungation, extensive scarring from prior unplanned procedures, and robust edema distally due to local lymphatic and venous compression from the tumor bulk

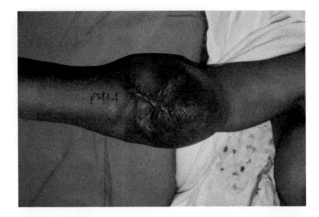

Fig. 9.15 Axial chest CT showing metastatic pulmonary synovial cell sarcoma

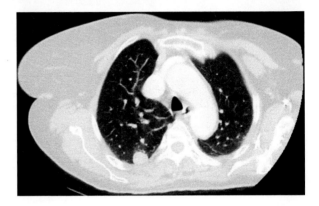

a diagnosis of synovial cell sarcoma; staging studies revealed numerous metastatic pulmonary nodules (Fig. 9.15).

Given her age and cardiac history, she was not an appropriate candidate for first-line, high-dose, cytotoxic chemotherapy. Therefore, her prognosis was very grave given the clinical stage and limited treatment options. Further, because of the size and location of the tumor, she had extensive distal upper extremity lymphedema and neurologic deficits, leaving a heavy, painful, non-functioning arm.

As a result of her many surgeries and prolonged time to referral allowing increased growth, the entire elbow was infiltrated with tumor (Fig. 9.16). After a thorough discussion with the multidisciplinary team, she underwent successful above-elbow amputation as a palliative measure. She went on to heal very well (Fig. 9.17) with excellent shoulder function and required no pain medication. She was subsequently treated with palliative chemotherapy and is still alive at 6 months postoperatively. However, it is likely that she will not experience complete disease remission in her remaining life [86].

With a massive, infiltrative tumor leaving behind a painful, non-functioning limb, amputation can provide an excellent outcome [87]. However, with the likelihood of dying of her disease, living her remaining life without her dominant upper extremity is certainly morbid and function limiting. Given the size and stage of

Fig. 9.16 Sagittal fat-saturated T2-weighted MRI of a 69-year-old female with confirmed synovial cell sarcoma following multiple unplanned resections over a several year course showing extensive lobular local infiltration of disease including involvement of the radiocapitellar joint

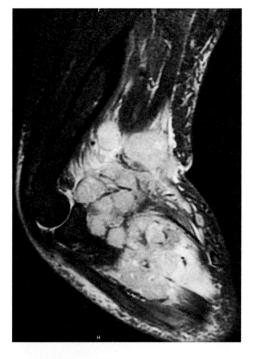

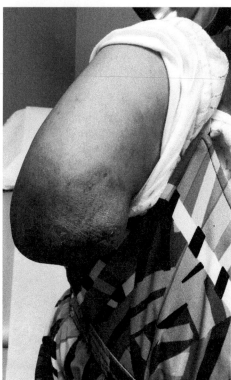

Fig. 9.17 Clinical photograph at 6 month follow-up following above elbow amputation showing excellent local wound healing

the tumor coupled with the length of time and multiple surgeries between initial presentation and the time when she was finally referred to orthopedic oncology, it is quite possible that a local limb-sparing resection may have been initially possible. Likewise, the chance for cure would have been much higher if the tumor had not spread to the lungs yet at that time. However, the sad part of care for patients experiencing unplanned resections of sarcoma is that these suppositions will never be known with any certainty.

Case 5: *Death*

This case was briefly mentioned in a previous publication regarding unplanned resection of sarcoma [5] but will be discussed in greater detail here. It involves an otherwise healthy 48-year-old female who presented initially to the orthopedic oncologist's outpatient office in a wheelchair with failure to ambulate. History revealed a mass found in her left thigh after "bumping" into her bathroom counter 6 months previous. She presented at that time to a community orthopedic surgeon who presumed a hematoma and aspirated 500 mL of fluid from the thigh. The fluid collection rapidly reaccumulated over a few weeks, and she was then taken to the operating room for an evacuation, irrigation, and debridement. Following that procedure, she reaccumulated the mass and began to show signs of wound infection. She was taken back to the operating room for a second debridement and application of a wound vacuum-assisted closure (VAC). After 2 months of failure of the VAC to cure her infection, she was referred to musculoskeletal oncology due to the complexity of the condition. No imaging was done, and none of the aspirated or evacuated tissues were ever sent for pathologic analysis or culture.

Physical examination at the orthopedic oncology clinic revealed a hot, edematous thigh with intense rubor and a wound VAC apparatus over a 5 cm wound on the anterolateral left mid-thigh. She was slightly tachycardic and was direct admitted to the hospital for monitoring and workup. Overnight she went into septic shock and gross purulence was seen at the VAC site.

She was taken urgently to the operating room for irrigation and debridement, culture, and biopsy of the large, suspicious mass seen on the imaging done upon admission (Fig. 9.18). Cultures of the wound revealed polymicrobial growth with mixed bacterial and fungal organisms, including *Candida tropicalis*, vancomycin-resistant *Enterococcus*, and *Escherichia coli*, and she was begun on appropriate parenteral antibiotics and antifungals in accordance with infectious disease consultation. Biopsy revealed a high-grade hemorrhagic extraskeletal osteosarcoma. Staging was then done that revealed a solitary pulmonary metastasis (Fig. 9.19a).

This case was discussed at the multidisciplinary sarcoma conference, with a plan to begin chemotherapy once the infection was adequately treated. However, the

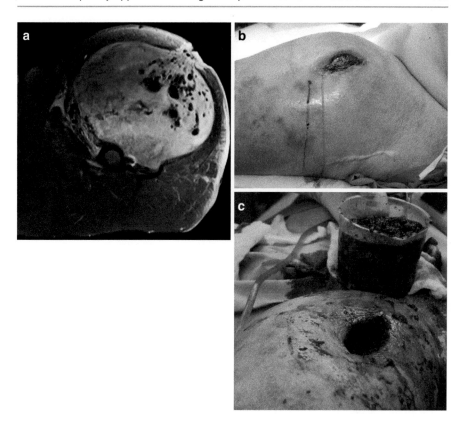

Fig. 9.18 (**a**) Axial T2 fat saturated MRI image of a massive, infected left thigh sarcoma with extensive intratumoral emphysema and cutaneous fungation in a 48-year-old female treated for over 6 months at an outside institution with repeated aspirations and surgical debridements for presumed hematoma. No advanced imaging or biopsy was done prior to her presentation at the authors' institution. (**b**) Clinical image of the fungating thigh wound and (**c**) purulent myonecrosis removed at first attempt to eradicate her infection. (Reprinted with permission from Tedesco NS, Henshaw RM. J Am Acad Orthop Surg 2016;24(3):150-159.)

patient continued to show signs of infection after several days of systemic antibiotics and was thus taken for wide resection of the entire infected tumor cavity. This unfortunately necessitated a massive radical anterior thigh compartment resection along with the tumor (Fig. 9.20). The patient continued to decline and serial imaging demonstrated rapid progression of her pulmonary disease (Fig. 9.19b, c). She was never able to regain her ambulatory status and was never medically stable enough to begin systemic cytotoxic chemotherapy. She succumbed to respiratory failure and anemia as a result of her pulmonary disease and recurrent malignant pleural effusions despite several procedures by the cardiothoracic surgery team.

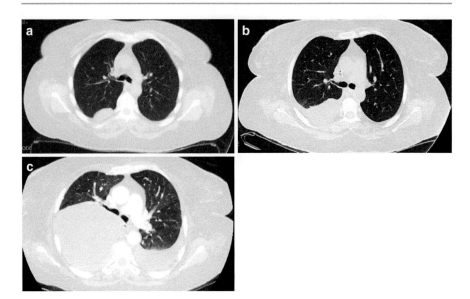

Fig. 9.19 Rapid progression of pulmonary metastatic disease in the 48-year-old female with extraskeletal osteosarcoma (**a**) at initial presentation to the authors' institution, (**b**) one month later, and (**c**) two months after initial presentation and immediately prior to death. (Reprinted with permission from Tedesco NS, Henshaw RM. J Am Acad Orthop Surg 2016; 24(3):150-159.)

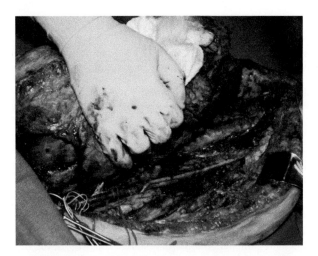

Fig. 9.20 Intraoperative resection of the same 48-year-old female's infected left thigh sarcoma and entire anterior thigh muscular compartment after serial debridements and systemic polyantimicrobial agents failed to clear her infection. The vessel loops surround the superficial femoral artery and vein and the exposed femur can be seen deep to the distal end of the tumor being elevated by the surgeon. (Reprinted with permission from Tedesco NS, Henshaw RM. J Am Acad Orthop Surg 2016; 24(3):150-159.)

A retrospective look at the pulmonary disease and how rapidly it progressed over her 2-month hospital stay suggests it is possible her initial presentation 6 months prior may not have demonstrated any evidence of pulmonary disease. However, if she did have metastatic spread at that time, she would have been a candidate for neoadjuvant chemotherapy with pulmonary metastectomy that could potentially save or at least prolong her life. Further, radiation could have been used as a local adjuvant to help avoid removal of her entire anterior thigh that may have allowed her to ambulate safely.

This case is a sober reminder of the diligence required for adequate initial workup and planned treatment of a potential sarcoma. Had the initial general orthopedist recognized the presenting mass or worked it up appropriately, a lot of the issues with this case could have been avoided. Recognition that a 500 mL hematoma should not occur in a young, healthy individual after insignificant trauma is paramount to raising index of suspicion for a tumor. Had the initial treating surgeon recognized this, it is quite likely her life could have been spared.

9.8 Summary

Unplanned resection of sarcoma has been a major problem for patients and physicians involved in sarcoma care alike. Since these issues were first reported in the 1980s, there has been little to no progress in the way the medical community views, evaluates, and treats patients presenting with a mass involving the trunk, extremities, spine, or retroperitoneum. This is all despite the fact that, however rare, sarcoma is always in the differential diagnosis of an extremity mass until proven otherwise.

Primum non nocere ("first, do no harm") is the credo by which all physicians and allied healthcare professionals live, but it appears that this platitude has been largely ignored when it comes to care of tumors and tumor-like conditions of the musculoskeletal system. This is no more evidenced than by the literature exposing the harm done with unplanned resections, including increased costs to the patients and healthcare system, increased morbidity and mortality for the patient, increased psychological distress for both the patient and treating physician, and the medicolegal ramifications to the treating physician involved in such a "whoops" surgery. Yet, unplanned resections continue to happen at an alarming rate and may even be more common than planned resections.

Treatment of these patients poses many dilemmas for tertiary referral centers involved with regular sarcoma care. Salvage of these situations is predicated on restoring oncologic prognosis to identical that of a similar presentation with a planned resection, while maximizing functional and emotional outcomes. This requires strict focus of a multispecialty, multidisciplinary team adept at dealing with these issues, organizing workup and treatment in an efficient manner, and providing the best collective experience available for each situation on a case-by-case basis.

In the future of sarcoma care, a coordinated, multidisciplinary, international effort should be employed to develop an educational curriculum and referral guidelines for community physicians who may encounter a tumor involving the musculoskeletal system. Education of the medical community at large will need to begin at an early stage in each care provider's career. Techniques of tumor resection, appropriate workup of a mass, knowledge of sarcoma, and focus on both classic and non-classic sarcoma presentations will be required if unplanned resections are to be abated. Caution with interpretation of "group" studying of these cases (i.e., combining into the same cohort of "unplanned resections" an unplanned, small, subcutaneous tumor excision and a reamed, intramedullary nailing of a fracture in a bone with missed sarcoma) should be taken. Ideally, future studies on the subject should be aimed at direct comparison of matched tumor presentations with the only variable being the unplanned resection to elucidate the true effect of the unplanned sarcoma resection.

References

1. Mukherjee S. The new friends of chemotherapy. In: The emperor of all maladies: a biography of cancer. New York: Scribner; 2010.
2. Lokich JJ. Primer of cancer management. Boston: G.K. Hall; 1978.
3. Giuliano AE, Eilber FR. The rationale for planned reoperation after unplanned total excision of soft tissue sarcomas. J Clin Oncol. 1985;3:1344–8.
4. Noria S, Davis A, Kandel R, Levesque J, O'Sullivan B, Wunder J, Bell R. Residual disease following unplanned excision of a soft-tissue sarcoma of an extremity. J Bone Joint Surg Am. 1996;78(5):650–5.
5. Tedesco NS, Henshaw RM. Unplanned resection of sarcoma. J Am Acad Orthop Surg. 2015;24(3): 150–9.
6. Fletcher CDM. WHO classification of tumours of soft tissue and bone. Lyon: IARC; 2013.
7. Siegel R, Naishadham D, Jemal A. Cancer statistics. CA Cancer J Clin. 2013;63(1):11–30.
8. FY 2012 research funding by cancer type. Research Funding Statistics for FY 2012 Cancer Type. National Cancer Institute. 2013. http://fundedresearch.cancer.gov/nciportfolio/search/funded;jsessionid=5349A969354D79D99204658AD784AC4F?fy=PUB2012&type=site. Accessed 23 Feb 2015.
9. Grimer R, Athanasou N, Gerrand C, Judson I, Lewis I, Morland B, Peake D, Seddon B, Whelan J. UK guidelines for the management of bone sarcomas. Sarcoma. 2010;2010:317462.
10. Kim MS, Lee SY, Cho WH, Song WS, Koh JS, Lee JA, Yoo JY, Shin DS, Jeon DG. Prognostic effect of inadvertent curettage without treatment delay in osteosarcoma. J Surg Oncol. 2009;100:484–7.
11. Wang TI, Wu PK, Chen CF, Chen WM, Yen CC, Hung GY, Liu CL, Chen TH. The prognosis of patients with primary osteosarcoma who have undergone unplanned therapy. Jpn J Clin Oncol. 2011;41(11):1244–50.
12. Biau DJ, Weiss KR, Bhumbra RS, Davidson D, Brown C, Griffin A, Wunder JS, Ferguson PC. Monitoring the adequacy of surgical margins after resection of bone and soft-tissue sarcoma. Ann Surg Oncol. 2013;20:1858–64.
13. Ayerza MA, Muscolo DL, Aponte-Tinao LA, Farfalli G. Effect of erroneous surgical procedures on recurrence and survival rates for patients with osteosarcoma. Clin Orthop Relat Res. 2006;452:231–5.
14. Puri A, Shah M, Agarwal MG, Jambhekar NA, Basappa P. Chondrosarcoma of bone: Does the size of the tumor, the presence of a pathologic fracture, or prior intervention have an impact on local control and survival? J Cancer Res Ther. 2009;5(1):14–9.

15. Wong CK, Lam YL, So YC, Ngan KC, Wong KY. Management of extremity soft tissue sarcoma after unplanned incomplete resection: Experience of a regional musculoskeletal tumour Centre. Hong Kong Med J. 2004;10(2):117–22.
16. Venkatesan M, Richards CJ, McCulloch TA, Perks AGB, Raurell A, Ashford RU. Inadvertent surgical resection of soft tissue sarcomas. Eur J Surg Oncol. 2012;38:346–51.
17. Potter BK, Adams SC, Pitcher JD, Temple HT. Local recurrence of disease after unplanned excisions of high-grade soft tissue sarcomas. Clin Orthop Relat Res. 2008;466:3093–100.
18. Rehders A, Stoecklein NH, Poremba C, Alexander A, Knoefel WT, Peiper M. Reexcision of soft tissue sarcoma: Sufficient local control but increased rate of metastasis. World J Surg. 2009;33:2599–605.
19. Fiore M, Casali PG, Miceli R, Mariani L, Bertulli R, Lozza L, Collini P, Olmi P, Mussi C, Gronchi A. Prognostic effect of re-excision in adult soft tissue sarcoma of the extremity. Ann Surg Oncol. 2006;13(1):110–7.
20. Alamanda VK, Delisa GO, Mathis SL, Archer KR, Ehrenfeld JM, Miller MW, Homlar KC, Halpern JL, Schwartz HS, Holt GE. The financial burden of reexcising incompletely excised soft tissue sarcomas: A cost analysis. Ann Surg Oncol. 2013;20:2808–14.
21. Alamanda VK, Delisca GO, Archer KR, Song Y, Schwartz HS, Holt GE. Incomplete excisions of extremity soft tissue sarcomas are unaffected by insurance status or distance from a sarcoma center. J Surg Oncol. 2013;108:477–80.
22. Qureshi YA, Huddy JR, Miller JD, Strauss DC, Thomas JM, Hayes AJ. Unplanned excision of soft tissue sarcoma results in increased rates of local recurrence despite full further oncological treatment. Ann Surg Oncol. 2012;19:871–7.
23. Sawamura C, Matsumoto S, Shimoji T, Tanizawa T, Ae K. What are risk factors for local recurrence of deep high-grade soft-tissue sarcomas? Clin Orthop Relat Res. 2012;470:700–5.
24. Manoso MW, Frassica DA, Deune EG, Frassica FJ. Outcomes of re-excision after unplanned excisions of soft-tissue sarcomas. J Surg Oncol. 2005;91:153–8.
25. Davis AM, Kandel RA, Wunder JS, Unger R, Meer J, O'Sullivan B, Catton CN, Bell RS. The impact of residual disease on local recurrence in patients treated by initial unplanned resection for soft tissue sarcoma of the extremity. J Surg Oncol. 1997;66:81–7.
26. Morii T, Aoyagi T, Tajima T, Yoshiyama A, Ichimura S, Mochizuki K. Unplanned resection of a soft tissue sarcoma: Clinical characteristics and impact on oncological and functional outcomes. J Orthop Sci. 2015;20(2):373–9.
27. Lewis JJ, Leung D, Espat J, Woodruff JM, Brennan MF. Effect of reresection in extremity soft tissue sarcoma. Ann Surg. 2000;231:655–63.
28. Davies AM, Mehr A, Parsonage S, Evans N, Grimer RJ, Pynsent PB. MR imaging in the assessment of residual tumour following inadequate primary excision of soft tissue sarcomas. Eur Radiol. 2004;14(3):506–13.
29. Goodlad JR, Fletcher CDM, Smith MA. Surgical resection of primary soft-tissue sarcoma: Incidence of residual tumor in 95 patients needing re-excision after local resection. J Bone Joint Surg Br. 1996;78B(4):658–61.
30. Chandrasekar CR, Wafa H, Grimer RJ, Carter SR, Tillman RM, Abudu A. The effect of unplanned excision of a soft-tissue sarcoma on prognosis. J Bone Joint Surg Br. 2008;90B(2):203–8.
31. Zagars GK, Ball MT, Pisters PWT, Pollock RE, Patel SR, Benjamin RS. Surgical margins and reresection in the management of patients with soft tissue sarcoma using conservative surgery and radiation therapy. Cancer. 2003;97(10):2544–53.
32. Temple HT, Worman DS, Mnaymneh WA. Unplanned surgical excision of tumors of the foot. Cancer Control. 2001;8(3):262–8.
33. Nishimura A, Matsumine A, Asanuma K, Matsubara T, Nakamura T, Uchida A, Kato K, Sudo A. The adverse effect of an unplanned surgical excision of foot soft tissue sarcoma. World J Surg Oncol. 2011;9:160.
34. Sawamura C, Springfield DS, Marcus KJ, Perez-Atayde AR, Gebhardt MC. Factors predicting local recurrence, metastasis, and survival in pediatric soft tissue sarcoma in extremities. Clin Orthop Relat Res. 2010;468:3019–27.

35. Chui CH, Spunt SL, Liu T, Pappo AS, Davidoff AM, Rao BN, Shochat SJ. Is reexcision in pediatric nonrhabdomyosarcoma soft tissue sarcoma necessary after an initial unplanned resection? J Pediatr Surg. 2002;37(10):1424–9.
36. Rougraff BT, Davis K, Cudahy T. The impact of previous surgical manipulation of subcutaneous sarcoma on oncologic outcome. Clin Orthop Relat Res. 2005;438:85–91.
37. Pretell-Mazzini J, Barton Jr MD, Conway SA, Temple HT. Unplanned excision of soft-tissue sarcomas: Current concepts for management and prognosis. J Bone Joint Surg. 2015;97(7): 597–603.
38. Mochizuki K. How should orthopaedic oncologists prevent unplanned resections of soft tissue sarcomas by general practitioners? J Orthop Sci. 2012;17(4):339–40.
39. Karakousis CP, Driscoll DL. Treatment and local control of primary extremity soft tissue sarcomas. J Surg Oncol. 1999;71(3):155–61.
40. Gronchi A, Miceli R, Fiore M, Collini P, Lozza L, Grosso F, Mariani L, Casili PG. Extremity soft tissue sarcoma: Adding to the prognostic meaning of local failure. Ann Surg Oncol. 2007; 14(5):1583–90.
41. Alamanda VK, Crosby SN, Archer KR, Song Y, Schwartz HS, Holt GE. Primary excision compared with re-excision of extremity soft tissue sarcomas – is anything new? J Surg Oncol. 2012;105(7):662–7.
42. Umer HM, Umer M, Qadir I, Abbasi N, Masood N. Impact of unplanned excision on prognosis of patients with extremity soft tissue sarcoma. Sarcoma. 2013;2013:498604.
43. Siegel HJ, Brown O, Lopez-Ben R, Siegal GP. Unplanned surgical excision of extremity soft tissue sarcomas: Patient profile and referral patterns. J Surg Orthop Adv. 2009;18(2):93–8.
44. Hoshi M, Ieguchi M, Takami M, Aono M, Taguchi S, Kuroda T, Takaoka K. Clinical problems after initial unplanned resection of sarcoma. Jpn J Clin Oncol. 2008;38(10):701–9.
45. Sugiura H, Takahashi M, Katagiri H, Nishida Y, Nakashima H, Yonekawa M, Iwata H. Additional wide resection of malignant soft tissue tumors. Clin Orthop Relat Res. 2002;394:201–10.
46. Jeon DG, Lee SY, Kim JW. Bone primary sarcomas undergone unplanned intralesional procedure–The possibility of limb salvage and their oncologic results. J Surg Oncol. 2006;94:592–8.
47. Picci P, Sangiorgi L, Bahamonde L, Aluigi P, Bibiloni AJ, Zavatta M, MercuriM BA, Campanacci M. Risk factors for local recurrences after limb-salvage surgery for high-grade osteosarcoma of the extremities. Ann Oncol. 1997;8:899–903.
48. Kepka L, Suit HD, Goldberg SI, Rosenberg AE, Gebhardt MC, Hornicek FJ, Delaney TF. Results of radiation therapy performed after unplanned surgery (without re-excision) for soft tissue sarcomas. J Surg Oncol. 2005;92:39–45.
49. Kang S, Han I, Lee SA, Cho HS, Kim HS. Unplanned excision of soft tissue sarcoma: The impact of the referring hospital. Surg Oncol. 2013;22:e17–22.
50. Han I, Kang HG, Kang SC, Choi JR, Kim HS. Does delayed reexcision affect outcome after unplanned excision of soft tissue sarcoma? Clin Orthop Relat Res. 2011;469:877–83.
51. Siebenrock KA, Hertel R, Ganz R. Unexpected resection of soft tissue sarcoma: More mutilating surgery, higher local recurrence rates, and obscure prognosis as consequences of improper surgery. Arch Orthop Trauma Srug. 2000;120(1–2):65–9.
52. Kaste SC, Hill A, Conley L, Shidler TJ, Rao BN, Neel MM. Magnetic resonance imaging after incomplete resection of soft-tissue sarcoma. Clin Orthop. 2002;397:204–11.
53. Wodajo FM, Gannon F, Murphey MD. Diagnostic features of bone tumors. In: Visual guide to musculoskeletal tumors: a clinical, radiologic, histologic approach. 1st ed. Philadelphia: Saunders/Elsevier; 2010. p. 3–18.
54. Maheshwari AV, Cheng EY. Ewing sarcoma family of tumors. J Am Acad Orthop Surg. 2010;18(2):94–107.
55. Leddy LR, Holmes RE. Chondrosarcoma of bone. Cancer Treat Res. 2014;162:117–30.
56. Arai E, Nishida Y, Tsukushi S, Wasa J, Ishiguro N. Clinical and treatment outcomes of planned and unplanned excisions of soft tissue sarcomas. Clin Orthop Relat Res. 2010;468(11):3028–34.
57. Zornig C, Peiper M, Schroder S. Re-excision of soft tissue sarcoma after inadequate initial operation. Br J Surg. 1995;82(2):278–9.

58. Peiper M, Knoefel WT, Izbicki JR. The influence of residual tumor on local recurrence after unplanned resection of soft tissue sarcoma. Dtsch Med Wochenschr. 2004;129(5):183–7.
59. Morii T, Yabe H, Morioka H, Anazawa U, Suzuki Y, Toyama Y. Clinical significance of additional wide resection for unplanned resection of high grade soft tissue sarcoma. Open Orthop J. 2008;2:126–9.
60. Bierman JS. Orthopedic knowledge update: musculoskeletal tumors, vol. 3. Rosemont: American Academy of Orthopaedic Surgeons; 2013.
61. Estourgie SH, Nielsen GP, Ott MJ. Metastatic patterns of extremity myxoid liposarcoma and their outcome. J Surg Oncol. 2002;80(2):89–93.
62. Newman EN, Jones RL, Hawkins DS. An evaluation of [F-18]-fluorodeoxy-D-glucose positron emission tomography, bone scan, and bone marrow aspiration/biopsy as staging investigations in Ewing sarcoma. Pediatr Blood Cancer. 2013;60(7):1113–7.
63. Federico SM, Spunt SL, Krasin MJ, Billup CA, Wu J, Shulkin B, Mandell B, McCarville MB. Comparison of PET-CT and conventional imaging in staging pediatric rhabdomyosarcoma. Pediatr Blood Cancer. 2013;60(7):1128–34.
64. Combemale P, Valeyrie-Allanore L, Giammarile F, Pinson S, Guillot B, Goulart DM, Wolkenstein P, Blay JY, Mognetti T. Utility of 18F-FDG PET with a semi-quantitative index in the detection of sarcomatous transformation in patients with neurofibromatosis type 1. PLoS One. 2014;9(2):e85954.
65. Reid MM, Saunders PW, Bown N, Bradford CR, Maung ZT, Craft AW, Malcolm AJ. Alveolar rhabdomyosarcoma infiltrating bone marrow at presentation: The value to diagnosis of bone marrow trephine biopsy specimens. J Clin Pathol. 1992;45(9):759–62.
66. Schwartz HS, Spengler DM. Needle tract recurrences after closed biopsy for sarcoma: Three cases and review of the literature. Ann Surg Oncol. 1997;4(3):228–36.
67. Mankin HJ, Lange TA, Spanier SS. The hazards of biopsy in patients with malignant primary bone and soft-tissue tumors. J Bone Joint Surg. 1982;64:1121–7.
68. Enneking WF, Maale GE. The effect of inadvertent tumor contamination of wounds during the surgical resection of musculoskeletal neoplasms. Cancer. 1988;62(7):1251–6.
69. Mayerson JL, Scharschmidt TJ, Lewis VO, Morris CD. Diagnosis and management of soft tissue masses. J Am Acad Orthop Surg. 2014;22(11):742–50.
70. Mesko NW, Mesko JL, Gaffney LM, Halpern JL. Schwartz.HS, Holt GE. Medical malpractice and sarcoma care–a thirty-three year review of case resolutions, inciting factors, and at risk physician specialties surrounding a rare diagnosis. J Surg Oncol. 2014;110:919–29.
71. Delaney TF, Kepka L, Goldberg SI, Hornicek FJ, Gebhardt MC, Yoon SS, Springfield DS, Raskin KA, Harmon DC, Kirsch DG, Mankin HJ, Rosenberg AE, Nielsen GP, Suit HD. Radiation therapy for control of soft-tissue sarcomas resected with positive margins. Int J Radiat Oncol Biol Phys. 2007;67(5):1460–9.
72. Roberge D, Skamene T, Nahal A, Turcotte RE, Powell T, Freeman C. Radiological and pathological response following pre-operative radiotherapy for soft-tissue sarcoma. Radiother Oncol. 2010;97(3):404–7.
73. Jones DA, Shideman C, Yuan J, Dusenbery K, Manivel JC, Ogilvie C, Clohisy DR, Cheng EY, Shanley R, Cho LC. Management of unplanned excision for soft-tissue sarcoma with preoperative radiotherapy followed by definitive resection. Am J Clin Oncol. 2016;39(6):586–92.
74. Dumont SN, Araujo DM, Munsell MF, Salganick JA, Dumont AG, Raymond KA, Linassier C, Patel S, Benjamin RS, Trent JC. Management and outcome of 239 adolescent and adult rhabdomyosarcoma patients. Cancer Med. 2013;2(4):553–63.
75. Gerber NK, Wexler LH, Singer S, Alektiar KM, Keohan ML, Shi W, Zhang Z, Wolden S. Adult rhabdomyosarcoma survival improved with treatment on multimodality protocols. Int J Radiat Oncol Biol Phys. 2013;86(1):58–63.
76. Oberlin O, Rey A, Sanchez de Toledo J, Martelli H, Jenney ME, Scopinaro M, Bergeron C, Merks JH, Bouvet N, Ellershaw C, Kelsey A, Spooner D, Stevens MC. Randomized comparison of intensified six-drug versus standard three-drug chemotherapy for high-risk nonmetastatic rhabdomyosarcoma and other chemotherapy-sensitive childhood soft tissue sarcomas:

Long-term results from the International Society of Pediatric Oncology MMT95 study. J Clin Oncol. 2012;30(20):2457–65.
77. Mirabello L, Troisi RJ, Savage SA. Osteosarcoma incidence and survival rates from 1973 to 2004: Data from the surveillance, epidemiology, and end results program. Cancer. 2009;115(7): 1531–43.
78. Demetri GD, Antonia S, Benjamin RS, Bui MM, Casper ES, Conrad 3rd EU, DeLaney TF, Ganjoo KN, Heslin MJ, Hutchinson RJ, Kane 3rd JM, Letson GD, McGarry SV, O'Donnell RJ, Paz IB, Pfeifer JD, Pollock RE, Randall RL, Riedel RF, Schupak KD, Schwartz HS, Thornton K, von Mehren M, Wayne J. National comprehensive cancer network soft tissue sarcoma panel. Soft tissue sarcoma. J Natl Compr Cancer Netw. 2010;8(6):630–74.
79. Hohenberger P, Kasper B, Ahrar K. Surgical management and minimally invasive approaches for the treatment of metastatic sarcoma. Am Soc Clin Oncol Educ Book 2013;457–64.
80. Cazzato RL, Buy X, Grasso RF, Luppi G, Faiella E, Quattrocchi CC, Pantano F, Beomonte Zobel B, Tonini G, Santini D, Palussiere J. Interventional Radiologist's perspective on the management of bone metastatic disease. Eur J Surg Oncol. 2015;41(8):967–74.
81. Edwards B, Clarke V. The psychological impact of a cancer diagnosis on families: The influence of family functioning and patients' illness characteristics on depression and anxiety. Psychooncology. 2004;13(8):562–76.
82. Dionne-Odom JN, Azuero A, Lyons KD, Hull JG, Tosteson TD, Li Z, Li Z, Frost J, Dragnev KH, Akyar I, Hegel MT, Bakitas MA. Benefits of early versus delayed palliative care to informal family caregivers of patients with advanced cancer: Outcomes from the ENABLE III randomized controlled trial. J Clin Oncol. 2015;33(13):1446–52.
83. Bakitas MA, Tosteson TD, Li Z, Lyons KD, Hull JG, Li Z, Dionne-Odom JN, Frost J, Dragnev KH, Hegel MT, Azuero A, Ahles TA. Early versus delayed initiation of concurrent palliative oncology care: Patient outcomes in the ENABLE III randomized controlled trial. J Clin Oncol. 2015;33(13):1438–45.
84. Kuzel P, Mahmood MN, Metelitsa AI, Salopek TG. A clinicopathologic review of a case series of dermatofibrosarcoma protuberans with fibrosarcomatous differentiation. J Cutan Med Surg. 2015;19(1):28–34.
85. Socoliuc C, Zurac S, Andrei R, Staniceanu F. A review of morphological aspects in dermatofibrosarcoma protuberans with clinicopathological correlations. Rom J Intern Med. 2014;52(4):239–50.
86. D'Angelo SP, Tap WD, Schwartz GK, Carvajal RD. Sarcoma immunotherapy: Past approaches and future directions. Sarcoma. 2014;2014:391967.
87. Puhaindran ME, Chou J, Forsberg JA, Athanasian EA. Major upper-limb amputations for malignant tumors. J Hand Surg [Am]. 2012;37(6):1235–41.

Radiation Therapy for Sarcomas

10

Keith Unger, Marie Gurka, and K. William Harter

10.1 Soft Tissue Sarcoma of the Extremity and Superficial Trunk

Historically, amputation was the treatment of choice for soft tissue sarcomas (STS) of the extremity [1, 2]. Advances made throughout the latter half of the last century have led to local control rates approaching 90%, utilizing a multimodality approach that allows for functional limb preservation in the vast majority of cases [3]. Recent progress in radiation therapy includes personalization of adjuvant radiation therapy, utilization of preoperative radiation therapy in selected cases, and the application of novel treatment techniques to improve outcomes.

10.1.1 Adjuvant Radiation Therapy

While surgery is the foundation of treatment for STS, the addition of adjuvant radiation therapy to the treatment paradigm improves outcomes in selected patients. The evidence suggests that radiation therapy reduces local recurrence in the setting of limb-sparing surgery and occasionally after amputation [4–7], yet no trial has demonstrated a clear survival benefit.

Amputation was the standard treatment for STS of the extremity until small, nonrandomized studies of limb-preserving surgery followed by radiation demonstrated local control rates of approximately 80% or greater [8–10]. These results led

K. Unger, M.D. (✉)
Department of Radiation Medicine, Georgetown University, Washington, DC, USA
e-mail: KXU2@gunet.georgetown.edu

M. Gurka, M.D.
Radiation Oncology, University of Louisville, Louisville, KY, USA

K. William Harter, M.D.
Department of Radiation Medicine, Georgetown University, Washington, DC, USA

© Springer International Publishing Switzerland 2017
R.M. Henshaw (ed.), *Sarcoma*, DOI 10.1007/978-3-319-43121-5_10

to a landmark randomized trial conducted at the NCI (National Cancer Institute) comparing amputation to limb-preserving surgery plus postoperative radiation therapy (PORT) in patients with high-grade extremity STS [11]. The radiation dose was 50 Gy to the entire anatomic area at risk for local spread and 60–70 Gy to the tumor bed. All participants received adjuvant chemotherapy. While patients had a higher rate of local recurrence with limb-sparing therapy, four vs. none, the disease-free survival and overall survival were not significantly different between the two arms. This established that amputation was not necessary in most cases.

Two additional randomized trials have examined the role of adjuvant radiation therapy after limb-sparing surgery. In a follow-up randomized trial at the NCI, limb-sparing surgery alone was compared to surgery followed by radiation in patients with high- and low-grade STS [4]. Patients with high-grade sarcoma also received adjuvant chemotherapy. Radiation was given postoperatively as 45 Gy delivered to a wide field followed by an 18 Gy boost to the tumor bed. Postoperative radiation was found to significantly decrease local recurrence in both high-grade and low-grade sarcomas. At a median follow-up of almost 10 years, local recurrence rates in the PORT arms were 0% and 4% for high grade and low grade, respectively. In patients not receiving radiation, they were 19% and 33%, respectively. However, this was at the expense of worse limb strength, increased edema, and decreased range of motion. Fortunately, these deficits were often transient and rarely impacted activities of daily life or global quality of life.

Recently, a 20-year update of this trial focusing on the quality of life outcomes was published [12]. The authors reported that there was a trend toward increased rate of pathologic fracture, wound complications, and edema with adjuvant radiation. There was a nonsignificant difference in OS favoring PORT; however, the study was not powered to detect a survival difference. In summary, both studies concluded that the use of adjuvant external beam radiation therapy (EBRT) for patients at low risk of recurrence should be selective. It is important to recall that these conclusions are made based on older radiation techniques. Newer modalities, such as intensity-modulated radiation therapy (IMRT), have improved sparing of critical structures; therefore, long-term results of contemporary trials may have lower fracture and complication rates after radiation as discussed below [13].

The only other randomized study comparing limb sparing surgery (LSS) alone to surgery plus radiation utilized brachytherapy. In the study by Pisters et al., en bloc resection alone was compared to resection plus brachytherapy. A total dose of 42–45 Gy was delivered by an iridium-192 implant over 4–6 days. With a median follow-up of 6.3 years, the local control rate with high-grade lesions was 89% in the brachytherapy group and 66% without adjuvant radiation ($P = 0.0025$). Adjuvant brachytherapy had no impact on local control in patients with low-grade lesions ($P = 0.49$). Furthermore, radiation did not impact survival in either group [5].

In a later update of this paper, with a median follow-up of 100 months, there was a reported 24% wound complication rate with brachytherapy. This included patients requiring reoperation, persistent seroma requiring repeat aspirations, wound separation greater than 2 cm, hematoma greater than 25 mL, or purulent wound discharge. Larger resection specimens were associated with an increased complication rate [14]. In the NCI study of adjuvant external beam radiation, the

Table 10.1 Results of randomized trials with adjuvant radiation therapy for soft tissue sarcoma of the extremity and superficial trunk

Study	Study schema	Number of patients	Radiation dose	Chemotherapy	Local control
NCI (*Rosenberg et al. 1982* [11])	Amputation vs	16	–	Doxorubicin, cyclophosphamide, and methotrexate	100%
	LSS + EBRT	27	50 Gy + 10 to 20 Gy boost		85%
NCI (*Yang et al. 1998* [4])	LSS Alone	44 (HG)	–	Doxorubicin and cyclophosphamide	80%
	LS + EBRT	47 (HG)	45 Gy + 18 Gy boost		100%
	LSS Alone	24 (LG)	–	–	67%
	LSS + EBRT	26 (LG)	45 Gy + 18 Gy boost		96%
MSKCC (*Pisters et al. 1996* [5])	LSS	63 (HG)	–	Doxorubicin-based in selected patients	70%
	LSS + Brachytherapy	56 (HG)	42–45 Gy (Ir-192)		91%
	LSS	23 (LG)	–	–	74%
	LSS + Brachytherapy	22 (LG)	42–45 Gy (Ir-192)		64%

Abbreviations: *LSS* limb sparing surgery, *EBRT* external beam radiation therapy, *HG* high grade, *LG* low grade, *Ir-* Iridium

rate of similar wound complications was 17% [4]. These three randomized trials are summarized in Table 10.1.

Additional large, nonrandomized series have supported the benefit of adjuvant radiation therapy for extremity STS. In a systematic review by the Swedish Council of Technology Assessment in Health Care, adjuvant radiotherapy improved the local control rate in combination with limb-preserving surgery in the treatment of STS of extremities and trunk with local control rates equal to or approaching 90% [3]. This has also been supported by a large retrospective review performed by the Scandinavian sarcoma group study [15]. Lastly, an overall survival benefit in favor of PORT for patients with high-grade sarcomas was demonstrated in a recent SEER analysis with a hazard ratio 0.67, 95% confidence interval 0.57–0.79. There was no overall survival benefit in patients with low-grade sarcomas [16].

10.1.2 Preoperative Radiation Therapy

There are several potential advantages to preoperative as compared to postoperative radiation therapy for STS of the extremity including: (1) reduced radiation dose to a smaller target volume resulting in fewer long-term complications [17, 18], (2) facilitation of surgical resection by means of tumor regression and reducing the possibility of microscopic tumor seeding at the time of surgery [19], and (3) easier delineation of target volumes.

However, concerns with preoperative therapy include delays in surgery, while radiation is being administered and prolonged wound healing afterward. To verify that oncologic outcomes were not different between preoperative and postoperative radiation, a randomized trial was conducted in Canada, which was stopped early due to increased postoperative wound complication with preoperative therapy. A total of 190 patients were enrolled. Preoperative radiation was given as a wide field of 50 Gy in 2 Gy fractions with an additional 16 Gy to 20 Gy to the tumor plus a 2 cm expansion after resection if the margins were positive. Patients in the adjuvant (PORT) arm received 66 Gy in 33 fractions. The wound complication rates were 35% vs. 17% in the neoadjuvant and PORT groups, respectively ($P = 0.01$), with most complications occurring in patients with lower extremity sarcomas. Moreover, limb function at 6 weeks postsurgery was worse in the neoadjuvant group ($P = 0.01$) [20]. At 5 years, both arms had comparable local control rates (93% vs. 92%) and OS (73 vs. 67%, $P = 0.48$). Of the 129 patients evaluated for limb function at 21 to 27 months after surgery, limb function was similar, but there was a statistical trend for less fibrosis in the neoadjuvant radiation group ($P = 0.07$) [21].

A meta-analysis consisting of mainly retrospective studies supported the finding that delaying surgery does not lead to a detriment in survival with preoperative radiation therapy [22]. This paper confirmed that preoperative therapy increased wound healing complications, while postoperative treatment had higher rates of late fibrosis and decreased limb function. In general, a preoperative approach should be strongly considered for large lesions and high-grade tumors, in order to downstage the tumor, decrease treatment fields, and allow easier treatment planning. This is particularly applicable for large, myxoid liposarcomas, which respond well to radiation compared to other histological subtypes [23] (Fig. 10.1).

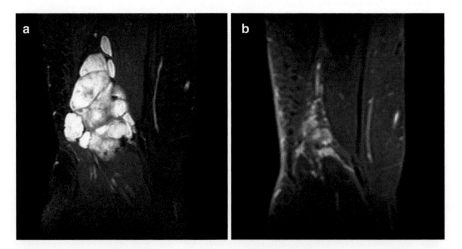

Fig. 10.1 A 52 year old woman with a large, recurrent myxoid liposarcoma, who was treated with pre-operative radiation therapy to a total dose of 45 Gy. (**a**) Pre-treatment coronal MRI demonstrating the mass in the popliteal fossa measuring 10 cm cranial-caudal by 6 cm transverse by 7 cm anterior-posterior. (**b**) MRI after pre-operative radiation therapy, which demonstrates the mass has markedly diminished in size, measuring 4.5 cm cranial-caudal by 2.7 cm transverse by 4.4 cm anterior-posterior

10.1.3 Neoadjuvant Radiation Therapy Combined with Chemotherapy

Early reports utilizing doxorubicin (Adriamycin) with neoadjuvant radiation therapy for STS of the extremity had promising local recurrence rates of <10% and survival rates of 74% in Stage III tumors [24]. More intensive chemotherapy with mesna, Adriamycin, ifosfamide, and dacarbazine (MAID) combined with radiation, followed by resection [25], was also encouraging, and the RTOG conducted a phase II cooperative trial based on this regimen. Oncologic outcomes were satisfactory, but 5% of patients experienced a treatment-related death, deeming this regimen too toxic [26].

The advent of targeted therapies may produce more effective, but less toxic treatment regimens when chemotherapy and radiation are combined. Vascular endothelial growth factor (VEGF), a promoter of angiogenesis, is overexpressed by most malignant tumors, including soft tissue sarcomas [27]. A small phase II has demonstrated promising outcomes, with three complete responses out of 20 patients, who received bevacizumab with radiation prior to resection [28].

10.1.4 Patient Selection

Due to the increased risk of long-term morbidity from radiation after surgery, efforts have been made to identify patients that may not benefit from adjuvant radiation. Most of these data originate from single-institution experiences at large centers. In a retrospective series that included patients from 1970 to 1994, 74 of 242 patients with localized STS of the trunk and extremity were treated with limb-sparing surgery without radiation. The 10-year local control rate was excellent, reaching 100% for patients with resection margins ≥1 cm regardless of tumor grade, size, site (truncal v extremity), or depth (superficial v deep) [29].

A more recent prospective trial also reported high local control rates for selected patients with T1 STS of the extremity and trunk treated with LSS alone. Postoperative external beam radiation was employed only for patients with microscopically positive surgical margins. Of the 88 patients enrolled, 74 (84%) underwent R0 resection and were, therefore, treated by surgery alone. The median follow-up was 75 months. The cumulative incidence rates of local recurrence after an R0 resection at 5 and 10 years were 7.9% and 10.6%, respectively. [30]. In a retrospective series from Memorial Sloan Kettering Cancer Center, there was no benefit with adjuvant radiation for STS < 5 cm in size [31]. Subcutaneous or intramuscular high-grade sarcomas less than 5 cm in size or for low-grade sarcoma of any size can be treated with surgery alone and are adequate if wide excision with a 1 cm margin of surrounding tissue can be obtained. However, it is important to note that data supporting these guidelines are from large, high-volume, and experienced centers.

10.1.5 Margin Status

Re-excision is preferred if margins are not clear after initial surgery. Several studies have noted higher recurrence rates after adjuvant radiation when margins are positive [32, 33]. A review of 100 patients with high-grade sarcoma and positive margins treated with surgery alone or surgery plus adjuvant radiation reported local recurrence rates of 56% and 74%, respectively [32]. Although adjuvant radiation reduces the recurrence risk in the setting of positive margins, the local control rate is inferior to what is observed in large series in which most patients underwent R0 resections [4, 5]. If a positive margin cannot be re-excised, it is recommended that the adjuvant radiation dose be escalated to a minimum of 64 Gy due to statistically significant improvements in local control, disease-free survival, and overall survival [33].

10.1.6 Radiation Therapy Alone for Unresectable Disease

In circumstances where surgery is precluded, radiation therapy may offer palliation in regard to local control. An early report by Tepper reported a 5-year local control rate of 33% in patients treated with external beam radiation therapy with doses ranging from 64 to 66 Gy [34]. This series was updated and the most recent report includes 112 patients that have been treated with definitive radiation therapy for gross disease. The 5-year local control rate was dependent on tumor size and dose. For lesions <5 cm, 5–10 cm, and >10 cm, the local control rates at 5 years were 51%, 45%, and 9%, respectively. In patients who received more than 63 Gy, the 5-year local control rate was 60% compared to 22% in patients receiving lower doses. Furthermore, higher dose resulted in improved 5-year DFS and OS. However, increasing the dose to >68 Gy was also associated with a higher rate of treatment complications (26% vs. 8%, $p = 0.02$) [35].

10.1.7 Specific Radiation Modalities

Brachytherapy and Intraoperative Radiation Therapy. Other radiation modalities, such as brachytherapy and intraoperative radiation therapy (IORT), are also effective in decreasing local recurrence after limb-sparing surgery. Brachytherapy is appealing due to its superior conformality compared to 2D and 3D radiation therapy and decreased treatment time compared to external beam radiation.

In general, reported rates of local control have been slightly lower than those reported with EBRT. At experienced centers the 5-year local control rates range from 82 to 84% [5, 36]. Other single institutions report slightly inferior local control rates (67–75%) [37–39]. Due to concerns that highly conformal treatment such as brachytherapy and IORT alone may not effectively treat subclinical areas at risk or areas of extra compartmental spread, some have examined the use of brachytherapy or IORT as a boost in combination with EBRT. Together these series demonstrate

5-year local control rates of 63–91.5% with wound healing complication rates of 12–34%. [30, 40–42].

IMRT/IGRT. Advances in treatment planning and delivery, such as intensity-modulated radiation therapy (IMRT), allow many centers the ability to deliver highly conformal treatment. A recent comparison of IMRT to brachytherapy found that IMRT provided improved 5-year local control rates in high-grade STS, 92% compared with 81% ($p = 0.04$), respectively. Yet the rate of significant wound complications was 19% with IMRT compared to 11% with brachytherapy. Complications requiring reoperation were observed in 2% of patients treated with IMRT compared with 6% for those treated with brachytherapy. Neither of these complication rates were significantly different [43].

10.2   Retroperitoneal Sarcomas

Retroperitoneal (RPS) and intra-abdominal soft tissue sarcomas account for approximately 14% of soft tissue sarcomas [44]. Therefore, one can estimate that up to 1200 retroperitoneal sarcomas occur annually in the United States. Sarcomas arising in the retroperitoneum are often large at the time of diagnosis. The relatively large size of these tumors along with frequently involved nearby critical organs often precludes a R0 resection, although in modern series complete resection (R0-R1) rates range from 80 to 90% [45–48]. Local failure is the predominant pattern of relapse and cause of morbidity and death in this disease [49].

10.2.1 Adjuvant Radiation

Radiation in either the pre- or postoperative setting is an appealing treatment modality due to the high local failure rates after surgery alone, which ranges from approximately 40 to 60% [45, 46, 48]. Adjuvant radiation therapy has been proven to be highly effective in STS of the extremity, and efforts have been made to translate this into the management of retroperitoneal sarcomas [50]. Technical concerns in delivering an effective dose of external beam radiation to the retroperitoneum postoperatively include uncertainty in the target volume, potential delays due to recovery from surgery, and dose limitations due to nearby structures such as the bowel or kidneys [51]. Therefore, postoperative trials have generally involved a combination of IORT or brachytherapy with EBRT.

In a small randomized trial that included 35 patients, 20 Gy IORT in combination with postoperative EBRT (35 to 40 Gy) was compared with postoperative EBRT alone (50 to 55 Gy). With a median follow-up of 8 years, there was no difference in overall survival, but local recurrences were more common with external beam radiation therapy alone at 80% compared to 40% in patients who received IORT [52]. In a single-institution prospective trial, 32 patients with primary or recurrent RPS were treated with maximal tumor resection, IORT, and postoperative EBRT when feasible. IORT was given to a dose of 12–15 Gy high-dose rate (HDR), and 78% of patients received additional EBRT to a dose of 45–50.4 Gy. The 5-year actuarial local control rate for the whole group was 62%. For patients with primary disease, the local control rate was 74% compared to 54% in patients with recurrent disease. The most frequent treatment complications included gastrointestinal obstruction (18%) followed by fistula formation (9%), peripheral neuropathy (6%), hydronephrosis (3%), and wound complication (3%) [53].

More recently, aggressive surgical approaches, mostly done in Europe, have improved local control rates [48, 54]. Since the implementation of frontline aggressive surgery (en bloc resection of tumor and involved organs), one center has reported a decrease in 5-year local recurrence rate from 48 to 28% [48]. Despite this more aggressive surgery, PORT has been shown to significantly improve recurrence-free survival at 5 years compared to surgery alone, 60% vs. 47%, respectively, with an adjusted hazard ratio of recurrence of 0.43 (95% CI, 0.20–0.88, $P = 0.02$).

10.2.2 Neoadjuvant Radiation

Preoperative radiation is an attractive option since it reduces the risk of tumor seeding at the time of resection and may improve the rate of gross total resection [55]. Furthermore, having the tumor in place allows better delineation of treatment volumes and targets, while the tumor itself displaces the bowel away from the high-dose area. A combined analysis of two prospective single-arm trials demonstrated that preoperative EBRT followed by surgical resection of RPS is feasible and safe. In addition, patients with intermediate- or high-grade RPS treated with preoperative radiation and surgery had a median survival >60 months, which compares favorably to historical controls [56–61]. Although the 5-year local recurrence-free survival rate was 60%, local failure remained the predominant pattern of recurrence [62].

Improvements in treatment delivery, such as the utilization of IMRT, allow preoperative dose escalation utilizing a dose-painting technique. In a report by Tzeng, patients received 45 Gy to the entire tumor with an integrated boost to the posterior retroperitoneal tumor margin of 57.5 Gy. The 2-year local control rate was 80%, with two recurrences out of 16 patients [63]. More novel approaches for dose escalation include the placement of mesh spacers to displace critical organs [64].

Due to the success of preoperative radiation with extremity sarcoma and results of the previously mentioned trials, accrual for phase III trials has been initiated. Unfortunately, ACOSOG Z-9031 was closed early due to poor accrual. The EORTC has an ongoing randomized trial which will hopefully further elucidate the role of preoperative radiation in RPS.

10.3 Desmoid Tumors/Aggressive Fibrosis

Complete excision, when possible, is the primary treatment for desmoid tumors [65, 66]. For small, asymptomatic aggressive fibromatosis, radiation therapy is often applied when the risk of recurrence or tumor growth would result in functional limitations [67, 68]. Factors influencing recurrence include tumor size, location (intra-abdominal vs. extremity), patient age, and margin status [68–70]. Albeit, margin status is controversial as some have demonstrated an increased risk of recurrence with positive margins [70–72] and others have not [69, 73, 74].

Definitive radiation therapy alone can be used in the setting of inoperable desmoid tumors of the extremity, head and neck, and superficial trunk as opposed to amputation. Local control at 3 years after external beam doses of at least 50 Gy ranges from 81.5 to 92% [73, 75]. The response to radiation therapy can be slow with tumor regression seen after 3 years [75]. In the absence of prior radiation, doses of 54–58 Gy should be used. Radiation is generally not recommended for retroperitoneal or intra-abdominal desmoid tumors.

10.4   Sarcomas of the Head and Neck

As in other sites, the mainstay of treatment for sarcomas of the head and neck is surgery. Postoperative radiation should be applied for low-grade tumors when margins are close (<1 cm) or positive and for all high-grade tumors [76]. Radical resection results in a high rate of local control for soft tissue sarcomas, but achieving this in the head and neck area is often not possible [29]. Wide margins may be obtained, but nevertheless the recurrence rates for high-grade STS after a wide local excision still approach 50% in several series [77–79]. Consequently, most patients are treated with adjuvant radiation, including those with low-grade lesions.

Patients who would likely have gross residual disease after surgery are appropriate candidates for upfront radiation treatment. If the lesion is likely to be resectable, the dose is 50 Gy followed by surgery 4–6 weeks after. One advantage of preoperative radiation treatment is that the risk of late complications may be decreased because a lower dose is applied. This is highly pertinent if radiation treatment is near the eyes or optic apparatus. If surgery will not be feasible, definitive radiation therapy to high doses should be used. In this event, the use of IMRT or proton beam therapy may reduce the risk of late complications when the tumor is in close proximity to dose-limiting normal tissues [80]. The outcomes for radiation alone for unresectable sarcomas are poor [34, 35].

10.5   Radiation for Salvage Treatment and Metastatic Disease

10.5.1   Salvage Treatment

In patients, who have an isolated local recurrence after surgery alone, multimodality aggressive therapy can be safely administered. Re-irradiation with external beam radiation combined with surgery for local recurrence should be used cautiously due to the high risk of complications and poor results. In a series of 62 patients treated with EBRT and surgery after previous irradiation, there was no benefit in regard to local control with the addition of radiation. Furthermore, complication rates were very high in patients who received re-irradiation compared to those who did not (80% vs. 17%, $p < 0.001$), and the amputation rate was also higher (35% with radiation vs. 11% without, $p = 0.05$) [81].

Re-irradiation with brachytherapy is a safer option. Twenty-six patients, who previously received external beam irradiation, were treated with surgery and brachytherapy. The mean dose of radiation prescribed at the implant procedure was 47.2 Gy +/− 1.6 Gy (range, 11.0–50.0 Gy). The 5-year local recurrence-free, distant recurrence-free, disease-free, and overall survival rates after brachytherapy were 52%, 75%, 33%, and 52%, respectively. Complications occurred in five patients: three had wound breakdown, one with osteonecrosis, and one with neuralgia [82]. Another series, with shorter follow-up, reported a local control rate of 100% at a median follow-up of 24 months after re-irradiation with brachytherapy [83].

10.5.2 Metastatic Disease

Radiation mainly plays a role in the palliation of metastatic disease for painful bony lesions. Fractionated stereotactic radiation therapy or radiosurgery has been demonstrated to be effective modalities for lung and spine metastases with local control rates ranging from 82 to 88% [84–86].

10.6 Bone Sarcomas

Primary malignancies of the bone are rare and represent less than 0.2% of all cancers [87]. Osteosarcoma, chondrosarcoma, and Ewing's sarcoma are the most common bone sarcomas. Bone sarcomas exhibit a wide range of clinical behaviors and have heterogeneous histologic and molecular profiles. Osteosarcoma is the most common primary malignancy of bone, occurring mainly during childhood and adolescence, which is concomitant with the period of most active skeletal growth. Osteosarcomas that occur in patients older than 40 years are typically associated with pre-existing conditions, such as Paget's disease or prior radiation exposure. Chondrosarcomas occur primarily in patients over 40 years of age.

Primary and metastatic bone tumors should be managed by a multidisciplinary team with the necessary expertise in surgical, radiation, and medical oncology. Surgery is the mainstay of treatment for most malignant bone tumors. Advances in surgical techniques including soft tissue and bone transfer, prostheses, and chemotherapy agents have contributed to the routine use of limb-sparing approaches rather than amputation. Local control for osteosarcomas and chondrosarcomas is typically incumbent upon wide excision with negative surgical margins. Radiation therapy is generally not used in the primary management of osteosarcomas and chondrosarcomas, but can be used for tumors not amenable to surgical resection or in the setting of positive margins. Palliative radiation therapy can be considered for unresectable metastatic or symptomatic local disease. Radiation therapy for unresectable osteosarcomas and chondrosarcomas requires high doses to limited treatment volumes while sparing surrounding normal tissues. Advanced techniques should be considered, including intensity-modulated radiation therapy and proton beam treatment.

10.6.1 Osteosarcoma

Historical experiences in the pre-chemotherapy era have demonstrated that high doses of radiation therapy can provide definitive treatment for osteosarcoma. In 1955, Cade reported complete responses to radiation therapy with subsequent delayed amputation for those who did not develop metastases [88]. Similarly, high doses of preoperative radiation therapy were shown to result in complete histologic responses in six of seven patients in a series reported in 1973 [89]. A dose response has been reported in one series, with all lesions controlled with doses greater than 90 Gy [90].

The current standard of care for osteosarcomas involves neoadjuvant chemotherapy followed by resection and additional chemotherapy. Definitive, adjuvant, and preoperative radiation therapy has been applied in highly selected cases, including when the tumor is subtotally resected, resected with positive margins, or when surgery would result in undue morbidity. In a study by Machak et al., 31 patients with extremity osteosarcomas were treated with induction chemotherapy followed by definitive radiation therapy after refusing surgical resection [91]. The 5-year local progression-free survival and overall survival were 56% and 61%, respectively. Local control was correlated with response to induction chemotherapy. Delaney reported their experience with 41 patients treated with radiation therapy for osteosarcomas that were not resected or excised with close or positive margins [92]. The local control rate at 5 years following gross total resection, subtotal resection, and biopsy alone was 78%, 78%, and 25%, respectively.

Radiation therapy has been applied for the management of osteosarcomas arising in anatomic sites in which wide surgical resection would result in loss of structural or functional integrity. The Cooperative Osteosarcoma Study Group reported their experience with 67 patients with pelvic osteosarcomas, including 30 patients who underwent intralesional surgery or no resection [93]. They reported improved survival in patients treated with radiation therapy if radical, wide, or marginal resections were not possible. In a study of 111 patients with mandibular osteosarcoma, 25 patients received postoperative radiation, including 13 patients who had incomplete resections [94]. There was no significant benefit of postoperative radiation after R1 resection, though the doses were less than 55 Gy in many cases which the authors concluded were inadequate. In contrast, Laskar found improved overall survival with the addition of radiation therapy following R1 or R2 resection for osteosarcomas of the head and neck [95].

10.6.2 Chondrosarcoma

Although chondrosarcomas are considered relatively radioresistant tumors, radiation therapy is used to maximize local control in selected situations. Radiation therapy can be indicated for chondrosarcomas when radical surgery is not possible or in the adjuvant setting following incomplete resections. Goda reported on 60 patients with extracranial chondrosarcomas treated with pre- or postoperative radiation therapy [96]. The median preoperative dose was 50 Gy and the median postoperative dose was 60 Gy. Following R0, R1, and R2 resections, the local control rates were 100%, 94%, and 42%, respectively. In a series from MD Anderson, 5 of 11 patients had local control with definitive radiation therapy with 40–70 Gy [97]. In a study using the National Cancer Database, 400 patients were treated for chondrosarcomas of the head and neck, of which 84 patients received combined surgery and radiation therapy, typically in the setting of positive margins. The disease-specific survival at 5 and 10 years for the entire cohort was 87% and 71%, respectively [98].

Proton beam and particle radiation therapy has been shown to result in high rates of local control and survival in resected chondrogenic tumors of the skull base and axial spine [99, 100]. Due to anatomic constraints in these areas, complete microscopic resection is often not feasible and adjuvant radiation is typically recommended. Proton therapy has the advantage of minimal dose in the exit beam, allowing for relative sparing of adjacent critical organs such as the spinal cord and brainstem. A series from Massachusetts General Hospital included 229 patients with chondrosarcomas of the skull base treated with a combination of photon and proton radiation therapy with doses of 66 to 83 cobalt gray equivalent (CGE) resulting in a 10-year local control rate of 94% [101]. Ares reported on 22 patients with skull base chondrosarcomas treated with proton radiation therapy with a 5-year local control rate of 94% and a 5-year freedom from high-grade toxicity rate of 94% [102]. Local control rates greater than 90% have also been reported using carbon ion radiation therapy [103, 104].

Since particle therapy is not universally available, stereotactic radiosurgery (SRS) and stereotactic body radiation therapy (SBRT) are alternative techniques for the treatment of skull base and spine chondrosarcomas [105]. In a study from Jiang, 16 patients with 12 cranial and 8 spinal lesions were treated with SRS or SBRT using 1–5 fractions to 22–30 Gy [106]. The 3-year actuarial control rate was 80% for primary tumors and 50% for recurrent tumors. Lower control rates were associated with metastatic, recurrent, and spinal tumors as well as tumors treated with lower doses. An example of a primary myxoid chondrosarcoma of the lumbar spine after resection and adjuvant SBRT is shown in (Fig. 10.2).

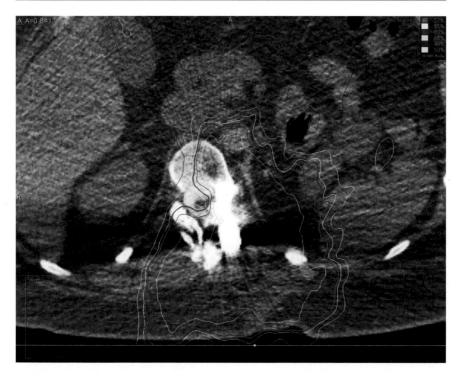

Fig. 10.2 A stereotactic body radiation therapy (SBRT) plan for a myxoid chondrosarcoma of the lumbar spine after resection and stabilization. A CT myelogram was used for planning. The pre-scription isodose line (red) was treated to 3000 cGy in 5 fractions. Note the conformality of the isodose lines around the spinal cord

10.7   Radiation Therapy Techniques

Due to the number of anatomic sites involved by sarcomas and the settings in which radiation therapy is indicated, a diversity of radiation therapy techniques must be utilized. These techniques include three-dimensional (3D) conformal planning, intensity-modulated radiation therapy (IMRT), particle beam radiation therapy, brachytherapy, intraoperative radiation therapy (IORT), and stereotactic body radiation therapy or stereotactic radiosurgery. Knowledge of the patterns of spread of sarcomas and the associated anatomic compartments is essential to radiation planning.

10.7.1 Treatment Volumes

Radiation therapy target volumes for sarcomas are primarily based on the physical examination, operative findings, radiology studies, and patterns of spread. Standardized target volume may not be suitable for all sarcoma histologies, and anatomic sites must be considered when defining target volumes. CT-based

Table 10.2 Suggested external beam radiation therapy treatment guidelines for extremity soft tissue sarcomas

Setting	Phase	Clinical target volume (CTV)	Dose (Gy)
Preoperative	Phase I	GTV + 4 cm longitudinal and 1.5 cm radial	50–50.4
	Phase II[a]	Original GTV + 2 cm longitudinal and 1.5 cm radial	16–26
Postoperative	Phase I	Surgical bed + 4 cm longitudinal and 1.5 cm radial[b]	45–50.4
	Phase II	Surgical bed + 2 cm longitudinal and 1.5 cm radial	10–16

GTV gross tumor volume
[a]If indicated for positive margins in the adjuvant setting
[b]Modified to include the surgical scar and drain exit scar if indicated

radiation therapy planning techniques are required. In the preoperative setting for extremity sarcomas, gross tumor volume (GTV) is optimally delineated based on the co-registration between a contrast-enhanced T1-weighted MRI and the planning CT scan since MRI better defines soft tissue as compared to CT [107]. The clinical tumor volume (CTV) is defined as the GTV plus a margin to account for subclinical disease spread. The optimal margin used to form the CTV has yet to be established, and the risks of missing tumor cells must be weighed against the risks of late toxicity. Peritumoral edema visualized on T2-weighted MRI images has been found to harbor tumor cells in a small study of patients reported by White [108]. The CTV has been previously defined as the GTV plus 3–4 cm longitudinal margins and 1.5 cm radial margins, which likely covers suspicious peritumoral edema in the majority of cases [109, 110]. The CTV should be edited based on clinical judgment if the suspicious edema extends beyond these margins. The CTV should also be modified to not extend beyond the end of the compartment in the longitudinal direction or the intact fascial or bone barriers. See Table 10.1. The CTV to planning target volume (PTV) expansion is dependent on the immobilization of the patient, treatment site, and daily imaging techniques. This margin should be individualized by institutions based on the setup variability that is observed.

For extremity sarcomas treated in the postoperative setting, a "shrinking field technique" is commonly used in which the tumor bed is targeted with a margin followed by a reduced field to the tumor bed with a smaller margin. See Table 10.2. The optimal margin around the tumor bed is the subject of controversy. Traditionally, a 5–7 cm margin in longitudinal direction around the tumor bed is utilized to field edge [9, 111]. The radial margins are typically 2–3 cm to the field edge and the surgical scar and drain sites are included. However, low local recurrence rates have been reported with more limited treatment volumes that exclude the scar using brachytherapy [5]. If the scar is being irradiated, bolus should be applied to ensure full dosing of the scar. Elective nodal radiation therapy is not routinely used given the low risk of lymph node involvement in most sarcomas. Regional lymph node radiation should be considered for epithelioid sarcoma, clear cell sarcoma, high-grade rhabdomyosarcoma, and synovial sarcoma.

Circumferential irradiation of the extremity should be avoided and at least 1 cm of tissue should be spared to reduce the risk of edema. At least half of the cross section of underlying weight-bearing bone should be spared and irradiating the entire joint should be avoided if possible. Treatment of the hand, foot, and forearm by high-energy photons may require the use of bolus or other techniques to ensure uniform dosing [112].

10.7.2 Dose

For adjuvant radiation therapy of extremity sarcomas, the initial treatment volume is usually irradiated to 45–50 Gy followed by an additional 10 Gy boost for negative margins or 16–18 Gy for microscopically positive margins. In the setting of gross residual disease, a boost of 20–26 Gy is often utilized if normal tissue can be adequately spared. See Table 10.2. Several studies have indicated a benefit for dose escalation, while others have failed to demonstrate an association [113–115]. In a retrospective series of 775 patients with soft tissue sarcomas treated with adjuvant radiation therapy, doses ≥64 Gy vs. < 64 Gy were independently associated with improved local control [116]. Local control rates were specifically improved with doses of 64–68 Gy for recurrent disease, head and neck or deep trunk tumor sites, and positive or uncertain margin status; higher doses did not completely abrogate the effects of positive margins. In the preoperative setting, 45–50 Gy is typically used for extremity sarcomas. A boost using external beam radiation therapy or IORT should be considered for positive margins if re-resection is not possible; however, investigators have questioned the benefit of a boost [117, 118]. With external beam radiation therapy, a boost of 16–18 Gy is used for microscopic disease and 20–26 Gy for gross residual disease.

10.7.3 Selected Techniques

Brachytherapy may be used as a stand-alone treatment or in combination with external beam radiation therapy following resection for sarcomas. Brachytherapy has also been used for re-irradiation after local recurrence [82]. Techniques include low-dose rate (LDR) brachytherapy with iridium-192 or iodine-125, fractionated high-dose rate (HDR) brachytherapy, or IORT high-dose rate therapy. HDR or LDR catheters are placed at intervals of 1–1.5 cm at the time of surgery to encompass the CTV with a margin, typically using a single-plane implant [119]. For LDR brachytherapy as monotherapy, doses of 45–50 Gy at 0.45 Gy per hour are used between 5 and 14 days after wound closure. When LDR brachytherapy is used as a boost to external beam radiation therapy, doses of 15–25 Gy at 0.45 Gy per hour are used. Intermediate- or high-grade sarcomas of the extremity or superficial trunk can be treated with brachytherapy as adjuvant monotherapy when the surgical margins are negative [38, 39, 119]. However, adjuvant brachytherapy alone should not be used if the CTV cannot be encompassed by the implant; if normal tissue tolerance cannot be met; in the setting of positive margins; or if there is evidence of cutaneous tumor spread. Adjuvant brachytherapy alone has been previously shown to not improve outcomes for low-grade sarcomas and is therefore not recommended [120].

IMRT has been increasingly utilized for the treatment of sarcomas, as it can spare normal tissue in close proximity to the tumor volume. In contrast to conventional radiation therapy techniques, IMRT enables variations in the radiation intensity within each beam by using advanced computer planning algorithms typically delivered using multileaf collimators on the treatment machine. Image-guided radiation therapy (IGRT) is another technology that has emerged that can reduce dose to the surrounding normal tissue. IGRT relies on daily imaging of the patient in the treatment position to improve targeting and reduce setup errors. IGRT allows for a reduction in the treatment volume since large fields are often required due to the uncertainty in treating sarcomas, especially in sites where rigid immobilization is not possible. Encouraging results have been demonstrated using IMRT and IGRT in the pre- and postoperative setting for sarcomas, and further study is warranted in larger patient cohorts [13, 43, 121]. See (Fig. 10.3a–b).

Stereotactic radiosurgery (SRS) and stereotactic body radiation therapy (SBRT) have a role in the treatment of sarcomas. SRS and SBRT utilize highly accurate and precise techniques to deliver high doses over a few number of treatment sessions, while sparing surrounding normal tissue. SRS refers to treatment in a single fraction, while SBRT is typically delivered in 2–5 fractions. These techniques are often delivered using a modified linear accelerator, which includes the CyberKnife (Accuray, Inc., Sunnyvale, CA). Studies have applied SRS or SBRT for metastatic sarcoma to the brain [122, 123], lung [85, 124], and spine [125–127].

10.7.4 Treatment Complications

Complication rates following radiation therapy for sarcomas can vary drastically and are related to the treatment site, tumor type, patient age, and patient medical history. The acute effects of radiation therapy typically include dermatitis, moist desquamation, and risks of wound complications. Patients are indefinitely at risk for late radiation-related sequelae, though the majority will develop within 5 years [128, 129]. Late complications include fibrosis, edema, bone fracture, decreased range of motion, lymphedema, and internal organ injuries.

Pre- or postoperative radiation therapy is associated with a risk of wound complications. See Table 10.3. In a National Cancer Institute of Canada (NCIC) study of 182 extremity sarcoma patients randomized to preoperative or postoperative radiation therapy, preoperative treatment resulted in a 35% wound complication rate as compared to 17% with postoperative radiation [20]. Factors associated with risks of wound complications following preoperative radiation therapy include lower extremity tumor location, increased age, and brachytherapy boost [130]. Adjuvant brachytherapy alone increased wound complication rates in a study of 105 patients with extremity and superficial truncal sarcomas to 44% as compared to 14% with surgery alone [131]. In contrast, adjuvant brachytherapy showed no significant

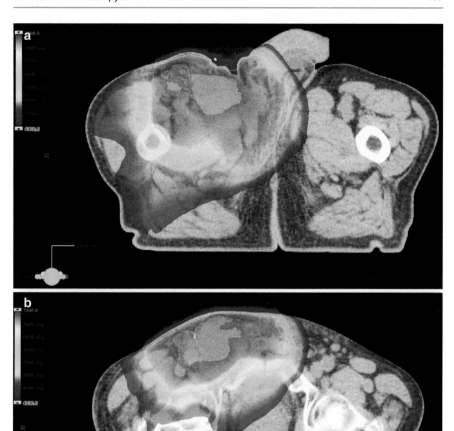

Fig. 10.3 (**a, b**) An intensity modulated radiation therapy (IMRT) plan for the adjuvant treatment of a recurrent high-grade spindle sarcoma of the groin. The gross tumor specimen measured 13 × 12 × 6 cm and was resected with microscopically positive margins. The prescribed cumulative dose was 6660 cGy over 37 fractions at 180 cGy per fraction using 6 MV photons. The treatment was delivered using daily image-guidance. The dose is depicted using a color wash; note the relative sparing of the adjacent critical structures including the genitalia and bone

difference in wound complications as compared to surgery alone when the brachytherapy was delayed until the fifth postoperative day [5].

In patients undergoing limb preservation surgery for soft tissue sarcomas with or without adjuvant radiation therapy, approximately 50% of patients have significant

Table 10.3 Wound complication rates associated with radiation therapy for soft tissue sarcomas

Treatment	Study	Patient (n)	RT dose (Gy)	Wound complications (%)
Preoperative RT	O'Sullivan et al. [20]	88	50	35
	Cannon et al. [137]	269	50 (range, 44–70)	34
	Pisters et al. [138]	26	50	23
Postoperative RT	O'Sullivan et al. [20]	94	66	17
	Cannon et al. [137]	143	60 (range, 50–72)	16
	Beane et al. [12]	70	63	17
Brachytherapy	Ormsby et al. [139]	21	45	14[a]
	Arbeit et al. [131]	54	30–50	44

RT radiation therapy, *NA* not applicable
[a]Wound complications defined as requiring operative intervention

functional impairments, but the frequency of disability is less [132]. The NCIC randomized trial reported higher rates of grade 2 or higher fibrosis (48% vs. 32%) and nonsignificantly increased rates of edema (23% vs. 15%) and joint stiffness (23% or 18%) in patients receiving postoperative radiation as compared to preoperative radiation. Field size predicted for fibrosis, joint stiffness, and edema [21]. Stinson found that treatment of more than 50% of the joint was associated with joint contracture, and doses greater than 63 Gy in the lower extremity were associated with increased moderate to severe edema rates [133]. Bone fractures can occur in 3–10% of patients following radiation therapy and limb preservation surgery [12, 134–136]. Pak found a dose-volume relationship that predicted for femoral neck fractures and found no fractures when the mean dose was under 40 Gy [136]. Novel radiation therapy techniques, including preoperative IGRT and IMRT, are being evaluated to minimize the risks of acute and late radiation-related complications.

10.8 Multidisciplinary Care

An experienced multidisciplinary team composed of members from radiation oncology, surgery, medical oncology, radiology, and pathology is required for management and selection of therapy for bone and soft tissue sarcomas. Additionally, the multidisciplinary sarcoma team facilitates greater staging accuracy and improved coordination of care. Modern radiation therapy techniques, such as IMRT, necessitate using advanced imaging modalities to aid in treatment planning. An MRI scan co-registered with CT simulation images should be used for planning preoperative radiation therapy for extremity STS to accurately account for the extent of disease. Consultation with an experienced radiologist can further aid the radiation oncologist in target delineation. Collaboration between the radiation oncologist and the surgeon is critical in the preoperative and postoperative setting to identify anatomic regions which are at high risk for recurrence to ensure appropriate targeting. In the postoperative setting, this includes leaving surgical clips to identify the operative bed for subsequent radiation therapy. A phase II study reported decreased wound and treatment morbidity by using the planned skin flaps identified by the surgeon as an avoidance structure for preoperative IMRT [13]. Given the complexity of radiation therapy for bone cancers and STS, multidisciplinary collaboration is essential.

References

1. Cantin J, et al. The problem of local recurrence after treatment of soft tissue sarcoma. Ann Surg. 1968;168(1):47–53.
2. Gerner RE, Moore GE, Pickren JW. Soft tissue sarcomas. Ann Surg. 1975;181(6):803–8.
3. Strander H, Turesson I, Cavallin-Stahl E. A systematic overview of radiation therapy effects in soft tissue sarcomas. Acta Oncol. 2003;42(5–6):516–31.
4. Yang JC, et al. Randomized prospective study of the benefit of adjuvant radiation therapy in the treatment of soft tissue sarcomas of the extremity. J Clin Oncol. 1998;16(1):197–203.
5. Pisters PW, et al. Long-term results of a prospective randomized trial of adjuvant brachytherapy in soft tissue sarcoma. J Clin Oncol. 1996;14(3):859–68.
6. Peiper M, Zurakowski D, Zornig C. Local recurrence of soft tissue sarcoma of the extremities and trunk. Langenbecks Arch Chir. 1995;380(6):333–9.
7. Keus RB, et al. Limb-sparing therapy of extremity soft tissue sarcomas: treatment outcome and long-term functional results. Eur J Cancer. 1994;30A(10):1459–63.
8. Suit HD, Russell WO, Martin RG. Sarcoma of soft tissue: clinical and histopathologic parameters and response to treatment. Cancer. 1975;35(5):1478–83.
9. Lindberg RD, et al. Conservative surgery and postoperative radiotherapy in 300 adults with soft-tissue sarcomas. Cancer. 1981;47(10):2391–7.
10. McNeer GP, et al. Effectiveness of radiation therapy in the management of sarcoma of the soft somatic tissues. Cancer. 1968;22(2):391–7.
11. Rosenberg SA, et al. The treatment of soft-tissue sarcomas of the extremities: prospective randomized evaluations of (1) limb-sparing surgery plus radiation therapy compared with amputation and (2) the role of adjuvant chemotherapy. Ann Surg. 1982;196(3):305–15.
12. Beane JD, et al. Efficacy of adjuvant radiation therapy in the treatment of soft tissue sarcoma of the extremity: 20-year follow-up of a randomized prospective trial. Ann Surg Oncol. 2014;21(8):2484–9.
13. O'Sullivan B, et al. Phase 2 study of preoperative image-guided intensity-modulated radiation therapy to reduce wound and combined modality morbidities in lower extremity soft tissue sarcoma. Cancer. 2013;119(10):1878–84.
14. Alektiar KM, Zelefsky MJ, Brennan MF. Morbidity of adjuvant brachytherapy in soft tissue sarcoma of the extremity and superficial trunk. Int J Radiat Oncol Biol Phys. 2000;47(5):1273–9.
15. Jebsen NL, et al. Radiotherapy to improve local control regardless of surgical margin and malignancy grade in extremity and trunk wall soft tissue sarcoma: a Scandinavian sarcoma group study. Int J Radiat Oncol Biol Phys. 2008;71(4):1196–203.
16. Koshy M, Rich SE, Mohiuddin MM. Improved survival with radiation therapy in high-grade soft tissue sarcomas of the extremities: a SEER analysis. Int J Radiat Oncol Biol Phys. 2010;77(1):203–9.
17. Clarkson P, Ferguson PC. Primary multidisciplinary management of extremity soft tissue sarcomas. Curr Treat Options Oncol. 2004;5(6):451–62.
18. Davis AM, et al. Function and health status outcomes in a randomized trial comparing preoperative and postoperative radiotherapy in extremity soft tissue sarcoma. J Clin Oncol. 2002;20(22):4472–7.

19. Maples WJ, Buskirk SJ. Multimodality treatment of upper extremity bone and soft tissue sar-comas. Hand Clin. 2004;20(2):vi. 221-5

20. O'Sullivan B, et al. Preoperative versus postoperative radiotherapy in soft-tissue sarcoma of the limbs: a randomised trial. Lancet. 2002;359(9325):2235–41.

21. Davis AM, et al. Late radiation morbidity following randomization to preoperative versus post-operative radiotherapy in extremity soft tissue sarcoma. Radiother Oncol. 2005;75(1):48–53.

22. Al-Absi E, et al. A systematic review and meta-analysis of oncologic outcomes of pre- ver-sus postoperative radiation in localized resectable soft-tissue sarcoma. Ann Surg Oncol. 2010;17(5):1367–74.

23. Chung PW, et al. Radiosensitivity translates into excellent local control in extremity myxoid liposarcoma: a comparison with other soft tissue sarcomas. Cancer. 2009;115(14):3254–61.

24. Eilber F, Eilber F, Giuliano A, Huth J, Mirra J, Rosen G, Morton D. Neoadjuvant chemo-therapy, radiation, and limited surgery for high grade soft tissue sarcoma of the extremity. In: Ryan JR, Baker LO, editors. Recent concepts in sarcoma treatment (proceedings of Internat Symp on sarcomas, Tarpan Springs, Florida, 1987). Dordrecht: Springer; 1988. p. 115–22.

25. DeLaney TF, et al. Neoadjuvant chemotherapy and radiotherapy for large extremity soft-tissue sarcomas. Int J Radiat Oncol Biol Phys. 2003;56(4):1117–27.

26. Kraybill WG, et al. Phase II study of neoadjuvant chemotherapy and radiation therapy in the management of high-risk, high-grade, soft tissue sarcomas of the extremities and body wall: Radiation Therapy Oncology Group Trial 9514. J Clin Oncol. 2006;24(4):619–25.

27. Yoon SS, et al. Angiogenic profile of soft tissue sarcomas based on analysis of circulating fac-tors and microarray gene expression. J Surg Res. 2006;135(2):282–90.

28. Yoon SS, et al. Phase II study of neoadjuvant bevacizumab and radiotherapy for resectable soft tissue sarcomas. Int J Radiat Oncol Biol Phys. 2011;81(4):1081–90.

29. Baldini EH, et al. Long-term outcomes after function-sparing surgery without radiotherapy for soft tissue sarcoma of the extremities and trunk. J Clin Oncol. 1999;17(10):3252–9.

30. Pisters PW, et al. Long-term results of prospective trial of surgery alone with selective use of radiation for patients with T1 extremity and trunk soft tissue sarcomas. Ann Surg. 2007;246(4):675–81. discussion 681-2

31. Geer RJ, et al. Management of small soft-tissue sarcoma of the extremity in adults. Arch Surg. 1992;127(11):1285–9.

32. Alektiar KM, et al. Adjuvant radiotherapy for margin-positive high-grade soft tissue sarcoma of the extremity. Int J Radiat Oncol Biol Phys. 2000;48(4):1051–8.

33. Delaney TF, et al. Radiation therapy for control of soft-tissue sarcomas resected with positive margins. Int J Radiat Oncol Biol Phys. 2007;67(5):1460–9.

34. Tepper JE, Suit HD. Radiation therapy alone for sarcoma of soft tissue. Cancer. 1985;56(3):475–9.

35. Kepka L, et al. Results of radiation therapy for unresected soft-tissue sarcomas. Int J Radiat Oncol Biol Phys. 2005;63(3):852–9.

36. Alektiar KM, et al. Adjuvant brachytherapy for primary high-grade soft tissue sarcoma of the extremity. Ann Surg Oncol. 2002;9(1):48–56.

37. Habrand JL, et al. Twenty years experience of interstitial iridium brachytherapy in the manage-ment of soft tissue sarcomas. Int J Radiat Oncol Biol Phys. 1991;20(3):405–11.

38. Chaudhary AJ, Laskar S, Badhwar R. Interstitial brachytherapy in soft tissue sarcomas. The Tata Memorial Hospital experience. Strahlenther Onkol. 1998;174(10):522–8.

39. Rosenblatt E, et al. Low dose-rate interstitial brachytherapy in soft tissue sarcomas. Sarcoma. 1999;3(2):101–5.

40. Beltrami G, et al. Limb salvage surgery in combination with brachytherapy and external beam radiation for high-grade soft tissue sarcomas. Eur J Surg Oncol. 2008;34(7):811–6.

41. Delannes M, et al. Low-dose-rate intraoperative brachytherapy combined with external beam irradiation in the conservative treatment of soft tissue sarcoma. Int J Radiat Oncol Biol Phys. 2000;47(1):165–9.

42. Niewald M, et al. Intraoperative radiotherapy (IORT) combined with external beam radiother-apy (EBRT) for soft-tissue sarcomas—a retrospective evaluation of the homburg experience in the years 1995-2007. Radiat Oncol. 2009;4:32.

43. Alektiar KM, Brennan MF, Singer S. Local control comparison of adjuvant brachytherapy to intensity-modulated radiotherapy in primary high-grade sarcoma of the extremity. Cancer. 2011;117(14):3229–34.
44. Brennan MF, et al. The role of multimodality therapy in soft-tissue sarcoma. Ann Surg. 1991;214(3):328–36. discussion 336-8
45. Strauss DC, et al. Surgical management of primary retroperitoneal sarcoma. Br J Surg. 2010;97(5):698–706.
46. Bonvalot S, et al. Aggressive surgery in retroperitoneal soft tissue sarcoma carried out at high-volume centers is safe and is associated with improved local control. Ann Surg Oncol. 2010;17(6):1507–14.
47. Perez EA, et al. Retroperitoneal and truncal sarcomas: prognosis depends upon type not location. Ann Surg Oncol. 2007;14(3):1114–22.
48. Gronchi A, et al. Aggressive surgical policies in a retrospectively reviewed single-institution case series of retroperitoneal soft tissue sarcoma patients. J Clin Oncol. 2009;27(1):24–30.
49. Ballo MT, et al. Retroperitoneal soft tissue sarcoma: an analysis of radiation and surgical treatment. Int J Radiat Oncol Biol Phys. 2007;67(1):158–63.
50. Swallow CJ, Catton CN. Local management of adult soft tissue sarcomas. Semin Oncol. 2007;34(3):256–69.
51. Stucky CC, et al. Excellent local control with preoperative radiation therapy, surgical resection, and intra-operative electron radiation therapy for retroperitoneal sarcoma. J Surg Oncol. 2014;109(8):798–803.
52. Sindelar WF, et al. Intraoperative radiotherapy in retroperitoneal sarcomas. Final results of a prospective, randomized, clinical trial. Arch Surg. 1993;128(4):402–10.
53. Alektiar KM, et al. High-dose-rate intraoperative radiation therapy (HDR-IORT) for retroperitoneal sarcomas. Int J Radiat Oncol Biol Phys. 2000;47(1):157–63.
54. Bonvalot S, et al. Primary retroperitoneal sarcomas: a multivariate analysis of surgical factors associated with local control. J Clin Oncol. 2009;27(1):31–7.
55. Zlotecki RA, et al. Adjuvant radiation therapy for resectable retroperitoneal soft tissue sarcoma: the University of Florida experience. Am J Clin Oncol. 2005;28(3):310–6.
56. Jaques DP, et al. Management of primary and recurrent soft-tissue sarcoma of the retroperitoneum. Ann Surg. 1990;212(1):51–9.
57. Lewis JJ, et al. Retroperitoneal soft-tissue sarcoma: analysis of 500 patients treated and followed at a single institution. Ann Surg. 1998;228(3):355–65.
58. Stoeckle E, et al. Prognostic factors in retroperitoneal sarcoma: a multivariate analysis of a series of 165 patients of the French Cancer Center Federation Sarcoma Group. Cancer. 2001;92(2):359–68.
59. Karakousis CP, et al. Retroperitoneal sarcomas and their management. Arch Surg. 1995;130(10):1104–9.
60. Ferrario T, Karakousis CP. Retroperitoneal sarcomas: grade and survival. Arch Surg. 2003;138(3):248–51.
61. Chiappa A, et al. Primary and recurrent retroperitoneal sarcoma: factors affecting survival and long-term outcome. Hepatogastroenterology. 2004;51(59):1304–9.
62. Pawlik TM, et al. Long-term results of two prospective trials of preoperative external beam radiotherapy for localized intermediate- or high-grade retroperitoneal soft tissue sarcoma. Ann Surg Oncol. 2006;13(4):508–17.
63. Tzeng CW, et al. Preoperative radiation therapy with selective dose escalation to the margin at risk for retroperitoneal sarcoma. Cancer. 2006;107(2):371–9.
64. Yoon SS, et al. Surgical placement of biologic mesh spacers prior to external beam radiation for retroperitoneal and pelvic tumors. Pract Radiat Oncol. 2013;3(3):199–208.
65. Lev D, et al. Optimizing treatment of desmoid tumors. J Clin Oncol. 2007;25(13):1785–91.
66. Ballo MT, et al. Desmoid tumor: prognostic factors and outcome after surgery, radiation therapy, or combined surgery and radiation therapy. J Clin Oncol. 1999;17(1):158–67.
67. Bonvalot S, et al. Extra-abdominal primary fibromatosis: aggressive management could be avoided in a subgroup of patients. Eur J Surg Oncol. 2008;34(4):462–8.

68. Fiore M, et al. Desmoid-type fibromatosis: a front-line conservative approach to select patients for surgical treatment. Ann Surg Oncol. 2009;16(9):2587–93.
69. Gronchi A, et al. Quality of surgery and outcome in extra-abdominal aggressive fibromatosis: a series of patients surgically treated at a single institution. J Clin Oncol. 2003;21(7):1390–7.
70. Peng PD, et al. Management and recurrence patterns of desmoids tumors: a multi-institutional analysis of 211 patients. Ann Surg Oncol. 2012;19(13):4036–42.
71. Huang K, et al. Prognostic factors for extra-abdominal and abdominal wall desmoids: a 20-year experience at a single institution. J Surg Oncol. 2009;100(7):563–9.
72. Stoeckle E, et al. A critical analysis of treatment strategies in desmoid tumours: a review of a series of 106 cases. Eur J Surg Oncol. 2009;35(2):129–34.
73. Gluck I, et al. Role of radiotherapy in the management of desmoid tumors. Int J Radiat Oncol Biol Phys. 2011;80(3):787–92.
74. Crago AM, et al. A prognostic nomogram for prediction of recurrence in desmoid fibromatosis. Ann Surg. 2013;258(2):347–53.
75. Keus RB, et al. Results of a phase II pilot study of moderate dose radiotherapy for inoperable desmoid-type fibromatosis—an EORTC STBSG and ROG study (EORTC 62991-22998). Ann Oncol. 2013;24(10):2672–6.
76. Balm AJ, et al. Report of a symposium on diagnosis and treatment of adult soft tissue sarcomas in the head and neck. Eur J Surg Oncol. 1995;21(3):287–9.
77. Enneking WF, Spanier SS, Goodman MA. Current concepts review. The surgical staging of musculoskeletal sarcoma. J Bone Joint Surg Am. 1980;62(6):1027–30.
78. Simon MA, Enneking WF. The management of soft-tissue sarcomas of the extremities. J Bone Joint Surg Am. 1976;58(3):317–27.
79. Parsons JT, et al. The role of radiotherapy and limb-conserving surgery in the management of soft-tissue sarcomas in adults. Hematol Oncol Clin North Am. 2001;15(2):377–88. vii
80. Mendenhall WM, et al. Adult head and neck soft tissue sarcomas. Head Neck. 2005;27(10):916–22.
81. Torres MA, et al. Management of locally recurrent soft-tissue sarcoma after prior surgery and radiation therapy. Int J Radiat Oncol Biol Phys. 2007;67(4):1124–9.
82. Pearlstone DB, et al. Re-resection with brachytherapy for locally recurrent soft tissue sarcoma arising in a previously radiated field. Cancer J Sci Am. 1999;5(1):26–33.
83. Catton C, et al. Soft tissue sarcoma of the extremity. Limb salvage after failure of combined conservative therapy. Radiother Oncol. 1996;41(3):209–14.
84. Folkert MR, et al. Outcomes and toxicity for hypofractionated and single-fraction image-guided stereotactic radiosurgery for sarcomas metastasizing to the spine. Int J Radiat Oncol Biol Phys. 2014;88(5):1085–91.
85. Dhakal S, et al. Stereotactic body radiotherapy for pulmonary metastases from soft-tissue sarcomas: excellent local lesion control and improved patient survival. Int J Radiat Oncol Biol Phys. 2012;82(2):940–5.
86. Stragliotto CL, et al. A retrospective study of SBRT of metastases in patients with primary sarcoma. Med Oncol. 2012;29(5):3431–9.
87. Siegel R, Naishadham D, Jemal A. Cancer statistics, 2013. CA Cancer J Clin. 2013;63(1):11–30.
88. Cade S. Osteogenic sarcoma; a study based on 133 patients. J R Coll Surg Edinb. 1955;1(2):79–111.
89. Allen CV, Stevens KR. Preoperative irradiation for osteogenic sarcoma. Cancer. 1973;31(6):1364–6.
90. Gaitan-Yanguas M. A study of the response of osteogenic sarcoma and adjacent normal tissues to radiation. Int J Radiat Oncol Biol Phys. 1981;7(5):593–5.
91. Machak GN, et al. Neoadjuvant chemotherapy and local radiotherapy for high-grade osteosarcoma of the extremities. Mayo Clin Proc. 2003;78(2):147–55.
92. DeLaney TF, et al. Radiotherapy for local control of osteosarcoma. Int J Radiat Oncol Biol Phys. 2005;61(2):492–8.
93. Ozaki T, et al. Osteosarcoma of the pelvis: experience of the Cooperative Osteosarcoma Study Group. J Clin Oncol. 2003;21(2):334–41.

94. Thariat J, et al. Osteosarcomas of the mandible: multidisciplinary management of a rare tumor of the young adult a cooperative study of the GSF-GETO, Rare Cancer Network, GETTEC/REFCOR and SFCE. Ann Oncol. 2013;24(3):824–31.
95. Laskar S, et al. Osteosarcoma of the head and neck region: lessons learned from a single-institution experience of 50 patients. Head Neck. 2008;30(8):1020–6.
96. Goda JS, et al. High-risk extracranial chondrosarcoma: long-term results of surgery and radiation therapy. Cancer. 2011;117(11):2513–9.
97. McNaney D, et al. Fifteen year radiotherapy experience with chondrosarcoma of bone. Int J Radiat Oncol Biol Phys. 1982;8(2):187–90.
98. Koch BB, et al. National cancer database report on chondrosarcoma of the head and neck. Head Neck. 2000;22(4):408–25.
99. Noel G, et al. Radiation therapy for chordoma and chondrosarcoma of the skull base and the cervical spine. Prognostic factors and patterns of failure. Strahlenther Onkol. 2003;179(4):241–8.
100. Austin-Seymour M, et al. Fractionated proton radiation therapy of cranial and intracranial tumors. Am J Clin Oncol. 1990;13(4):327–30.
101. Munzenrider JE, Liebsch NJ. Proton therapy for tumors of the skull base. Strahlenther Onkol. 1999;175(Suppl 2):57–63.
102. Ares C, et al. Effectiveness and safety of spot scanning proton radiation therapy for chordomas and chondrosarcomas of the skull base: first long-term report. Int J Radiat Oncol Biol Phys. 2009;75(4):1111–8.
103. Schulz-Ertner D, et al. Carbon ion radiotherapy of skull base chondrosarcomas. Int J Radiat Oncol Biol Phys. 2007;67(1):171–7.
104. Schulz-Ertner D, et al. Results of carbon ion radiotherapy in 152 patients. Int J Radiat Oncol Biol Phys. 2004;58(2):631–40.
105. Iyer A, et al. Stereotactic radiosurgery for intracranial chondrosarcoma. J NeuroOncol. 2012;108(3):535–42.
106. Jiang B, et al. CyberKnife radiosurgery for the management of skull base and spinal chondrosarcomas. J Neuro-Oncol. 2013;114(2):209–18.
107. Wang D, et al. Variation in the gross tumor volume and clinical target volume for preoperative radiotherapy of primary large high-grade soft tissue sarcoma of the extremity among RTOG sarcoma radiation oncologists. Int J Radiat Oncol Biol Phys. 2011;81(5):e775–80.
108. White LM, et al. Histologic assessment of peritumoral edema in soft tissue sarcoma. Int J Radiat Oncol Biol Phys. 2005;61(5):1439–45.
109. Bahig H, et al. Agreement among RTOG sarcoma radiation oncologists in contouring suspicious peritumoral edema for preoperative radiation therapy of soft tissue sarcoma of the extremity. Int J Radiat Oncol Biol Phys. 2013;86(2):298–303.
110. Haas RL, et al. Radiotherapy for management of extremity soft tissue sarcomas: why, when, and where? Int J Radiat Oncol Biol Phys. 2012;84(3):572–80.
111. O'Sullivan B, et al. The local management of soft tissue sarcoma. Semin Radiat Oncol. 1999;9(4):328–48.
112. Talbert ML, et al. Conservative surgery and radiation therapy for soft tissue sarcoma of the wrist, hand, ankle, and foot. Cancer. 1990;66(12):2482–91.
113. Mundt AJ, et al. Conservative surgery and adjuvant radiation therapy in the management of adult soft tissue sarcoma of the extremities: clinical and radiobiological results. Int J Radiat Oncol Biol Phys. 1995;32(4):977–85.
114. Pao WJ, Pilepich MV. Postoperative radiotherapy in the treatment of extremity soft tissue sarcomas. Int J Radiat Oncol Biol Phys. 1990;19(4):907–11.
115. Robinson M, et al. Treatment of extremity soft tissue sarcomas with surgery and radiotherapy. Radiother Oncol. 1990;18(3):221–33.
116. Zagars GK, Ballo MT. Significance of dose in postoperative radiotherapy for soft tissue sarcoma. Int J Radiat Oncol Biol Phys. 2003;56(2):473–81.
117. Tanabe KK, et al. Influence of surgical margins on outcome in patients with preoperatively irradiated extremity soft tissue sarcomas. Cancer. 1994;73(6):1652–9.

118. Al Yami A, et al. Positive surgical margins in soft tissue sarcoma treated with preoperative radiation: is a postoperative boost necessary? Int J Radiat Oncol Biol Phys. 2010;77(4):1191–7.
119. Nag S, et al. The American Brachytherapy Society recommendations for brachytherapy of soft tissue sarcomas. Int J Radiat Oncol Biol Phys. 2001;49(4):1033–43.
120. Pisters PW, et al. A prospective randomized trial of adjuvant brachytherapy in the management of low-grade soft tissue sarcomas of the extremity and superficial trunk. J Clin Oncol. 1994;12(6):1150–5.
121. Alektiar KM, et al. Impact of intensity-modulated radiation therapy on local control in primary soft-tissue sarcoma of the extremity. J Clin Oncol. 2008;26(20):3440–4.
122. Flannery T, et al. Gamma knife radiosurgery as a therapeutic strategy for intracranial sarcomatous metastases. Int J Radiat Oncol Biol Phys. 2010;76(2):513–9.
123. Powell JW, et al. Gamma Knife surgery in the management of radioresistant brain metastases in high-risk patients with melanoma, renal cell carcinoma, and sarcoma. J Neurosurg. 2008;109(Suppl):122–8.
124. Mehta N, et al. Safety and efficacy of stereotactic body radiation therapy in the treatment of pulmonary metastases from high grade sarcoma. Sarcoma. 2013;2013:360214.
125. Gill B, et al. Fiducial-free CyberKnife stereotactic body radiation therapy (SBRT) for single vertebral body metastases: acceptable local control and normal tissue tolerance with 5 fraction approach. Front Oncol. 2012;2:39.
126. Chang UK, et al. Stereotactic radiosurgery for primary and metastatic sarcomas involving the spine. J Neuro-Oncol. 2012;107(3):551–7.
127. Levine AM, Coleman C, Horasek S. Stereotactic radiosurgery for the treatment of primary sarcomas and sarcoma metastases of the spine. Neurosurgery. 2009;64(2 Suppl):A54–9.
128. Zagars GK, Mullen JR, Pollack A. Malignant fibrous histiocytoma: outcome and prognostic factors following conservation surgery and radiotherapy. Int J Radiat Oncol Biol Phys. 1996;34(5):983–94.
129. Jung H, et al. Quantification of late complications after radiation therapy. Radiother Oncol. 2001;61(3):233–46.
130. Bujko K, et al. Wound healing after preoperative radiation for sarcoma of soft tissues. Surg Gynecol Obstet. 1993;176(2):124–34.
131. Arbeit JM, Hilaris BS, Brennan MF. Wound complications in the multimodality treatment of extremity and superficial truncal sarcomas. J Clin Oncol. 1987;5(3):480–8.
132. Davis AM. Functional outcome in extremity soft tissue sarcoma. Semin Radiat Oncol. 1999;9(4):360–8.
133. Stinson SF, et al. Acute and long-term effects on limb function of combined modality limb sparing therapy for extremity soft tissue sarcoma. Int J Radiat Oncol Biol Phys. 1991;21(6):1493–9.
134. Dickie CI, et al. Bone fractures following external beam radiotherapy and limb-preservation surgery for lower extremity soft tissue sarcoma: relationship to irradiated bone length, volume, tumor location and dose. Int J Radiat Oncol Biol Phys. 2009;75(4):1119–24.
135. Livi L, et al. Late treatment-related complications in 214 patients with extremity soft-tissue sarcoma treated by surgery and postoperative radiation therapy. Am J Surg. 2006;191(2):230–4.
136. Pak D, et al. Dose—effect relationships for femoral fractures after multimodality limb-sparing therapy of soft-tissue sarcomas of the proximal lower extremity. Int J Radiat Oncol Biol Phys. 2012;83(4):1257–63.
137. Cannon CP, et al. Complications of combined modality treatment of primary lower extremity soft-tissue sarcomas. Cancer. 2006;107(10):2455–61.
138. Pisters PW, et al. Phase I trial of preoperative doxorubicin-based concurrent chemoradiation and surgical resection for localized extremity and body wall soft tissue sarcomas. J Clin Oncol. 2004;22(16):3375–80.
139. Ormsby MV, et al. Wound complications of adjuvant radiation therapy in patients with soft-tissue sarcomas. Ann Surg. 1989;210(1):93–9.

Chemotherapy and Multidisciplinary Approaches to Pediatric Sarcomas

AeRang Kim, Jeffrey S. Dome, and Holly J. Meany

Collectively, sarcomas represent 12% of cancers occurring in individuals between birth and 19 years of age; 60% are soft tissue sarcomas and 40% are bone sarcomas [1]. Soft tissue sarcomas may be broadly divided into two groups: rhabdomyosarcoma (RMS) and non-rhabdomyosarcoma soft tissue sarcomas (NRSTS). The two most common malignant primary bone sarcomas are osteosarcoma (OS) and Ewing sarcoma (ES). The incidence of sarcomas rises sharply from early childhood into adolescence, as shown in Fig. 11.1. An exception is a peak during infancy, largely explained by the occurrence of fibrosarcoma and other NRSTS in this age group. RMS occurs throughout a broad age range, with a peak incidence between age 1 and 4 years. NRSTS demonstrates the aforementioned peak in infancy followed by a nadir during the first decade of life and then an increase in adolescence and young adulthood. The peak incidence of both OS and ES is in the second decade of life.

The treatment of sarcomas has been a vexing challenge in the field of pediatric oncology. There has not been a demonstrable improvement in 5-year survival in any pediatric sarcoma type since 1990 [2]. Survival rates for patients with metastatic sarcomas have been especially disappointing despite the conduct of clinical trials that have introduced new chemotherapy agents into standard backbones of therapy. This chapter provides an overview of the workup and multidisciplinary treatment of the common pediatric bone and soft tissue sarcomas.

A. Kim, M.D., Ph.D. (✉) J.S. Dome, M.D., Ph.D. H.J. Meany, M.D.
Divisions of Hemaology and Oncology, George Washington Univeristy School of Medicine and Health Sciences, Children's National Health System, Washington, DC, USA
e-mail: aekim@childrensnational.org

© Springer International Publishing Switzerland 2017
R.M. Henshaw (ed.), *Sarcoma*, DOI 10.1007/978-3-319-43121-5_11

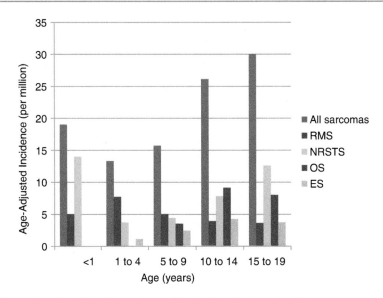

Fig. 11.1 Age-adjusted incidence (per million) of pediatric and adolescent sarcomas. *RMS* rhabdomyosarcoma, *NRSTS* non-rhabdomyosarcoma soft tissue sarcoma, *OS* osteosarcoma, *ES* Ewing sarcoma

11.1 Multidisciplinary Management of Sarcomas

The successful treatment of sarcomas involves numerous specialists, ideally working together in a coordinated manner. The need for a multidisciplinary approach begins at the time of diagnosis and extends through the treatment course. The diagnosis is typically made after a patient presents with symptoms and is referred for a radiology study. The radiologist can help distinguish between a benign or malignant process and advise on appropriate imaging studies to delineate the extent of disease. The diagnosis is confirmed via surgical biopsy or resection, performed by an orthopedic oncologist, general surgeon, or interventional radiologist, depending on the tumor site. The surgical approach should be planned with the medical and radiation oncologists, who can advise on the indications for neo-adjuvant therapy. Additionally, the pathologists should be apprised of the clinical and imaging features, so that an appropriate histologic and molecular workup may be undertaken. As described in the sections below, the therapy of sarcomas is multimodal, involving surgery, chemotherapy, and radiation therapy, so the different specialists have continued involvement throughout the treatment course. A successful functional and emotional outcome is also optimized by inclusion of nurses, physical therapists, social workers, psychologists, and child life specialists.

Recognizing the importance of a multidisciplinary approach, we established a Multidisciplinary Sarcoma Program at the Children's National Health System several years ago. The program includes oncologists, surgeons, radiologists, radiation oncologists, pathologists, nurses, physical therapists, biologists, social workers, and a genetic counselor. We hold bimonthly clinics that begin with a preclinic conference that includes a journal club, followed by radiology review and discussion of the patients who will be seen that day. Aside from fostering collaborative medical planning, the sarcoma clinic provides a logistical benefit for patients and families, who are able to have a "one-stop shopping" experience and see several specialists in a single clinic visit.

11.2   Bone Sarcomas

11.2.1 Osteosarcoma

OS is the most common primary bone cancer of childhood and adolescence. It is a tumor of malignant connective tissue that, by definition, produces osteoid. The World Health Organization (WHO) classification system recognizes the following histologic subtypes: conventional (osteoblastic, chondroblastic, and fibroblastic), telangiectatic, small cell, low-grade central, secondary, parosteal, periosteal, and high-grade surface [3]. Conventional OS, a high-grade tumor, is the most common variant seen in children and adolescents. With the exception of the low-grade central and parosteal types, all types of OS are treated with a combination of surgical resection and chemotherapy. The value of chemotherapy in the treatment of periosteal OS is an area of controversy.

11.2.1.1 Clinical Presentation and Evaluation
The most common sites of OS in children and adolescents are the femur (50%), tibia (26%), and humerus (10%) [4]. The axial skeleton may be involved, particularly in older individuals. Pain, which may be intermittent, is the most frequent presenting symptom. Swelling is another sign of OS, which may be minimal at first but becomes progressively worse over time. Approximately 10–20% of patients with newly diagnosed OS have distant metastases detectable on imaging studies. The lungs are by far the most common site of metastatic disease, followed by the bone. Other reported, but infrequent, locations of tumor spread include lymph nodes, the liver, the brain, and soft tissue [4–6].

The diagnostic workup of OS involves several imaging modalities. Plain films of the affected bone are a valuable initial tool. Typical radiologic features of OS include lytic, sclerotic, or mixed lesions that may be confined to the medullary canal but often destroy the cortex and elevate soft tissue. Osteoid produced by tumor cells appears cloudlike with ill-defined margins. Periosteal reaction, appearing as triangular-shaped elevations called Codman triangle, occurs frequently. The major limitation of plain films is their insensitivity in delineating the extent of tumor involvement. Magnetic resonance imaging (MRI) is more accurate in defining tumor extent, including skip lesions in distant areas of the affected bone, and anatomic relationships with muscle, nerves, and vessels. Computed tomography (CT) is also accurate in determining tumor extent, but MRI is recommended because it does not involve ionizing radiation [7, 8]. Radiologic studies are also critical to assess for distant metastases. Chest CT is the most sensitive way to detect lung metastases, though CT sometimes underestimates the burden of lung metastatic disease and, conversely, can detect nodules that are not confirmed to be tumor by biopsy. Bone scintigraphy, using technetium-99m-methylene diphosphonate (MDP), is the most commonly used technique to detect distant bone metastases. A comparison of fluorodeoxyglucose positron emission tomography (FDG-PET) with MDP bone scans found that for OS, the two techniques have similar sensitivity in detecting bone metastases [9]. However, for ES, PET scan was more sensitive. Functional imaging modalities, such as PET scans and dynamic contrast-enhanced MRI, have been used to predict OS responsiveness to chemotherapy, but this has not been adopted as standard of care at most centers [10–12].

Distinguishing between OS and other tumors or conditions requires a biopsy. The choice between open and percutaneous biopsy varies according to institutional preference. Open biopsies provide the greatest quantity of tissue for microscopic examination and the conduct of biology studies. Percutaneous biopsies, either core or needle, are less invasive and can be performed by an interventional radiologist with rapid recovery time. With either type of biopsy, the biopsy site should be planned with the orthopedic oncologist so that the biopsy tract can be excised at the time of definitive resection.

11.2.1.2 Surgery

Surgery was the first available therapy for OS and remains the centerpiece of treatment today. Once the diagnosis of OS is established, the current standard is to administer neo-adjuvant chemotherapy to treat micrometastatic disease and facilitate subsequent surgical resection. The surgical options for treating bone tumors are described in other chapters, but most patients undergo limb salvage procedures in which the affected portion of the bone is removed and replaced with an artificial implant (endoprosthesis), cadaveric bone graft (allograft), or both (allograft-prosthetic composite). A significant challenge in young patients is the small size of the limb and vessels and the amount of remaining skeletal growth. Approximately 5% of patients undergo amputation, usually when tumor resection cannot be accomplished with a limb salvage procedure. Another surgical option is rotationplasty, which involves resecting the distal femur but leaving an intact neurovascular bundle to the tibia. The tibia is then rotated so that the foot is inverted and fixated to the remaining femur, resulting in a functional joint (the ankle) to replace the knee. A removable prosthesis may then be fitted with good results. Regardless of the procedure performed, it is critically important to achieve complete surgical resection with negative margins, if possible.

Surgery also plays an important role in the treatment of pulmonary metastases. Although the outcome for patients with pulmonary metastases has traditionally been poor, surgical resection of both primary and metastatic diseases combined with chemotherapy has increased disease-free survival rates to 20–40%. After relapse, resection of metastases may significantly extend the survival time.

11.2.1.3 Radiation Therapy

OS is a radioresistant tumor that requires very high doses to achieve local control. As such, radiation therapy does not play a major role in initial management. However, there are settings in which radiation therapy may be employed to complement surgery in the setting of positive microscopic margins. Radiation therapy may be useful in the setting of unresectable tumors (especially of the spine) and for palliative care, to curtail tumor growth and alleviate symptoms [13].

11.2.1.4 Chemotherapy

Before the era of chemotherapy, 80% of patients with localized OS would develop pulmonary metastases despite complete tumor resection via radical amputation. In the 1970s, it was recognized that high-dose methotrexate, doxorubicin, and cisplatin have activity against osteosarcoma (reviewed in [14]). In 1978, the Mayo Clinic reported improved survival without chemotherapy, which was attributed to improved surgical techniques or a change in the natural history of OS [15]. As a result, adjuvant chemotherapy was not the definitive standard of care until prospective randomized trials firmly established the benefit of chemotherapy [16, 17]. In the mid-1970s, the Memorial Sloan Kettering Cancer Center pioneered the use of preoperative neoadjuvant chemotherapy with response-based chemotherapy after definitive surgical resection [18]. Purported advantages of this approach included the more immediate treatment of micrometastatic disease and the facilitation of surgical resection. Additionally, assessing tumor response to chemotherapy provided prognostic information such that poor histologic responders were found to have survival rates of only 40–50% compared to good responders, with survival rates >70% [4, 19]. However, attempts to improve the survival rate by increasing pre- or postoperative chemotherapy or changing chemotherapy agents after surgery have been unsuccessful [20].

Today, the most commonly used chemotherapy regimens for osteosarcoma include high-dose methotrexate, doxorubicin, and cisplatin (MAP), with or without ifosfamide. For localized disease, current regimens have resulted in durable event-free survival (EFS) estimates of 60–70% [4, 21, 22]. For metastatic disease, durable EFS is only 20–40% [4, 23, 24]. Table 11.1 summarizes impactful cooperative group trials for osteosarcoma that were reported in the past 10 years.

Recent clinical trials have evaluated novel approaches to improve outcomes. The INT-0133 study, conducted by the Children's Cancer Group (CCG) and the Pediatric Oncology Group (POG), posed two questions. The first question was to evaluate the benefit of adding muramyl tripeptide phosphatidyl ethanolamine (MTP-PE) to a chemotherapy backbone of MAP. MTP-PE, also called mifamurtide, is a synthetic lipophilic analogue of a mycobacterial cell wall component that potentiates the immune system by activating monocytes and macrophages. Mifamurtide showed activity against OS in preclinical models and in early-phase clinical trials. The second question was to evaluate the benefit of adding ifosfamide to the standard MAP backbone (MAPI). The study was conducted using a 2×2 factorial design resulting in four treatment arms: MAP±mifamurtide and MAPI±mifamurtide. The initial findings of the study found that adding ifosfamide made no difference in event-free survival (EFS) for patients with localized OS [19]. Addition of mifamurtide made no difference in EFS in the MAP arm but seemed to improve EFS in the MAPI arm. This suggested an interaction between ifosfamide and mifamurtide. However, longer-term follow-up did not observe this interaction [21]. Longer follow-up confirmed that adding ifosfamide had no impact on EFS or overall survival (OAS).

Table 11.1 Recent cooperative group chemotherapeutic trials in patients with osteosarcoma

Study	Hypothesis	Patients	Results	Conclusion
INT-0133 [21, 24]	Randomized study to test whether ifosfamide or mifamurtide improves outcome of patients with osteosarcoma treated with methotrexate, doxorubicin, and cisplatin (MAP)	Localized: n = 662	−Ifos: 6 years EFS: 63%	Ifosfamide did not improve EFS or OAS
			+Ifos: 4 years EFS: 64%	For localized disease, mifamurtide showed a statistically significant improvement in OAS and a trend toward improvement in EFS
			−Ifos: 6 years OAS: 73%	
			+Ifos: 6 years OAS: 75%	
			−mifamurtide: 6 years EFS: 61%	
			+mifamurtide: 6 years EFS: 67%	
			−mifamurtide: 4 years OAS: 70%	
			+ mifamurtide: 4 years OAS: 78%	
		Metastatic: n = 91	−Ifos: 4 years EFS: 35%	
			+Ifos: 4 years EFS: 34%	
			−Ifos: 4 years OAS: 52%	
			+Ifos: 4 years OAS: 43%	
			−mifamurtide: 5 years EFS: 26%	
			+mifamurtide: 5 years EFS: 42%	
			−mifamurtide: 5 years OAS: 40%	
			+mifamurtide: 5 years OAS: 53%	

Table 11.1 (continued)

Study	Hypothesis	Patients	Results	Conclusion
EURAMOS [20, 25]	**Good histologic response (>90% necrosis):** randomized study of maintenance therapy with pegylated interferon in addition to MAP	Good histologic response (localized and resectable metastatic): $n = 716$	MAP: 3 years EFS: 74%	Neither interferon nor ifosfamide/ etoposide improved outcomes
			MAP-IFN: 3 years EFS: 77%	
			MAP: 5 years OAS: 81%	
			MAP-IFN: 5 years OAS: 84%	
	Poor histologic response (<90% necrosis): randomized study of ifosfamide/etoposide in addition to MAP	Poor histologic Response (localized and resectable metastatic): $n = 615$	MAP: 3 years EFS: 54%	
			MAPIE: 3 years EFS: 52%	
			MAP: 5 years OAS: 68%	
			MAPIE: 5 years OAS: 66%	
SFOP-OS94 [145]	Randomized comparison of pre-op chemotherapy with MTX/Dox versus Ifos/etoposide/MTX for localized disease. Good histologic response continued same therapy post-op. Poor histologic responders had post-op therapy altered to include other active agents	Localized disease: $n = 234$	5 years EFS: 62%	MTX/Ifos/etoposide yielded a higher rate of good histologic responders than MTX/Dox. There was no significant difference in survival between the arms, but a trend toward improved EFS in the MTX/Ifos/etoposide arm
			5 years OAS: 76%	
ISG-OS1 [22]	Randomization for patients with nonmetastatic OS to receive preoperative MAP chemotherapy versus MAP with ifosfamide. Postoperatively, patients in the MAP arm received Ifos only for poor histologic response. Patients in the MAPI arm received ifosfamide postoperatively regardless of response	Localized disease: $n = 246$	MAP: 5 years EFS: 64%	Ifosfamide did not provide a benefit for EFS or OAS
			MAPI: 5 years EFS: 55%	
			MAP: 5 years OAS: 73%	
			MAPI: 5 years OAS: 74%	

EFS event-free survival, *OAS* overall survival, *MTX* methotrexate, *Dox* doxorubicin, *Ifos* ifosfamide, *MAP* methotrexate/doxorubicin/cisplatin, *MAPI* methotrexate/doxorubicin/cisplatin/ifosfamide *IFN* interferon

However, there was a suggestion that mifamurtide modestly improved EFS (6-year EFS 67% versus 61%, $p = 0.08$) and OAS (6-year OAS 78% versus 70%). For metastatic disease, the pattern of benefit for ifosfamide and mifamurtide was the same: there was clearly no benefit for ifosfamide, but there was a suggestion, though not statistically significant, that mifamurtide improved EFS and OAS [24]. Mifamurtide has been approved for use in Europe, but is not approved by the Food and Drug Administration in the United States.

The recently completed EURAMOS study, an international collaboration between the Children's Oncology Group (COG), German-Austrian-Swiss Cooperative Osteosarcoma Group (COSS), European Osteosarcoma Intergroup (EOI), and Scandinavian Sarcoma Group (SSG), also addressed two questions. Patients with a good histologic response to chemotherapy, defined as a necrosis rate >90% after 10 weeks of preoperative MAP chemotherapy, continued MAP for a total of 29 weeks of therapy and were randomized to stop therapy or receive a maintenance phase with pegylated interferon alfa-2b [25]. The study showed no improvement in EFS with interferon, though many patients discontinued interferon early. Patients with a poor histologic response to chemotherapy were randomized to continue MAP therapy or receive MAP with ifosfamide and etoposide (MAPIE) [20]. There was no EFS or OS benefit with the MAPIE arm, though more toxicity and second malignancies were observed.

11.2.1.5 Experimental Therapeutics/Targeted Agents

Phase 2 trials for OS included studies of topotecan, imatinib, oxaliplatin, ixabepilone, docetaxel, iproplatin, irinotecan, and rebeccamycin [26]. Aside from docetaxel, which produced 1 complete response and 1 partial response among 21 evaluable patients, there were no objective responses [27]. Several case series have reported objective responses in recurrent OS to the gemcitabine/docetaxel combination, and this combination is commonly used in the treatment of recurrent OS [28–30]. Phase 2 studies of trastuzumab, an anti-HER2 antibody, and inhaled granulocyte-monocyte stimulating factor (GM-CSF) did not show evidence of activity for metastatic or recurrent OS, respectively [31, 32]. Current studies are evaluating the bisphosphonate zoledronic acid for metastatic OS. A previous study found that administration of zoledronic acid with chemotherapy is feasible [33]. Current and future studies will evaluate the activity of eribulin (novel microtubule inhibitor), denosumab (monoclonal antibody directed against receptor activator of nuclear factor kappa B ligand, RANKL), dinutuximab (anti-GD2 antibody), and glembatumumab vedotin (targets a transmembrane glycoprotein) [26].

11.2.1.6 Recurrent Disease

Most recurrences of OS occur in the lungs (~75%), followed by distant bone (~15%) and local bone (~10%) [34]. Durable survival rates following recurrence are only 20–35% [35, 36]. Surgery plays a crucial role in the management of recurrence. Numerous studies have confirmed the benefit of resecting pulmonary metastases, both in terms of OAS rate and duration of survival [37]. In some cases, multiple thoracotomies are necessary to achieve a long-term cure. Although responses to chemotherapy are observed, the effect of chemotherapy on long-term survival in recurrent OS remains undefined.

11.2.2 Ewing Sarcoma

First described by James Ewing in 1921, Ewing sarcoma (ES) is a tumor derived from mesenchymal cells. ES is the second most common primary malignant bone cancer with approximately 225 new cases diagnosed annually in patients less than 20 years of age in North America. Compared to osteosarcoma, ES tends to occur more frequently in the axial skeleton and arise from the diaphyseal region of the bone but may also arise in the soft tissues. The most common primary tumor sites are the long bones of the lower extremities, pelvic bones, and the bones of the chest wall. Metastatic disease, present in approximately 25% of patients with ES, typically involves the lungs, bone, bone marrow, or a combination of these sites.

The most common age of diagnosis is the second decade of life, although 20%–30% of cases are diagnosed in the first decade, with a slight male predominance. ES more frequently affects Caucasian patients as compared to Asians, African-Americans, or Africans [38–42].

11.2.2.1 Clinical Presentation and Evaluation

Local pain followed by swelling or a palpable mass is often the initial presenting symptom though, based on the affected site, specific symptoms will vary. Fever, fatigue, loss of appetite, weight loss, and other nonspecific symptoms may occur but are more common in more advanced or metastatic disease.

Initial imaging should include plain radiographs of the involved region, which classically demonstrate a lamellated or "onionskin" periosteal reaction. A lytic lesion with spiculated periosteal reaction or detachment of the periosteum from the bone (Codman triangle) can also be associated with ES. Additional evaluation of the primary site with MRI delineates the full extent of bone and soft tissue involvement as well as the relationship of the tumor to surrounding structures.

Tissue biopsy is the preferred method to confirm the diagnosis. Histologically, ES is a small round blue cell tumor characterized by membrane expression of CD99 with positivity for vimentin by immunohistochemical analysis. A reciprocal chromosomal translocation involving the *EWS* gene on chromosome 22 and an *ETS*-type gene, most commonly the *FLI 1* gene on chromosome 11 [t(11;22) (q24;q12)], is present in greater than 85% of Ewing tumors. These pathognomonic translocations can be detected using fluorescence in situ hybridization and/or reverse transcription-polymerase chain reaction and add confirmation to the histologic diagnosis.

Patients with ES are classified as having either localized or metastatic disease. Metastatic evaluation includes bone scintigraphy, bone marrow aspirates and biopsies, and a chest CT scan. FDG-PET imaging is more frequently being incorporated into the metastatic workup for patients with ES as it has been shown to provide important diagnostic information as well as correlation to response to chemotherapy and outcome [43–46]. Current cooperative group clinical trials are prospectively evaluating the utility of FDG-PET.

The presence of metastatic disease, older age at diagnosis, axial primary tumor, and larger tumor size have been shown to be independent negative prognostic factors in multivariate analysis [47, 48]. Other studies have suggested features such as male sex, fever, anemia, high-serum LDH level, and type of chemotherapy regimen may also be prognostic [49]. For the group of patients with metastatic disease, there was a trend for better survival in those with lung involvement compared with those with bone metastases or a combination of lung and bone metastases [50].

11.2.2.2 Treatment Overview

Treatment for ES includes systemic, multi-agent chemotherapy as well as local control with surgical resection, radiation therapy, or a combination of these two modalities. An interdisciplinary team including medical oncology, orthopedic surgery, and radiation oncology is advisable to determine the optimal treatment plan aiming to maximize antitumor effect and minimize acute and late adverse effects [41]. Patients with localized ES have a 5-year overall survival of 65% to 75%. Patients with metastatic disease have a significantly lower 5-year overall survival of <30%, with the exception of those with isolated pulmonary metastasis where overall survival ranges 30–50% [40, 50].

11.2.2.3 Surgery

Surgery is the most commonly used form of local control. Patients with an isolated, resectable tumor after induction chemotherapy typically go on to have surgical resection of their primary tumor, a limb salvage procedure in the case of extremity bone lesions. The aim of surgery is resection with negative margins defined in pediatric protocols as bony margins of at least 1 cm, with a 2–5 cm margin recommended. For soft tissue tumors, at least 5 mm in fat or muscle with 2 mm through fascial planes is required. When complete surgical resection with pathologically negative margins is achieved, postoperative radiation therapy is not required.

11.2.2.4 Radiation Therapy

Radiation therapy is an effective method of local control for patients in ES [51–53]. Typically radiation is utilized for patients in whom surgical resection with negative margins cannot be achieved or when surgical resection would be deforming or particularly morbid. Radiation is recommended for metastatic sites that are not completely resected, including whole-lung radiation for patients with pulmonary disease at diagnosis and radiation to involved, unresected lymph nodes. The ongoing Euro-Ewing study is randomizing patients with lung metastases to receive high-dose therapy with autologous stem cell transplant (ASCT) versus pulmonary radiation.

11.2.2.5 Chemotherapy

Early trials demonstrated chemotherapy regimens incorporating vincristine, doxorubicin, cyclophosphamide, and actinomycin D to be active in patients with ES, particularly for localized disease (Table 11.2) [54]. The addition of ifosfamide

Table 11.2 Recent chemotherapeutic trials in patients with Ewing sarcoma

Study	Hypothesis	Patients		Results	Conclusion
United Kingdom Children's Cancer Study Group (UKCCSG) and the Medical Research Council Bone Sarcoma Working Party Ewing's Tumour Study (ET-1), 1978–1986 [54]	Vincristine, cyclophosphamide, doxorubicin, actinomycin D with radiotherapy ± surgery to the primary tumor	120 patients with localized disease		45 remain alive (median follow-up 11.2 years)	Long-term survival has improved in patients treated for ES
		22 patients with metastatic disease		2 remain alive	
Cooperative Ewing's Sarcoma Study (CESS) 86, 1986–1991 [55]	Vincristine, cyclophosphamide, doxorubicin, actinomycin D in standard-risk patients, and ifosfamide in place of cyclophosphamide in high-risk patients (large or central axis tumors)	301 patients with localized disease	Standard-risk group $n = 52$	10-year EFS = 52%	High-risk patients seem to have benefited from intensified treatment that included ifosfamide
			High-risk group $n = 241$	10-year EFS = 51%	
National Cancer Institute protocol INT-0091 (CCG-7881 and POG-8850), 1988–1992 [56]	Randomized trial adding ifosfamide and etoposide to standard chemotherapy (doxorubicin, vincristine, cyclophosphamide, dactinomycin) in patients with ES	398 patients with localized disease	Standard therapy group $n = 200$	5-year EFS = 54 ± 4%	The addition of ifosfamide and etoposide significantly improved outcome for patients with localized disease
				5-year OAS =61 ± 3.6%	
			Experimental therapy group $n = 198$	5-year EFS = 69 ± 3%	
				5-year OAS = 72 ± 3.4%	
		120 patients with metastatic disease	Standard therapy group $n = 62$	5-year EFS = 22 ± 6%	
				5-year OAS = 35%	
			Experimental therapy group $n = 58$	5-year EFS = 22 ± 5%	
				5-year OAS = 34%	

(continued)

Table 11.2 (continued)

Study	Hypothesis	Patients		Results	Conclusion
Children's Oncology Group phase 3 protocol AEWS0031, 2001–2005 [57]	Randomized controlled trial of intensification through interval-compressed chemotherapy (vincristine-doxorubicin-cyclophosphamide and ifosfamide-etoposide) in patients with localized ES	568 patients with localized disease	Standard therapy group $n = 284$	5-year EFS = 65%	Intensification through interval-compressed chemotherapy is more effective than chemotherapy administered every 3 weeks, without increase in toxicity
			Intensified therapy group $n = 284$	5-year EFS = 73% ($p = 0.048$)	

EFS event-free survival, *OAS* overall survival

[55] and, later, ifosfamide and etoposide [56] significantly improved outcomes for patients with localized disease, even those considered at higher risk (central axis primary tumor location and large initial tumor volume). A recent Children's Oncology Group (COG) randomized phase 3 trial evaluated chemotherapy dose intensification through interval compression in patients with localized ES. Patients received cycles of vincristine, doxorubicin, and cyclophosphamide alternating with ifosfamide and etoposide administered every 21 days (standard therapy arm) or every 14 days (intensified therapy arm). Local control included surgery and/or radiation therapy. A statistically significant difference was observed in the 5-year EFS between the standard and intensified arms, 65% and 73%, respectively ($p = 0.048$). Importantly the toxicity of the regimens was similar [57]. This interval-compressed backbone is now considered the standard therapy for localized disease in North America.

ES patients with metastatic disease at presentation and patients with disease recurrence remain a challenge. High-dose chemotherapy with ASCT has been evaluated in these groups, but results are inconclusive. Select studies suggest benefit in small patient cohorts, but with significant toxicity [58–60]. A larger European study demonstrated a 3-year EFS of 27% and 3-year OAS of 34% in patients with metastatic ES following induction chemotherapy, local control, then high-dose chemotherapy with busulfan and melphalan, and ASCT [61]. A risk-stratified treatment approach for high-dose therapy was developed from this study based on prognostic factors.

In an effort to improve outcomes, clinical trials for patients with newly diagnosed ES are ongoing. In the COG AEWS1031 study, patients with localized disease receive the standard interval-compressed backbone of vincristine, doxorubicin, cyclophosphamide, ifosfamide, and etoposide, with a randomization to receive or not receive vincristine, topotecan, and cyclophosphamide.

11.2.2.6 Experimental Therapeutics/Targeted Agents

In patients with metastatic ES, a phase 2 randomized trial will compare disease response following a standard therapy arm of interval-compressed multi-agent chemotherapy to an experimental arm with interval-compressed multi-agent chemotherapy and the addition of ganitumab (AEWS1221). Ganitumab is a fully human monoclonal antibody directed against the insulin-like growth factor receptor 1 (IGF-1R). Early studies have demonstrated response in ES following single-agent IGF-1R therapy [62, 63].

Other therapies are undergoing evaluation in patients with recurrent ES including antiangiogenesis agents (bevacizumab), small-molecule tyrosine kinase inhibitors (cabozantinib), inhibitors of the insulin receptor and IGF-1R (linsitinib), poly (ADP-ribose) polymerase (PARP) inhibitors (olaparib), and immunotherapeutic approaches such as anti-GD2 monoclonal antibody therapy and cancer vaccine trials.

11.3   Soft Tissue Sarcomas

11.3.1 Rhabdomyosarcoma

RMS is the most common sarcoma in children less than 20 years of age and accounts for approximately 40% of all pediatric soft tissue sarcomas [64]. Although RMS can arise anywhere in the body, certain locations can be more common based on age and subtype, and clinical signs and symptoms correlate with site of disease. The overwhelming majority of RMS occurs sporadically with no known predisposing factors; however, the development of RMS has been associated with tumor predisposition syndromes such as Li-Fraumeni Syndrome [65], neurofibromatosis type 1 [66], Costello syndrome [67], and DICER1 mutations [68].

The WHO describes four subtypes of RMS, embryonal (ERMS), alveolar (ARMS), pleomorphic, and spindle cell/sclerosing [3]. Each type has distinct molecular, genetic, and clinical features. The majority of ARMS are characterized by translocations between the FOXO1 gene on chromosome 13 and either the PAX3 gene on chromosome 2 [t(2;13) (q35;q14)] or PAX7 gene on chromosome 1 [t(1;13) (p36;q14)] [69]. ERMS is characterized by LOH at the 11p15 locus suggesting tumorigenesis by inactivation of a tumor suppressor gene [70]. Genes with recurring mutations include those in the RAS pathway, observed in one-third of cases [71]. Identifying translocations may be of prognostic significance as there are data that demonstrate that ARMS carrying translocation behaves differently from ARMS that does not and from ERMS [72, 73]. In young children, the spindle cell subtype has recurring chromosomal rearrangements involving the *NCOA2* gene and is associated with favorable outcome [74]. Importantly, gene expression of tumors will likely play important roles in classification, stratification of treatment, and identification of new potential therapies.

General principles of RMS therapy begin with histologic diagnosis (± molecular subtyping), primary site and extent of disease, and extent of surgical resection [75]. Cooperative groups have defined risk-adapted treatments requiring a multidisciplinary approach including surgery, chemotherapy, and usually radiation. The two major staging systems developed by the Intergroup Rhabdomyosarcoma Study Group (IRSG) are site-modified TNM staging system (stage) and pathologic extent of resection (group) detailed in Tables 11.3 and 11.4 [76, 77]. The COG Soft Tissue Sarcoma (STS) Committee defines low-, intermediate-, and high-risk groups based on the clinical stage, group, and histology (Table 11.5) [78].

11.3.1.1 Surgery

The aim of surgery should be for complete surgical resection whenever possible at diagnosis without causing major function or cosmetic defects [75]. This is not feasible for many RMS, particularly when located in parameningeal, orbital, and genitourinary areas. For tumors where complete surgical resection is not possible due to location, size, or invasion, biopsy should be undertaken to determine histology.

Table 11.3 Intergroup Rhabdomyosarcoma Study Group (IRSG) staging system [12, 13]

Stage	Sites	Tumor size	Lymph node	Metastasis
1	Orbit, non-PM	Any	N0, N1	M0
	Head/neck			
	GU-non-bladder/prostate			
	Biliary tract/liver			
2	All other	≤ 5 cm	N0	M0
3	All other	≤ 5 cm	N1	M0
		>5 cm	N0 or N1	
4	Any	Any	N0 or N1	M1

Abbreviations: *N0* no regional lymph nodes clinically involved, *N1* regional lymph nodes clinical involved, *M0* no distant metastasis, *M1* distant metastasis

Table 11.4 Intergroup Rhabdomyosarcoma Study Group (IRSG) grouping system [12]

Group	Extent of disease and surgical result
I	Localized tumor, completely resected
II	Localized tumor, grossly removed with
	(a) Microscopic margins
	(b) Involved regional lymph nodes
	(c) Both a and b
III	Localized tumor with gross residual disease or biopsy only
IV	Distant metastasis present at diagnosis (including positive cytology in CSF/pleural/peritoneal fluid) regardless of surgical approach

Table 11.5 COG rhabdomyosarcoma risk groups [14]

Risk	5-year FFS %	Stage	Group	Histology
Low, subset 1	90	1 or 2	I or II	ERMS
		1	III orbit	ERMS
Low, subset 2	87	1	III non-orbit	ERMS
		3	I or II	ERMS
Intermediate	65–73	2 or 3	III	ERMS
		1, 2, or 3	I, II, or III	ARMS
High	<30	4	IV	ERMS/ARMS

Abbreviations: *FFS* failure-free survival, *ERMS* embryonal rhabdomyosarcoma, *ARMS* alveolar rhabdomyosarcoma

There does not appear to be significant benefit in debulking operations on progression free or overall survival in RMS [79]. For tumors that are incompletely resected upfront, but have potential for complete resection, primary re-excision is often recommended as improvement in survival can be produced by primary surgical re-excision if feasible [80].

Surgery may also be used in a delayed primary excision (DPE) or as second-look surgery either during or at the end of therapy. DPE following induction chemotherapy may allow for reduced doses of radiation therapy without affecting local control outcomes [81]. Second-look surgeries of residual tumor either during or at the end of therapy have previously been evaluated. Persistence of radiographic masses at the end of therapy is well known, but biologic potential is uncertain, and resection of residual masses at the end of therapy has not been associated with improved outcome [82]. However, second-look surgeries may demonstrate whether viable tumor is present, which has decreased failure-free survival compared to those without viable tumor [83]. One challenge is to determine which residual masses warrant second-look procedures that may alter treatment and mitigate response. Further study evaluating imaging modalities such as FDG-PET may have a role in the future.

In addition to the primary site, careful attention should be made to regional lymph node assessment. Specific guidelines of histologic or radiologic assessment vary among cooperative groups. The COG requires ipsilateral retroperitoneal lymph node dissection for boys ≥10 years of age with paratesticular tumors, whether or not nodes are enlarged by imaging studies. This requirement is based on results from the IRS-IV trial, which showed inferior outcome for boys ≥10 years of age classified as Group I based on imaging alone [84]. In patients with extremity tumors, approximately half have regional lymph node involvement [85], and surgical sampling of clinically negative regional lymph nodes is recommended in current trials. The role of FDG-PET and less aggressive surgical sampling with sentinel node biopsy is of ongoing interest [86].

11.3.1.2 Radiation Therapy

There is a clear role for radiation in non-resected/residual RMS; however, the extent and dose vary depending on cooperative group. The COG STS has historically based radiation doses on the amount of tumor that remains after initial surgery and pre-chemotherapy [87, 88]. The European cooperative groups have allowed for radiation dose reduction and elimination based on the amount of tumor remaining after chemotherapy initiation with or without DPE [89]. The COG STS has evaluated RT dose reduction after DPE, which demonstrated no significant change in EFS or OAS compared to historical controls, but this was only applicable to patients who are eligible for DPE [81].

Current RT guidelines have evolved and reducing toxicity associated with radiotherapy remains an important goal in RMS therapy [90–94]. COG STS currently recommends a cumulative dose of between 36 and 41.4 Gy for microscopic residual disease, whereas higher cumulate RT doses between 50.4 and 54 Gy (45 for orbital tumors) are used for gross residual disease. The use of "cone down" has been used for patients who initially presented with unresectable tumors who have responded to neoadjuvant chemotherapy. Advances in radiation technology and growing use of intensity-modulated RT (IMRT) [95, 96] and proton beam therapy [97, 98] continue to be evaluated in order to minimize dose received by normal surrounding tissue. Survival data suggest comparable outcome with potential for reductions of late effects [99]; but ongoing research is needed.

11.3.1.3 Chemotherapy

All patients with RMS should receive chemotherapy for both local and systemic therapies. Chemotherapy has primarily been given in combination with regimens containing vincristine, actinomycin D, and cyclophosphamide (VAC) [75]. Duration and intensity have varied depending on risk stratification as outlined in Table 11.5. The primary strategy for low-risk patients who generally have excellent survival outcomes has been to reduce acute and long-term toxicities associated with therapy. In the most recent COG low-risk RMS study (ARST0331), shorter duration that included lower-dose cyclophosphamide and RT did not compromise the failure-free survival with subset-one low-risk ERMS [100]. For intermediate-risk patients, no significant improvement in failure-free survival was seen with additional chemotherapeutic agents systematically introduced in randomized trials beyond that achieved with VAC therapy [76, 101, 102]. The initial data from the recently completed ARST0531 study showed that the addition of vincristine and irinotecan (VI) to VAC may have reduced acute toxicity without compromise in survival [102]. High-risk patients are currently treated on intensive multidrug regimen (additional agents with doxorubicin, ifosfamide, etoposide, irinotecan) where early outcome data showed an improved failure-free survival at 18 months that is 20% higher than previous studies, longer term follow up did not demonstrate improvement in survival [103].

11.3.1.4 Experimental Therapeutics/Targeted Agents

With the increasing understanding in the pathogenesis and genomics of RMS and growing repertoire of molecularly targeted agents in development, early clinical trials evaluating these agents for recurrent RMS have become available. Agents targeting the RAS pathway [71], angiogenesis [104, 105], and immune pathways [106] are being explored in both preclinical and clinical settings. Whether these agents have clinical promise, how genomic alterations will be evaluated, and ultimately how these will be incorporated into current therapy will be key to improving outcome and decreasing the acute and late effects of current multimodal therapy.

11.3.1.5 Recurrent Disease

The long-term prognosis for patients with recurrent or progressive RMS remains poor [107]. Metastatic recurrence, prior radiation therapy, initial tumor size >5 cm, and time to relapse <18 months are unfavorable prognostic features for survival after recurrence [108]. The selection of further treatment depends on many factors such as site(s) of recurrence and previous treatments, which should be evaluated and planned in a multidisciplinary approach. For patients with regional or local recurrence, therapy may include aggressive surgical removal and/or local radiotherapy. Adjuvant chemotherapy will be needed for further disease control, and previous agents used may direct choice of relapsed regimen therapy.

11.3.2 Non-rhabdomyosarcoma Soft Tissue Sarcomas

Pediatric NRSTS are a rare and heterogeneous group of tumors with over 50 distinct histologic subtypes with a wide spectrum of local aggressiveness and metastatic potential [109]. In children, synovial sarcoma, fibrosarcoma, fibrohistiocytic tumors, and malignant peripheral nerve sheath tumors are the most common histologies [110, 111]. NRSTS are much more common in adolescents and adults and much knowledge regarding diagnosis; prognosis and therapy are based on sarcoma treatment in adults [112, 113]. However, there are differences that must be appreciated. Some histologic subtypes may behave differently in children, and local control measures, such as surgery and radiation, have to take into consideration the patient age, long-term function, and complications [114]. A multidisciplinary team of surgeons, pathologists, medical oncologists, and radiation oncologists is instrumental in the diagnosis and treatment of this heterogeneous group of sarcomas.

Similar to RMS, NRSTS can arise anywhere in the body, with the most common sites being extremities and trunk [115, 116]. Clinical signs and presentation will depend on site of disease. Due to the rarity of disease, accurate diagnosis of NRSTS is complex, and diagnoses are based on multiple evaluations including morphology, immunohistochemistry, cytogenetics, and molecular factors [117, 118]. Many are now defined by specific chromosomal translocations, cytogenetic abnormalities, and molecular studies (Table 11.6). Factors that most influence survival in pediatric NRSTS are presence of metastasis, histologic grade, size of primary tumor, and extent of surgical resection [115]. Based on these factors, prognosis and survival

Table 11.6 Frequent chromosomal aberrations in select non-rhabdomyosarcoma soft tissue sarcomas [53]

Histology	Chromosomal aberration	Gene involved
Alveolar soft part sarcoma	t(x;17) (p11.2;q25)	ASPL/TFE3
Clear cell sarcoma	t(12;22) (q13;q12), t(2;22) (q33;q12)	ATF1/EWS, EWSR1/CREB1
Congenital (infantile) fibrosarcoma	t(12;15) (p13,q25)	ETV-NTRK3
Dermatofibrosarcoma protuberans	t(17;22) (q22;q13)	COL1A1/PDGFB
Desmoplastic small round cell tumors	t(11;22) (p13;q12)	EWS/WT1
Epithelioid hemangioendothelioma	t(1;3) (p36;q25)	WWTR1/CAMTA1
Epithelioid sarcoma	Inactivation SMARCB1	SMARCB1
Inflammatory myofibroblastic tumor	t(1;2) (q23;q23), t(2;19) (q23;q13), t(2;17) (q23;q23), t(2;2) (p23;q13), t(2;11) (p23;p15)	TPM3/ALK, TPM4/ALK, CLTC/ALK, RANBP2/ALK, CARS/ALK
Synovial sarcoma	t(x;18) (p11.2;q11.2)	SYT/SSX
Tenosynovial giant cell tumor	t(1;2) (p13;q35)	CSF1

estimates can be classified into low-, intermediate-, and high-risk groups [119]. Individualized therapy may vary depending on clinical presentation and histology, as some tumors may be more chemotherapy and radiation sensitive than others; in-depth discussion for each type of pediatric NRSTS is beyond the scope of this chapter. Caring for a pediatric NRSTS patient must be done in a multidisciplinary manner for the best outcome.

11.3.2.1 Surgery

Local control is key and the first consideration in the treatment of pediatric NRSTS. Only a small percentage of patients with NRSTS presents with metastatic disease at presentation [120]. Surgery remains the principal therapeutic modality in pediatric NRSTS. Whenever possible, a complete surgical resection of the primary tumor with adequate margins is recommended, with re-excision recommended for residual disease or inadequate margins if feasible as tumors with <1 cm margins have higher rate of recurrence [121]. The ability for complete resection is a crucial prognostic factor with the estimated 5-year survival rate for patients with complete resection, unresected disease, and metastatic disease as 86%, 52%, and 17%, respectively [116]. Adequate margins or resection with wide margins is not always feasible, in particular in pediatric patients and depending on location of disease.

Lymph node sampling or dissection is not routine for pediatric NRSTS but should be considered for certain histologies such as clear cell sarcoma [122] and epithelioid sarcoma [123], as these histologies have greater tendency for regional lymph node metastasis. Pulmonary disease is the most common site of metastasis for NRSTS, and in adults about 20% of NRSTS will develop evidence of metastatic disease [124]. The principles of surgery remain, with complete surgical resection of all sites required for cure, and yet the long-term survival remains dismal in these patients [124].

11.3.2.2 Radiation Therapy

There are no standardized guidelines for radiation therapy (RT) in pediatric NRSTS, and much of the framework is adapted from adult STS experience [125, 126]. The extent of surgery, histologic grade, and size seem to play the most important in determining the need for adjuvant radiation therapy [127, 128]. Preoperative radiation should also be considered in particular for patients with high-grade, large tumors for which adjuvant radiation will be given regardless, as the total volume and dose of RT can be significantly lower in these cases [129]. Although preoperative RT may affect wound healing, there may be some advantage to minimizing long-term late effects [130, 131]. These decisions again should be considered in a multidisciplinary fashion.

11.3.2.3 Chemotherapy

The role of chemotherapy varies for pediatric NRSTS, and again there is no standardized guideline. Certain histologies such as synovial sarcoma [132] have greater chemosensitivity than others. The two chemotherapeutic agents that have shown clinical benefit with objective tumor shrinkage in a variety of NRSTS are doxorubicin and ifosfamide [133]. For most pediatric NRSTS, chemotherapy may be most indicated in unresectable or metastatic disease, although tumor response and ultimate survival may only be modestly improved with chemotherapy [116]. In an updated large meta-analysis in the outcome of over 1900 adults treated on 18 trials comparing local therapy alone to local therapy plus chemotherapy, adjuvant chemotherapy demonstrated a modest increase in the overall recurrence-free interval (10%) and slight reduction in absolute risk of death (HR 0.77, 95% CI 0.64–0.93, $p = 0.01$) [134]. There are differences in the distribution of histologies in adult versus pediatric NRSTS, so direct extrapolation is not always possible, and whenever feasible, medical therapy for pediatric NRSTS should be done within the context of a clinical trial.

Fibrosarcoma is one histology highlighted here due to the stark differences between pediatric and adult types. Fibrosarcoma represents about 30% of the soft tissue malignancies in children less than 1 years of age, and because this specific entity has been found to be less aggressive and more curable than fibrosarcoma in older children and adults, it is typically called infantile fibrosarcoma (IFS) [114, 135, 136]. IFS is characterized by specific translocation t(12,13) involving the *ETV6-NTRK3* genes, which is also seen in cellular mesoblastic nephroma, differentiating it from adult fibrosarcomas [137]. Clinical presentation also differs in that in infants, it typically presents in an extremity site and with rapid growth. They are typically quite responsive to chemotherapy, with the most common agents used being vincristine and actinomycin with or without cyclophosphamide [135, 138]. Patients may have good prognosis and long-term survival even in the setting of marginal or subtotal resection [135, 138, 139]. Radiation is typically not required and often avoided due to the very young age of these children.

11.3.2.4 Experimental Therapeutics/Targeted Agents

Pediatric NRSTS are histologically diverse, many with pathognomonic translocations on molecular characterization. With the increasing understanding in the pathogenesis of these tumors and the increasing pipeline of targeted agents for cancer therapy, targeted agents may have a significant role in the future treatments of these malignancies. There is evidence to support the role of the mTOR pathway in malignant peripheral nerve sheath tumors [140, 141], angiogenesis inhibitors in alveolar soft part sarcoma [142], and other tyrosine kinases expressed in a range of NRSTS [143, 144]. Many of these developments have led to clinical trials evaluating these novel compounds in the clinical setting.

In conclusion, pediatric NRSTS are a diverse group of malignancies for which treatment primarily consists of surgery for local control with radiation and/or chemotherapy to aid in local control. However, the actual treatment plans vary depending on the age, location, clinical presentation, and histology such that these tumors should be treated at expert centers with a multidisciplinary team of surgeons, oncologists, radiation oncologists, and pathologists.

References

1. Howlader N, et al. SEER cancer statistics review, 1975–2011. 2014.
2. Smith MA, et al. Declining childhood and adolescent cancer mortality. Cancer. 2014;120(16): 2497–506.
3. Fletcher CDM, et al. WHO classification of tumours of soft tissue and bone. In: Pathology and genetics of tumours of soft tissue and bone. IARC Press: Lyon; 2013.
4. Bielack SS, et al. Prognostic factors in high-grade osteosarcoma of the extremities or trunk: an analysis of 1,702 patients treated on neoadjuvant cooperative osteosarcoma study group protocols. J Clin Oncol. 2002;20(3):776–90.
5. Goorin AM, et al. Phase II/III trial of etoposide and high-dose ifosfamide in newly diagnosed metastatic osteosarcoma: a pediatric oncology group trial. J Clin Oncol. 2002;20(2):426–33.
6. Bacci G, et al. Neoadjuvant chemotherapy for osteosarcoma of the extremities with metastases at presentation: recent experience at the Rizzoli Institute in 57 patients treated with cisplatin, doxorubicin, and a high dose of methotrexate and ifosfamide. Ann Oncol. 2003;14(7): 1126–34.
7. Panicek DM, et al. CT and MR imaging in the local staging of primary malignant musculoskeletal neoplasms: report of the radiology diagnostic oncology group. Radiology. 1997;202(1): 237–46.
8. Meyer JS, et al. Imaging guidelines for children with Ewing sarcoma and osteosarcoma: a report from the Children's Oncology Group bone tumor committee. Pediatr Blood Cancer. 2008;51(2):163–70.
9. Volker T, et al. Positron emission tomography for staging of pediatric sarcoma patients: results of a prospective multicenter trial. J Clin Oncol. 2007;25(34):5435–41.
10. Kaste SC. Imaging pediatric bone sarcomas. Radiol Clin N Am. 2011;49(4):749–65, vi–vii.
11. Uhl M, et al. Evaluation of tumour necrosis during chemotherapy with diffusion-weighted MR imaging: preliminary results in osteosarcomas. Pediatr Radiol. 2006;36(12):1306–11.
12. Hamada K, et al. Evaluation of chemotherapy response in osteosarcoma with FDG-PET. Ann Nucl Med. 2009;23(1):89–95.
13. Rahn III DA, et al. Clinical outcomes of palliative radiation therapy for children. Pract Radiat Oncol. 2015;5(3):183–7.
14. Dome JS, Schwartz CL. Osteosarcoma. Cancer Treat Res. 1997;92:215–51.

15. Taylor WF, et al. Trends and variability in survival among patients with osteosarcoma: a 7-year update. Mayo Clin Proc. 1985;60(2):91–104.
16. Link MP, et al. The effect of adjuvant chemotherapy on relapse-free survival in patients with osteosarcoma of the extremity. N Engl J Med. 1986;314(25):1600–6.
17. Eilber F, et al. Adjuvant chemotherapy for osteosarcoma: a randomized prospective trial. J Clin Oncol. 1987;5(1):21–6.
18. Rosen G, et al. Chemotherapy, en bloc resection, and prosthetic bone replacement in the treatment of osteogenic sarcoma. Cancer. 1976;37(1):1–11.
19. Meyers PA, et al. Osteosarcoma: a randomized, prospective trial of the addition of ifosfamide and/or muramyl tripeptide to cisplatin, doxorubicin, and high-dose methotrexate. J Clin Oncol. 2005;23(9):2004–11.
20. Marina N, et al. MAPIE vs. MAP as postoperative chemotherapy in patients with a poor response to preoperative chemotherapy for newly-diagnosed osteosarcoma: results from EURAMOS-1. In: Connective Tissue Oncology Society meeting 2014, Berlin, Germany.
21. Meyers PA, et al. Osteosarcoma: the addition of muramyl tripeptide to chemotherapy improves overall survival—a report from the Children's Oncology Group. J Clin Oncol. 2008;26(4):633–8.
22. Ferrari S, et al. Neoadjuvant chemotherapy with methotrexate, cisplatin, and doxorubicin with or without ifosfamide in nonmetastatic osteosarcoma of the extremity: an Italian sarcoma group trial ISG/OS-1. J Clin Oncol. 2012;30(17):2112–8.
23. Kager L, et al. Primary metastatic osteosarcoma: presentation and outcome of patients treated on neoadjuvant cooperative Osteosarcoma Study Group protocols. J Clin Oncol. 2003;21(10):2011–8.
24. Chou AJ, et al. Addition of muramyl tripeptide to chemotherapy for patients with newly diagnosed metastatic osteosarcoma: a report from the Children's Oncology Group. Cancer. 2009;115(22):5339–48.
25. Bielack SS, et al. Methotrexate, doxorubicin, and cisplatin (MAP) plus maintenance pegylated interferon Alfa-2b versus map alone in patients with resectable high-grade osteosarcoma and good histologic response to preoperative MAP: first results of the EURAMOS-1 good response randomized controlled trial. J Clin Oncol. 2015;33(20):2279–87.
26. Isakoff MS, et al. Osteosarcoma: current treatment and a collaborative pathway to success. J Clin Oncol. 2015;33(27):3029–35.
27. Zwerdling T, et al. Phase II investigation of docetaxel in pediatric patients with recurrent solid tumors: a report from the Children's Oncology Group. Cancer. 2006;106(8):1821–8.
28. Navid F, et al. Combination of gemcitabine and docetaxel in the treatment of children and young adults with refractory bone sarcoma. Cancer. 2008;113(2):419–25.
29. Gosiengfiao Y, et al. Gemcitabine with or without docetaxel and resection for recurrent osteosarcoma: the experience at Children's Memorial Hospital. J Pediatr Hematol Oncol. 2012;34(2):e63–5.
30. Song BS, et al. Gemcitabine and docetaxel for the treatment of children and adolescents with recurrent or refractory osteosarcoma: Korea Cancer Center Hospital experience. Pediatr Blood Cancer. 2014;61(8):1376–81.
31. Ebb D, et al. Phase II trial of trastuzumab in combination with cytotoxic chemotherapy for treatment of metastatic osteosarcoma with human epidermal growth factor receptor 2 overexpression: a report from the Children's Oncology Group. J Clin Oncol. 2012;30(20):2545–51.
32. Arndt CA, et al. Inhaled granulocyte-macrophage colony stimulating factor for first pulmonary recurrence of osteosarcoma: effects on disease-free survival and immunomodulation. A report from the Children's Oncology Group. Clin Cancer Res. 2010;16(15):4024–30.
33. Goldsby RE, et al. Feasibility and dose discovery analysis of zoledronic acid with concurrent chemotherapy in the treatment of newly diagnosed metastatic osteosarcoma: a report from the Children's Oncology Group. Eur J Cancer. 2013;49(10):2384–91.
34. Chi SN, et al. The patterns of relapse in osteosarcoma: the Memorial Sloan-Kettering experience. Pediatr Blood Cancer. 2004;42(1):46–51.

35. Kempf-Bielack B, et al. Osteosarcoma relapse after combined modality therapy: an analysis of unselected patients in the Co-operative Osteosarcoma Study Group (COSS). J Clin Oncol. 2005;23(3):559–68.
36. Chou AJ, et al. Treatment of osteosarcoma at first recurrence after contemporary therapy: the Memorial Sloan-Kettering cancer center experience. Cancer. 2005;104(10):2214–21.
37. Bielack SS, et al. Second and subsequent recurrences of osteosarcoma: presentation, treatment, and outcomes of 249 consecutive Cooperative Osteosarcoma Study Group patients. J Clin Oncol. 2009;27(4):557–65.
38. Bernstein M, et al. Ewing's sarcoma family of tumors: current management. Oncologist. 2006;11(5):503–19.
39. Meyers PA. Malignant bone tumors in children: Ewing's sarcoma. Hematol Oncol Clin North Am. 1987;1(4):667–73.
40. Gaspar N, et al. Ewing sarcoma: current management and future approaches through collaboration. J Clin Oncol. 2015;33(27).
41. Meyers PA, Levy AS. Ewing's sarcoma. Curr Treat Options in Oncol. 2000;1(3):247–57.
42. Pizzo P, Poplack D. Principles and practice of pediatric oncology. 6th ed. Philadelphia: Lippincott, Williams and Wilkins; 2010.
43. Guimaraes JB, et al. The importance of PET/CT in the evaluation of patients with Ewing tumors. Radiol Bras. 2015;48(3):175–80.
44. Quartuccio N, et al. Pediatric bone sarcoma: diagnostic performance of (1, 8)F-FDG PET/CT versus conventional imaging for initial staging and follow-up. AJR Am J Roentgenol. 2015;204(1):153–60.
45. Raciborska A, et al. Response to chemotherapy estimates by FDG PET is an important prognostic factor in patients with Ewing sarcoma. Clin Transl Oncol. 2016;18(2):189–95.
46. Hawkins DS, et al. [18F] Fluorodeoxyglucose positron emission tomography predicts outcome for Ewing sarcoma family of tumors. J Clin Oncol. 2005;23(34):8828–34.
47. Zang J, et al. Ewing's sarcoma of bone: treatment results and prognostic factors. Zhonghua Wai Ke Za Zhi. 2010;48(12):896–9.
48. Karski EE, et al. Identification of discrete prognostic groups in Ewing sarcoma. Pediatr Blood Cancer. 2016;63(1):47–53.
49. Bacci G, et al. Prognostic factors in nonmetastatic Ewing's sarcoma of bone treated with adjuvant chemotherapy: analysis of 359 patients at the Istituto Ortopedico Rizzoli. J Clin Oncol. 2000;18(1):4–11.
50. Cotterill SJ, et al. Prognostic factors in Ewing's tumor of bone: analysis of 975 patients from the European Intergroup Cooperative Ewing's Sarcoma Study Group. J Clin Oncol. 2000;18(17):3108–14.
51. La TH, et al. Radiation therapy for Ewing's sarcoma: results from Memorial Sloan-Kettering in the modern era. Int J Radiat Oncol Biol Phys. 2006;64(2):544–50.
52. Lopez JL, et al. Role of radiation therapy in the multidisciplinary management of Ewing's sarcoma of bone in pediatric patients: an effective treatment for local control. Rep Pract Oncol Radiother. 2011;16(3):103–9.
53. Perez CA, et al. Radiation therapy in the multimodal management of Ewing's sarcoma of bone: report of the Intergroup Ewing's Sarcoma Study. Natl Cancer Inst Monogr. 1981;56:263–71.
54. Craft AW, et al. Long-term results from the first UKCCSG Ewing's Tumour Study (ET-1). United Kingdom Children's Cancer Study Group (UKCCSG) and the Medical Research Council Bone Sarcoma Working Party. Eur J Cancer. 1997;33(7):1061–9.
55. Paulussen M, et al. Localized Ewing tumor of bone: final results of the cooperative Ewing's Sarcoma Study CESS 86. J Clin Oncol. 2001;19(6):1818–29.
56. Grier HE, et al. Addition of ifosfamide and etoposide to standard chemotherapy for Ewing's sarcoma and primitive neuroectodermal tumor of bone. N Engl J Med. 2003;348(8):694–701.
57. Womer RB, et al. Randomized controlled trial of interval-compressed chemotherapy for the treatment of localized Ewing sarcoma: a report from the Children's Oncology Group. J Clin Oncol. 2012;30(33):4148–54.
58. Hartmann O, et al. [Role of high-dose chemotherapy followed by bone marrow autograft in the treatment of metastatic Ewing's sarcoma in children]. Bull Cancer. 1990;77(2):181–7.

59. McTiernan A, et al. High dose chemotherapy with bone marrow or peripheral stem cell rescue is an effective treatment option for patients with relapsed or progressive Ewing's sarcoma family of tumours. Ann Oncol. 2006;17(8):1301–5.
60. Meyers PA, et al. High-dose melphalan, etoposide, total-body irradiation, and autologous stem-cell reconstitution as consolidation therapy for high-risk Ewing's sarcoma does not improve prognosis. J Clin Oncol. 2001;19(11):2812–20.
61. Ladenstein R, et al. Primary disseminated multifocal Ewing sarcoma: results of the Euro-EWING 99 trial. J Clin Oncol. 2010;28(20):3284–91.
62. Tolcher AW, et al. Phase I, pharmacokinetic, and pharmacodynamic study of AMG 479, a fully human monoclonal antibody to insulin-like growth factor receptor 1. J Clin Oncol. 2009;27(34):5800–7.
63. Tap WD, et al. Phase II study of ganitumab, a fully human anti-type-1 insulin-like growth factor receptor antibody, in patients with metastatic Ewing family tumors or desmoplastic small round cell tumors. J Clin Oncol. 2012;30(15):1849–56.
64. Ognjanovic S, et al. Trends in childhood rhabdomyosarcoma incidence and survival in the United States, 1975–2005. Cancer. 2009;115(18):4218–26.
65. Li FP, Fraumeni Jr JF. Rhabdomyosarcoma in children: epidemiologic study and identification of a familial cancer syndrome. J Natl Cancer Inst. 1969;43(6):1365–73.
66. Felix CA, et al. Frequency and diversity of p53 mutations in childhood rhabdomyosarcoma. Cancer Res. 1992;52(8):2243–7.
67. Gripp KW. Tumor predisposition in Costello syndrome. Am J Med Genet C Semin Med Genet. 2005;137C(1):72–7.
68. Doros L, et al. DICER1 mutations in embryonal rhabdomyosarcomas from children with and without familial PPB-tumor predisposition syndrome. Pediatr Blood Cancer. 2012;59(3):558–60.
69. Barr FG. Gene fusions involving PAX and FOX family members in alveolar rhabdomyosarcoma. Oncogene. 2001;20(40):5736–46.
70. Koufos A, et al. Loss of heterozygosity in three embryonal tumours suggests a common pathogenetic mechanism. Nature. 1985;316(6026):330–4.
71. Shern JF, et al. Comprehensive genomic analysis of rhabdomyosarcoma reveals a landscape of alterations affecting a common genetic axis in fusion-positive and fusion-negative tumors. Cancer Discov. 2014;4(2):216–31.
72. Missiaglia E, et al. PAX3/FOXO1 fusion gene status is the key prognostic molecular marker in rhabdomyosarcoma and significantly improves current risk stratification. J Clin Oncol. 2012;30(14):1670–7.
73. Sorensen PH, et al. PAX3-FKHR and PAX7-FKHR gene fusions are prognostic indicators in alveolar rhabdomyosarcoma: a report from the Children's Oncology Group. J Clin Oncol. 2002;20(11):2672–9.
74. Mosquera JM, et al. Recurrent NCOA2 gene rearrangements in congenital/infantile spindle cell rhabdomyosarcoma. Genes Chromosomes Cancer. 2013;52(6):538–50.
75. Gosiengfiao Y, Reichek J, Walterhouse D. What is new in rhabdomyosarcoma management in children? Paediatr Drugs. 2012;14(6):389–400.
76. Raney RB, et al. The Intergroup Rhabdomyosarcoma Study Group (IRSG): major lessons from the IRS-I through IRS-IV studies as background for the current IRS-V treatment protocols. Sarcoma. 2001;5(1):9–15.
77. Lawrence Jr W, et al. Pretreatment TNM staging of childhood rhabdomyosarcoma: a report of the Intergroup Rhabdomyosarcoma Study Group. Children's Cancer Study Group. Pediatric Oncology Group. Cancer. 1997;80(6):1165–70.
78. Malempati S, Hawkins DS. Rhabdomyosarcoma: review of the Children's Oncology Group (COG) Soft-Tissue Sarcoma Committee experience and rationale for current COG studies. Pediatr Blood Cancer. 2012;59(1):5–10.
79. Cecchetto G, et al. Biopsy or debulking surgery as initial surgery for locally advanced rhabdomyosarcomas in children? The experience of the Italian Cooperative Group studies. Cancer. 2007;110(11):2561–7.
80. Hays DM, et al. Primary reexcision for patients with 'microscopic residual' tumor following initial excision of sarcomas of trunk and extremity sites. J Pediatr Surg. 1989;24(1):5–10.

81. Rodeberg DA, et al. Delayed primary excision with subsequent modification of radiotherapy dose for intermediate-risk rhabdomyosarcoma: a report from the Children's Oncology Group Soft Tissue Sarcoma Committee. Int J Cancer. 2015;137(1):204–11.
82. Rodeberg DA, et al. Prognostic significance of tumor response at the end of therapy in group III rhabdomyosarcoma: a report from the Children's Oncology Group. J Clin Oncol. 2009;27(22):3705–11.
83. Raney B, et al. Impact of tumor viability at second-look procedures performed before completing treatment on the intergroup rhabdomyosarcoma study group protocol IRS-IV, 1991-1997: a report from the Children's Oncology Group. J Pediatr Surg. 2010;45(11):2160–8.
84. Wiener ES, et al. Controversies in the management of paratesticular rhabdomyosarcoma: is staging retroperitoneal lymph node dissection necessary for adolescents with resected paratesticular rhabdomyosarcoma? Semin Pediatr Surg. 2001;10(3):146–52.
85. Neville HL, et al. Preoperative staging, prognostic factors, and outcome for extremity rhabdomyosarcoma: a preliminary report from the Intergroup Rhabdomyosarcoma Study IV (1991–1997). J Pediatr Surg. 2000;35(2):317–21.
86. De Corti F, et al. Does surgery have a role in the treatment of local relapses of non-metastatic rhabdomyosarcoma? Pediatr Blood Cancer. 2011;57(7):1261–5.
87. Crist W, et al. The third intergroup rhabdomyosarcoma study. J Clin Oncol. 1995;13(3):610–30.
88. Crist WM, et al. Intergroup rhabdomyosarcoma study-IV: results for patients with nonmetastatic disease. J Clin Oncol. 2001;19(12):3091–102.
89. Stevens MC, et al. Treatment of nonmetastatic rhabdomyosarcoma in childhood and adolescence: third study of the International Society of Paediatric Oncology–SIOP Malignant Mesenchymal Tumor 89. J Clin Oncol. 2005;23(12):2618–28.
90. Wolden SL, et al. Indications for radiotherapy and chemotherapy after complete resection in rhabdomyosarcoma: a report from the Intergroup Rhabdomyosarcoma Studies I to III. J Clin Oncol. 1999;17(11):3468–75.
91. Mandell L, et al. Radiocurability of microscopic disease in childhood rhabdomyosarcoma with radiation doses less than 4,000 cGy. J Clin Oncol. 1990;8(9):1536–42.
92. Breneman J, et al. Local control with reduced-dose radiotherapy for low-risk rhabdomyosarcoma: a report from the Children's Oncology Group D9602 study. Int J Radiat Oncol Biol Phys. 2012;83(2):720–6.
93. Heyn R, et al. Late effects of therapy in orbital rhabdomyosarcoma in children. A report from the Intergroup Rhabdomyosarcoma Study. Cancer. 1986;57(9):1738–43.
94. Donaldson SS, et al. Hyperfractionated radiation in children with rhabdomyosarcoma—results of an Intergroup Rhabdomyosarcoma Pilot Study. Int J Radiat Oncol Biol Phys. 1995;32(4):903–11.
95. Lin C, et al. Effect of radiotherapy techniques (IMRT vs. 3D-CRT) on outcome in patients with intermediate-risk rhabdomyosarcoma enrolled in COG D9803—a report from the Children's Oncology Group. Int J Radiat Oncol Biol Phys. 2012;82(5):1764–70.
96. McDonald MW, et al. Intensity-modulated radiotherapy with use of cone-down boost for pediatric head-and-neck rhabdomyosarcoma. Int J Radiat Oncol Biol Phys. 2008;72(3):884–91.
97. Cotter SE, et al. Proton radiotherapy for pediatric bladder/prostate rhabdomyosarcoma: clinical outcomes and dosimetry compared to intensity-modulated radiation therapy. Int J Radiat Oncol Biol Phys. 2011;81(5):1367–73.
98. Childs SK, et al. Proton radiotherapy for parameningeal rhabdomyosarcoma: clinical outcomes and late effects. Int J Radiat Oncol Biol Phys. 2012;82(2):635–42.
99. Ladra MM, et al. Preliminary results of a phase II trial of proton radiotherapy for pediatric rhabdomyosarcoma. J Clin Oncol. 2014;32(33):3762–70.
100. Walterhouse DO, et al. Shorter-duration therapy using vincristine, dactinomycin, and lower-dose cyclophosphamide with or without radiotherapy for patients with newly diagnosed low-risk rhabdomyosarcoma: a report from the Soft Tissue Sarcoma Committee of the Children's Oncology Group. J Clin Oncol. 2014;32(31):3547–52.
101. Arndt CA, et al. Vincristine, actinomycin, and cyclophosphamide compared with vincristine, actinomycin, and cyclophosphamide alternating with vincristine, topotecan, and

cyclophosphamide for intermediate-risk rhabdomyosarcoma: Children's Oncology Group Study D9803. J Clin Oncol. 2009;27(31):5182–8.
102. Hawkins DS, et al. Vincristine, dactinomycin, cyclophosphamide (VAC) versus VAC/V plus irinotecan (VI) for intermediate risk rhabdomyosarcoma (IRRMS): a report from the Children's Oncology Group Soft Tissue Sarcoma Committee. J Clin Oncol. 2014;32(5 s):suppl; abstr 10004.
103. Weigel B, et al. Intensive multiagent therapy, including dosecompressed cycles of ifosfamide/etoposide and vincristine/doxorubicin/cyclophosphamide, irinotecan, and radiation, in patients with high-risk rhabdomyosarcoma: a report from the Children's Oncology Group. J Clin Oncol. 2016;34(2):117–22.
104. Kim A, et al. Phase 2 trial of sorafenib in children and young adults with refractory solid tumors: a report from the Children's Oncology Group. Pediatr Blood Cancer. 2015;62(9):1562–6.
105. Hashimoto A, et al. Effective treatment of metastatic rhabdomyosarcoma with pazopanib. Gan To Kagaku Ryoho. 2014;41(8):1041–4.
106. Roberts SS, Chou AJ, Cheung NK. Immunotherapy of childhood sarcomas. Front Oncol. 2015;5:181.
107. Pappo AS, et al. Survival after relapse in children and adolescents with rhabdomyosarcoma: a report from the Intergroup Rhabdomyosarcoma Study Group. J Clin Oncol. 1999;17(11): 3487–93.
108. Chisholm JC, et al. Prognostic factors after relapse in nonmetastatic rhabdomyosarcoma: a nomogram to better define patients who can be salvaged with further therapy. J Clin Oncol. 2011;29(10):1319–25.
109. Doyle LA. Sarcoma classification: an update based on the 2013 World Health Organization classification of tumors of soft tissue and bone. Cancer. 2014;120(12):1763–74.
110. Ferrari A, et al. Non-metastatic unresected paediatric non-rhabdomyosarcoma soft tissue sarcomas: results of a pooled analysis from United States and European groups. Eur J Cancer. 2011;47(5):724–31.
111. Spunt SL, Skapek SX, Coffin CM. Pediatric nonrhabdomyosarcoma soft tissue sarcomas. Oncologist. 2008;13(6):668–78.
112. Rosenberg SA, et al. Prospective randomized evaluation of the role of limb-sparing surgery, radiation therapy, and adjuvant chemoimmunotherapy in the treatment of adult soft-tissue sarcomas. Surgery. 1978;84(1):62–9.
113. Pisters PW, O'Sullivan B, Maki RG. Evidence-based recommendations for local therapy for soft tissue sarcomas. J Clin Oncol. 2007;25(8):1003–8.
114. Spunt SL, Pappo AS. Childhood nonrhabdomyosarcoma soft tissue sarcomas are not adult-type tumors. J Clin Oncol. 2006;24(12):1958–9; author reply 1959–60.
115. Spunt SL, et al. Prognostic factors for children and adolescents with surgically resected nonrhabdomyosarcoma soft tissue sarcoma: an analysis of 121 patients treated at St Jude Children's Research Hospital. J Clin Oncol. 1999;17(12):3697–705.
116. Ferrari A, et al. Adult-type soft tissue sarcomas in pediatric-age patients: experience at the Istituto Nazionale Tumori in Milan. J Clin Oncol. 2005;23(18):4021–30.
117. Bridge JA. The role of cytogenetics and molecular diagnostics in the diagnosis of soft-tissue tumors. Mod Pathol. 2014;27(Suppl 1):S80–97.
118. Marino-Enriquez A. Advances in the molecular analysis of soft tissue tumors and clinical implications. Surg Pathol Clin. 2015;8(3):525–37.
119. Waxweiler TV, et al. Non-rhabdomyosarcoma soft tissue sarcomas in children: a surveillance, epidemiology, and end results analysis validating cog risk stratifications. Int J Radiat Oncol Biol Phys. 2015;92(2):339–48.
120. Pappo AS, et al. Metastatic nonrhabdomyosarcomatous soft-tissue sarcomas in children and adolescents: the St. Jude Children's Research Hospital experience. Med Pediatr Oncol. 1999; 33(2):76–82.
121. Blakely ML, et al. The impact of margin of resection on outcome in pediatric nonrhabdomyosarcoma soft tissue sarcoma. J Pediatr Surg. 1999;34(5):672–5.
122. Bianchi G, et al. Clear cell sarcoma of soft tissue: a retrospective review and analysis of 31 cases treated at Istituto Ortopedico Rizzoli. Eur J Surg Oncol. 2014;40(5):505–10.

123. Casanova M, et al. Epithelioid sarcoma in children and adolescents: a report from the Italian Soft Tissue Sarcoma Committee. Cancer. 2006;106(3):708–17.
124. Billingsley KG, et al. Pulmonary metastases from soft tissue sarcoma: analysis of patterns of diseases and postmetastasis survival. Ann Surg. 1999;229(5):602–10; discussion 610–2.
125. Wolden SL. Radiation therapy for non-rhabdomyosarcoma soft tissue sarcomas in adolescents and young adults. J Pediatr Hematol Oncol. 2005;27(4):212–4.
126. Strander H, Turesson I, Cavallin-Stahl E. A systematic overview of radiation therapy effects in soft tissue sarcomas. Acta Oncol. 2003;42(5-6):516–31.
127. Smith KB, et al. Adjuvant radiotherapy for pediatric and young adult nonrhabdomyosarcoma soft-tissue sarcoma. Int J Radiat Oncol Biol Phys. 2011;81(1):150–7.
128. Paulino AC, Ritchie J, Wen BC. The value of postoperative radiotherapy in childhood non-rhabdomyosarcoma soft tissue sarcoma. Pediatr Blood Cancer. 2004;43(5):587–93.
129. El-Bared N, Wong P, Wang D. Soft tissue sarcoma and radiation therapy advances, impact on toxicity. Curr Treat Options in Oncol. 2015;16(5):19.
130. Wang D, et al. Significant reduction of late toxicities in patients with extremity sarcoma treated with image-guided radiation therapy to a reduced target volume: results of Radiation Therapy Oncology Group RTOG-0630 Trial. J Clin Oncol. 2015;33(20):2231–8.
131. O'Sullivan B, et al. Preoperative versus postoperative radiotherapy in soft-tissue sarcoma of the limbs: A randomised trial. Lancet. 2002;359(9325):2235–41.
132. Pappo AS, et al. Phase II trial of neoadjuvant vincristine, ifosfamide, and doxorubicin with granulocyte colony-stimulating factor support in children and adolescents with advanced-stage nonrhabdomyosarcomatous soft tissue sarcomas: a Pediatric Oncology Group Study. J Clin Oncol. 2005;23(18):4031–8.
133. Edmonson JH, et al. Randomized comparison of doxorubicin alone versus ifosfamide plus doxorubicin or mitomycin, doxorubicin, and cisplatin against advanced soft tissue sarcomas. J Clin Oncol. 1993;11(7):1269–75.
134. Pervaiz N, et al. A systematic meta-analysis of randomized controlled trials of adjuvant chemotherapy for localized resectable soft-tissue sarcoma. Cancer. 2008;113(3):573–81.
135. Loh ML, et al. Treatment of infantile fibrosarcoma with chemotherapy and surgery: results from the Dana-Farber Cancer Institute and Children's Hospital, Boston. J Pediatr Hematol Oncol. 2002;24(9):722–6.
136. Cecchetto G, et al. Fibrosarcoma in pediatric patients: results of the Italian Cooperative Group studies (1979–1995). J Surg Oncol. 2001;78(4):225–31.
137. Adem C, et al. ETV6 rearrangements in patients with infantile fibrosarcomas and congenital mesoblastic nephromas by fluorescence in situ hybridization. Mod Pathol. 2001;14(12): 1246–51.
138. Orbach D, et al. Infantile fibrosarcoma: management based on the European experience. J Clin Oncol. 2010;28(2):318–23.
139. Sulkowski JP, Raval MV, Browne M. Margin status and multimodal therapy in infantile fibrosarcoma. Pediatr Surg Int. 2013;29(8):771–6.
140. Johansson G, et al. Effective in vivo targeting of the mammalian target of rapamycin pathway in malignant peripheral nerve sheath tumors. Mol Cancer Ther. 2008;7(5):1237–45.
141. Johannessen CM, et al. TORC1 is essential for NF1-associated malignancies. Curr Biol. 2008;18(1):56–62.
142. Vistica DT, et al. Therapeutic vulnerability of an in vivo model of alveolar soft part sarcoma (ASPS) to antiangiogenic therapy. J Pediatr Hematol Oncol. 2009;31(8):561–70.
143. Hawkins DS, et al. Children's Oncology Group's 2013 blueprint for research: soft tissue sarcomas. Pediatr Blood Cancer. 2013;60(6):1001–8.
144. Ray A, Huh WW. Current state-of-the-art systemic therapy for pediatric soft tissue sarcomas. Curr Oncol Rep. 2012;14(4):311–9.
145. Le Deley MC, et al. SFOP OS94: a randomised trial comparing preoperative high-dose methotrexate plus doxorubicin to high-dose methotrexate plus etoposide and ifosfamide in osteosarcoma patients. Eur J Cancer. 2007;43(4):752–61.

Chemotherapy and Other Systemic Approaches to Adult Sarcomas

12

Dennis A. Priebat

12.1 Overview

Sarcomas are rare, mesenchymal tumors of the soft tissue and bone that exhibit a marked heterogeneity in their clinical presentation, biologic behavior, and histologic and molecular features. Approximately 15,610 new cases are diagnosed annually, 12,310 of which arise from the soft tissues (50–60% of which involve the extremities) and 3300 from bones [1]. Major advances in the treatment of these tumors have been limited by an inability to accumulate sufficient numbers of similar patients to perform prospective randomized clinical trials with results that can achieve statistical significance.

Until the 1970s, surgery was the accepted method for the primary management of most soft tissue and bone sarcomas of the extremities. However, surgery alone, especially wide resection, was associated with a high incidence of local recurrences. Even when local control was achieved, more than 50% of patients with soft tissue sarcoma (STS) and 80% of patients with skeletal sarcoma (osteogenic and Ewing's sarcoma) eventually developed distant metastasis and died, usually within 2 years.

Nonsurgical treatment modalities (i.e., radiation therapy and chemotherapy) were subsequently found to exhibit reproducible antitumor effects against these neoplasms. Initially used only in the treatment of metastatic disease, they were later used as a part of combined modality therapy in the adjuvant (postoperative) setting and then as preoperative (neoadjuvant, induction) therapy in an attempt to preserve limb function and/or increase long-term survival. More recently, molecular targeted therapies have been developed, which for the most part have a more favorable toxicity profile but have thus far yielded limited results, (except for gastrointestinal stromal tumors {GISTs}).

D.A. Priebat, M.D.
Medical Oncology, Washington Cancer Institute at MedStar Washington Hospital Center, Washington, DC, USA
e-mail: Dennis.A.Priebat@medstar.net

© Springer International Publishing Switzerland 2017   223
R.M. Henshaw (ed.), *Sarcoma*, DOI 10.1007/978-3-319-43121-5_12

12.2 Soft Tissue Sarcoma (STS)

Despite the development of successful therapeutic modalities for local tumor control (e.g., limb-sparing surgery and radiation therapy), 40–50% of patients, particularly those with high-grade, large, deep tumors, will have local recurrences and die from metastases that were not apparent at presentation. An additional 10% of patients will have metastasis (usually the lung) at the time of initial diagnosis. Consequentially, chemotherapy was used initially to treat metastatic disease. It was later used to attempt to increase survival after local treatment and to also possibly maximize the number of candidates for limb-sparing surgery.

12.2.1 Chemotherapy Development

Only two single agents, doxorubicin and ifosfamide, have shown a reproducible response that is greater than 20% for soft tissue sarcomas. The largest experience with single-agent chemotherapy in this disease is with doxorubicin. A steep dose-response relationship can be seen, as was first demonstrated in the Southwest Oncology Group (SWOG) study in the 1970s, in which a dose of 75 mg/m^2 given every 3 weeks was shown to have a superior response rate to doses of 60 and 45 mg/m^2 [2]. Further evidence of a dose response has come from other studies of doxorubicin administered alone, as well as in conjunction with ifosfamide [3]. Unfortunately, doxorubicin is associated with dose-limiting cardiotoxicity, which can be reduced without altering the drug's effectiveness by administering it as a continuous IV infusion over 72–96 h via a central venous catheter or by concomitant use of dexrazoxane (a cardioprotectant) [4]. To obtain an optimal response, it appears to be important to achieve a dose intensity of at least 70 mg/m^2 every 3 weeks.

Analogues of doxorubicin have been developed in an effort to reduce the potential for cardiotoxicity that exists at higher cumulative doses. Epirubicin has been the most extensively studied. The EORTC Sarcoma Group compared equitoxic doses of doxorubicin 75 mg/m^2 and epirubicin 150 mg/m^2 (given as a single bolus or fractioned over 3 days). An overall response rate of 18% was obtained. No difference was seen between the three study arms; however, myelosuppression was greater for epirubicin than for doxorubicin. The incidence of cardiotoxicity was similar for both agents. Unfortunately, none of the currently available anthracycline analogues show any advantage over doxorubicin for patients with soft tissue sarcomas [5]. Liposomal doxorubicin has demonstrated activity in soft tissue sarcomas (especially angiosarcoma, Kaposi sarcoma, and desmoid tumors) [6, 7, 8]. However, for most other STS, the response rates are not equivalent to doxorubicin, and doses greater than 50 mg/m^2 are fraught with debilitating mucocutaneous toxicity (hand-foot syndrome) [9].

Alkylating agents have also been studied extensively, but only ifosfamide has shown activity equivalent to that of doxorubicin. There was debate over its activity compared with that of cyclophosphamide. In the 1980s, the EORTC performed a randomized trial comparing a 24-h continuous infusion of cyclophosphamide 1.5 g/m^2 vs. ifosfamide 5 g/m^2 (chosen to produce a comparable degree of myelosuppression) [10]. The response rate for ifosfamide in previously untreated patients with sarcoma was 25 vs. 13% for cyclophosphamide. In addition, ifosfamide showed activity in previously treated patients and in patients who were resistant to cyclophosphamide. There were no responses observed in patients crossed over to cyclophosphamide, indicating an incomplete cross-resistance between the two agents. Leukopenia was much less common in patients who received ifosfamide, suggesting that further dose escalation would be possible.

Both the dosage and scheduling appear to be important factors for the use of ifosfamide in soft tissue sarcomas. Doses of less than or equal to 8 g/m^2 demonstrated clinical activity in numerous studies in the 1980s. But it was only in the 1990s that a dose-response relationship was recognized and fully evaluated [11]. There appeared to be further antitumor activity of high-dose ifosfamide (12–14 g/m^2) in patients who did not respond to lower doses or who relapsed after standard dose ifosfamide-containing regimens. Several dose-intensified studies have shown higher clinical response rates than conventional dose regimens. When ifosfamide is used as a single-agent therapy, several experts recommend that a dose of ≥ 10 g/m^2 be the minimum needed to obtain an optimal response for patients with soft tissue sarcomas. With the availability of mesna (M), which protects against urothelial toxicity (i.e., hemorrhagic cystitis), the clinical use of this agent became practical. The scheduling of ifosfamide appears to be clinically important. Studies by Antman et al. [12] and Patel et al. [11] have suggested that a 2–4-h IV bolus schedule appears to have approximately twice the response rate as a continuous IV infusion. An EORTC randomized trial that compared two different dose schedules of ifosfamide (5 g/m^2 over 24 h vs. 3 g/m^2 over 4 h, day 1–3) demonstrated an advantage for the IV bolus intensive regimen in terms of response (10 vs. 25%) [13]. This same group also evaluated ifosfamide given at 12 g/m^2 as a 72-h continuous IV infusion every four weeks which yielded an overall response rate of only 14% [14].

Ifosfamide has been shown to have significant activity against synovial cell sarcoma. With the availability of mesna, it is much safer to use, but it still has dose-limiting myelosuppression, renal, and Central Nervous System (CNS) toxicity. Vigorous hydration with electrolytes and bicarbonate/acetate must be utilized to prevent severe metabolic acidosis and to reduce the risk of significant neurotoxicity. Central nervous system toxicity usually presents as a metabolic encephalopathy that may include confusion, blurred vision, mutism, auditory or visual paranoid hallucinations, seizures, and rarely, coma. The exact mechanism for this toxicity is not known, but it may be related to the accumulation of chloroacetaldehyde, one of ifosfamide's metabolites. Patients who are particularly prone to renal and CNS toxicity include those with a poor performance status, low serum albumin level (< 3 gm/dL), renal dysfunction (as indicated by a prior nephrectomy, clinical or subclinical renal tubular dysfunction, or previous treatment with cisplatinum), and bulky pelvic disease, as well as those over the age of 65 [15].

Neurotoxicity is usually self-limited. Methylene blue (50 mg IV) and diazepam (5 mg IV) have been reported to reverse the encephalopathy; however, methylene blue should not be given to patients who are glucose-6-phosphate dehydrogenase (G6PD) deficient. Both agents can be given prophylactically in subsequent cycles to prevent neurotoxicity (i.e., methylene blue 65 mg tablets four times per day). Hematologic toxicity in terms of myelosuppression has been lessened using the hematopoietic growth factors G- or GM-CSF, but patients still can develop dose-limiting thrombocytopenia [15–17].

Dacarbazine (DTIC) has also been used extensively for soft tissue sarcomas, but it has a response rate under 20% as a single agent. Emesis, a major side effect, can be reduced when the drug is given as a continuous IV infusion. A similar oral formulation, with similar efficacy, temozolomide (undergoes conversion to 3-methyl-(triazen-1-yl) imidazole-4-carboxamide {MTIC}), has also been developed [18]. Of note, it has shown specific activity against non-gastrointestinal leiomyosarcoma. Administering this at night and utilizing a daily low-dose scheme (75 mg/m^2 by mouth) reduce the incidence of emesis and enhance tolerability.

12.2.2 Combination Therapy in the Treatment of Advanced Disease

Given the modest results of single-agent chemotherapy in the treatment of soft tissue sarcomas, several combination chemotherapy regimens have been explored. There is still controversy as to whether single-agent doxorubicin or a multiagent regimen that includes doxorubicin is better for the treatment of advanced disease. Based on its activity in refractory and relapsed soft tissue sarcoma, ifosfamide with mesna has been studied in combination with doxorubicin.

Patel and colleagues at MD Anderson Cancer Center (MDACC) escalated the doses of doxorubicin and ifosfamide and have reported the highest observed response rates for STS. They conducted two pilot studies to evaluate the feasibility and activity of doxorubicin at either 75 or 90 mg/m^2 combined with ifosfamide at 10 g/m^2 (2 g/m^2 for 5 days), with G-CSF support. The overall objective response rate in 79 evaluable patients was 65%. There was no further benefit in response in the higher doxorubicin dose arm, but about 50% of patients experienced grade 3–4 thrombocytopenia within the first two cycles and virtually all patients by cycle three. This higher dose therapy is felt to be feasible only for selected patients (i.e., age less than 65, ECOG performance status 0–1, no prior chemotherapy, and radiation therapy to less than 20% of the bone marrow) [19].

To try to conclusively answer the question of whether the combination of doxorubicin plus ifosfamide produces superior outcomes, the EORTC performed a randomized phase III study of doxorubicin 75 mg/m^2 and ifosfamide 10 g/m^2 over 4 days with growth factor support vs. doxorubicin 75 mg/m^2 alone. There was no significant difference in overall survival (median 12.8 vs. 14.3 months, HR = 0.83, $p = 0.076$). However, median progression-free survival was significantly longer for the combination (7.4 vs. 4.6 months, HR = 0.74, $p = 0.003$), and the objective response rate (ORR) was doubled (26 vs. 14%, $p < 0.006$) [20]. Not surprisingly, toxicity was substantially higher for the combination. Thus, it was concluded that doxorubicin remains the standard first-line chemotherapy for most patients with advanced soft tissue sarcomas. However, in young (<65 years), good performance status patients with symptomatic and/or small-volume disease where a response may render the tumor resectable and the patient disease-free, the use of the combination therapy should be considered and discussed with the patient due to the expected higher response rate.

An improved response rate may be more clinically important in the neoadjuvant setting for young, good performance status patients with a high-grade, borderline resectable lesion or for patients with pulmonary metastases who are borderline candidates for metastasectomy. A significant response could facilitate subsequent surgery and/or radiation therapy, and render the patient disease-free. For palliation, particularly in older or poor performance status patients, and in those with low- to intermediate-grade tumors, doxorubicin or doxorubicin/DTIC regimens seem preferable. Toxicity can be reduced by giving this regimen as a continuous IV infusion.

Although early studies suggested a very low response rate in soft tissue sarcomas for gemcitabine, the MD Anderson group described a higher response rate, confirming the importance for timed delivery of gemcitabine, i.e., rate of 10 mg/m^2/min. Hensley et al. combined gemcitabine (900 mg/m^2) as a 90-min intravenous infusion on days 1 and 8 with docetaxel, 100 mg/m^2 intravenous on day 8, and granulocyte growth factor support in patients with leiomyosarcoma [21].

After others confirmed activity in different sarcomas, the SARC group performed a randomized study comparing single-agent equimyelosuppressive doses and timed infusion of gemcitabine vs. gemcitabine/docetaxel. A Bayesian adaptive randomization design was used. Results reported by Maki et al. showed a statistically significant benefit for the combination in terms of response rate and progression-free survival [22]. Overall responses were seen more often in leiomyosarcoma, undifferentiated pleomorphic sarcoma/malignant fibrous histiocytoma, and angiosarcoma. Based on this study and others, some have utilized this combination regimen as first-line treatment instead of a doxorubicin-containing regimen [23]. However, a recent prospective phase III GEDDIS study compared the doublet of gemcitabine/docetaxel vs. doxorubicin as a first-line treatment in 257 patients with advanced unresectable or metastatic STS [24]. Patients were stratified by tumor histiotype (uterine LMS, synovial sarcoma, pleomorphic sarcoma, other). There was no difference in progression-free relapse at 24 weeks (46.1 vs. 46.0%) or median overall survival (71 vs. 63 weeks). In a planned subgroup analysis, there was no evidence of benefit for leiomyosarcoma vs. non-leiomyosarcoma ($p = 0.326$) or uterine vs. non-uterine leiomyosarcoma ($p = 0.38$). In addition, gemcitabine/docetaxel was found to have more toxicity. This study further confirmed that single-agent doxorubicin should remain the standard of care for most patients with advanced unresectable or metastatic soft tissue sarcoma.

Although frontline chemotherapy for STS has been a doxorubicin +/− ifosfamide-containing regimen for many years, there is increasing evidence suggesting that tailoring chemotherapy choices based upon specific sarcoma histiotypes is beneficial due to different response profiles to a range of drugs. Other single agents that have been found to be more specific to certain tumor subtypes include paclitaxel [25, 26] and other taxanes for angiosarcoma [27–29], irinotecan for small cell sarcomas, and dacarbazine (or temozolomide) for leiomyosarcoma [30].

12.2.3 Newer Approved Drugs for Soft Tissue Sarcoma

Pazopanib is a multitargeted, orally-active inhibitor of several tyrosine kinases (TKIs), including vascular endothelial growth factor receptor (VEGFR). The European Organisation for Research and Treatment of Cancer (EORTC) performed a worldwide, randomized, double-blind phase III study (PALETTE trial) comparing 800 mg pazopanib vs. placebo in 369 patients with a variety of sarcoma subtypes (but excluding adipocytic sarcomas based on previous phase II data) whose disease had progressed during or after first-line chemotherapy (including an anthracycline) [31, 32]. Median progression-free survival was found to be significantly higher in the pazopanib arm (4.6 vs. 1.6 months, HR 0.31, $p < 0.0001$), and benefit was seen across all histologic subtypes. Partial responses were 6 vs. 0%, and stable disease was 67 vs. 38%. There was no significant difference in overall survival (12.5 vs. 10.7 months HR 0.86). The most common grade III/IV treatment-related toxicities included fatigue, hypertension, anorexia, diarrhea, and a transient elevation of liver function tests. There was also an increased drop in left ventricular ejection fraction, venous thromboembolism, and pneumothorax seen in the pazopanib group. Based on these results, pazopanib was approved by the FDA in April 2012 for treatment of patients with advanced STS (excluding adipocytic sarcomas). Close monitoring is recommended during the first 9 weeks because of the small risk of fatal hepatotoxicity, and concomitant use of drugs that raise the gastric pH are to be avoided (proton pump inhibitors and histamine H2 receptor antagonists) since an elevated gastric pH may decrease bioavailability.

Trabectedin, originally isolated from a Caribbean sea sponge (but now synthesized), has been shown to be an active agent for patients with advanced leiomyosarcoma and myxoid/round cell liposarcoma and has been available in the European Union and other countries for more than 5 years [33]. It appears to cause apoptosis by poisoning the DNA nucleotide excision repair machinery. This drug was recently approved in the United States, based on the results of a phase III multicenter trial [34] of trabectedin (1.5 mg/m^2 over 24 h) vs. dacarbazine, (1000 mg/m^2), both given every 3 weeks [35–37]. While the primary endpoint median overall survival was not significantly different (12.4 vs. 12.9 months), there was a significant improvement seen in progression-free survival (median 4.2 vs. 1.5 months, HR 0.56, $p < 0.0001$) and in overall clinical benefit (34 vs. 19%). Significant benefit was seen for both uterine and non-uterine leiomyosarcomas and in the myxoid/round cell liposarcoma group as well. The most common grade III/IV toxicities were neutropenia, thrombocytopenia, anemia, and elevation of hepatic enzymes. Trabectedin carries a risk of severe and fatal neutropenic sepsis, rhabdomyolysis, hepatotoxicity, extravasation soft tissue necrosis, and heart failure. Pretreatment with intravenous dexamethasone is recommended to ameliorate the hepatotoxicity [38]. Patients most at risk for life threatening toxicity are those with liver function tests that show an obstructive pattern with elevation of alkaline phosphatase.

Eribulin, previously approved for breast cancer, inhibits microtubules through a distinct mechanism separate from other microtubule agents (e.g., taxanes, vinca alkaloids). A recent multicenter phase III trial of eribulin (1.4 mg/m^2 Days 1 and 8) vs. dacarbazine (850–1200 mg/m^2), both administered every 3 weeks, led to its recent FDA approval for liposarcoma with a similar median progression-free survival, but a median overall survival benefit of 15.6 vs. 8.4 months (HR 0.77, p = 0.017) [39, 40].

Most recently, the safety and efficacy of olaratumab (platelet-derived growth factor receptor-alpha blocking antibody) were evaluated [41] in a randomized phase II clinical trial of 133 patients with multiple subtypes of metastatic soft tissue sarcoma; patients received either olaratumab (OLA) and doxorubicin (DOX) or doxorubicin alone. The objective response rate for combined OLA + DOX was 18.2 vs. 7.5% for DOX alone; median progression-free survival was 8.2 months for the combination and 4.4 months for DOX alone (HR 0.74). However, there was a highly significant benefit in median overall survival, 26.5 months for OLA + DOX compared to 14.7 months for DOX alone (HR 0.46, p = 0.0003). Although the proportion of some DOX associated toxicities were higher for the OLA arm (neutropenia and mucositis), this did not result in a higher rate of febrile neutropenia, infections, hospital admissions, or treatment-related mortality. There was also no significant difference in cardiac toxicity. The number of infusion-related reactions with olaratumab was 13% (8/64 patients), but this led to its discontinuation in only two patients (3%). The overall percentage of patients who discontinued treatment related to an adverse event was lower for the combined group (13%, 8/64) than in the DOX alone group (18%, 12/65). Based on the striking improvement in median overall survival (11.8 months) with an acceptable safety profile, olaratumab with doxorubicin was granted accelerated FDA approval [42]. Pending its use in more patients with metastatic soft tissue sarcomas (i.e., larger phase III trial), this will probably lead to a potential paradigm shift in the standard of care of treatment for many patients with metastatic STS [41, 42].

12.2.4 Other Molecular Targeted Drugs

Based on the success of molecular targeted therapy for GIST, other driver targets and inhibitors have been found for several rare sarcomas. Imatinib is now approved for dermatofibrosarcoma protuberans (DFSP), where there is a characteristic $t(17;22)$ translocation in which the co1A1 gene is juxtaposed to platelet-derived growth factor gene (PDGF), leading to upregulation of the PDGF receptor [43, 44]. Both sunitinib and cediranib have been shown to have activity against alveolar soft part sarcoma (ASPS), a highly vascular but inherently chemoresistant sarcoma [45, 46]. Solitary fibrous tumor/hemangiopericytoma (SFT/HPC) is another rare, slow-growing vascular tumor where it has been shown that several antiangiogenic agents have durable activity (i.e., bevacizumab with DTIC or temozolomide, sorafenib, and sunitinib) [47–49]. An extremely rare tumor, perivascular epithelioid cell tumors (PEComas), in which the mTOR signaling pathway is activated, appears to respond to sirolimus (an mTOR inhibitor) [50]. Crizotinib has been shown to have activity in inflammatory myofibroblastic tumor (IMFT) in which rearrangements of the anaplastic lymphoma kinase (ALK) gene occur in 50% of patients [51, 52].

Soft Tissue Sarcoma	Targeted therapy
DFSP	Imatinib
ASPS	Cediranib
	Sunitinib
SFT/HPC	Bevacizumab/temozolomide
	Sorafenib
	Sunitinib
PEComas	Sirolimus
IMFT	Crizotinib

Table 12.1 Molecular targeted therapies for specific rare soft tissue sarcomas

Table 12.1 lists several rare soft tissue sarcomas and their corresponding targeted therapy.

Early findings of activity in these rare sarcoma subsets are encouraging. However, despite these hopeful successes, further work is needed for the more common sarcomas. Unfortunately, these are often associated with multiple and different molecular abnormalities, where specific molecular targets have not yet been identified. Even when a known molecular target is identified, the response to targeted therapy is often short-lived, likely due to the development of resistance from activation of other cellular pathways. Future efforts to harness immune therapy, either alone or combined with targeted molecular therapy, will hopefully overcome such resistance and lead to more sustained responses.

12.2.5 Adjuvant Chemotherapy

Although the role of adjuvant chemotherapy is well established in the treatment of several sarcomas that occur predominantly in children (i.e., rhabdomyosarcoma, osteosarcoma, and Ewing's sarcoma), as well as in GIST, its use in patients with a high risk of recurrence of adult-type soft tissue sarcomas (e.g., liposarcoma, leiomyosarcoma, synovial sarcoma, etc.) remains controversial and unresolved. Published articles range from retrospective reviews of outcome at single institutions, to prospective nonrandomized studies, to formal randomized trials.

Most of these studies have enrolled too few patients (less than 100), have used different patient inclusion criteria, and/or have had an imbalance between the two arms with respect to pathologic grade, histologic subtype, and anatomic site or utilized different drugs, doses, and schedules (some with suboptimal doses and/or a delayed start). Several have an extremely short follow-up period, while others included patients with good risk factors (i.e., small, less than 5 cm and low-grade tumors). For these reasons, it is hard to draw definitive conclusions on the benefit of adjuvant chemotherapy.

Resection of pulmonary metastases and the use of preoperative chemotherapy may also affect overall survival. Furthermore, it is difficult to detect small but potentially clinically important differences in survival, when only moderately effective chemotherapy regimens are used. Several single-arm studies show adjuvant chemotherapy to be beneficial when compared with historical controls; however, in nearly all prospective randomized trials with an observation arm, there is no difference in overall survival. Both the treated and observation (control) arms do better than previous historical controls. Most studies show a trend toward longer disease-free survival but no significant increase in overall survival.

Tierney et al. of the MRC Cancer Trials Office and the Sarcoma Meta-analysis Collaboration published an individual patient data meta-analysis (IPD-MA) of updated outcomes of 1568 patients from 14 randomized trials of doxorubicin-based adjuvant chemotherapy vs. observation control [53]. The median follow-up period was 9.4 years. Soft tissue sarcomas of all sites, sizes, grades, and histologies were included. Only 59% of the histologic subtypes and 25% of the grading had been reviewed at the time of its publication. This IPD-MA showed a significant improvement for adjuvant chemotherapy with respect to time to recurrence (local and distant) and disease-free survival but only a trend for benefit in overall survival. However, in the subset of patients with extremity soft tissue sarcoma ($n = 886$), there was a significant (7%) absolute benefit in overall survival at 10 years ($p = 0.029$). Caution must be taken in interpreting the survival benefit as extremity STS was not included as part of the initial randomization and analysis, and there can be inherent dangers in the later evaluation of patient subsets [53]. Additionally, this early IPD meta-analysis is not fully relevant for present medical practice, since it did not include adjuvant studies containing ifosfamide or use hematopoietic growth factors to maintain dose intensity.

Frustaci et al. reported on the Italian Cooperative Soft Tissue Sarcoma Group's randomized adjuvant trial of 104 patients with high-risk (i.e., high-grade, deep, and greater than 5 cm) extremity soft tissue sarcomas utilizing high doses of epirubicin and ifosfamide with G-CSF support. At a median follow-up of 24 months (range, 5–57 months), there was a significant difference in favor of the chemotherapy arm for both disease-free ($p = 0.001$) and overall ($p = 0.005$) survival [54]. At interim analysis, after only half of the planned number of patients had been randomized, the investigators decided to stop accrual, even though follow-up was short. No evaluation of toxicity was reported. Unfortunately, with further follow-up, the benefit in overall survival was lost [55].

A larger 351-patient randomized EORTC 62931 trial of five cycles of doxorubicin (75 mg/m^2) and ifosfamide (5 g/m^2) plus lenograstim (GM-CSF) showed no benefit in relapse-free survival or overall survival vs. placebo [56]. This has been criticized for using a lower ifosfamide dose (5 g/m^2 instead of 9 g/m^2) than was utilized in the Frustaci study and for having 24% of patients with tumors <5 cm in size.

A later updated meta-analysis of randomized trials (including 2145 patients) [57], added to the previous IPDM reported by Tierney, also suggested that there was a small but appreciable benefit for patients receiving adjuvant chemotherapy (HR 0.86, $p = 0.02$). Unfortunately, the confidence intervals are too wide to draw any definitive conclusions. An updated individual patient data meta-analysis would more reliably allow for the exact determination of benefit of adjuvant chemotherapy.

Since the survival of patients with high-grade extremity soft tissue sarcomas is already 50–70% at several centers, it will be increasingly difficult to show a statistically significant difference in randomized adjuvant trials [58]. More patients will be needed to show small differences in survival, a challenging proposition for such a rare disease. Patients with low-grade sarcomas should not be given adjuvant chemotherapy because of their inherently low rate of metastatic spread and excellent prognosis. In addition, small (less than 5 cm), superficial, high-grade primary extremity sarcomas should not be included in chemotherapy trials, since studies also suggest that these patients have an excellent survival. Despite their limitations, the IPD-MA, the Italian study, and the updated meta-analysis all suggest that adjuvant chemotherapy may be beneficial for select patients with extremity soft tissue sarcoma. Future randomized trials should include only patients at high-risk for metastases (i.e., large, high-grade, deep-seated tumors and a good performance status) with a reasonable likelihood of local control (radical resection or resection with uninvolved margins and radiotherapy) [59]. The recent National Comprehensive Cancer Network (NCCN) Practice Guidelines recommend considering adjuvant chemotherapy with an aggressively dosed ifosfamide/doxorubicin regimen for patients with AJCC Stage IIB or III extremity sarcomas who have undergone optimal resection, with or without radiation therapy [60].

Our present approach is to consider adjuvant chemotherapy for patients on an individual basis, based upon the patient's performance status, comorbid medical problems, age (usually under 65), tumor location and size, histologic subtype (chemosensitive), and grade. For many years, we have utilized an every 3-week AIM regimen, consisting of doxorubicin (75 mg/m^2) given as a continuous IV infusion through a double lumen central venous catheter with ifosfamide (2.25 g/m^2/day) given intravenously over 3 h for 4 days (total 9 g/m^2), with pegylated G-CSF support afterwards.

12.2.6 Neoadjuvant Chemotherapy

Neoadjuvant (also referred to as induction or preoperative) chemotherapy for soft tissue sarcomas of the extremities evolved as a result of studies initially performed for osteogenic sarcoma. Routes of administration have included IV bolus, continuous IV infusion, and intra-arterial regional therapy, with or without concomitant radiation therapy, and have also included isolated limb perfusion. Neoadjuvant therapy has primarily been utilized for patients with large primary or recurrent sarcomas, usually with the goal of permitting a limb-sparing operation in patients in whom amputation may otherwise have been necessary or for converting a marginally resectable tumor to one that can be adequately resected with preservation of extremity function. Other theoretical advantages include early treatment of micrometastases, an in vivo assessment of the effectiveness of the chemotherapy, and improved patient survival. Although initial local tumor control and limb salvage rates appear very good, most studies have enrolled only small numbers of patients and have short follow-up. Therefore, the effect of neoadjuvant therapy on disease-free and overall survival rates is not fully known. There have been no prospective phase III randomized trials comparing preoperative and postoperative chemotherapy for patients with soft tissue sarcoma. Nevertheless, patients with large, deep-seated, high-grade lesions of the extremities are a high-risk group that is an optimal target population for investigating the effectiveness of multimodality treatment strategies.

A randomized phase II EORTC study (62874) randomizing 150 patients to either three cycles of neoadjuvant doxorubicin at 50 mg/m^2 and ifosfamide at 5 g/m^2 vs. surgery alone failed to show a survival benefit for the chemotherapy arm [61]. This trial suffered from slow accrual and was stopped early, before expansion into a phase III study. The low-dose intensity of both drugs may have contributed to this negative result (5-year disease-free survival 56 vs. 52%, $p = $ NS).

When induction therapy is being considered for a patient with a large, high-grade, extremity sarcoma, radiotherapy alone or with concomitant sequential chemotherapy may also be utilized. Preoperative radiation therapy is usually associated with a higher rate of wound complications, while late tissue fibrosis is seen with postoperative adjuvant radiation therapy [62–64].

Hyperthermic isolated limb perfusion with melphalan and tumor necrosis factor (TNF) has been used at a limited number of centers in patients with large soft tissue extremity sarcomas that are close to bone, nerve, and/or blood vessels and in whom amputation would otherwise be necessary. A high limb salvage rate (> 80%) has been reported [65]. Nevertheless, this is a localized treatment when used alone, and there has been no control of or reduction in the recurrence of systemic disease, with patients dying from distant metastases. Further impeding study of this modality is the fact that TNF is not available in the United States.

Chemotherapy with regional hyperthermia (RHT) has also been utilized. The pleotropic effects of heat on the malignant cells and tumor stroma are felt to reduce tumor growth and progression, and heat stress-induced mechanisms may play a role in the initiation of antitumor immunity. An updated analysis of an EORTC-ESHO Intergroup randomized phase III trial of RHT combined with neoadjuvant chemotherapy vs. neoadjuvant chemotherapy alone showed a significantly improved long-term overall survival for the RHT chemotherapy arm [66].

In general, neoadjuvant chemotherapy for large, high-grade soft tissue sarcomas of the extremities is feasible and associated with good local control and survival. Limb-sparing surgery is often possible for most of these patients. More aggressive regimens appear to reduce local recurrence and result in a high complete pathologic response rate. The best regimen, in terms of specific drugs or drug/radiation sequence, is not known at this time; also unknown is whether radiation therapy is necessary for all patients. However, neoadjuvant chemotherapy should be considered for patients who have traditionally been thought to be at high risk for local recurrence (i.e., patients with large, deep-seated, high-grade, extremity sarcomas and a good performance status). We believe that amputation should rarely be performed for large, high-grade extremity soft tissue sarcomas without first considering a trial of neoadjuvant therapy.

We utilize the same AIM regimen as previously mentioned in the adjuvant chemotherapy section. NCCN guidelines suggest that preoperative radiation therapy alone, preoperative chemotherapy (with postoperative adjuvant radiation therapy), and preoperative chemoradiotherapy are all acceptable options [60]. In Europe, there is also the availability of neoadjuvant chemotherapy combined with regional hyperthermia. It is recommended that these patients be managed at a center with multidisciplinary expertise [67].

12.3   Bone Sarcomas

Sarcomas of the bone are typically classified by the type of matrix produced by the tumor; osteosarcomas are bone-producing tumors, chondrosarcomas produce cartilage, and fibrosarcomas have a fibrous matrix (a notable exception is Ewing's sarcoma). Although the incidence of bone sarcoma is much lower than that for soft tissue sarcoma, the role and value of chemotherapy in the treatment of bone sarcoma have been better studied and established compared to STS.

12.3.1 Osteosarcoma

Although osteosarcoma is a rare tumor, it is the most common malignant tumor of bone in adolescents and young adults. Approximately 900 new cases occur each year in the United States. It is more prevalent in males and has a strong predilection for the distal femur, proximal tibia, and proximal humerus. About 80% of patients have localized disease at the time of diagnosis. The most common sites of metastasis are the lung and other bones.

Prior to 1970, the primary treatment of nonmetastatic osteosarcoma of the extremities consisted of surgical removal (usually amputation) and/or high-dose radiation therapy of the primary tumor. The 5-year disease-free survival rate was no more than 20%; lung metastases were the most common reason for treatment failures, even after radical amputation. Early investigations of chemotherapy for osteosarcoma were unrewarding, and it was considered a chemoresistant tumor.

By the early 1970s, and continuing through the 1980s, reports began to emerge of effective drugs for the treatment of osteosarcoma, i.e., doxorubicin, high-dose methotrexate with calcium leucovorin rescue, cisplatinum, and later ifosfamide. It was demonstrated that these agents could eradicate overt metastatic disease and improve disease-free survival, and they have since been incorporated into modern chemotherapy regimens in varying combinations. The major advances made over the past several decades in the treatment of osteosarcoma are a consequence of the development of effective chemotherapy. The introduction of these agents into multidisciplinary treatment strategies has allowed for more conservative and limb-sparing procedures to be performed and has resulted in improved overall patient survival.

12.3.1.1 Chemotherapy Development

There has been a wide variation in reported response rates to methotrexate (e.g., 0–80%), leading several investigators to question its effectiveness. The activity of methotrexate appears to be dose dependent, given that dose escalation has been associated with responses in patients previously unresponsive to lower doses [68]. It has the significant advantage of being nonmyelosuppressive, but it is expensive and needs to be used with care and appropriate monitoring, especially in older patients. It should only be considered for children, adolescents, and adults under age 40. Rosen and others believed the variable response rates reported with methotrexate were directly related to improper drug administration [69, 70]. Several studies have shown that for methotrexate to be effective in osteosarcoma, one must achieve a minimum peak serum concentration of greater than 1000 μmol (10^{-3} M) at the completion of a 4-h infusion (700 μmol after a 6-h infusion) [71]. To attain these drug levels, it is necessary to give a dose of at least 8–12 g/m². Furthermore, excessive amounts of intravenous hydration should not be administered during the first 24 h, to limit urine output to less than 1400 cc/m².

There also appears to be a steep dose-response rate for doxorubicin; i.e., doses ≥70 mg/m² have more activity than lower doses. Whether carboplatinum can be substituted for cisplatinum is still controversial. Carboplatinum has reduced renal and ototoxicity but produces more myelosuppression (including thrombocytopenia) and may be less active than cisplatinum. Initial reports indicated that the combination of bleomycin, cyclophosphamide, and dactinomycin (BCD) was effective in the treatment of metastatic disease, and in several early preoperative studies, this regimen was given with other known active agents. However, subsequent studies failed to confirm the activity of BCD when given alone, consequently it is not included in most modern chemotherapy regimens.

Ifosfamide appears to have significant activity for the treatment of both primary and recurrent osteosarcoma. It also has a clear dose-dependent response curve (with responses occurring at doses of 12–18 g/m² in patients who had failed with previous doses below 10 g/m²). It has been given alone, or in a lower dose in combination with etoposide [72, 73].

How to best combine these known active drugs is still unknown, and there is still debate over what constitutes optimum chemotherapy. While most institutions utilize an intensive multiagent regimen, some have questioned the merits of prolonged and complicated schemes over regimens that include fewer drugs given over a shorter time frame.

A study by the European Osteosarcoma Intergroup (EOI) explored whether the intensive use of two active agents, cisplatinum and doxorubicin, administered in six cycles over 18 weeks, is better than a more complex, multiagent-modified Memorial Sloan Kettering Cancer Center (MSKCC) T10-like regimen given over 44 weeks [74, 75]. There was poor patient compliance and a reduction in dose intensity with the multidrug regimen. The shorter, two-drug combination was found to have equivalent survival outcomes to that observed with the modified T10 program, the 5-year progression-free and overall survival rates for both groups being only 44 and 55%, respectively. Unfortunately, these results are somewhat lower than that achieved in other previous studies.

12.3.1.2 Adjuvant Chemotherapy

Once chemotherapy had been found to be effective against metastatic disease, investigations were initiated to determine the efficacy of these agents in destroying micrometastases, which are thought to be present in most patients at the time of initial primary surgery (i.e., adjuvant or postoperative chemotherapy). In 1286 patients collected from the world literature between 1946 and 1971 (prechemotherapy era), there was a 5-year mean survival rate of 19.7% (range 16–23%) [76, 77]. Eighty percent of patients developed metastases despite amputation, suggesting the presence of micrometastatic disease in most cases.

In the 1970s, early uncontrolled adjuvant trials of single and multiagent chemotherapy regimens documented relapse-free survival rates of 35–60%. However, the contribution of adjuvant chemotherapy was then questioned by researchers from the Mayo Clinic, where the outcome with surgery alone was found to be improved (13% disease-free survival for patients treated in the 1960s compared with 42% for patients in the 1970s) [78, 79]. A randomized adjuvant chemotherapy trial at the Mayo Clinic of moderate-dose methotrexate (considered inadequate by today's standards) vs. surgery alone indicated no benefit for adjuvant chemotherapy. The relapse-free survival of the surgery-alone group was 44%, more than twice what was expected based on the historical experience.

The exact role of adjuvant chemotherapy was heatedly debated. Some felt that an increased survival for osteosarcoma patients had occurred over time, due to diagnostic advances in staging, earlier detection of metastases, and improvements in surgical techniques and supportive care. Two subsequent prospective randomized trials conducted by the Multi-Institutional Osteosarcoma Study (MIOS) Group and the UCLA group resolved this controversy when they confirmed the significant favorable impact of adjuvant chemotherapy on outcome. They also corroborated the poor prognosis for patients treated with surgery alone (Table 12.2) [80–82].

Adjuvant chemotherapy has been shown to reduce the number of pulmonary metastases and to delay their appearance, thus possibly facilitating surgical removal. Interestingly, it has also changed the natural history of this neoplasm; more patients develop extrapulmonary metastases (e.g., to the skin, brain, and/or heart). Most trials of adjuvant chemotherapy now report event-free survival rates of 45–65%. Even with the increased use of preoperative chemotherapy to induce tumor necrosis, intensive additional adjuvant chemotherapy is still believed to be needed for optimal results.

12.3.1.3 Induction Chemotherapy

Simultaneous advances with chemotherapy and improved techniques of primary surgical resection have reduced the need for amputation. New limb-sparing procedures often required that surgery be delayed 2–3 months for the manufacture of a custom-made endoprosthesis. In the mid-1970s, Rosen et al. at MSKCC designed a strategy to use induction (neoadjuvant) chemotherapy to treat patients who were awaiting manufacture of their prosthesis in an effort to prevent progression of their disease during this time [83].

Table 12.2 Osteogenic sarcoma—randomized adjuvant chemotherapy studies

Adjuvant chemo. vs. observation	Patients, n	RFS, %	OS, %
MAYO [79]			
HDMTX+VCR	38	40	
		$P = $ NS	
vs. No adjuvant therapy		44	
MIOS [82]		6 years	
BCD+HDMTX ADRIA+CDDP	36 random	63	71
	165 nonrandom		
		$P = 0.001$	$P = 0.04$
vs. No adjuvant therapy		12	48
UCLA [80]		2 years	
BCD+HDMTX+VCR+ADRIA (+intra-arterial ADRIA+XRT)	59	55	80
		$P = 0.004$	$P = 0.04$
vs. No adjuvant therapy		20	48
Neoadjuvant vs. adjuvant POG#8651 [86]			
Chemotherapy	*5-year survival*		
	DFS		*OS*
Neoadjuvant	63.2		79.7
	$P = 0.60$		$P = 0.41$
Adjuvant	65.5		75.3

RFS relapse free survival, *OS* overall survival, *NS* not significant, *HDMTX* high-dose methotrexate, *VCR* vincristine, *BCD* bleomycin, cytoxan, dactinomycin-D, *ADRIA* adriamycin, *CDDP* cis-platinum, *XRT* radiation therapy

Adapted from data tables published in Priebat et al. 1992 [84, 167]

The induction therapy approach had other potential benefits as well. It was felt to be an early defense against the possible presence of pulmonary metastases and had the theoretical advantage of being able to reduce the emergence of drug-resistant tumor cells. It was also thought to help downstage a tumor by reducing the size of any accompanying soft tissue mass and forming a surrounding reactive rim that would confine the tumor within a calcified periosteum. These effects could possibly lead to better tumor demarcation and permit successful tumor removal with a limb-sparing resection. In addition, it provided an opportunity to test chemotherapy sensitivity in vivo based on the initial histologic response, which could then be used to customize or tailor adjuvant chemotherapy.

When intensive multiagent regimens were used, induction chemotherapy trials have often produced better relapse-free survival rates (42–82%) than those reported for patients undergoing immediate surgery followed by adjuvant chemotherapy [84–92]. Most modern induction protocols include a multidrug regimen, given for 6–18 weeks, followed by resection of the primary tumor, and then by 3–6 months of adjuvant IV chemotherapy. Drugs used in these regimens include cisplatinum and doxorubicin with or without high-dose methotrexate. Patients need to be followed closely, since a small number may be completely insensitive to induction chemotherapy and the tumor may continue to progress while on treatment. These patients need to be identified early so that they can be either switched to another chemotherapeutic regimen or have immediate surgical resection.

In conjunction with improvements in surgical technique and prosthetic devices, there was growing enthusiasm for limb-sparing surgery by orthopedic surgeons, which led to the more frequent use of induction chemotherapy. However, there were concerns about the development of resistant cells and/or an increase in growth of micrometastatic disease during treatment. The Pediatric Oncology Group (POG 8651) performed a randomized trial of induction vs. adjuvant chemotherapy in 100 patients under age 30 with nonmetastatic high-grade osteosarcoma [86]. Patients were randomized to immediate surgery or to presurgical treatment with two cycles (10-week duration) of high-dose methotrexate, cisplatinum, and doxorubicin. Except for timing, postsurgical chemotherapy (methotrexate, cisplatinum, doxorubicin, and BCD), given over 44 weeks, was the same in both arms.

The survival rate for the group receiving induction chemotherapy was no better than that of the adjuvant chemotherapy-alone group (61 vs. 65%, $p = 0.8$), as were the limb salvage rates (50 vs. 55%). Poor responders in the induction arm were not crossed over to other agents; thus, the strategy of salvage (tailoring) therapy was not evaluated. The study has been criticized for the small number of patients randomized over a 7-year period at 37 institutions (suggesting a bias of patient selection), the relatively low rate of limb-sparing surgery in both groups, and the inclusion of BCD chemotherapy as a component of the regimen. Some have used this study as a reason not to give induction chemotherapy since there was no improvement in patient survival or limb salvage rate. However, for many others, the results suggest that induction chemotherapy did not compromise overall survival, as was initially feared, and it was felt that a more efficacious regimen would further improve the limb salvage rate [86].

Based on the POG study results and the input of most orthopedic oncologists, the use of preoperative (neoadjuvant) chemotherapy has become widely accepted due to the advantages of increased surgical planning time, potential of improved or more complete tumor removal, and the ability to assess the histologic response to chemotherapy.

12.3.1.4 Histologic Assessment of Chemotherapy Response

The response of osteosarcoma to preoperative chemotherapy may be assessed by clinical, laboratory, radiologic, and pathologic parameters. Clinical responses are noted with a decrease in pain, swelling, and heat. On laboratory analysis, there can be a reduction of an elevated alkaline phosphatase. With plain radiography and computerized tomography scan, one can see a reduction or complete disappearance of any associated soft tissue mass, revisualization of the fat planes between muscle bundles, healing of pathologic fractures, and organized deposition of calcium within the neoplastic bone (calcified periosteum). An arteriogram can offer a more objective means of assessing a tumor response, as manifest by a diminution or a disappearance of tumor vascularity. Assessment by thallium three-phase scintigraphy or PET scan can also be helpful.

Despite the utility of these various findings, the histologic appearance of the resected primary tumor specimen after induction chemotherapy has emerged as the gold standard for evaluating and measuring a therapeutic response. Several pathologic grading systems for assessing the effect of induction chemotherapy have been developed, all of which are based on the degree of tumor cellularity and necrosis found within the resected specimen. Grading systems can be imprecise, subjective, and prone to sampling errors. Nevertheless, with careful attention to adequate and fastidious sectioning from many sites of the surgical specimen, a determination of response can be assessed which appears to correlate with patient outcome.

Most institutions now define a good pathologic response as >90% tumor necrosis and a poor response as ≤90% tumor necrosis. Certain subtypes, i.e., chondroblastic osteosarcoma, have lower reported rates of necrosis but show no difference in outcome for good vs. poor responders. For all other subtypes, histologic response correlates with patient prognosis [93–95].

12.3.1.5   Tailoring Adjuvant Therapy

The concept of tailoring adjuvant therapy, based on the histologic response of the primary tumor to induction chemotherapy, was first proposed by Rosen et al. and tested in the MSKCC T10 protocol [87]. This was formulated on the hypothesis that the responsiveness of the primary tumor to chemotherapy will predict the responsiveness of micrometastases. Thus, a good-responding patient receives the same drugs after surgery as before surgery, while the postoperative regimen of a patient who has responded poorly to induction chemotherapy is changed. Early results from the T10 protocol reported an excellent disease-free survival rate for poor-responding patients as well, suggesting that they could be salvaged with a modified adjuvant (postoperative) treatment.

The T10 protocol was a model for many trials launched in the 1980s, virtually all of which featured induction chemotherapy and the individualization of postoperative therapy based on the pathologic responsiveness of the primary tumor. Unfortunately, later studies from several groups, including the Children's Cancer Study Group (CCSG), German-Austrian-Swiss Cooperative Osteosarcoma Study Group (COSS-82), and Rizzoli Institute, failed to confirm an improved prognosis for poor responders treated with alternative postoperative chemotherapy regimens [88–91]. Furthermore, an update of the MSKCC T10 protocol, reported by Meyers et al. [92], indicated that Rosen's promising preliminary results were not sustained over time. With longer follow-up, the efficacy of tailored treatment was not demonstrated.

However, a study by Benjamin et al. from MDACC suggested that the addition of postoperative ifosfamide significantly improved the 5-year disease-free survival of poor-responding patients over that seen in their previous treatment regimens (67 vs. 34%, respectively, $p = 0.015$) [96]. Other studies incorporating ifosfamide also documented better survival rates.

12.3.1.6 Duration and Intensification of Induction Chemotherapy

There is considerable variability in the duration of induction chemotherapy. Most studies use an arbitrary time of 6–18 weeks with the administration of two to six cycles of chemotherapy. Some investigators have attempted to adjust surgical intervention to the time of maximal response to induction chemotherapy. Longer duration intensified chemotherapy regimens may be associated with a higher proportion of good histologic responses; however, as the duration of induction chemotherapy is prolonged, the value of using its effect on histologic response as a predictor of patient outcome may be lost. Thus, regimens of longer duration may result in a better histologic response which do not necessarily translate into improved patient survival. Meyers et al. have suggested that the rate of a good histologic response may be related to the duration of induction chemotherapy but that the duration of chemotherapy does not correlate with relapse-free overall survival [97].

Dose compression was evaluated by the European Osteosarcoma Intergroup (EOI) with chemotherapy given every 2 weeks with G-CSF support compared to every 3 weeks. Again, there was enhanced tumor necrosis seen, but with no survival advantage [98].

12.3.1.7 Intra-arterial Chemotherapy

To improve the results of induction IV systemic chemotherapy, to further downstage tumors, and to augment the rate of successful limb-sparing procedures, several investigators began to administer induction chemotherapy via the IA route [84]. This allows for a higher concentration of chemotherapy to be delivered to the primary tumor, with possible improved penetration of drug across the cell membrane. Pharmacological studies have confirmed an increase in regional drug concentration, drug uptake, and tumor destruction when the IA route is utilized. Furthermore, the concentration of chemotherapy reaching the systemic circulation after initial intra-arterial passage has been found to be similar to that attained via the IV route and therefore should be enough to destroy any microscopic pulmonary metastases.

Jaffe et al. established the use of IA cisplatinum as a single agent for the treatment of osteosarcoma in the pediatric population [99, 100]. IA cisplatinum has been given concurrently with different IV systemic agents. Small single-institution studies suggested that this allows for more limb-sparing procedures to be performed and does not substantially increase the risk of local recurrence or the development of metastatic disease. Such an approach has been associated with a higher tumor necrosis rate, perhaps making it possible to convert a marginal resection to a wide resection and to allow for a safer surgical procedure to be performed. Relapse or disease-free survival (DFS) rates for single-institution IA studies appear to be similar to those using IV induction chemotherapy.

The use of IA chemotherapy has been limited to centers with excellent angiographic support and facilities. However, the cost, complexity, time commitment, and morbidity associated with this approach may not be justifiable. A prospective randomized study from the Rizzoli Institute reported that patients who received induction IA cisplatinum had a significantly higher proportion of good histologic responses than those who received similar doses of IV cisplatinum, but there was no difference between the two groups in the number of limb-sparing procedures or survival [101].

Proof of benefit of IA induction chemotherapy will require prospective randomized investigation. To date, it has not appeared to make a significant difference in terms of disease-free and overall survival.

12.3.1.8 Addition of Other Agents

The CCG/POG INT-0133 trial evaluated in a 2 × 2 factorial design whether the addition of ifosfamide and/or mifurmatide (muramyl tripeptide-phosphatidyl ethanolamine, MTPE) to a standard MAP regime (high-dose methotrexate, doxorubicin, and cisplatin) would improve outcome [102–104]. The results have been difficult to interpret, with an assumed interaction between the two added agents based on event-free survival, precluding statistical analysis. In a later follow-up publication, there appeared to be no interaction with a benefit in overall survival only for mifurmatide, regardless of regimen. There is continued controversy as to whether there was enough statistical evidence to support the addition of mifurmatide. It has been approved in Europe, but not by the FDA, and is not available in the United States. No benefit for ifosfamide was found [105].

More recently, in an effort to perform larger-scale and statistically significant randomized trials for this rare tumor, a multisite, multinational, intergroup collaboration was developed; i.e., the European and American Osteosarcoma Study Group (EURAMOS). Their first study, EURAMOS-1, was a prospective randomized trial to evaluate response-guided treatment modification ("tailoring"), both for good and poor histologic responding patients [106]. The addition of maintenance treatment with 2 years of pegylated interferon alpha-2b following completion of adjuvant chemotherapy was assessed in good responding patients. While for poor responders, the addition of high-dose ifosfamide and etoposide to postoperative (adjuvant) chemotherapy was evaluated [106].

For the good responder cohort, there was no significant benefit in survival with the addition of pegylated interferon to postoperative MAP chemotherapy when compared to MAP alone. Interestingly, a quarter of patients were never started on interferon, and 45% of patients who received interferon stopped the treatment early, due to the toxicity of the interferon [107]. In the poor responder group, there was no improvement in outcome with the addition of high-dose ifosfamide and etoposide when compared to continuing MAP alone [108]. However, there was an increase in toxicity and a higher rate of second malignancies [109].

Therefore, at the present time, there is no proven benefit of tailoring chemotherapy based on the pathologic response to neoadjuvant chemotherapy. Nonetheless, the creation of the EURAMOS group will serve as a model for further international collaboration with a resulting infrastructure for future joint efforts and trials [110–112].

12.3.2 Relapsed Osteosarcoma

At present, there are few other agents with efficacy, after the aforementioned drugs, to be utilized for relapsed osteosarcoma. Patients with only a few pulmonary nodules can benefit from an aggressive surgical approach (metastasectomy). Gemcitabine alone or with docetaxel has been shown to have some benefit [113]. High-dose chemotherapy with stem cell support has been ineffective. Sorafenib has been noted to have efficacy by nonstandard criteria, usually decreased activity on PET imaging, changes in CT tumor density, and improved clinical symptoms, but the responses have usually been of short duration with a 6 month PFS of only 29% [114]. More recently, an mTOR inhibitor was combined with sorafenib in order to overcome mTOR C2 resistance, resulting in a 45% 6-month PFS (thus showing prolonged stabilization of disease but not meeting the defined study endpoint of 50%) [115, 116].

When evaluating new therapeutic agents in the treatment of osteosarcoma, Response Evaluation Criteria in Solid Tumors (RECIST) criteria may not always be a meaningful endpoint. Osteosarcoma does not always shrink in response to chemotherapy (especially if lacking a soft tissue component). This is because of the residual bone in the primary tumor and because the residual extracellular tumor matrix does not disappear despite tumor cell death. Patients with pulmonary metastases can have tumor cell necrosis but with resultant residual calcification and minimal tumor shrinkage. PET/CT can be helpful in assessing tumor activity as well as tumor extent. RECIST response can therefore be misleading and should not be solely used as response criteria for osteosarcoma [116].

Other agents in trial include eribulin [110, 117, 118], denosumab (RANK ligand antibody) [119], glembatumumab (novel antibody-auristatin conjugate) that targets the transmembrane glycoprotein GPNMB gene (osteoactivin) [120, 121], and an anti-GD2 (disialoganglioside) antibody [122].

In summary, the prognosis for patients with osteosarcoma of the extremities had markedly improved by the end of the twentieth century. More than two-thirds of patients who present with nonmetastatic disease are now cured. These advances are mainly due to the use of intensive multiagent chemotherapy. The impact of adjuvant chemotherapy is now indisputable, and it has become part of standard treatment. It is not clear which combination or duration schedule of chemotherapy is the best (among cisplatinum, doxorubicin, and high-dose methotrexate).

Limb-salvage surgery is now an accepted practice by orthopedic oncologists for most osteosarcoma patients. Most centers administer induction chemotherapy in order to enhance limb salvage opportunities, although its role in further improving patient survival remains uncertain. Dose intensification and/or dose compression has not resulted in improved survival outcomes. The benefit of tailoring adjuvant chemotherapy based on the histologic response of the primary tumor to induction chemotherapy has not been substantiated. New biomarkers are needed that can conclusively predict the histologic response and prognosis of patients at diagnosis, prior to induction chemotherapy, such that patients can be stratified into high- and low-risk subgroups.

Finally, despite the enormous initial progress that has been made, we are still faced with limitations in the options for chemotherapy because of the small number of modestly active chemotherapeutic agents. There is a need for new drugs and strategies to treat those patients already known to have a poor prognosis (e.g., chondroblastic subtype, metastases at presentation) earlier in the course of their treatment and for patients who recur later with metastatic disease.

12.3.3 Ewing's Sarcoma

Ewing's sarcoma is a rare, aggressive small cell sarcoma of the bone that may also arise from the soft tissues. It has a peak incidence occurring in adolescence and young adults. It is part of a spectrum of tumors known as the Ewing's family of tumors (ESFT). Even when localized, it should be considered as a systemic disease with a high likelihood of recurrence and metastases after local treatment alone [124].

The treatment of Ewing's sarcoma (ES) requires a multidisciplinary approach, combining risk-adapted intensified chemotherapy (neoadjuvant and adjuvant) with surgery and/or radiation therapy for control of both local and metastatic disease, requiring close coordination and communication between the treating physicians. Local treatment should be judiciously interposed in between and should not compromise or delay systemic chemotherapy. The dose and timing of chemotherapy are critical for improving outcome. Surgery is preferred if there is a function-preserving surgical option or a lesion arising in dispensable bones. Radiation therapy is utilized for inadequate surgical margins or an unresectable/nonfunctional preserving option because of tumor extent and/or location. This approach maximizes the chance of cure.

Although overall survival for patients with localized disease now approaches 65–75%, patients with metastatic disease at clinical presentation do much worse with a 5-year overall survival of less than 30%. When there is isolated lung involvement amenable to surgical resection, it can approach 50%. Both acute and long-term toxicities from intensified therapy have occurred in long-term survivors.

Improvements in multimodality therapeutic strategies have been the result of several national and international group collaborations involving treatment of the pediatric and young adult group population. Initially, there were successive first-line trials assessing the efficacy of vincristine, actinomycin D, cyclophosphamide (VAC), and doxorubicin (D). These were followed by studies involving alternating the VDC with ifosfamide/etoposide (IE). Then both dose intensification and interval compression/dose density were evaluated. More recent studies attempted to refine treatments based on prognostic factors to further improve outcomes.

Fewer than 5% of ES arise in adults older than 40 years of age. There are no clinical trials that address treatment for adult patients with most published studies excluding older individuals [123, 124]. Furthermore, adults more often have pelvic or extraskeletal primary disease, both of which are associated with a poor prognosis [125]. The treatment for adult patients with ES is guided by the general principles of treatment in children and adolescents [126–128].

In the 1970s, the Intergroup Ewing's Sarcoma Study (IESS-1) combined VAC with doxorubicin, resulting in an improved survival for ES patients. The importance of doxorubicin dose intensity was established from the IESS-2 trial and eventually replaced actinomycin D in the VDC regimen [129, 130].

In the 1980s, the combination of ifosfamide/etoposide was found to have activity as a second-line treatment for ES [131]. This was then incorporated into the INT-0091 first-line trial, alternating IE with VDC vs. VDC alone and showing a significant benefit in survival for the alternating regimen in those patients with localized disease, thereby establishing this as the standard of care [132, 133].

The introduction of hematopoietic growth factors allowed for the testing of dose intensification of the alkylating agents contained in the alternating regimen or shortening the treatment interval of each treatment cycle [134]. The INT-0154 COG study randomized dose-intensified cyclophosphamide and ifosfamide vs. the standard dose for VDC/IE, but with the same cumulative dose given. No benefit was found [135]. The next COG trial AEWS0031 tested the interval compression concept with VDC/IE given every 2 weeks vs. the standard cycle of every 3 weeks [136]. The dose dense 2-week regimen had a superior 5-year overall survival (73 vs. 65%, $p = 0.048$), with no increase in toxicity. However, further subgroup evaluation showed that the benefit was seen only for patients 17 years of age and younger, establishing this dose dense regimen as the new standard of care in North America for patients with localized ES under 18 years of age.

High-dose chemotherapy with stem cell mobilization rescue has been utilized for patients with poor prognostic factors (metastases, recurrent and progressive disease, etc.). Several single-arm studies have suggested a benefit, but there has been no randomized study to definitively confirm a better outcome. Its beneficial role is controversial; therefore, its use has remained investigational [137–141].

The prognosis for patients with refractory or recurrent ES remains poor. To date, there is no standard second-line treatment. Several combinations have shown activity mostly in small studies, (i.e., topotecan/cyclophosphamide [142, 143], temozolomide/irinotecan [144], and gemcitabine/docetaxel [113]).

With a better understanding of the molecular biology of ES and the critical role of the EWRS1 fusion oncogenes in its pathogenesis, strategies to target the fusion gene and/or its gene protein product have commenced, i.e., TK216 [145, 146]. Other approaches include the use of insulin-like growth factor receptors (IGF-IR monoclonal antibodies) [147–150], mTOR inhibitors, poly(ADP)-ribose polymerase (PARP) inhibitors, etc. [151, 152].

The treatment for patients with localized ES is improved but has plateaued with a cure rate of 65–75%. Patients with metastases and other poor prognostic factors have a much worse survival rate. New approaches for treatment, specifically those with a profile of reduced toxicity, are needed.

12.3.4 Chondrosarcoma

Conventional chondrosarcomas (by far the most common) are resistant to standard chemotherapy regardless of grade, and therefore, surgery, when feasible, has been the principle treatment. Two aggressive variants of chondrosarcoma are associated with significant mortality, and for these, chemotherapy may be helpful.

Mesenchymal chondrosarcoma has a high-grade small cell (Ewing's-like) component and can respond to treatment with a Ewing's type of chemotherapy treatment [153, 154]. Dedifferentiated chondrosarcoma is associated with a high-grade osteosarcoma or undifferentiated pleomorphic sarcoma (UPS) component in addition to a low-grade component and should be treated as an osteosarcoma [155, 156].

12.3.5 Malignant Fibrous Histiocytoma/Undifferentiated Pleomorphic Sarcoma of the Bone

This entity, in which there is no osteoid matrix being produced by the malignant cells, should be considered as a high-grade variant of osteosarcoma. It should be treated with an osteosarcoma-like regimen. However, results are somewhat inferior compared to patients with conventional osteosarcoma.

12.3.6 Giant Cell Tumor of the Bone (GCTB)

GCTB is a relatively rare benign (but locally aggressive) tumor of bone that is associated with a high rate of local recurrence and a small risk (<5%) of pulmonary metastases (usually slow growing). Curettage with local adjuvants is the preferred treatment. For more advanced and recurrent disease, joint salvage may not be feasible and resection could be indicated.

RANK ligand has been found to be overexpressed in GCTB [157]. Recent work has suggested that the use of denosumab, a fully-human monoclonal antibody to RANK ligand, blocks osteoclast maturation and resultant bone destruction. It has been used for cytoreduction in order to allow for potential intralesional surgery, therefore avoiding more invasive surgery. It has also been utilized as treatment for unresectable local disease and rare pulmonary metastases [158]. Unfortunately, interruption of treatment can be followed by regrowth; therefore, treatment usually needs to be maintained. It is usually well tolerated with an acceptable toxicity profile with side effects consisting of headache and bone pain (1–10%), osteonecrosis of the jaw (1–2%), hypocalcemia, and hypophosphatemia (<0.1%). It was recently FDA approved (2013) for advanced or unresectable disease where surgery would result in severe morbidity. The long-term effects of treatment for GCTB are not known [159–161].

Conclusions

Much of the progress in systemic therapy for sarcomas occurred in the last quarter of the twentieth century. Between the 1970s and 1980s, various chemotherapeutic agents were developed and tested with some evolving into standards of practice. With the availability of hematopoietic growth factors and improved supportive care, dose intensification became possible, thereby allowing for the maximum potential of active combination regimens and/or high-dose single-agent use.

However, by the beginning of the twenty-first century, a plateau in efficacy for available agents was reached. New and mechanistically different therapies were needed to enhance the therapeutic index and further improve patient outcomes. Encouraged by the significantly positive results seen with imatinib for gastrointestinal stromal tumors (GISTs) and the continued advances in molecular genomics, several newer targeted therapies have shown modest success in other sarcomas [162]. Nevertheless, for most sarcomas with complex genomic profiles, results have been limited due to a lack of identifiable specific driver growth pathways and actionable targets. It is hoped that with continued improvements in genetic sequencing and with the reintroduction of immunotherapy for other solid tumors, new treatments will be forthcoming [163–166]. The expanding understanding of cancer immunology and more precise and directed immune modulation (i.e., checkpoint inhibitors, etc.) may lead to more successful long-lasting treatment approaches, which could possibly change the sarcoma treatment paradigm.

As we have entered the new millennium, the treatment of patients with sarcomas will become more individualized. Based on their rarity and heterogeneity, this will require further collaboration among a variety of different health disciplines and researchers. A multidisciplinary, multicenter, and international approach will need to be further promoted for the future development of new therapies and the rapid and efficient accrual to randomized studies. This will enable physicians to achieve the goal of optimum function, minimal morbidity and toxicity, and improved long-term survival for our patients with these rare neoplasms.

References

1. Siegel RL, Miller KD, Jemal A. Cancer statistics, 2016. CA Cancer J Clin. 2016;66(1):7–30.
2. O'Bryan RM, Luce JK, Talley RW, Gottlieb JA, Baker LH, Bonadonna G. Phase II evaluation of adriamycin in human neoplasia. Cancer. 1973;32(1):1–8.
3. Wang B, Yu X, Xu S, Xu M. Combination of cisplatin, ifosfamide, and adriamycin as neoadjuvant chemotherapy for extremity soft tissue sarcoma: a report of twenty-eight patients. Medicine (Baltimore). 2016;95(4):2611.
4. Huh WW, Jaffe N, Durand JB, Munsell MF, Herzog CE. Comparison of doxorubicin cardiotoxicity in pediatric sarcoma patients when given with dexrazoxane versus as continuous infusion. Pediatr Hematol Oncol. 2010;27(7):546–57.
5. Nielsen OS, Dombernowsky P, Mouridsen H, et al. Epirubicin is not superior to doxorubicin in the treatment of advanced soft tissue sarcomas. The experience of the EORTC Soft Tissue and Bone Sarcoma Group. Sarcoma. 2000;4(1–2):31–5.

6. Judson IRJ, Harris M, Blay JY, van Hoesel Q, le Cesne A. Randomised phase II trial of pegylated liposomal doxorubicin (DOXIL/CAELYX) versus doxorubicin in the treatment of advanced or metastatic soft tissue sarcoma: a study by the EORTC Soft Tissue and Bone Sarcoma Group. Eur J Cancer. 2001;37(7):870–7.
7. Skubitz K. Phase II trial of pegylated-liposomal doxorubicin (Doxil) in sarcoma. Cancer Invest. 2003;21(2):167–76.
8. Skubitz KM, Haddad PA. Paclitaxel and pegylated-liposomal doxorubicin are both active in angiosarcoma. Cancer. 2005;104(2):361–6.
9. Lorusso D, Di Stefano A, Carone V, Fagotti A, Pisconti S, Scambia G. Pegylated liposomal doxorubicin-related palmar-plantar erythrodysesthesia ('hand-foot' syndrome). Ann Oncol. 2007;18(7):1159–64.
10. Bramwell VH, Mouridsen H, Santoro A, et al. Cyclophosphamide versus ifosfamide: final report of a randomized phase II trial in adult soft tissue sarcomas. Eur J Cancer Clin Oncol. 1987;23(3):311–21.
11. Patel SR, Vadhan-Raj S, Papadopolous N, et al. High-dose ifosfamide in bone and soft tissue sarcomas: results of phase II and pilot studies—dose-response and schedule dependence. J Clin Oncol. 1997;15:2378.
12. Antman K, Crowley J, Balcerzak SP, et al. An intergroup phase III randomized study of doxo-rubicin and dacarbazine with or without ifosfamide and mesna in advanced soft tissue and bone sarcomas. J Clin Oncol. 1993;11(7):1276–85.
13. Lorigan P, Verweij J, Papai Z, et al. Phase III trial of two investigational schedules of ifos-famide compared with standard dose doxorubicin. J Clin Oncol. 2007;25:3144–50.
14. Nielsen OS, Judson I, van Hoesel Q, et al. Effect of high-dose ifosfamide in advanced soft tissue sarcomas. A multicentre phase II study of the EORTC Soft Tissue and Bone Sarcoma Group. Eur J Cancer. 2000;36(1):61–7.
15. David KA, Picus J. Evaluating risk factors for the development of ifosfamide encephalopathy. Am J Clin Oncol. 2005;28(3):277–80.
16. Hansen HO, Yuen C. Aprepitant-associated ifosfamide neurotoxicity. J Oncol Pharm Pract. 2010;16:137–8.
17. Patel PN. Methylene blue for management of ifosfamide-induced encephalopathy. Ann Pharmacother. 2006;40(2):299–303.
18. Talbot SM, Keohan ML, Hesdorffer M, et al. A phase II trial of temozolomide in patients with unresectable or metastatic soft tissue sarcoma. Cancer. 2003;98:1942–6.
19. Patel SR, Vadhan-Raj S, Burgess MA, et al. Results of two consecutive trials of dose-intensive chemotherapy with doxorubicin and ifosfamide in patients with sarcomas. Am J Clin Oncol. 1998;21(3):317–21.
20. Judsen I, Verweij J, Gelderblom H, et al. Doxorubicin alone versus intensified doxorubicin plus ifosfamide for first-line treatment of advanced or metastatic soft-tissue sarcoma: a ran-domised controlled phase 3 trial. Lancet Oncol. 2014;15:4:415–23
21. Hensley ML, Blessing JA, Mannel R, Rose PG. Fixed-dose rate gemcitabine plus docetaxel as first-line therapy for metastatic uterine leiomyosarcoma: a Gynecologic Oncology Group phase II trial. Gynecol Oncol. 2008;109(3):329–34.
22. Maki RG, Wathen JK, Patel SR, et al. Randomized phase II study of gemcitabine and docetaxel compared with gemcitabine alone in patients with metastatic soft tissue sarcomas: results of sarcoma alliance for research through collaboration study 002 [corrected]. J Clin Oncol. 2007;25:2755–63.
23. Maki RG, Hensley ML, Wathen JK, et al. A SARC multicenter phase III study of gemcitabine (G) vs. gemcitabine and docetaxel (G + D) in patients (pts) with metastatic soft tissue sarcomas (STS). J Clin Oncol (Meeting Abstracts). 2006;24(18 Suppl):523S.
24. Seddon B, Whelan J, Strauss SJ, Leahy MG, et al. GeDDiS: a prospective randomised con-trolled phase III trial of gemcitabine and docetaxel compared with doxorubicin as first-line treatment in previously untreated advanced unresectable or metastatic soft tissue sarcomas (EudraCT 2009-014907-29). J Clin Oncol. 2015;33(S1):abstract 10500.

25. Penel N, Bui B, Bay J-O, et al. Phase II trial of weekly paclitaxel for unresectable angiosarcoma: the ANGIOTAX Study. J Clin Oncol. 2008;26(32):5269–74.
26. Italiano A, Cioffi A, Penel N, et al. Comparison of doxorubicin and weekly paclitaxel efficacy in metastatic angiosarcomas. Cancer. 2012;118:3330–6.
27. The ESMO/European Sarcoma Network Working Group. Soft tissue and visceral sarcomas: ESMO clinical practice guidelines. Ann Oncol. 2014;25(Suppl 3):iii102–12.
28. Hensley M, Maki R, Venkatraman E, et al. Gemcitabine and docetaxel in patients with unresectable leiomyosarcoma: results of a phase II trial. J Clin Oncol. 2002;20:2824–31.
29. Garcia-del-Muro X, Lopez-Pousa A, Maurel J, et al. Randomized phase II study comparing gemcitabine plus dacarbazine versus dacarbazine alone in patients with previously treated soft tissue sarcoma: a Spanish Group for Research on Sarcomas Study. J Clin Oncol. 2011;29:2528–33.
30. Garcia-del-Muro X, Lopez-Pousa A, Martin J, et al. A phase II trial of temozolomide as a 6-week, continuous, oral schedule in patients with advanced soft tissue sarcoma: a study by the Spanish Group for Research on Sarcomas. Cancer. 2005;104(8):1706–12.
31. van der Graaf WT, Blay JY, Chawla SP, et al. Pazopanib for metastatic soft-tissue sarcoma (PALETTE): a randomised, double-blind, placebo-controlled phase 3 trial. Lancet. 2012;379(9829):1879–86.
32. Sleijfer S, Ray-Coquard I, Papai Z, et al. Pazopanib, a multikinase angiogenesis inhibitor, in patients with relapsed or refractory advanced soft tissue sarcoma: a phase II study from the European Organisation for Research and Treatment of Cancer–Soft Tissue and Bone Sarcoma Group (EORTC study 62043). J Clin Oncol. 2009;27:3126–32.
33. Blay JYIA, Italiano A, Ray-Coquard I, et al. Long-term outcome and effect of maintenance therapy in patients with advanced sarcoma treated with trabectedin: an analysis of 181 patients of the French ATU compassionate use program. BMC Cancer. 2013;13:64.
34. FDA approves Trabectedin for two soft tissue sarcomas: Medscape, October 23, 2015.
35. Samuels BL, Chawla S, Patel S, et al. Clinical outcomes and safety with trabectedin therapy in patients with advanced soft tissue sarcomas following failure of prior chemotherapy: results of a worldwide expanded access program study. Ann Oncol. 2013;24:1703–9.
36. Demetri GD, von Mehren M, Jones RL, et al. Efficacy and safety of trabectedin or dacarbazine for metastatic liposarcoma or leiomyosarcoma after failure of conventional chemotherapy: results of a phase III randomized multicenter clinical trial. J Clin Oncol. 2016;34(8):786–93.
37. Schwartz GK. Trabectedin and the L-sarcomas: a decade-long odyssey. J Clin Oncol. 2016;34:769–71.
38. Paz-Ares L, López-Pousa A, Poveda A, et al. Trabectedin in pre-treated patients with advanced or metastatic soft tissue sarcoma: a phase II study evaluating co-treatment with dexamethasone. Invest New Drugs. 2012;30(2):729–40.
39. Schöffski P, Ray-Coquard IL, Cioffi A. Activity of eribulin mesylate in patients with soft-tissue sarcoma: a phase 2 study in four independent histological subtypes. Lancet Oncol. 2011;12(11):1045–52.
40. Schoffski P, Maki RG, Italiano A, et al. Randomized, open-label, multicenter, phase III study of eribulin versus dacarbazine in patients (pts) with leiomyosarcoma (LMS) and adipocytic sarcoma (ADI). J Clin Oncol. 2015;33:Abstract 10502.
41. Tap WD, Jones RL, Van Tine BA, et al. Olaratumab and doxorubicin versus doxorubicin alone for treatment of soft-tissue sarcoma: an open-label phase 1b and randomised phase 2 trial. Lancet. 2016;388(10043):488–97.
42. FDA Approval. Olaratumab October 19, 2016. http://www.fda.gov/Drugs/InformationOnDrugs/ApprovedDrugs/ucm526087.htm
43. Rutkowski P, Van Glabbeke M, Rankin CJ, et al. Imatinib mesylate in advanced dermatofibrosarcoma protuberans: pooled analysis of two phase II clinical trials. J Clin Oncol. 2010;28(10):1772–9.
44. Ugurel S, Mentzel T, Utikal J, et al. Neoadjuvant imatinib in advanced primary or locally recurrent dermatofibrosarcoma protuberans: a multicenter phase II DeCOG trial with long term follow-up. Clin Cancer Res. 2014;20(2):499–510.

45. Stacchiotti S, Negri T, Zaffaroni N. Sunitinib in advanced alveolar soft part sarcoma: evidence of a direct antitumor effect. Ann Oncol. 2011;7:1682–90.
46. Kummar S, Allen D, Monks A, et al. Cediranib for metastatic alveolar soft part sarcoma. J Clin Oncol. 2013;31(18):2296–302.
47. Park M, Patel SR, Ludwig JA, et al. Activity of temozolomide and bevacizumab in the treatment of locally advanced, recurrent, and metastatic hemangiopericytoma and malignant solitary fibrous tumor. Cancer. 2011;117(21):4939–47.
48. Stacchiotti S, Tortoreto M, Bozzi F, et al. Dacarbazine in solitary fibrous tumor: a case series analysis and preclinical evidence vis-a-vis temozolomide and antiangiogenics. Clin Cancer Res. 2013;19(18):5192–201.
49. Stacchiotti S, Negri T, Libertini M, et al. Sunitinib malate in solitary fibrous tumor (SFT). Ann Oncol. 2012;23(12):3171–9.
50. Wagner AJ, Malinowska-Kolodziej I, Morgan JA. Clinical activity of mTOR inhibition with sirolimus in malignant perivascular epithelioid cell tumors: targeting the pathogenic activation of mTORC1 in tumors. J Clin Oncol. 2010;28(5):835–40.
51. Gadgeel SM, Bepler G. Crizotinib: an anaplastic lymphoma kinase inhibitor. Future Oncol. 2011;7(8):947–53.
52. Butrynski JE, D'Adamo DR, Hornick JL, et al. Crizotinib in ALK-rearranged inflammatory myofibroblastic tumor. N Engl J Med. 2010;363(18):1727–33.
53. Tierney J. Adjuvant chemotherapy for localised resectable soft-tissue sarcoma of adults: meta-analysis of individual data. Sarcoma meta-analysis collaboration. Lancet. 1997;350:1647–54.
54. Frustaci S, Gherlinzoni F, De Paoli A, et al. Adjuvant chemotherapy for adult soft tissue sarcomas of the extremities and girdles: results of the Italian randomized cooperative trial. J Clin Oncol. 2001;19:1238–47.
55. Frustaci S, De Paoli A, Bidoli E, et al. Ifosfamide in the adjuvant therapy of soft tissue sarcomas. Oncology. 2003;65(Supplement 2):80–4.
56. Woll PJ, Reichardt P, Le Cesne A, et al. Adjuvant chemotherapy with doxorubicin, ifosfamide, and lenograstim for resected soft-tissue sarcoma (EORTC 62931): a multicentre randomised controlled trial. Lancet. Oncology 2012;13(10):1045–54.
57. Afonso SL, Ramos LA, Viani GA, et al. Improvement in the survival for adult soft tissue sarcoma with adjuvant anthracycline chemotherapy combination: a meta-analysis and metaregression. J Clin Oncol. 2010;28(ASCO Pubs 15):10042.
58. Gronchi A, Frustaci S, Mercuri M, et al. Short, full-dose adjuvant chemotherapy in high-risk adult soft tissue sarcomas: a randomized clinical trial from the Italian Sarcoma Group and the Spanish Sarcoma Group. J Clin Oncol. 2012;30:850–6.
59. D'Adamo A. Is adjuvant chemotherapy useful for soft-tissue sarcomas? Lancet Oncol. 2012;13(10):968–70.
60. National Comprehensive Cancer Network. Soft Tissue Sarcoma (Version 2016). https://www.nccn.org/professionals/physician_gls/PDF/sarcoma.pdf
61. Gortzak E, Rouesse J, Verwey J. Randomized phase II study of neoadjuvant chemotherapy in soft tissue sarcomas in adults. Protocol 62874. Eur J Cancer. 1993;29(6):S183.
62. O'Sullivan B, Davis AM, Turcotte R, et al. Preoperative versus postoperative radiotherapy in soft-tissue sarcoma of the limbs: a randomised trial. Lancet. 2002;359(9325):2235–41.
63. Davis AM, O'Sullivan B, Turcotte R, et al. Late radiation morbidity following randomization to preoperative versus postoperative radiotherapy in extremity soft tissue sarcoma. Radiother Oncol. 2005;75:48–53.
64. Pisters PW, O'Sullivan B, Maki RG. Evidence-based recommendations for local therapy for soft tissue sarcomas. J Clin Oncol. 2007;25:1003–8.
65. Verhoef C, de Wilt JH, Grunhagen DJ, et al. Isolated limb perfusion with melphalan and TNF-α in the treatment of extremity sarcoma. Curr Treat Options Oncol. 2007;8(6): 417–27.
66. Issels RD, Lindner LH, Verweij J, et al. Neo-adjuvant chemotherapy alone or with regional hyperthermia for localised high-risk soft-tissue sarcoma: a randomised phase 3 multicentre study. Lancet Oncol. 2010;11(6):561–70.

67. Issels RD, Lindner LH. Regional hyperthermia for high-risk soft tissue sarcoma treatment: present status and next questions. Curr Opin Oncol. 2016;28:447–52.
68. Grem JL, King SA, Wittes RE, et al. The role of methotrexate in osteosarcoma. J Natl Cancer Inst. 1988;80:626–55.
69. Rosen G, Nirenberg A. Chemotherapy for osteogenic sarcoma: an investigative method, not a recipe. Cancer Treat Rep. 1982;66:1687–97.
70. Rosen G, Eilber FC, Eckhardt J. Guidelines for chemotherapy of osteosarcoma. Second Osteosarcoma Research Conference. Bologna, Italy, 1996.
71. Jaffe N, Gorlick R. High-dose methotrexate in osteosarcoma: let the questions surcease—time for final acceptance. J Clin Oncol. 2008;26(27):4365–6.
72. Miser JS, Kinsella TJ, Triche TJ, et al. Ifosfamide with mesna uroprotection and etoposide: an effective regimen in the treatment of recurrent sarcomas and other tumors of children and young adults. J Clin Oncol. 1987;5(8):1191–8.
73. Marti C, Kroner T, Remagen W, Berchtold W, Cserhati M, Varini M. High-dose ifosfamide in advanced osteosarcoma. Cancer Treat Rep. 1985;69:115–7.
74. Bramwell VH, Burgers M, Sneath R, Souhami R. A comparison of two short intensive adjuvant chemotherapy regimens in operable osteosarcoma of limbs in children and young adults: the first study of the European Osteosarcoma Intergroup. J Clin Oncol. 1992;10(10): 1579–91.
75. Souhami RL, Craft AW, Van der Eijken JW. Randomised trial of two regimens of chemotherapy in operable osteosarcoma: a study of the European Osteosarcoma Intergroup. Lancet. 1997;350(9082):911–7.
76. Malawer M, Link MP, Donaldson SS. Sarcomas of bone. In: Devita H, Rosenberg SA, editors. Cancer: principles and practice of oncology. Philadelphia: Lippincott-Raven; 1997. p. 1789–852.
77. Link MP, Eilber F. Osteosarcoma. In: Poplack DG, Pizzo PA, editors. Principles and practice of pediatric oncology. Philadelphia: Lippincott-Raven; 1997. p. 889–920.
78. Carter S. Adjuvant chemotherapy in osteogenic sarcoma: the triumph that isn't? J Clin Oncol. 1984;2:147–8.
79. Taylor WE, Ivins JC, Pritchard DI, et al. Trends and variability in survival among patients with osteosarcoma. A 7-year update. Mayo Clin Proc. 1985;60:91–104.
80. Eilber F, Giuliano A, Eckhardt J et al. Adjuvant chemotherapy for osteosarcoma. A randomized prospective trial. J Clin Oncol. 1987;5:21–26.
81. Link MP, Goorin AM, Miser AW, et al. The effect of adjuvant chemotherapy on relapse-free survival in patients with osteosarcoma of the extremity. N Engl J Med. 1986;314:1600–6.
82. Link MP, Goorin AM, Horowitz M, et al. Adjuvant chemotherapy of high grade osteosarcoma of the extremity: updated results of the multi-institutional osteosarcoma study. Clin Orthop Relat Res. 1991;270:8–14.
83. Rosen G, Marcove RC, Caparros B. Primary osteosarcoma. The rationale for preoperative chemotherapy and delayed surgery. Cancer. 1979;43:2163–77.
84. Priebat DA, Trehan PS, Malawer MM, et al. Induction chemotherapy for sarcomas of the extremities. In: Sugarbaker PH, Malawer MM, editors. Musculoskeletal surgery for cancer. New York, NY: Thieme; 1992. p. 96–120.
85. Epelman S, Siebel N, Melaragno R, et al. Treatment of newly diagnosed high-grade osteosarcoma with ifosfamide, Adriamycin, and cisplatin without high-dose methotrexate. Proc Am Soc Clin Oncol. 1995;14:439.
86. Goorin AM, Schwartzentruber DJ, Devidas M, et al. Presurgical chemotherapy compared with immediate surgery and adjuvant chemotherapy for nonmetastatic osteosarcoma, Pediatric Oncology Group Study, POG-8651. J Clin Oncol. 2003;21:1574–80.
87. Rosen G, Caparros B, Huvos AG, et al. Preoperative chemotherapy for osteosarcoma. Selection of postoperative adjuvant chemotherapy based on response of primary tumor to preoperative chemotherapy. Cancer. 1982;49:1221–39.
88. Winkler K, Beron G, Delling G, et al. Neoadjuvant chemotherapy of osteosarcoma: results of a randomized cooperative trial (COSS-82) with salvage chemotherapy based on tumor response. J Clin Oncol. 1988;6:329–37.

89. Gherlinzoni M, Mercuri M, Avella M, et al. Surgical implications of neoadjuvant chemotherapy the experience at the Instituto Orthopedico Rizzoli in osteosarcoma and malignant fibrous histiocytoma. In: Jacquillat C, Weil M, Khayat D, editors. Neoadjuvant chemotherapy John Libbey Eurotext; 1988. p. 541–4.
90. Bacci G, Picci P, Ferrari S, et al. Primary chemotherapy and delayed surgery for nonmetastatic osteosarcoma of the extremities. Cancer. 1993;72:3227–38.
91. Provisor AJ, Ettinger LJ, Nachman JB, et al. Treatment of nonmetastatic osteosarcoma of the extremity with preoperative and postoperative chemotherapy: a report from the Children's Cancer Group. J Clin Oncol. 1997;15:76–84.
92. Meyers PA, Heller G, Healey J, et al. Chemotherapy for non-metastatic osteogenic sarcoma: the Memorial Sloan Kettering experience. J Clin Oncol. 1992;10:5–15.
93. Bacci G, Bertoni F, Longhi A, et al. Neoadjuvant chemotherapy for high-grade central osteosarcoma of the extremity. Histologic response to preoperative chemotherapy correlates with histologic subtype of the tumor. Cancer. 2003;97(12):3068–75.
94. Hauben EI, Weeden S, Pringle J, Van Marck EA, Hogendoorn PC. Does the histological subtype of high-grade central osteosarcoma influence the response to treatment with chemotherapy and does it affect overall survival? A study on 570 patients of two consecutive trials of the European Osteosarcoma Intergroup. Eur J Cancer. 2002;38(9):1218–25.
95. Bielack SS, Kempf-Bielack B, Delling G. Prognostic factors in high-grade osteosarcoma of the extremities or trunk: an analysis of 1,702 patients treated on neoadjuvant cooperative osteosarcoma study group protocols. J Clin Oncol. 2002;20(3):776–90.
96. Benjamin RS, Patel S, Armen CH, et al. The value of ifosfamide in postoperative neoadjuvant chemotherapy of osteosarcoma. Proc Am Soc Clin Oncol. 1995;14:1690a.
97. Meyers PA, Gorlick R, Heller G, et al. Intensification of preoperative chemotherapy for osteogenic sarcoma: results of the Memorial Sloan Kettering T-12 protocol. J Clin Oncol. 1998;16:2452–8.
98. Lewis IJ, Nooij MA, Whelan J, et al. Improvement in histologic response but not survival in osteosarcoma patients treated with intensified chemotherapy: a randomized phase III trial of the European Osteosarcoma Intergroup. J Natl Cancer Inst. 2007;99:112–28.
99. Jaffe N, Knapp J, Chuang VP, et al. Osteosarcoma: intraarterial treatment of the primary tumor with cisdiammine dichloroplatinum II (CDP). Angiographic, pathologic, and pharmacologic studies. Cancer. 1983;51:402–7.
100. Jaffe N, Raymond AK, Ayala A, et al. Effect of cumulative courses of intraarterial cis-diammine-dichloroplatinum II on the primary tumor in pediatric osteosarcoma. J Clin Oncol. 1985;3:1101–4.
101. Bacci G, Picci P, Avella M, et al. Effect of intraarterial versus intravenous cisplatinum in addition to systemic Adriamycin and high-dose methotrexate on histologic tumor response of osteosarcoma of the extremities. J Chemother. 1992;4:189–95.
102. Meyers PA, Schwartz CL, et al. Osteosarcoma: a randomized, prospective trial of the addition of ifosfamide and/or muramyl tripeptide to cisplatin, doxorubicin, and high-dose methotrexate. J Clin Oncol. 2005 Mar 20;23(9):2004-11.
103. Meyers PA, Schwartz CL, Krailo MD, et al. Osteosarcoma: the addition of muramyl tripeptide to chemotherapy improves overall survival—a report from the Children's Oncology Group. J Clin Oncol. 2008;26(4):633–8.
104. Chou AJ, Kleinerman ES, Krailo MD, et al. Addition of muramyl tri-peptide to chemotherapy for patients with newly diagnosed metastatic osteosarcoma: a report from the Children's Oncology Group. Cancer. 2009;115:5339–48.
105. Shafer E. FDA panel rejects mifamurtide for osteosarcoma in children. HemOnc Today 2007 (June 1).
106. Whelan JS, Bielack SS, Marina N, et al. EURAMOS-1. An international randomised study for osteosarcoma: results from prerandomisation treatment. Ann Oncol. 2015;26(2): 407–14.
107. Bielack SS, Smeland S, Whelan JS, et al. Methotrexate, doxorubicin, and cisplatin (MAP) plus maintenance pegylated interferon alfa-2b versus MAP alone in patients with resectable high-grade osteosarcoma and good histologic response to preoperative MAP: first

results of the EURAMOS-1 good response randomized controlled trial. J Clin Oncol. 2015;33(20):2279–87.

108. Marina NM, Smeland SS, Bielack SS, et al. Comparison of MAPIE versus MAP in patients with a poor response to preoperative chemotherapy for newly diagnosed high-grade osteosarcoma (EURAMOS-1): an open-label, international, randomised controlled trial. Lancet Oncol. 2016;17(10):1396–408.

109. Kleinerman E. Maximum benefit of chemotherapy for osteosarcoma achieved-what are the next steps? Lancet Oncol. 2016;17(10):1340–2.

110. Isakoff MS, Bielack SS, Meltzer P, Grlick R. Osteosarcoma: current treatment and a collaborative pathway to success. J Clin Oncol. 2015;33:3029–35.

111. Luetke A, Meyers PA, Lewis I, Juergens H. Osteosarcoma treatment—where do we stand? A state of the art review. Cancer Treat Rev. 2013;40(4):523–32.

112. Marina N, Bielack S, Whelan J. International collaboration is feasible in trials for rare conditions: the EURAMOS experience. Cancer Treat Rep. 2009;152:339–53.

113. Fox E, Patel S, Wathen JK. Phase II study of sequential gemcitabine followed by docetaxel for recurrent Ewing sarcoma, osteosarcoma, or unresectable or locally recurrent chondrosarcoma: results of sarcoma alliance for research through collaboration study 003. Oncologist. 2012;17(3):321.

114. Grignani G, Palmerini E, Dileo P, et al. A phase II trial of sorafenib in relapsed and unresectable high-grade osteosarcoma after failure of standard multimodal therapy. An Italian Sarcoma Group study. Ann Oncol. 2011;23:508–16.

115. Grignani G, Palmerini E, Ferraresi V, et al. Sorafenib and everolimus for patients with unresectable high-grade osteosarcoma progressing after standard treatment: a non-randomised phase 2 clinical trial. Lancet Oncol. 2015;16(1):98–107.

116. Benjamin R. Osteosarcoma: better treatment through better trial design. Lancet Oncol.16(1): 12-13. 2015.

117. Kolb EA, Gorlick R, Reynolds CP. Initial testing (stage 1) of eribulin, a novel tubulin binding agent, by the pediatric preclinical testing program. Pediatr Blood Cancer. 2013;60(8): 1325–32.

118. Schoffski P, Ray-Coquard IL, Cioffi A, et al. Activity of eribulin mesylate in patients with soft-tissue sarcoma: a phase 2 study in four independent histological subtypes. Lancet Oncology 12;11:1045-1052, 2011.

119. Zoledronic acid and combination chemotherapy in treating patients with newly diagnosed metastatic osteosarcoma. Children's Oncology Group-National Cancer Institute. ClinicalTrials. gov Identifier: NCT00742924. https://clinicaltrials.gov/ct2/show/NCT00742924. Accessed 4 June 2014.

120. Kolb EA, Gorlick R, Billups CA. Initial testing (stage 1) of glembatumumab vedotin (CDX-011) by the pediatric preclinical testing program. Pediatr Blood Cancer. 2014;61(10):1816–21.

121. Roth M, Barris DM, Piperdi S, et al. Targeting glycoprotein NMB with antibody-drug conjugate, Glembatumumab vedotin, for the treatment of osteosarcoma. Pediatr Blood Cancer. 2016;63(1):32–8.

122. Roth M, Linkowski M, Tarim J, et al. Ganglioside GD2 as a therapeutic target for antibody-mediated therapy in patients with osteosarcoma. Cancer. 2014;120(4):548–54.

123. Balamuth NJ, Womer RB. Ewing's sarcoma. Lancet Oncol. 2010;11(2):184–92.

124. Gaspar N, Hawkins DS, Dirksen U, et al. Ewing sarcoma: current management and future approaches through collaboration. J Clin Oncol. 2015;33(27):3036–46.

125. Karski EE, Matthay KK, Neuhaus JM, Goldsby RE, Dubois SG. Characteristics and outcomes of patients with Ewing sarcoma over 40 years of age at diagnosis. Cancer Epidemiol. 2013;37(1):29–33.

126. Verrill MWJI, Wiltshaw E. The use of paediatric chemotherapy protocols at full dose is both a rational and feasible treatment strategy in adults with Ewing's family tumours. Ann Oncol. 1997;8(11):1099–105.

127. Ahmed SK, Robinson SI, Okuno SH, Rose PS, Laack NN. Adult Ewing sarcoma: survival and local control outcomes in 102 patients with localized disease. Sarcoma. 2013;2013:681425.
128. Ahmed SK, Robinson SI, Okuno SH, Rose PS, Issa Laack NN. Adult Ewing sarcoma: survival and local control outcomes in 36 patients with metastatic disease. Am J Clin Oncol. 2014;37(5):423–9.
129. Razek A, Perez CA, Tefft M, et al. Intergroup Ewing's Sarcoma Study: local control related to radiation dose, volume, and site of primary lesion in Ewing's sarcoma. Cancer. 1980;46(3):516–21.
130. Burgert Jr EO, Nesbit ME, Garnsey LA, et al. Multimodal therapy for the management of nonpelvic, localized Ewing's sarcoma of bone: intergroup study IESS-II. J Clin Oncol. 1990;8(9):1514–24.
131. Wexler LH, TF DL, Tsokos M, et al. Ifosfamide and etoposide plus vincristine, doxorubicin, and cyclophosphamide for newly diagnosed Ewing's sarcoma family of tumors. Cancer. 1996;78(4):901–11.
132. Yock TI, Krailo M, Fryer CJ, et al. Local control in pelvic Ewing sarcoma: analysis from INT-0091—a report from the Children's Oncology Group. J Clin Oncol. 2006;24:3838–43.
133. Grier HE, Krailo M, Tarbell NJ, et al. Addition of ifosfamide and etoposide to standard chemotherapy for Ewing's sarcoma and primitive neuroectodermal tumor of bone. Cancer. 2003;348(8):694–701.
134. Womer RB, Daller RT, Fenton JG, Miser JS. Granulocyte colony stimulating factor permits dose intensification by interval compression in the treatment of Ewing's sarcomas and soft tissue sarcomas in children. Eur J Cancer. 2000;36(1):87–94.
135. Granowetter L, Womer R, Devidas M, et al. Dose-intensified compared with standard chemotherapy for nonmetastatic Ewing sarcoma family of tumors: a Children's Oncology Group Study. J Clin Oncol. 2009;27(15):2536–41.
136. Womer RB, West DC, Krailo MD. Randomized controlled trial of interval-compressed chemotherapy for the treatment of localized Ewing sarcoma: a report from the Children's Oncology Group. J Clin Oncol. 2012;30(33):4148–54.
137. Rasper MJS, Jabar S, Ranft A, Jürgens H, Amler S, Dirksen U. The value of high-dose chemotherapy in patients with first relapsed Ewing sarcoma. Pediatr Blood Cancer. 2014;61(8): 1382–6.
138. Oberlin O, Rev A, Desfachelles AS. Impact of high-dose busulfan plus melphalan as consolidation in metastatic Ewing tumors: a study by the Société Française des Cancers de l'Enfant. J Clin Oncol. 2006;24(24):3997–4002.
139. Laurence V, Pierga J, Barthier S, et al. Long-term follow up of high-dose chemotherapy with autologous stem cell rescue in adults with Ewing tumor. Am J Clin Oncol. 2005;28:301–9.
140. Burdach S, van Kaick B, Laws HJ, et al. Allogeneic and autologous stem-cell transplantation in advanced Ewing tumors. An update after long-term follow-up from two centers of the European intergroup study EICESS. Stem-cell transplant programs at Düsseldorf University Medical Center, Germany and St. Anna Kinderspital, Vienna, Austria. Ann Oncol. 2000;11(11):1451–62.
141. Dirksen U, LeDeley M-C, Brennan B, et al. Efficacy of busulfan-melphalan high dose chemotherapy consolidation (BuMel) compared to conventional chemotherapy combined with lung irradiation in Ewing's Sarcoma (ES) with primary lung metastases: Results of EURO-EWING 99-R2 pulmonary randomized trial (EE9922R2pul). J Clin Oncol 34, 2016(Suppl; abstract 11001).
142. Saylors RL, Stine KC, Sullivan J, et al. Cyclophosphamide plus topotecan in children with recurrent or refractory solid tumors: a Pediatric Oncology Group Phase II Study. J Clin Oncol. 2001;19(15):3463–9.
143. Hunold A, Weddeling N, Paulussen M, et al. Topotecan and cyclophosphamide in patients with refractory or relapsed Ewing's tumors. Pediatr Blood Cancer. 2006;47(6):795–800.

144. Casey DA, Wexler LH, Merchant MS, et al. Irinotecan and temozolomide in patients with relapsed and refractory Ewing's sarcoma. Pediatr Blood Cancer. 2009;53:1029–34.
145. Song SH, Youbi SE, Hong SP, et al. Pharmacokinetic modeling optimizes inhibition of the 'undruggable' EWS-FLI1 transcription factor in Ewing sarcoma. Oncotarget. 2014;5(2):338–50.
146. Fidaleo M, De Paola E, Paronetto MP. The RNA helicase A in malignant transformation. Oncotarget. 2016;7(19):28711–23.
147. Strammiello R, Benini S, Manara MC, et al. Impact of IGF-I/IGF-IR circuit on the angiogenetic properties of Ewing's sarcoma cells. Horm Metab Res. 2003;35(11–12):675–84.
148. Pappo AS, Patel SR, Crowley J, et al. R1507, a monoclonal antibody to the insulin-like growth factor 1 receptor, in patients with recurrent or refractory Ewing sarcoma family of tumors: results of a phase II sarcoma alliance for research through collaboration study. J Clin Oncol. 2011;29(34):4541–7.
149. Tap WD, Demetri G, Barnette P, et al. Phase II study of Ganitumab, a fully human anti–type-1 insulin-like growth factor receptor antibody, in patients with metastatic Ewing family tumors or desmoplastic small round cell tumors. J Clin Oncol. 2012;15:1849–56.
150. Schwartz GK, Tap WD, Qin LX. Cixutumumab and temsirolimus for patients with bone and soft-tissue sarcoma: a multicentre, open-label, phase 2 trial. Lancet Oncol. 2013;14(4):371–82.
151. Ordóñez JL, Amaral AT, Carcaboso AM, et al. The PARP inhibitor olaparib enhances the sensitivity of Ewing sarcoma to trabectedin. Oncogene. 2015;6(22):18875–90.
152. Engert F, Schneider C, Weiß LM, Probst M, Fulda S. PARP inhibitors sensitize Ewing sarcoma cells to temozolomide-induced apoptosis via the mitochondrial pathway. Mol Cancer Ther. 2015;14(12):2818–30.
153. Dantonello TM, Int-Veen C, Leuschner I, Schuck A. Mesenchymal chondrosarcoma of soft tissues and bone in children, adolescents, and young adults: experiences of the CWS and COSS Study Groups. Cancer. 2008;112:2424–31.
154. Cesari M, Bertoni F, Bacchini P, et al. Mesenchymal chondrosarcoma. An analysis of patients treated at a single institution. Tumori. 2007;93:423–7.
155. Benjamin RS, Chu P, Patel SR, et al. Dedifferentiated chondrosarcoma: a treatable disease. Proc Am Assoc Cancer Res. 1995;36:243. [Abstract]
156. Yasko AW, Ravi V, Guadagnolo A. Chondrosarcoma. In: Lin PP, Patel S, editors. Bone sarcoma. New York: Springer; 2013.
157. Roudier MP, Kellar-Graney KL, Huang LY, et al. RANK and RANKL expression in giant cell tumors of the bone: an immunohistochemical study. In: 12th Annual Connective Tissue Oncology Society Meeting, Venice, Italy 2006.
158. Thomas D, Henshaw R, Skubitz K, et al. Denosumab in patients with giant-cell tumour of bone: an open-label, phase 2 study. Lancet Oncol. 2010;11(3):275–80.
159. Chawla S, Henshaw R, Seeger L, et al. Safety and efficacy of denosumab for adults and skeletally mature adolescents with giant cell tumour of bone: interim analysis of an open-label, parallel-group, phase 2 study. Lancet Oncol. 2013;14(9):901–8.
160. van der Heijden L, Dijkstra PD, van de Sande MA. The clinical approach toward giant cell tumor of bone. Oncologist. 2014;19:550–61.
161. Skubitz KM, Thomas DM, Chawla SP, et al. Response to treatment with denosumab in patients with giant cell tumor of bone (GCTB): FDG PET results from two phase 2 trials. J Clin Oncol. Asco Annual Meeting, 2014:abstract 10505.
162. Ludwig J, Trent JC. Targeted therapy of sarcoma. In: Kurzrock R, Markman M, editors. Targeted cancer therapy. Totowa, NJ: Humana Press; 2008. p. 317–29.
163. D'Angelo S, Tap WD, Schwartz GK, Carvajal RD. Sarcoma immunotherapy: past approaches and future directions. Sarcoma. 2014;2014(391967):1–13.
164. Lim J, Poulin NM, Nielsen TO. New strategies in sarcoma: linking genomic and immunotherapy approaches to molecular subtype. Clin Cancer Res. 2015;21(21):1–6.

165. Mitsis D, Francescutti V, Skitzki J. Current immunotherapies for sarcoma: clinical trials and rationale. Sarcoma. 2016;2016:9757219.
166. Lee A, Huang P, DeMatteo RP, Pollack SM. Immunotherapy for soft tissue sarcoma: tomorrow is only a day away. Am Soc Clin Oncol Educ Book. 2016;35:281–90.
167. Priebat DA. In: Markman M, editor. Atlas of cancer. Philadelphia: Current Medicine Group Lippincott, Williams, and Wilkins; 2003.

Salvage Therapy and Palliative Care for Metastatic Sarcoma

Matthew Wallace and Albert Aboulafia

13.1 Introduction

The fundamental difference between benign and malignant bone and soft tissue tumors is the ability to spread to other sites throughout the body. This ability to spread or metastasize often occurs in very specific patterns early in the disease (Table 13.1). However, once the metastatic process is advanced, multiple different sites are often involved.

Once a malignancy has metastasized, there is often a sense of dread or despair on the part of the patient and the healthcare team. Though a few patients may still be cured, in most patients there is a shift from treatment with curative intent to palliative care. The timing of the shift is usually predicated by the specific type of tumor and will be detailed in the discussion of the specific tumor types. Synchronous metastatic disease occurs when the staging evaluation reveals sites of metastatic disease at the initial presentation. In contrast, metachronous metastases occur when the initial staging evaluation was negative and a site of metastasis is discovered after treatment or a disease-free interval.

The care of a patient with metastatic disease involves multiple disciplines. One individual must be the designated leader and always be accessible to the patient and/or family. The medical oncologist often utilizes salvage chemotherapy regimens that balance both quality of life and deceleration of the progression of disease. The radiation oncologist plays an important role with the delivery of radiation to painful sites for palliation, and to sites that require greater local control to slow the disease down. When the disease has spread to the spine, the orthopedist or

M. Wallace, M.D., M.B.A. (✉)
National Center for Bone and Soft Tissue Tumors, MedStar Franklin Square Medical Center, Baltimore, MD, USA
e-mail: Matthew.t.wallace@medstar.net

A. Aboulafia, M.D., M.B.A.
Weinberg Cancer Institute, National Center for Bone and Soft Tissue Tumors, MedStar Franklin Square Medical Center, Baltimore, MD, USA

© Springer International Publishing Switzerland 2017
R.M. Henshaw (ed.), *Sarcoma*, DOI 10.1007/978-3-319-43121-5_13

Table 13.1 Patterns of metastases in common bone and soft tissue sarcomas

Osteosarcoma	Lung, bone
Ewing's tumor	Lung, bone, bone marrow
Chondrosarcoma	Lung, bone
Undifferentiated sarcoma of the bone (malignant fibrous histiocytoma)	Lung
Adamantinoma	Lungs, skin, lymph nodes
Undifferentiated soft tissue sarcoma (malignant fibrous histiocytoma)	Lung
Pleomorphic (high-grade) liposarcoma	Lung
Myxoid liposarcoma	Lung, retroperitoneum, other organs
Synovial sarcoma	Lungs, lymph nodes
Rhabdomyosarcoma	Lungs, lymph nodes
Epithelioid sarcoma	Lungs, lymph nodes
Alveolar soft part sarcoma	Lung, bone, brain, other organs

neurosurgeon aids in preventing paralysis or neurologic pain. A mental health professional may be necessary to treat reactive depression in both the patient and any family members and involved caretakers. The primary care physician often knows the patient and family best and may assist in pain control and the general health of all involved. Above all, a member of the healthcare team must manage the patient's pain. Although it may not be possible to cure the patient with metastatic sarcoma, all efforts should be made to control the patient's pain and optimize a patient's function for the remaining duration of their life.

13.2 Assessing for Metastatic Disease

Staging studies are performed to evaluate possible sites of metastatic disease. These studies may include computerized tomography (CT) scans, magnetic resonance imaging (MRI) scans, technetium bone scans, and positron emission scans coupled with computerized tomography (PET/CT scans) when applicable. When these studies are performed, it is very important that an open line of communication is present between the patient and health team providers. It is important to give results promptly to the patient and family.

13.2.1 Computerized Tomography Scans of the Chest (CT Chest)

The lung parenchyma is the most common site, and often is the initial site, of spread in patients with metastases from sarcoma. Although chest radiographs can be used to screen the patient for the development of pulmonary metastases, most clinicians routinely rely on computed tomography scans. The CT scan is usually done without contrast. There are many variations in restaging schedules, but a common plan for lung surveillance in patients with high-grade sarcomas is chest CT scans every 3 months for 3 years, every 6 months for 2 years, and then once a year for life. For certain patients such as children and young adults in whom lifetime radiation exposure is a concern, clinicians often opt to switch to plain chest radiographs or alternate between CT and radiographs when restaging imaging is stable for a period of time, typically 1 year. For low-grade sarcomas, a frequent used schedule is every 6 months for 5 years and then once a year for life.

Analysis of the CT scan can determine that (1) there is no evidence of metastatic disease or there are no nodules present; (2) there is no evidence of metastatic disease, but there is the presence of one or more pulmonary nodules that are less than 1 cm in size (indeterminate nodules); and (3) there is the presence of metastatic disease (nodules that have increased in size) or the presence of one or more nodules that are greater than 1 cm.

13.2.2 Magnetic Resonance Imaging (MRI) Scans

The MRI scan can be used to evaluate a site where the patient has pain or the clinician is suspicious that a metastatic focus is present. For example, a patient with a history of Ewing's sarcoma may have back pain. The radiographs of the area of the spine may be normal, but MRI can be utilized to definitively check the bone marrow and soft tissues in the region of pain. If the MRI shows no evidence of tumor, then there is no oncologic cause of the pain. Compared to X-rays and CT scans, MRI is very sensitive in evaluating the bone marrow of the vertebral bodies.

Whole-body MRI has also been advocated to evaluate patients who may have spread from sarcoma. MRI scans are very sensitive in detecting soft tissue masses and involvement of the bone marrow. However, the cost and substantial time in the scanner required for whole-body MRI make this impractical in clinical practice.

13.2.3 Technetium Bone Scans

Nuclear medicine bone scans are useful to detect sites of spread to bones throughout the skeleton. These scans are very sensitive but are not specific. To verify that there is bone destruction in areas of increased uptake, radiographs any identified areas of activity need to be performed. If there are multiple areas of increased uptake and if radiographs show a destructive process, then metastases have most likely occurred.

False-positive scans commonly occur, and areas of increased uptake must not be considered as positive unless confirmatory radiographs are performed. Increased uptake may be secondary to arthritis, prior fractures, current stress fractures, Paget's disease, infections, and several other causes. A new area of activity on subsequent scans is always concerning for the development of metastatic disease in the absence of trauma or surgery.

13.2.4 Positron Emission Scans/Computerized Tomography (PET/CT) Scans

PET/CT scans are a very sensitive method of localizing tumors. The PET scan detects areas of abnormal metabolic uptake of radiolabeled glucose (FDG). The advantage of a combined PET/CT scan is that the entire body is imaged. Very subtle areas of increased uptake can be identified and correlated with specific anatomy, with a resolution on computed tomography of approximately 1 cm. A major disadvantage is that not all areas which show increased activity are sites of metastasis (false positives), which often lead to further testing, greatly increasing patients' anxiety.

13.3 Techniques for Confirmation of Metastatic Disease

In some patients the presence of metastatic foci is very apparent, while in others the findings may be very subtle. In patients with widespread disease (involving multiple sites such as the brain, liver, lungs, etc.), confirmation with a tissue biopsy is generally not necessary. In contrast, when there is just one new site or if the site is small, tissue confirmation is often necessary. Cancer survivors, particularly childhood cancer survivors with radiation exposure or chemotherapy regimens that include alkylating agents, are at a higher risk of developing other primary cancers compared to the general population [1]. These malignancies may present several years after diagnosis and treatment. If a tissue diagnosis is needed, most tissue biopsies are done percutaneously by fine-needle aspiration (FNA) or core needle sampling. A small needle is directed utilizing guidance (computerized tomography, magnetic resonance imaging, fluoroscopy, or ultrasound) and a small piece of tissue is sampled.

Lung nodules are commonly encountered in sarcoma patients and may be indeterminate or normal findings, particularly in large urban areas. When nodules are large (over 6 mm) and/or multiple, it is often necessary to confirm that these nodules are indeed metastatic foci. There are a number of different approaches. If the primary tumor is responsive to chemotherapy, one option is to deliver that chemotherapy and see how the nodules respond over time, either disappearing, enlarging, or not demonstrating any significant change. If nodules enlarge, there is no question that a neoplasm is present. If nodules completely disappear, there may have been tumor present or the nodules were from a non-tumor etiology. An evaluation by a thoracic surgeon is often helpful and can be reassuring to the patient.

Solitary or oligometastases to the lung are still curable in about 20–25% of patients. The thoracic surgeon plays a very prominent role in patients with advanced disease. Removal of nodules can be both a diagnostic procedure (in regard to the confirmation of metastatic disease and the response to preoperative chemotherapy) and potentially curative if all the nodules can be removed.

There are many factors considered when planning a thoracotomy to remove nodules of metastatic disease. A careful staging evaluation is important. If extrathoracic disease is present or if the primary tumor is not controlled, then thoracotomy is often not employed. If, in carefully selected patients, both the pulmonary and extrathoracic metastases can be resected, cure is still possible (Blackman).

The disease-free interval is extremely important. When a long period exists between the appearance of pulmonary nodules and the occurrence of a primary tumor, the prognosis is much better in regard to the efficacy of thoracotomy. Another consideration is the number of pulmonary nodules and whether the nodules are bilateral or unilateral. When numerous small nodules are present in both lungs (greater than ten), the chance for cure is much lower [2]. When there are a small number of nodules (<5), removal may result in cure. If any disease is left behind following resection, cure is not possible. The presence of pleural seeding excludes thoracotomy.

13.4 Salvage of Patients with Metastatic Disease

13.4.1 Osteosarcoma, Ewing's Tumor, and Other Bone Sarcomas

Metastases can be found in patients with bone sarcomas in the following situations: (1) pulmonary metastases at presentation, (2) pulmonary and bone metastases at presentation, (3) pulmonary metastases after neoadjuvant chemotherapy and wide resection of the primary tumor, and (4) pulmonary and bone metastases after neoadjuvant chemotherapy and wide resection of the primary tumor. There are differences in the approach to these patients, so each scenario will be discussed separately.

1. Pulmonary metastases at initial presentation

Pulmonary nodules that are judged to be metastases at presentation signal advanced state of disease. Despite spread of the tumor to the lungs, cure may still be possible. For most sarcomas, the general approach at this point is preoperative chemotherapy followed by wide resection of the primary tumor. There are several scenarios following resection of the primary tumor:

(a) Complete resolution of the pulmonary nodules. In this situation, adjuvant chemotherapy follows, and one observes for further development of pulmonary metastases.
(b) Stability or diminution of the nodules but the nodules are still present. In this scenario, chemotherapy continues with a plan to resect the nodules that persist after completion of chemotherapy.
(c) Increase in size and number of the nodules; in this scenario, the chemotherapy agents are generally changed. Following several rounds of chemotherapy, the pulmonary nodules are removed if they are resectable. If the nodules are not resectable, one continues chemotherapy with the goal of reducing the pulmonary disease until the thoracic surgeon can safely resect the disease.

2. Pulmonary and bone metastases at presentation

If pulmonary and bone metastases are found on initial presentation, the situation is very grave. Although cure may be possible, the odds are markedly diminished. The approach for the pulmonary metastases is the same as when only pulmonary metastases are present. If there is a single bone metastasis present and the pulmonary disease is controllable by thoracotomy, then the bone metastasis is resected. If there is more than one bone metastasis, the general approach is to continue chemotherapy to see the response of the tumor. If the primary lesion and the pulmonary and bone metastases are resectable, then all sites of disease are removed.

3. Pulmonary metastases after neoadjuvant chemotherapy and wide resection of the primary tumor

The development of pulmonary metastases after a disease-free interval of at least 6 months is the most common situation the clinician, patient, and family have to face. It is essential that a plan be developed when the pulmonary metastases are discovered so that the patient and family understand that everything possible will be done. The computerized tomography scan is carefully studied to determine how many nodules are present. Chemotherapy is usually given initially to determine if the nodule will respond and to see if additional nodules develop. After one to three cycles of chemotherapy, if the remaining nodules are resectable, then surgery is performed. At 3-month intervals, the CT is repeated to detect the presence of further nodules. If more nodules develop, further chemotherapy is delivered. The agent of choice is dependent on the response of the nodules to the pre-thoracotomy chemotherapy. Multiple thoracotomies are sometimes necessary to achieve a cure, but patients with a higher disease burden (>5 lesions) and those requiring more than two metastasectomies fare worse [3].

4. Pulmonary and bone metastases after neoadjuvant chemotherapy and wide resection of the primary tumor

The development of pulmonary and bone metastases after preoperative chemotherapy and wide resection is a very ominous situation. If there is a single bone metastasis and resectable pulmonary disease, then a very aggressive approach with the goal of removing both the pulmonary metastases and bone metastasis is employed. If there are numerous bone metastases, then approach shifts to palliative care. While chemotherapy is given for the pulmonary and bone metastases, radiation may be delivered to sites of bone metastasis if these sites are symptomatic.

13.5 Special Note: Treatment-Resistant Sarcomas

Certain bone sarcomas, most notably the chondrosarcomas, are notoriously resistant to chemotherapy and radiotherapy. Surgical extirpation remains the mainstay of treatment for these diseases. Several series have shown a very modest disease response rate to chemotherapy and radiation for mesenchymal and dedifferentiated subtypes of chondrosarcoma, but overall survival numbers remain dismal [4, 5]. Investigational drug trials may be explored in these cases.

13.5.1 Soft Tissue Sarcomas

Soft tissue sarcomas (STS) are a very heterogeneous assortment of malignancies. While most bone sarcomas are high grade, there is a wide range in clinical behavior of soft tissue malignancies. High-grade STS will often metastasize very early (within 2 years), while low-grade tumors may have a very long disease-free interval (2–20 years). There are several scenarios which may need to be addressed:

1. Pulmonary metastases at presentation
2. Pulmonary and diffuse metastases at presentation
3. Pulmonary metastases after a disease-free interval
4. Pulmonary and diffuse metastases after a disease-free interval

1. Pulmonary metastases at presentation

The presentation of both a soft tissue malignancy and pulmonary metastases at presentation is a difficult problem. In this scenario, chemotherapy is usually necessary for lung involvement that implies systemic disease. In addition, radiotherapy is often needed for the primary tumor. The chemotherapy and radiotherapy can be interdigitated preoperatively. Following preoperative chemotherapy and radiation to the primary tumor, a new computerized tomography scan of the chest is performed to assess the response of the chemotherapy. The primary soft tissue tumor is then resected. Once surgical site healing occurs (generally within 3 weeks), the chemotherapy is then restarted. After one or two cycles, a new computerized tomography scan is performed, and if the nodules in the chest are resectable, they are removed.

At this point careful surveillance of the pulmonary system is necessary (every 3 months). If new pulmonary nodules appear and they are resectable, then the new nodules are removed. The decision for additional chemotherapy depends on whether the initial response to first-line agents was favorable or not. If the nodules are not responsive to chemotherapy, then surgical resection is the dominant form of therapy for the nodules.

2. Pulmonary and diffuse metastases at presentation

This is a very difficult problem and often portends a very poor prognosis for the patient. Although there is potential for cure if the disease is limited, the odds are far against long-term survival. Unless death from metastases is imminent, the approach is for interdigitated chemotherapy and radiation therapy to the primary tumor with the goal of resecting the primary tumor. Once the primary tumor is removed, a decision has to be made about the metastases. The patient undergoes restaging to identify all the sites of disease. Postoperative chemotherapy is often delivered if there was a positive response to the initial chemotherapy. After one to three cycles of chemotherapy, an assessment is made as to the resectability of the sites of metastasis. If there are diffuse metastases (lung, bone, and visceral sites such as the liver or brain), then there is a shift to palliative rather than curative therapy. If the sites of metastasis are all resectable, then they should be resected with a wide margin similar to treatment of the primary tumor. Chemotherapy is often given between resections so that the disease remains in check.

3. Pulmonary metastases after a disease-free interval

The discovery of pulmonary metastases after a disease-free interval (usually at least 6 months) is the most common scenario faced by patients, family members, and the healthcare team. Patients often feel a sense of despair for their survival. It is very important to emphasize to patients and family members that cure is still possible in about one quarter of patients. The medical oncologist and thoracic surgeon need to engage the patient so that a very aggressive treatment plan is outlined for the patient.

If the pulmonary disease is resectable, the nodules are often removed first. This approach provides both a diagnosis of metastatic sarcoma and renders the patient disease-free. At this point there are two options; the first is for observation only with serial CT scans of the chest, and the second is for systemic chemotherapy in addition to monitoring the chest. The older patient with comorbidities will often choose careful observation, while the younger patient may be more suitable and amenable to systemic chemotherapy and careful monitoring of the chest.

Multiple thoracotomies and cycles of chemotherapy may be necessary to control the disease. Cure may be possible as long as the metastases are restricted to the chest and are resectable [4].

4. Pulmonary and diffuse metastases after a disease-free interval

Pulmonary and diffuse metastasis after a disease-free interval portends a very advanced state of disease, and the prognosis is very poor. The patient, family, and healthcare team need to decide whether to proceed with palliative therapy or to try for cure despite the poor odds. The general plan is the same as noted above in patients with pulmonary and diffuse metastases at presentation.

13.6   Palliative Care in the Patient with Metastatic Sarcoma

Once metastatic disease is confirmed and treatment is no longer intended to be curative, appropriate palliative care requires an almost paradoxical intensification of specialty care across multiple disciplines. Collaboration must exist between surgical, medical, and radiation oncologists, with the support of interventional radiologists, primary care providers, rehabilitation specialists, psychiatrists, and other services as needed. Cross-communication between specialists is essential to coordinate care, as the timing of trials of chemotherapy, radiation treatments, and urgent surgical interventions may overlap.

The goals of palliative sarcoma care focus on the prevention and treatment of the side effects or symptoms of advancing disease, which include:

- Pain control: management of pain from mass effect, post-chemotherapy neuropathy, radiculopathy or neural compression in the spine, etc.
- Preservation of mobility: preventing or managing disease that threatens to compromise skeletal integrity or the ability of the patient to ambulate and perform tasks independently.
- Survival: promoting longevity to assist patients in meeting personal goals before death.
- Psychological/spiritual care: assisting patients and families in coping with a difficult circumstance. The role of supportive counseling from psychiatrists and all members of the oncologic team cannot be overstated.

Palliative care requires an individualized approach to the sarcoma patient. A multidisciplinary plan must take into account the relative benefits and toxicities of any treatment, disease-specific factors, and the patient's own personal goals of treatment.

13.6.1 Chemotherapy

Palliative chemotherapy for advanced and metastatic sarcoma may be administered to achieve tumor shrinkage with the goal of local downstaging and decreased mass effect. For patients with personal life goals or specific functional demands, the potential benefit to progression-free or overall survival, no matter how modest, may justify the risks and toxicities of a treatment. This should be considered on a case-by-case basis.

The agent of choice is selected based on the chemosensitivity profile of the specific subtype of sarcoma. The most common agents selected are doxorubicin and ifosfamide, followed by paclitaxel, gemcitabine, and Taxotere. A discussion of disease-specific chemotherapy options is featured below.

The intensity of treatment is subject to considerable variability and is influenced by the patient's age, performance status, medical comorbidities, and prior treatments. Several studies including a meta-analysis examining single-agent versus combination therapy for metastatic sarcomas have consistently shown a slight trend favoring combination therapy in terms of response rates and survival, but these trends do not reach statistical significance. Treatment toxicities were also higher in the combination therapy groups. In both treatment groups, advancing age, limited performance status, and number of metastatic sites were the only independent factors associated with overall survival [6–11].

Treatment-related toxicities are common in the palliative chemotherapy setting, and hospitalizations for grade 3 and 4 toxic events occur in approximately 13% of single-agent regimens and 38–46% of combination therapy regimens [6, 11]. These include hospitalizations for intractable nausea and vomiting, myelosuppression, bleeding and anemia, lymphopenia and infection, renal impairment, CNS toxicity, and complications of hypoalbuminemia. Drug-specific toxicities may also be limiting. Doxorubicin-related cardiotoxicity risk increases for every 50 mg/m^2 over the total dosage of 400 mg/m^2. These considerations are to be taken into account when determining duration of treatment and overall dose intensity.

13.6.2 Disease-Specific Palliative Chemotherapy: Bone Sarcomas

The introduction of chemotherapy agents in the treatment of osteosarcoma and Ewing's sarcoma in the 1970s has led to an increase in 5-year survival rates from approximately 15–20% to 60–80%, suggesting the presence of micrometastatic disease at the time of initial presentation [12, 13]. A combination of doxorubicin, cisplatin, and methotrexate is the commonly administered regimen for osteosarcoma. For patients with metastatic disease or those with poor histological response to conventional treatment, considered <90% tumor necrosis, the addition of second-line therapy with ifosfamide and/or etoposide has been advocated [14, 15].

Ewing's sarcoma is most commonly treated with VAC-D chemotherapy (vincristine, actinomycin D, cyclophosphamide, and doxorubicin). The addition of ifosfamide and etoposide has been found to work synergistically with VAC-D regimens, although this was not found to demonstrate a survival advantage in patients with metastatic disease at presentation [16]. Whereas the 5-year survival for patients with nonmetastatic disease approaches over 80%, those with relapsed and metastatic disease fare far worse; 5-year survival is approximately 29% with isolated lung metastasis, 19% for bone metastasis, and 8% for both lung and bone metastasis [17].

Malignant fibrous histiocytoma is a primary sarcoma of the bone in older patients typically over 40 years of age. Chemotherapy regimens similar to that of conventional osteosarcoma have been used with 50–60% clinical response rates [18–20].

In patients with refractory or metastatic osteosarcoma, Ewing's tumor, and MFH of the bone, second-line treatment with gemcitabine and docetaxel has been shown to have an overall objective response rate of 29% [21].

Unlike other primary sarcomas of the bone, chondrosarcomas are classically radioresistant and chemoresistant. A modest benefit to ifosfamide has been suggested in the setting of dedifferentiated chondrosarcoma, although this is a disease with a dismal prognosis (5-year survival 10–15%) [4]. Therefore, the primary palliative strategy in patients with metastatic chondrosarcoma remains surgical resection.

13.6.3 Disease-Specific Palliative Chemotherapy: Soft Tissue Sarcomas

Soft tissue sarcomas are a heterogeneous group of rare malignancies, with wide variations in histology, cytogenetics, and patient demographics. As such, disease-specific investigations are typically lacking in statistical power, disease-grouping studies suffer from substantial confounding variables, and a statistically significant survival benefit has not been demonstrated with routine chemotherapy for all soft tissue sarcomas. Rather, the complications of chemotherapy toxicity may actually confer a negative impact on survival in some patients [22, 23]. With local surgery and radiation, the 5-year rate of distant relapse-free survival of soft tissue sarcoma is approximately 50%, and this has changed very little since the 1970s, owing to the lack of proven systemic therapy [22]. A meta-analysis of 14 randomized trials estimates a treatment advantage of approximately 10% with either doxorubicin- or anthracycline-based therapy with ifosfamide [24]. Adjuvant chemotherapy generally should not be considered a first-line therapy in palliative treatment of metastatic soft tissue sarcoma [23, 25].

Despite the lack of evidence supporting chemotherapy for routine use, several histologic subtypes of soft tissue sarcomas demonstrate notable chemosensitivity. In leiomyosarcoma has shown a 17% response rate to Gemcitabine and docetaxel [26]. Angiosarcoma has shown variable sensitivity to doxorubicin, ifosfamide, and taxanes [27]. Synovial sarcoma shows particular responsiveness to regimens with ifosfamide, cisplatin, and doxorubicin, showing 70% partial and 30% complete treatment response in the setting of metastatic disease [28]. Pediatric rhabdomyosarcoma has a reported cure rate of 70% with multidisciplinary care that includes surgery and chemotherapy with vincristine, actinomycin, and cyclophosphamide [29].

13.6.4   Targeted Therapies

Enthusiasm for mutation analysis-based therapy with targeted agents is expanding in sarcoma oncology. The insulin-like growth factor 1 receptor (IGF1-R) and its downstream pathways such as mTOR have shown prominent roles in the development of osteosarcoma and Ewing's sarcoma, and multi-target inhibitors such as pazopanib and sorafenib with antiangiogenic VEGF, PDGFR, and c-KIT activity are being explored as second-line agents in soft tissue and select bone sarcomas. These agents and many other targeted therapies are being explored in phase II and other trials, but their efficacy has not been established [30–32]. Comprehensive molecular profiling with mutation-based therapy is currently in its infancy, with only small case series that have not shown dramatic results [33].

13.6.5   Palliative Radiation Therapy

Radiation therapy is an attractive option for local control in patients with unresectable disease, lesions in anatomic locations in which surgical resection might be particularly morbid, patients unable to tolerate surgery or chemotherapy, and specific diseases with known radiosensitivity. For instance, palliative radiotherapy has been demonstrated to have clinical response rates of 76–84% in Ewing's sarcoma and 54% in osteosarcoma [34, 35]. For soft tissue sarcomas, radiotherapy combined with surgery is a mainstay of local treatment, but the efficacy of radiation for metastatic disease depends on the radiosensitivity of the specific disease. Myxoid liposarcoma is perhaps the most radiosensitive soft tissue sarcoma, with clinical response rates close to 100% [36].

Stereotactic body radiosurgery (SBRT) is being increasingly utilized for palliation of disease in anatomically challenging locations such as the spine and pelvis, in tissues that have been previously irradiated, and for tumors that are known to be less radiosensitive. SBRT has the advantage of delivering higher doses of radiation to the target lesion with less damage to the uninvolved tissues. The treatment course of SBRT is also much shorter, three to five sessions on average. This is much less intrusive to the patient's schedule, which can be of particular importance in the palliative setting. In the setting of metastatic sarcoma, SBRT is generally safe, with toxicities typically occurring in re-irradiated fields and when delivered concurrently with chemotherapy [37]. For metastasis from primary sarcomas, Stragliotto et al. found that SBRT demonstrated an overall response rate of 88%, with a 3-year survival rate of 31% [38]. Specific to pulmonary metastases from soft tissue sarcoma, Dhakal et al. treated 15 patients with a median number of four lesions per patient and found a local response rate of 82%, with a median overall survival benefit of 1.5 years over non-radiated controls [39]. Toxicities can occur with SBRT and may include myonecrosis, avascular necrosis of the bone, pathologic fracture, and sacral plexopathy [37].

Systemic radiopharmaceuticals that localize to the bone and osteoblastic sites may provide targeted irradiation to metastatic deposits of osteosarcoma, which may be multifocal and a source of considerable pain and disability. Radioactive isotopes of iodine-131 and strontium-85, strontium-89, and strontium-90, while used in the laboratory to induce osteosarcomas in mice, have been found to localize to metastatic osteogenic sarcoma [40]. Strontium may be used in nuclear medicine imaging for localization of osteosarcoma metastases, but its increased oncogenic potential makes any therapeutic applications unclear [41]. Samarium-153-EDTMP and radium-223 are both bone-seeking radiopharmaceuticals that have been tested in patients with widely metastatic osteosarcoma. The hematopoietic toxicity of these chemicals typically requires autologous stem cell support after treatment, and clinical response to treatment has been observed to last an average of 1 month [42–44].

13.6.6 Palliative Percutaneous Ablation

The interventional radiologist can be a valuable contributor to the palliation of metastatic sarcoma. Minimally invasive, percutaneous techniques to deliver local adjuvant therapy for ablation of metastatic deposits may obviate the need for larger, more invasive surgery. Selective nerve root ablation may provide palliative pain control in selected patients. Arterial catheterization techniques include isolated limb perfusion therapy and mechanical or chemoembolization techniques. Embolization of highly hypervascular lesions may provide pain relief in over 80% of patients with advanced disease [45].

Thermal ablation techniques such as cryoablation and radiofrequency ablation may be used to induce local tumor necrosis and halt local progression of disease. With radiofrequency ablation techniques, long-term pain relief can be obtained in 70–83% of patients [46] and may confer an average survival benefit of 32 months in the setting of oligometastatic disease [47]. This may be due to simply diminishing the local mass effect of the lesion, but recent investigations have postulated a post-procedure release of antigens that may stimulate an antitumor immune response [48].

For metastatic lesions within the bone, the structural integrity of the bone must be considered when using percutaneous ablation techniques. The simultaneous insertion of mechanical augments, such as hardware and/or polymethyl methacrylate (PMMA) cement, may be combined with thermal ablation techniques to provide palliative treatment in the spine, pelvis, or other sites at risk for fracture. Pain relief with combined percutaneous treatment can be obtained in up to 81% of selected patients [49].

13.6.7 Palliative Surgery

Although not performed with curative intent, surgery in the setting of palliative care may still be feasible if significant gains can be made in terms of pain control, functional mobility, or quality of life. Resection of pulmonary metastases for survival benefit has been discussed previously, but metastases in the bone can also be a significant source of pain and disability. Percutaneous stabilization techniques, prophylactic nail fixation, resection of an involved segment of the bone, joint replacement, and even amputation can all be reasonable interventions to alleviate pain and maintain upright mobility in terminal patients. It is important that surgical procedures ideally should be planned in consultation with the rest of the oncologic team around other planned chemotherapy or radiation treatments so as to minimize the risk of avoidable perioperative complications [50].

13.7 Summary

Metastatic sarcoma is often devastating news to the patient and the oncology team and can provoke feelings of despair and personal or professional failure. When a sarcoma has recurred or metastasized after a long disease-free interval, this can be particularly disheartening. It is important for all parties involved to refocus and specifically re-evaluate and discuss the goals of treatment. In up to a quarter of patients with metastatic disease, surgical extirpation and long-term remission of disease are still possible. Younger patients, patients with resectable oligometastatic disease, and patients with a treatment-sensitive sarcoma subtype warrant a more aggressive treatment strategy.

When the goals of treatment shift toward palliative care, treatment should proceed with a focus on pain relief, functional mobility, and the physical, mental, and emotional quality of life of the patient. Palliative care remains a multidisciplinary undertaking, and frequent communication should exist between members of the oncology team to explore the potential chemotherapy, radiotherapy, percutaneous interventions, and surgical treatment options available to serve the patient.

References

1. Neglia JP, Friedman DL, Yasui Y, et al. Second malignant neoplasms in five-year survivors of childhood cancer: childhood cancer survivor study. J Natl Cancer Inst. 2001;93(8): 618–29.
2. Dossett LA, Toloza EM, Fontaine J, et al. Outcomes and clinical predictors of improved survival in patients undergoing pulmonary metastasectomy for sarcoma. J Surg Oncol. 2015; 112(1):103–6.
3. Matsubara E, Mori T, Koga T, et al. Metastasectomy of pulmonary metastases from osteosarcoma: prognostic factors and indication for repeat metastasectomy. J Resp Med. 2015;2015:570314. 5 pages
4. Kawaguchi S, Sun T, Lin PP, Deavers M, Harun N, Lewis VO. Does ifosfamide therapy improve survival of patients with dedifferentiated chondrosarcoma? Clin Orthop Relat Res. 2014;472(3):983–9.
5. Italiano A, Mir O, Cioffi A, et al. Advanced chondrosarcomas: role of chemotherapy and survival. Ann Oncol. 2013;24(11):2916–22.
6. Yousaf N, Harris S, Martin-Liberal J, et al. First-line palliative chemotherapy in elderly patients with advanced soft tissue sarcoma. Clin Sarcoma Res. 2015;5:10.
7. Karavasilis V, Seddon BM, Ashley S, et al. Significant clinical benefit of first-line palliative chemotherapy in advanced soft tissue sarcoma: retrospective analysis and identification of prognostic factors in 488 patients. Cancer. 2008;112(7):1585–91.
8. Garbay D, Maki RG, Blay JY, et al. Advanced soft-tissue sarcoma in elderly patients: patterns of care and survival. Ann Oncol. 2013;24(7):1924–30.
9. Iwata S, Ishii T, Kawai A, et al. Prognostic factors in elderly osteosarcoma patients: a multi-institutional retrospective study of 86 cases. Ann Surg Oncol. 2014;21(1):263–8.
10. Bramwell VH, Anderson D, Charette ML. Doxorubicin-based chemotherapy for the palliative treatment of adult patients with locally advanced or metastatic soft-tissue sarcoma: a meta-analysis and clinical practice guideline. Sarcoma. 2000;4(3):103–12.
11. Judson I, Verweij J, Gelderblom H, et al. Doxorubicin alone versus intensified doxorubicin plus ifosfamide for first-line treatment of advanced or metastatic soft-tissue sarcoma: a randomized controlled phase 3 trial. Lancet Oncol. 2014;15(4):415–23.
12. Dahlin DC, Coventry MB. Osteogenic sarcoma: a study of six hundred cases. J Bone Joint Surg Am. 1967;49(1):101–10.
13. Eilber F, Giuliano A, Eckhardt J, Patterson K, Moseley S, Goodnight J. Adjuvant chemotherapy for osteosarcoma: a randomized prospective trial. J Clin Oncol. 1987;5(1):21–6.
14. Bacci G, Farrar S, Bertoni F, et al. Long-term outcome for patients with nonmetastatic osteosarcoma of the extremity treated at the Istituto Ortopedico Rizzoli according to the osteosarcoma-2 protocol: an updated report. J Clin Oncol. 2000;18(24):4016–27.
15. Maki RG. Ifosfamide in the neoadjuvant treatment of osteogenic sarcoma. J Clin Oncol. 2012;3(17):2033–5.
16. Grier HE, Krailo MD, Tarbell NJ, et al. Addition of ifosfamide and etoposide to standard chemotherapy for Ewing's sarcoma and primitive neuroectodermal tumor of bone. N Engl J Med. 2003;348(8):694–701.
17. Cotterill SJ, Ahrens S, Paulussen M, et al. Prognostic factors in Ewing's tumor of bone: analysis of 975 patients from the European intergroup cooperative Ewing's sarcoma study group. J Clin Oncol. 2000;18(17):3108–14.

18. Campanna R, Bertoni F, Bacchini P, Bacci G, Guerra A, Campanacci M. Malignant fibrous histiocytoma of bone. The experience at the Rizzoli institute: report of 90 cases. Cancer. 1984; 54(1):177–87.
19. Bramwell VH, Steward WP, Nooij M, Whelan J, Craft AW, Grimer RJ, et al. Neoadjuvant chemotherapy with doxorubicin and cisplatin in malignant fibrous histiocytoma of bone: a European osteosarcoma intergroup study. J Clin Oncol. 1999;17(10):3260–9.
20. Jeon DG, Song WS, Kong CB, Kim JR, Lee SY. MFH of bone and osteosarcoma show similar survival and chemosensitivity. Clin Orthop Relat Res. 2001;469(2):584–90.
21. Navid F, Willert JR, McCarville MB, Furman W, Watkins A, Roberts W, Daw NC. Combination of gemcitabine and docetaxel in the treatment of children and young adults with refractory bone sarcoma. Cancer. 2008;113(2):419–25.
22. Casali PG, Picci P. Adjuvant chemotherapy for soft tissue sarcoma. Curr Opin Oncol. 2005;17(4): 361–5.
23. Courmier JN, Pollock RE. Soft tissue sarcomas. CA Cancer J Clin. 2004;54(2):94–109.
24. Sarcoma Meta-Analysis Collaboration. Adjuvant chemotherapy for localized resectable soft tissue sarcoma of adults: meta-analysis of individual data. Lancet. 1997;350(9092):1647–54.
25. Patrikidou A, Domont J, Cioffi A, Le Cesne A. Treating soft tissue sarcomas with adjuvant chemotherapy. Curr Treat Options Oncol. 2012;17(8):515–27.
26. Maki RG, Wathen JK, Patel SR, et al. Randomized phase II study of gemcitabine and docetaxel compared with gemcitabine alone in patients with metastatic soft tissue sarcomas: results of sarcoma alliance for research through collaboration study 002. J Clin Oncol. 2007;25(19):2755–63.
27. Penel N, Bui BN, Bay JO, et al. Phase II trial of weekly paclitaxel for unresectable angiosarcoma. J Clin Oncol. 2008;26(32):5269–74.
28. Rosen G, Forcher C, Lowenbraun S, et al. Synovial sarcoma: uniform response of metastases to high dose ifosfamide. Cancer. 1994;73(10):2506–11.
29. Arndt CA, Rose PS, Folpe AL, Laack NN. Common musculoskeletal tumors of childhood and adolescence. Mayo Clin Proc. 2012;87(5):475–87.
30. Okuno SH, Postel-Vinay S, Molife LR, Okuno SH, Schuetze SM, Paccagnella ML, et al. Safety, pharmacokinetics, and preliminary activity of the anti-IGF-1R antibody figitumumab (CP-751,871) in patients with sarcoma and Ewing's sarcoma: a phase 1 expansion cohort study. Lancet Oncol. 2010;11:129–35.
31. Dubois SG, Shusterman S, Ingle AM, Ahern CH, Reid JM, Wu B, et al. Phase I and pharmacokinetic study of sunitinib in pediatric patients with refractory solid tumours: a children's oncology group study. Clin Cancer Res. 2001;17:5113–22.
32. Keir ST, Morton CL, Wu J, Kurmasheva RT, Houghton PJ, Smith MA. Initial testing of the multitargeted kinase inhibitor pazopanib by the pediatric preclinical testing program. Pediatr Blood Cancer. 2012;59:586–8.
33. Subbiah V, Wagner MJ, McGuire MF, et al. Personalized comprehensive molecular profiling of high risk osteosarcoma: implications and limitations for precision medicine. Oncotarget. 2015;6(38):40642–54.
34. Rahn DA, Mundt AJ, Murphy JD, Schiff D, Adams J, Murphy KT. Clinical outcomes of palliative radiation therapy for children. Pract Radiat Oncol. 2014;5(3):183–7.
35. Koontz BF, Clough RW, Halperin EC. Palliative radiation therapy for metastatic Ewing sarcoma. Cancer. 2006;106(8):1790–3.
36. Chung PW, Deheshi BM, Ferguson PC, Wunder JS, Griffin AM, Catton CN, Bell RS, White LM, Kandel RA, O'Sullivan BO. Radiosensitivity translates into excellent local control in extremity Myxoid liposarcoma. Cancer. 2009;115(14):3254–61.
37. Brown LC, Lester RA, Grams MP, Haddock MG, Olivier KR, Arndt CA, Rose PS, Laack NN. Stereotactic body radiotherapy for metastatic and recurrent Ewing sarcoma and osteosarcoma. Sarcoma. 2014;2014:418270.
38. Stragliotto CL, Karlsson K, Lax I, Rutkowska E, Bergh J, Strander H, Blomgren H, Friesland S. A retrospective study of SBRT of metastases in patients with primary sarcoma. Med Oncol. 2012;29(5):3431–9.

39. Dhakal S, Corbin KS, Milano MT, Philip A, Sahasrabudhe D, Jones C, Constine LS. Stereotactic body radiotherapy for pulmonary metastases from soft-tissue sarcomas: excellent local lesion control and improved patient survival. Int J Radiat Oncol Biol Phys. 2012;82(2):940–5.
40. Eisenhut M. Iodine-131-labeled diphosphonates for the palliative treatment of bone metastases: I. Organ distribution and kinetics of I-131 BDP3 in rats. J Nucl Med. 1984;25(12):1356–61.
41. Blake GM, Zivanovic MA, McEwan AJ, Condon BR, Ackery DM. Strontium-89 therapy: strontium kinetics and dosimetry in two patients treated for metastasizing osteosarcoma. Br J Radiol. 1987;60(711):253–9.
42. Berger M, Grignani G, Giostra A, Ferrari S, Ferraresi V, et al. 153 samarium-EDTMP administration followed by hematopoietic stem cell support for bone metastases in osteosarcoma patients. Ann Oncol. 2012;23(7):1899–905.
43. Franzius C, Schuck A, Bielack SS. High-dose samarium-153 ethylene diamine tetramethylene phosphonate: low toxicity of skeletal irradiation in patients with osteosarcoma and bone metastases. J Clin Oncol. 2002;20(1):189–96.
44. Anderson PM, Subbiah V, Rohren E. Bone-seeking radiopharmaceuticals as targeted agents of osteosarcoma: samarium-153-EDTMP and radium-223. Adv Exp Med Biol. 2014;804:291–304.
45. Mavrogenis AF, Ross G, Altimari G, Calabro T, Angelini A, Palmerini E, Rimondi E, Ruggieri P. Palliative embolization for advanced bone sarcomas. Radiol Med. 2013;118(8):1344–59.
46. Sanou R, Bazin C, Krakowski I, Boccaccini H, Mathias J, Beot S, Marchal F, Regent D. Radiofrequency ablation for palliation of soft tissue tumor pain. J Radiol. 2010;91(3):281–6.
47. Falk AT, Moureau-Zabotto L, Quali M, Penel N, Italiano A, Bay J, et al. Effect on survival of local ablative treatment of metastases from sarcomas: a study of the French sarcoma group. Clin Oncol. 2015;27(1):48–55.
48. Bastianpillai C, Petrides N, Shah T, et al. Harnessing the immunomodulatory effect of thermal and non-thermal ablative therapies for cancer treatment. Tumour Biol. 2015;36(12):9137–46.
49. Clarencon F, Jean B, Pham HP, Cormier E, Bensimon G, Rose M, Maksud P, Chiras J. Value of percutaneous radiofrequency ablation with or without percutaneous vertebroplasty for pain relief and functional recover in painful bone metastases. Skeletal Radiol. 2013;42(1):25–36.
50. Aboulafia AJ, Levine AM, Schmidt D, Aboulafia D. Surgical therapy of bone metastases. Semin Oncol. 2007;34(3):206–14.

Pain Management for Sarcoma Patients

14

Lee Ann Rhodes

14.1   Introduction

Fear is inevitable when one faces the threat of pain. When this feeling arises, it puts the patient's treatment course in jeopardy. The undertreatment of cancer pain has been a global epidemic for a number of years [1–3]. At the time of their diagnosis, approximately 30–50% of cancer patients have experienced pain [2, 4–7]. This percentage rises to 50–70% of patients during their cancer treatment [8], while 65–90% of patients with advanced cancer are burdened with inadequate control of their pain [2, 6, 7, 9]. Consequences of unrelieved pain include loss of autonomy, social isolation, suffering, psychological distress, and the diminished ability to comply with the cancer treatment.

With so many strategies in place to ameliorate cancer pain, why is it that so many people are in pain? Many patients are simply undertreated due to lack of knowledge about medication titration and how to control side effects [4]. Traditionally, the control of pain has been given a lower priority than controlling or eliminating the malignancy [10]. Several barriers have been identified that impair the appropriate treatment of pain. The patients' family members and health-care providers each collectively may contribute to these obstacles [11–14]. Typically, oncology patients have several health-care providers. This may present some confusion as to which provider is assuming the role of prescribing pain medications; therefore, communication is paramount for successful treatment. Patients may underreport pain to their doctor for a variety of reasons. Often they do not want to be seen as complaining or feel that the focus of their treatment may take a more palliative path instead of curing the disease. Sixty percent of patients feel that a choice must be made between

L.A. Rhodes, M.D.
Department of Anesthesia, MedStar Washington Hospital Center, Washington, DC, USA
e-mail: LeeAnn.Rhodes@Medstar.net

© Springer International Publishing Switzerland 2017
R.M. Henshaw (ed.), *Sarcoma*, DOI 10.1007/978-3-319-43121-5_14

pain control and cancer treatment [4]. Religious and cultural perspectives on pain also influence the way a patient will respond to pain, with some feeling that they must endure pain as a punishment for their past bad deeds. Other patients may become hopeless that nothing can be done to relieve their pain. This is particularly important when treating patients with sarcoma. Many patients present with pain on diagnosis. An interdisciplinary approach benefits the patient in many aspects which include restoration of function and reduction of postoperative pain.

Misinformation is a leading barrier to pain control [15–17]. Up to 80% of patients fear they will become addicted to opioids [17]. Other barriers include those imposed by insurance companies, many requiring special authorization for opioids and limitation on the amount dispensed. Eighty-five percent of patients fear that the side effects associated with opioids cannot be controlled [17]. Lack of knowledge exists about comprehensive pain management, which is comprised of behavioral therapies, physical therapy and rehabilitation, and interventional nerve blocks. This limits the ability of attaining satisfactory pain control. Fortunately, many pain organizations throughout the world have disseminated information to both patients and their family members and provided continuing medical education to health-care providers to dispel the myths that contribute to these pain barriers. By creating dialogues between patients and health-care workers, these barriers can be effectively overcome.

This chapter will discuss the causes of and treatment of cancer pain along with a discussion of phantom limb pain.

14.2 Causes of Cancer Pain

Pain can be the result of the cancer itself, the treatment given to manage the cancer, or completely unrelated to the cancer. Up to 75% of chronic cancer pain is the direct result of the malignancy [18]. The tumor itself produces mediators of inflammation that propagate pain. The tumor may invade surrounding structures, including nerves, bones, soft tissue, ligaments, and fascia [4]. Metastasis of the tumor to the bones may result in pain. Only one-third of advanced cancer patients have pain from one source [19–21].

Approximately 17% of patients' pain is the result of treatment [19]. Surgical, chemotherapy, or radiation treatment of the tumor may result in painful conditions. Incisional pain may produce scar neuromas, with ectopic foci of pain. Some chemotherapeutic agents, such as cisplatin, taxanes, and vincristines, may lead to painful peripheral neuropathies [4, 22]. Radiation treatment may also inflict injury to peripheral nerves, which may occur months to years after treatment [10]. Plexopathies from radiation are more likely when the dose of radiation is greater than 60 Gy or 6000 rad cumulatively [22]. Also, there are cases of radiation-induced osteonecrosis (G4).

The types of pain are characterized as nociceptive, neuropathic, or mixed nociceptive-neuropathic. Identification of the type of pain is necessary since some agents that effectively control nociceptive pain, such as opioid analgesics, may have minimal effect on the treatment of neuropathic pain. Nociceptive pain is associated with tissue injury from surgery, trauma, inflammation, or tumor. This injury activates pain receptors in the cutaneous or deep musculoskeletal structures [4]. Nociceptive pain may be further divided into somatic and visceral pain. Somatic pain arises from injury to bones, tissues, or tendons and is mainly described as achy, dull, or stabbing. It is typically localized, and examples include tumor invading a bone, a pathological fracture, or postoperative incisional pain [4]. Visceral pain may occur from tumor stretching, invading, compressing, obstructing, or distending visceral structures. This type of pain usually presents as a poorly localized pain. Frequent descriptions of visceral nociceptive pain are deep, cramping, colicky, and squeezing, especially when an obstruction is present, and sharp and throbbing when an organ capsule is distended [23]. The pain may be referred to the shoulder if the diaphragm is irritated or to the patient's back [4].

Neuropathic pain results from abnormal somatosensory processing in the peripheral or central nervous system [10]. Neuropathic pain may be described as pins and needles, burning, numbness, lancinating, and electrical shock-like [4]. Examples of neuropathic pain include tumor invasion or compression of plexuses, nerves, or the spinal cord, peripheral neuropathies from chemotherapeutic agents, or radiation-induced nerve injury. Even a surgical scar may develop ectopic painful nerve processing postoperatively. Why some patients develop neuropathic pain and others do not is unknown [10].

14.3 Pain Assessment

In order to treat pain, routine assessment and reassessment following intervention must be accomplished. Reliable pain scales exist that may be verbal or visual [24–26]. The most common assessment tool uses a ten-point verbal or visual scale where zero is no pain and ten is the worst pain imaginable. Placing pain scores on the vital sign flow sheets of both inpatient and outpatient areas has been one of the many efforts undertaken to make pain more visible. This enables multiple health-care workers to see the results of their pain interventions. Pain assessments also incorporate the location of pain, radiation of pain, description of pain, and temporal features, including breakthrough pain, duration of pain, and aggravating and alleviating factors. Additional symptoms, such as fatigue and psychological distress along with the influence of pain on activities, sleep, work, quality of life, and relationships with others, should be asked. Previous pain therapies and the patient's response to treatment also are included in the assessment. It is not uncommon that the patient had been on an effective pain regimen only to have it discontinued when the patient changed physicians or due to unfounded concerns that addictions may occur from prolonged use. By collecting the necessary information during the pain assessment, the differential diagnosis can be formulated, and appropriate pain interventions can be formulated.

14.4 Treatment of Pain

Controlling pain is achieved by either reducing or eliminating the source of pain, blunting the perception of pain, or blocking the transmission of pain to the central nervous system [27]. A variety of treatments have been developed to accomplish this goal, and ultimately 85–95% of patients with cancer pain can have their pain controlled with a combination of pharmacotherapy, nonpharmacological therapy, and antineoplastic treatment [28–31]. The principle treatment of pain has been pharmacotherapy. This resulted in the development of a three-step "ladder" published in 1986 by the World Health Organization (WHO) to assist in cancer pain management. Prior to this, use of algorithms for opioid treatment of cancer pain was highly variable. The first step of the WHO ladder is aimed at the treatment of mild to moderate pain and recommends nonopioid analgesics such as acetaminophen and nonsteroidal anti-inflammatory agents (NSAIDs). The second step of the ladder focuses on the treatment of moderate pain and includes short-acting opioids such as codeine, hydrocodone, and oxycodone. These opioids are frequently combined with either acetaminophen, aspirin, or ibuprofen. Due to the addition of these, analgesia may be limited by the safe maximum doses of the nonopioid components. It is also appropriate to use these to treat mild pain if the patient either does not respond to or cannot tolerate Step 1 treatment [23].

Severe pain is addressed in the final third step of the ladder. Morphine, oxycodone, hydromorphone, fentanyl, oxymorphone, and methadone are examples of Step 3 opioids. Doses of these opioids generally do not have a ceiling or maximal dose, thus enabling escalation of doses that are only limited by side effects [30–34]. The dose needed to obtain adequate analgesia is patient specific and is achieved through a balance between analgesia and side effects. The WHO ladder also allows for the addition of adjuvant drugs, such as those used to treat neuropathic pain, bisphosphonates, steroids, and topical analgesics. With the use of this algorithm, pain relief has been achieved in up to 90% of patients [35].

The nonopioid analgesics fall into several categories. Acetaminophen may be a useful drug for mild pain. Although it provides analgesia through a central mechanism of action [36, 37], it does not confer anti-inflammatory properties [38]. Doses exceeding a total of 4 g a day should always be avoided in order to prevent hepatotoxicity. Use of concurrent alcohol further increases the risk of liver damage. Additionally, acetaminophen is not a good choice in patients with hepatic metastasis or existing liver abnormalities. Since acetaminophen is an agent that is frequently found in over-the-counter formulations, a careful inventory of the patient's entire medication list is necessary to prevent exceeding the recommended daily dose [22]. Finally, since chemotherapy may impact liver function, appropriate lab work should be reviewed and necessary changes be made in prescribing agents in those individuals with an impaired function.

NSAIDs have analgesic, anti-inflammatory, and antipyretic properties. They inhibit the enzyme cyclooxygenase and block the synthesis of prostaglandins which act as mediators of inflammation that activate peripheral nociceptors [39]. Endoscopic evidence of gastrointestinal bleeding can be found in as little as

1 week of nonspecific NSAID therapy [40]. Additional toxicities include, but are not limited to, impairment of renal function, worsening of hypertension, and an increased risk of cardiovascular events. There are many NSAIDs to choose from with no appreciable differences in effectiveness at equianalgesic dosing. Ketorolac is an injectable NSAID that has important opioid-sparing effects; however, administration should be limited to several days to prevent renal and other side effects. Celecoxib is an available COX-2-specific inhibitor that exhibits less gastrointestinal distress and bleeding, especially if not taken for prolonged periods of time.

As a nonopioid, aspirin is one of the oldest analgesics. Its use is limited in the oncology patient population because of its high incidence of gastrointestinal side effects and inhibition of platelet aggregation [41]. Nonacetylated salicylates such as choline magnesium trisalicylate have less effect on platelet aggregation and no effect on bleeding times and may serve as an alternative when an anti-inflammatory agent is desirable [23].

Tramadol is a unique analgesic that is generally used for mild to moderate pain. Tramadol is a centrally acting analgesic with a dual mechanism of action. It weakly binds to the mu opioid receptor and inhibits the reuptake of norepinephrine and serotonin [42, 43]. Although its release into the pharmaceutical market was after the WHO guidelines were established, tramadol has been considered a Step 2 agent. An immediate and a long-acting preparation are available [44]. Fifty milligrams of tramadol is equivalent to 60 mg of codeine [42, 43]. A typical starting dose is 50 mg given orally every 6 h. This can be titrated up to 100 mg every 6 h; however, the dose should not exceed 300 mg daily for those over 75 years of age or more than 50 mg twice a day for patients with significant liver disease. One study examined a group of oncology patients with neuropathic pain randomized to receive either placebo or tramadol. The tramadol was titrated as needed to control pain. A statistically significant decrease in pain was found in the tramadol group compared to the placebo group. This was independent of changes in anxiety and depression [45]. For patients with moderate to severe pain, a timed-release version of tramadol is available for once-a-day dosing. Doses are limited to a maximum of 300 mg per day. Since tramadol lowers the threshold for seizures, its use is not recommended in those with a history of seizures. Side effects include nausea, dizziness, sedation, constipation, and headache [45].

Despite mostly unsubstantiated concerns of addiction, opioids remain the gold standard of analgesia therapy for patients with moderate to severe pain. When a patient is first prescribed opioids, they, too, may raise concerns regarding addiction. At this time, it is imperative for the clinician to educate the patient on their concerns, emphasizing that opioids have resulted in addiction in some patients; this is not common. In addition, as health-care providers, assessments need to be made routinely regarding misuse of opioids. Care must be given when prescribing opioids to patients with a prior history of substance abuse or a family history of substance abuse. These patients may benefit from ongoing participation with behavioral therapists, 12-step treatment meetings where appropriate, pill counts from their opioid bottles, and urine toxicology screening.

Opioids are effective for many pain conditions and are relatively easy to titrate. Any patient who did not respond with adequate relief of their cancer pain with Step 1 drugs is a candidate for opioid therapy. Analgesia is achieved by binding to the mu, delta, and kappa receptors in the central and peripheral nervous system. Opioids used for cancer pain are typically full agonists as opposed to partial agonists or mixed agonists-antagonists, since there are no ceiling doses of these agents. It is critical to understand the individual attributes of each opioid in order to make the best selection for the individual patient. Treatment is contingent upon appropriate titration and management of side effects.

Short-acting opioids are recommended when the patient has intermittent pain, acute pain, or breakthrough pain. They have a relatively fast onset of action compared to timed-release opioids. One example of a Step 2 opioid is codeine. Codeine acts as an analgesic by its metabolism to morphine in the liver. The enzyme responsible for this conversion is absent in 10% of the Caucasian population in which case there is no analgesic effect [46].

Codeine is usually formulated with acetaminophen. A typical starting dose is 30 mg codeine given every 4 h. If a total dose of acetaminophen exceeds three grams per day, then a stronger opioid should be initiated and the codeine discontinued. Hydrocodone is also a Step 2 opioid. Hydrocodone is a semisynthetic opioid derived from codeine and thebaine. Hydrocodone is metabolized by the liver into several metabolites and has a serum half-life of 4 h [47]. The hepatic cytochrome P450 enzyme, CYP2D6, converts the hydrocodone into hydromorphone. CYP2D6 poor metabolizers (about 10% of the Caucasian population) lack this metabolic pathway, thus limiting its effectiveness. Hydrocodone is typically formulated with either acetaminophen or ibuprofen, and a usual starting dose is 5 mg of hydrocodone every 4 h. This can be increased, as needed, until the ceiling dose of the nonopioid is reached (3 g of acetaminophen or 2400 mg of ibuprofen). Oxycodone is a popular Step 2 agent. It is available in both a short-acting and long-acting formulation. In its short-acting form, it may or may not be combined with a nonopioid. The usual starting dose is 5 mg every 4 h and its half-life is 2–3 h [23].

For patients with severe pain or patients with pain uncontrolled with Step 2 drugs, Step 3 opioids are available. These include morphine, oxycodone, hydromorphone, oxymorphone, fentanyl, and methadone. Morphine is the most widely available opioid worldwide. It is available in both short-acting and long-acting preparations. It may be administered orally, rectally, subcutaneously, parentally, epidurally, or intrathecally. It is the opioid in which all other opioids are compared to in the determination of equianalgesic dosing. Morphine is subject to the first pass phenomena with a large percent metabolized by the liver. It is converted to morphine-3-glucuronide and morphine-6-glucuronide. Morphine-6-glucuronide can accumulate in the presence of renal insufficiency, making it a poor choice in those with renal disease. The half-life of morphine is 2–3 h. A typical starting dose for immediate-release morphine is 10 mg orally every 4 h in opioid-naïve patients. However, if the patient is suffering from chronic constant pain, then a timed-release formulation should be used. It is often recommended to establish analgesia with short-acting morphine and then convert the total daily dose to the long-acting formulation. Depending on the manufacturer, the recommended dose of extended-release morphine may be every 8 h to every 24 h. Short-acting morphine should be available for breakthrough pain during the titration of the long-acting morphine. The long-acting morphine's dose can be increased every 2–3 days as needed. As of 2007, 54 studies examined the efficacy of morphine in the treatment of oncology patients [47]. Many studies were conducted examining the various available timed-release morphine preparations. All of the studies confirmed morphine as a good opioid analgesic for the treatment of cancer pain. Side effects more specific to morphine include asthma and pruritus due to histamine release.

Another Step 3 opioid is oxycodone which is one of the most versatile of all the opioids. It is synthesized from the opium derivative thebaine. Timed-release oxycodone is formulated to have both an immediate- and long-acting component. Thirty-eight percent of the timed-release oxycodone is released immediately with a peak serum level at 37 min for the immediate-release component. An active liver metabolite, oxymorphone, accumulates in only a small amount in those with renal impairment [48]. Dosing of the timed-release formulation is every 12 h with a typical starting dose of 10 mg in the opioid-naïve patient, as defined by patients who are on at least 60 mg of morphine a day or fentanyl patch of 25 µg per hour or 30 mg of oxycodone a day or 8 mg of hydromorphone a day or 25 mg of oxymorphone. Timed-release oxycodone can be increased every 24 h as tolerated. Demonstrated effectiveness in reducing pain in oncology patients has been published [49–51].

Hydromorphone is a semisynthetic derivative of morphine with activity at the mu receptor but with low affinity at the kappa receptor. It is available in oral, rectal, and intravenous formulations. A timed-release version is available. The half-life of immediate-release hydromorphone is 2–3 h, with starting doses of 2–4 mg every 4 h in an opioid-naïve patient.

Oxymorphone is a Step 3 opioid that is available both as a short- and a long-acting opioid. It is an active metabolite of oxycodone. Oxymorphone produces analgesia by its effects at the mu and delta opioid receptor [52]. It has been shown to provide pain relief for moderate to severe cancer pain equivalent to morphine [53] but requiring less breakthrough pain medication than that needed with timed-release morphine. The short-acting formulation's half-life is 7–9 h with a typical dosing interval of 6 h [54]. It is metabolized in the liver to oxymorphone-3-glucuronide and 6-hydroxyoxymorphine, the latter being an active metabolite [54]. It is renally excreted; thus, caution must be used in the setting of renal insufficiency.

Fentanyl is a synthetic opioid that is a selective mu receptor agonist [55]. Preparations include a short-acting oral agent or transdermal long-acting opioid and are also available for parental, epidural, and intrathecal use. Fentanyl preparations are on the third step of the WHO ladder and have been extensively studied for use in oncology patients [56–58]. The transdermal long-acting fentanyl is a good choice for patients who cannot take oral medications or when compliance with multiple daily doses of opioids is poor [10]. It is metabolized in the liver to an inactive metabolite. When administered intravenously, fentanyl provides rapid analgesia with minimal effects on the hemodynamic state of the patient [55]. Initiation of fentanyl patches in patients who have been exposed to low-dose opioids commences at 25 µg per hour patch applied every 72 h. Analgesia with the patch occurs via transfer of this lipophilic drug through the skin into the circulation. Analgesia typically starts 12–24 h after initial application. If analgesia does not occur after 72 h, the dose can be increased; however, subsequent increases in dosage should occur every 6 days due to the prolonged length of time for this drug to reach a steady-state level. Several formulations of short-acting fentanyl exist. Oral transmucosal fentanyl citrate allows for 25% of the dose to be absorbed reaching the central nervous system within 3–5 min where it binds to the mu receptor. Maximum concentration is reached within 20–30 min after which time serum levels rapidly decrease. The starting dose is 200 µg, and this dose can be increased at the next administration if analgesia does not occur. There is no correlation between the amount of transmucosal fentanyl needed to treat breakthrough pain and the long-acting opioid dose that the patient is receiving [59]. Several other formulations of short-acting fentanyl are available. One buccal effervescent preparation results in 50% of the drug being absorbed, thus allowing for a decreased dose needed than with the oral transmucosal fentanyl citrate.

Methadone is a long-acting opioid that is used in Step 3 of the ladder. It offers a unique property not seen in other opioids in its ability to inhibit the N-methyl-D-aspartate receptor [60–62]. In a study of cancer patients with either uncontrolled pain or intolerable side effects, when switched to methadone, 80% of the patients had improvements of their pain [63]. Methadone is considered a difficult drug to use since its plasma half-life averages 24 h but ranges from 15 to 190 h [62]. This is due to methadone binding to extravascular sites and then being slowly released into the bloodstream. Despite this, its analgesia half-life is 4–6 h [64]. This confers a risk of delayed toxicity including sedation and respiratory depression. Therefore, if methadone is to be given, it must be started at a low dose and titrated very slowly. It is typically dosed two to three times a day. If changing from another long-acting opioid to methadone, it should be done by slowly initiating methadone at low doses while consecutively reducing the dose of the existing opioid. This reflects the variable equianalgesic ratio of methadone to other opioids. In doses above 300 mg, there is a risk of QT prolongation and torsades de pointes. Other risks include hypokalemia, hypomagnesemia, and congestive heart failure [65, 66]. Methadone is metabolized in the liver to inactive metabolites that are excreted in the urine and bile [67].

Although mixed agonist-antagonist opioid analgesics are typically not recommended for the treatment of oncology patients, one agent has demonstrated effectiveness in this patient population. Buprenorphine is a semisynthetic opioid derived from thebaine and is available as a transdermal patch. It is a partial agonist at the mu receptor and the kappa receptor, while a weak agonist at the sigma receptor. Buprenorphine binding and dissociation from the mu receptor is delayed, giving it a slow onset and long duration of action, which explains why it takes several days to reach stable steady state. The medication is delivered via a patch taking 12 h to produce analgesia. As opposed to the pure opioid agents, buprenorphine has a ceiling dose and is not appropriate for patients who are already on an equivalent of 300 mg of oral morphine per day. Analgesia has been demonstrated in the oncology patient population with moderate to severe pain. If placed on the WHO ladder, it most likely would be a Step 3 agent.

Not included in the original WHO ladder, tapentadol is a newer centrally acting analgesic that also has a dual mode of action. It is an agonist of the mu opioid receptor and a norepinephrine reuptake inhibitor. This agent is similar to tramadol but more potent. Phase III clinical studies revealed a comparable analgesic effect to immediate-release oxycodone but with a statistically significant lower incidence of nausea, vomiting, and constipation [68, 69]. A typical starting dose of tapentadol is 50 mg given every 4–6 h as needed. Dosing above 700 mg total for the first day and 600 mg afterwards is not recommended. Based on the attributes of this drug, it most likely would be a Step 3 agent.

Despite having multiple opioid analgesics available, comparative clinical trials have not demonstrated differences in efficacy and side effects among timed-release morphine, timed-release oxycodone, and transdermal fentanyl [70]. In order to achieve analgesia, familiarity must be gained with a broad group of analgesics so appropriate selection and titration is accomplished. Most oncology patients prefer oral analgesic therapy [30–34, 71]. If oral medication cannot be used, transdermal fentanyl is an option [72]. Intramuscular injections are not recommended due to pain inflicted from the injection [30, 33]. When changing from one opioid to another, equianalgesic conversion tables should serve as guidelines. The calculated dose should be reduced by 25–50% due to incomplete cross-tolerance between opioids [31, 32]. As discussed above, conversion to methadone requires a reduction up to 90% due to its ultra-long half-life and potential for side effects [73]. Although meperidine is a Step 3 opioid, its use in oncology is extremely limited due to its short duration of action and toxicity. It is rarely given, except in cases of postoperative shivering. If used, it is not recommended for more than 48 h not to exceed 600 mg per day [74]. Its active metabolite, normeperidine, may produce seizures, myoclonus, and twitches [75]. If renal insufficiency is present, this risk is further heightened.

If the patient has severe, uncontrolled pain, intravenous patient-controlled analgesia should be started. Once analgesia is achieved, an attempt can be made at converting to an opioid in a non-parental formulation. If parental opioids are not available, titration of the opioid, based on its individual properties, is necessary to achieve analgesia. Since breakthrough pain is present in up to two-thirds of oncology patients [76], breakthrough opioids are often needed. The dose typically given is one-sixth the dose of the total daily opioid.

Tolerance may develop to opioids, which require an increasing dose of opioid to achieve the same analgesic effect. Tolerance to long-acting opioids is most likely lower than for short-acting opioids. If a patient that had been stable on a constant dose of opioids develops worsening pain, it is necessary to evaluate for progression of the disease [77].

Initial administration of opioids, especially in the opioid-naïve patient, may result in side effects. Most side effects are manageable and diminish with time; however, it is necessary that clinicians are able to anticipate and treat these conditions. Nausea is a common side effect due to stimulation of opioid receptors in the medulla [9]. Nausea may occur with initiation of an opioid or with an increase in the opioid dose. The incidence is reported to be 40% when morphine is given [78]. If this occurs, treatment with an antiemetic is indicated until symptoms resolve. If nausea and/or vomiting persists despite treatment for several days, another opioid should be considered [30–32, 34]. If the nausea is not treated and a conversion to another opioid is made, there is a good chance that the nausea will persist. If nausea is the result of intestinal obstruction, then subcutaneous octreotide may be given [78].

Constipation is a side effect that persists for patients receiving daily opioids. It is the result of opioid receptor binding both centrally and peripherally. Forty percent of patients on oral morphine were constipated in one study [79]. No firm evidence exists that one opioid is less constipating than another in equianalgesic dosing. Once opioid treatment is started, the patient should receive a daily stool softener plus propellant, such as senna, and continued as long as loose stool or diarrhea is not present. Enemas should be avoided since there is a higher risk of neutropenia in the oncology patient population.

The majority of patients that experience sedation with opioids do so only for a brief period of time following the initiation or dose escalation of opioids. If sedation persists, then another opioid may be considered. If, despite changing the opioid, sedation is still bothersome, the addition of methylphenidate in the morning at 5–10 mg with a second dose in the afternoon is a reasonable treatment [80].

Although opioids can depress the rate and depth of respiration, this is more common in the opioid-naïve patient [81]. If standard guidelines are followed, this effect is extremely rare. This risk is also minimized by paying close attention to other drugs that the patient may be taking, such as benzodiazepines, barbiturates, alcohol, and other sedatives that may accentuate the respiratory depression [4]. In the event that it occurs, opioid-induced respiratory depression can be reversed with naloxone in 0.4–2 mg every 2–3 min until complete reversal of the opioid is made or to a maximum dose of 10 mg. During this time, the patient's airway should be assessed and protected if compromised.

Unsubstantiated concerns regarding psychological addiction have been a cause that has prevented many clinicians from either prescribing or appropriately titrating opioids [82]. Psychological addition is a primary, chronic neurobiological disease with genetic, psychosocial, and environmental factors. Warning signs of addiction include the inability to control how much opioid is consumed, preoccupation with opioids, and negative consequences from using opioids such as loss of relationships and employment [83, 84]. For example, behavioral changes, motor vehicle accidents, or personal injuries may result from obtaining opioids from multiple sources. The incidence of psychological addiction among the cancer patient population is 7.7% [85–88]. Confusion exists for many between the terms of physical addiction and physical dependence. Physical dependence occurs with multiple classes of drugs. It simply means that if a patient is maintained on drugs and the drug is abruptly discontinued, then signs of withdrawal would occur. In the case of opioids, this may be manifested with shakiness, lacrimation, goose skin flesh, abdominal cramping, tachycardia, hypertension, yawning, dilated pupils, and severe pain. Exhibiting signs of withdrawal does not confer an association to psychological addiction.

14.5   Neuropathic Pain

It is estimated that 40–50% oncology patients suffer with neuropathic pain. Although some patients with neuropathic pain respond to opioids, there are some that either do not respond or only respond to large doses of opioids [89]. It is quite common for a sarcoma patient to suffer from both neuropathic and nociceptive pain. Oftentimes they are discharged postoperatively with an opioid analgesic. However, in some cases, it becomes a challenge to wean off the opioids. In these cases, a thorough assessment is needed for the presence of neuropathic pain. The addition of a neuro-modulating agent and evaluation for nerve blocks will often lead to a significant reduction in pain. When neuropathic pain is present, mu opioid receptors are down-regulated in the dorsal spinal cord probably through activation of the NMDA receptors [90]. Much of the treatment of neuropathic pain focuses on the use of adjuvant agents, which are defined as drugs indicated for more than one condition. For example, antidepressants are frequently employed in the treatment of pain due to their mechanism of action even in the absence of depression in the patient for which it is prescribed. Much of the treatment of neuropathic pain is an extrapolation of large randomized placebo-controlled studies examining outcomes for patients with postherpetic neuralgia and diabetic peripheral neuropathy. These two neuropathic disease states are more frequently studied since they are relatively common, thus allowing for recruitment of sufficient number of patients. Although there are studies specifically focusing on oncologic neuropathic pain, many either have a small sample size or exist as case reports. Antidepressants have been used to treat a variety of neuropathic pain states [91, 92]. The type most widely studied has been the tricyclic antidepressants which produced analgesia as a result of serotonin and norepinephrine inhibition directly at the spinal cord level. The ability to decrease pain has been demonstrated even in the absence of comorbid depression [93]. Amitriptyline, nortriptyline, and desipramine are commonly used as a once-daily dose often starting as low as 10 mg to prevent side effects. They are typically titrated in 10 mg increments to doses of 75–100 mg, although there are some patients who either will require less or more. The dose needed to control pain is generally less than that to alleviate depression. Nonetheless, a period of 3 weeks is often needed before a response is observed. Anticholinergic side effects often limit the use of the tricyclic antidepressants with amitriptyline having the greatest amount of these side effects and desipramine the least. Examples of anticholinergic effects include tachycardia, constipation, orthostatic hypotension, sedation, dry mouth, and arrhythmias [94, 95]. Additionally, the tricyclic antidepressants are contraindicated in patients with glaucoma and urinary retention and with caution in those with cardiovascular disease [96].

Duloxetine is an antidepressant indicated for the treatment of painful diabetic neuropathy, fibromyalgia, chronic musculoskeletal pain, and depression, although its use has extended to neuropathic oncology pain. Initiation is with 20 mg daily increasing the dose weekly by 20 mg until a total daily dose of 60 mg is reached. There are case reports of irreversible hepatocellular necrosis and should not be prescribed to those with substantial alcohol intake or chronic liver disease.

Although antiepileptic agents have had a role in treating neuropathic pain, gabapentin and pregabalin have been the most commonly used agents. Both agents also have the added benefit of not interfering with hepatic enzymes [96]. Gabapentin has been approved for the treatment of postherpetic neuralgia. In addition to postherpetic neuralgia, pregabalin is approved for diabetic painful neuropathy and fibromyalgia [97–101]. Further support for the use of gabapentin specifically for the use in oncology neuropathic pain has been published [102, 103]. There are several formulations available, including once-a-day dosing. In addition, when opioids are combined with gabapentin, there often is a synergistic reduction of neuropathic pain [104].

Topical medications are one strategy aimed at targeting peripheral receptors. Transdermal lidocaine has been used for the treatment of postherpetic neuralgia and in patients with allodynia due to different neuropathic pain states [105]. Up to three patches may be applied to the painful area: 12 out of 24 h. Use of transdermal lidocaine has extended outside of postherpetic neuralgia, mostly for neuropathic pain but also for nociceptive musculoskeletal pain, and is generally well tolerated.

The NMDA receptor antagonist, ketamine, has been used to treat neuropathic pain. In one study, ketamine decreased pain by 20–30% in cancer neuropathic pain that was already treated with opioids. This also leads to a 25–50% reduction in opioid use [106].

In 2010, the European Federation of Neurological Societies Task Force established their guidelines for treatment of neuropathic pain. These guidelines were established using the Cochrane Database and Medicine Class I or II randomized controlled trials for treating neuropathic pain from a variety of sources. First-line treatment for neuropathic pain in the non-oncology patient was tricyclic antidepressants, gabapentin, and pregabalin, and first-line treatment for neuropathic pain in the oncology patient population was gabapentin, tricyclic antidepressants, tramadol, gabapentin combined with tricyclic antidepressant, and gabapentin combined with opioids [107].

In addition to neuropathic pain, there are several other categories of adjuvant agents that are frequently used with the oncology patient. Corticosteroids are used for a variety of conditions that may contribute to cancer pain. Examples include nerve compression, spinal cord compression, bone metastasis, distension of the liver capsule, increased intracranial pressure, lymphedema, superior vena cava syndrome, and plexopathies. This group of drugs is highly effective at inhibiting prostaglandin synthesis and reducing neural tissue edema [22, 108, 109]. Dosing may be 1–2 mg twice daily all the way up to 100 mg oral or intravenous dosing for true neurosurgical emergencies. Once the underlying situation has been stabilized, doses of 4–6 mg orally given every 6 h are typical [110]. The duration of steroid therapy is generally short to reduce the incidence of steroid-induced osteoporosis or proximal myopathy [34]. The bisphosphonate drugs ameliorate the pain from bone metastasis as well. Drugs such as pamidronate, zoledronic acid, and clodronate act by inhibiting osteoclast activity [111–113]. Opioid consumption has been reduced by 20–50% in patients with bone metastasis who received pamidronate [114, 115].

14.6 Phantom Limb Pain

One type of neuropathic pain syndrome that may be seen in the sarcoma patient population is phantom limb pain following major amputation or resection of peripheral nerves. Phantom limb pain is defined as a noxious sensation where the limb existed [116–119]. Descriptions of the pain vary widely: from lancinating, cramping, and burning to sharp, pins and needles, itching, aching, crushing, and grinding [117, 120, 121]. The pain typically occurs in the distal region of the phantom limb [121] and rarely follows the distribution of the severed nerve [116].

Many reports have been published regarding the incidence of phantom pain. In a survey of 590 veteran amputees, 55% reported phantom pain, and 56% reported pain in their stump [122]. Up to 88% of patients undergoing hip disarticulation or hemipelvectomy suffer from phantom limb pain, supporting Roth and Sugarbaker's finding that the higher the level of lower extremity amputation, the greater the incidence of moderate to severe pain [123, 124].

Phantom limb pain occurs soon after amputation and can last indefinitely [125]. One study found that phantom limb pain occurred within 8 days after amputation in 72% of adult patients [126]. It has been observed that the incidence of phantom pain did not decrease 6 months following amputation, although there was a decrease in the duration of their intermittent pain exacerbations [127]. In 3–10% of amputees, the pain is chronic and severe [122]. There are several factors that influence the development and severity of the pain. Preamputation pain is a risk factor, with pain experienced months or years before, now re-experienced as phantom pain [126]. Another factor that may be associated with phantom pain is chemotherapy, especially those agents known to cause peripheral neurotoxicity [128, 129]. In a study of pediatric amputees, the incidence of phantom pain was 74% in patients who received either vincristine or cis-platinum prior to amputation, compared to 44% in patients who began their chemotherapy postamputation [128].

Although children can experience phantom sensation, the incidence of phantom limb pain is lower in the pediatric population compared to adults [130]. In a retrospective study of 75 pediatric patients, 48% of those with amputations necessitated by cancer and 12% of those who had traumatic amputations reported phantom limb pain [128].

The establishment of analgesia prior to surgical incision (preemptive analgesia) may help control postoperative pain by preventing the transmission of noxious afferent input from the periphery to the spinal cord [131, 132]. Otherwise, a prolonged state of central neural sensitization and hyperexcitability could occur that would amplify future input from the amputated site [133]. Epidural and epineural analgesia, given perioperatively and postoperatively, have revolutionized the ability to manage the pain. With these techniques, the need for postoperative opioids, as well as their associated side effects, has decreased.

Epidural infusions of morphine, bupivacaine, and clonidine initiated preoperatively for 24–48 h and continued for at least 3 days postoperatively have decreased the incidence of phantom limb pain to 8%, compared to the 73% incidence in the control group [134]. Postamputation analgesia and prevention of lower extremity phantom limb pain have been investigated using infusions of local anesthetics placed into a nerve sheath via a catheter at the time of amputation [135, 136]. Regional anesthetic techniques offer many advantages of pain control during the perioperative and postoperative periods. A study by Malawer et al. demonstrated when local anesthetic is directly administered into the peripheral nerve sheath following an amputation, an 80% reduction in narcotic requirement ensued [136].

As with other causes of neuropathic pain, pharmacotherapy with anticonvulsants and antidepressants is frequently used to treat phantom limb pain. In addition, several infusion therapies have been reported. MacFarlane et al. found that five daily doses of intravenous lidocaine (3 mg/kg) given over 30 min may produce prolonged relief [121]. Jaeger and Maier found that 200 IU of salmon calcitonin given via an intravenous infusion decreased phantom pain, with some patients requiring a second infusion. At 1-year follow-up, 62% of amputees that received the calcitonin reported greater than a 75% reduction in pain. Pain relief extended to 2 years in 58% of patients [137].

A great deal of excitement has been generated regarding the use of NMDA antagonists in the treatment of neuropathic pain. The blockade of the NMDA receptor may reduce central hyperexcitability. In a randomized, double-blind study of patients with persistent phantom limb pain, the NMDA receptor antagonist, ketamine, was given intravenously as a 0.1 mg/kg bolus over 5 min followed by an infusion of 7 µg/kg/min for up to 45 min. During the infusion and in some cases up to three later, ketamine relieved the pain in the phantom limb [138].

Although the above treatments appear promising for the treatment of phantom limb pain, some of the studies lacked sufficient power to conclude definitive treatments for phantom limb pain. It was for this reason a systematic review of pharmacological treatment was published. Level 2 evidence is defined as conclusions based on one or more well-powered randomized controlled trials, whereas level 3 evidence is defined as retrospective studies, open-label trials, or pilot studies. In this systematic review, level 2 evidence exists for the use of gabapentin, morphine, tramadol, and intravenous and epidural ketamine. Level 3 evidence exists for dextromethorphan, topiramate, intravenous calcitonin, memantine, and continuous perineural catheter analgesia with ropivacaine [139].

14.7 Role of a Multidisciplinary Team

In order to successfully treat the sarcoma patient, improvements need to be made on the available treatments. Pain assessments and aggressive interventions can be instituted to enable improved compliance and quality of life. This needs to be considered throughout the entire process, whether it be at diagnosis or during the peri- and postoperative period. Neuropathic pain remains a challenge due to its difficulty to treat. With new drug development, this hurdle will likely be less of an obstacle.

For those sarcoma patients who require surgery, certain aspects of the enhanced recovery after surgery program can be considered. This program examines and individualizes pre-, intra-, and postoperative care in regard to nutrition, thromboprophylaxis, stimulation of gut motility, avoidance of salt, and water overload and maintenance of normothermia to reduce overall complications [140].

There are patients who either have pain despite pharmacotherapy or who exhibit side effects from their therapy where a lower dose would serve as an advantage. For this reason, interdisciplinary and comprehensive pain management has become an important aspect in the treatment of cancer pain. This serves as an addition to traditional treatment, not as an alternative. Rehabilitation programs enable the patient to gain strength and balance to preserve as much autonomy as possible. Psychologists and other behavioral medicine therapists not only assist with the psychological distress associated with cancer and pain but teach patients strategies to reduce pain such as biofeedback, hypnosis, and guided imagery. Finally, a referral to a radiation oncologist may be beneficial if the tumor is sensitive to radiation.

With so many specialties involved, it is imperative to have appropriate team communication. Without this, patients and their families can be overwhelmed with the number of health-care providers involved and may lack clarity regarding the roles individual providers provide. By instituting multidisciplinary conferences, appropriate treatment plans can be formulated and conveyed to the patient to facilitate the best chance of a pain-free outcome.

References

1. Cancer facts and figures. American Cancer Society; 1995.
2. Cleeland CS, Gonin R, Hatfield AK. Pain and its treatment in outpatients with metastatic cancer. N Engl J Med. 1994;330:592–6.
3. Zhukovsky DS, Gorowski E, Hausdorff J, Napolitano B, Lesser M. Unmet analgesic needs in cancer patients. J Pain Symptom Manage. 1995;10:113–9.
4. Christo PJ, Mazloomdoost D. Cancer pain and analgesia. Ann N Y Acad Sci. 2008;1138:278–98.
5. Coyle N, Adelhardt J, Foley KM, Portenoy RK. Character of terminal illness in the advanced cancer patient: pain and other symptoms during the last four weeks of life. J Pain Symptom Manage. 1990;5:83–93.
6. Portenoy RK, Miransky J, Thaler HT. Pain in ambulatory patients with lung or colon cancer: prevalence, characteristics, and effect. Cancer. 1992;70:1616–24.
7. Grond S, Zech D, Diefenbach C, Bischoff A. Prevalence and pattern of symptoms in patients with cancer pain: a prospective evaluation of 1635 cancer patients referred to a pain clinic. J Pain Symptom Manage. 1994;9:372–82.
8. Bonica J. The management of pain. 2nd ed. Philadelphia: Lea &Febiger; 1990. p. 1484–514.
9. McQuay H. Opioids in pain management. Lancet. 1999;353:2229–32.
10. Portenoy RK, Lesage P. Management of cancer pain. Lancet. 1999;353:1695–700.
11. Baltic TE, Whedon MB, Ahles TA, Fanciullo G. Improving pain relief in a rural cancer center. Cancer Pract. 2002;10:S39–44.

12. Lasch K. Why study pain? A qualitative analysis of medical and nursing faculty and students' knowledge of and attitudes to cancer pain management. J Palliat Med. 2002;5: 57–71.
13. Payne R. Chronic pain: challenges in the assessment and management of cancer pain. J Pain Symptom Manage. 2000;19:S12–5.
14. Ward S. Patient education in pain control. Support Care Cancer. 2001;9:148–55.
15. Gunnarsdottir S. Patient-related barriers to pain management: the Barriers Questionnaire II. Pain. 2002;99:385–96.
16. Ward S, Gatwood J. Concerns about reporting pain and using analgesics. A comparison of persons with and without cancer. Pain. 1993;52:319–24.
17. Ward SE, Goldberg V, Miller-McCauley V. Patient-related barriers to management of persons with and without cancer. Pain. 1993;52:319–24.
18. Cherny NI, Portenoy RK. Cancer pain: principles of assessment and syndromes. In: Wall PD, Melzck R, editors. Textbook of pain. 4th ed. Edinburg: Churchill Livingstone; 1999.
19. Dy SM. Evidence-based approaches to pain in advanced cancer. Cancer J. 2010;16:500–6.
20. Vorobeychik Y, Gordin V, Mao J, Chen L. Combination therapy for neuropathic pain: a review of current evidence. CNS Drugs. 2011;25:1023–34.
21. Vadalouca A, Raptis E, Moka E, Zis P, Sykioti P, Siafaka I. Pharmacological treatment of neuropathic cancer pain: a comprehensive review of the current literature. Pain Pract. 2012;12:219–51.
22. Shaiova L. Difficult pain syndrome: bone pain, visceral pain, and neuropathic pain. Cancer J. 2006;12:330–40.
23. Cherny NI, Portenoy RK. The management of cancer pain. CA Cancer J Clin. 1994;44:262–303.
24. Cleeland CS. The impact of pain on the patient with cancer. Cancer. 1984;54:2635–41.
25. Fishman B, Pasternak S, Wallenstein SL, House RW, Holland JC, Foley KM. The Memorial Pain Assessment Card: a valid instrument for the evaluation of cancer pain. Cancer. 1987;60:1151–8.
26. Au E, Loprinzi CL, Dhodapkar M. Regular use of a verbal pain scale improves the understanding of oncology inpatient pain intensity. J Clin Oncol. 1994;12:2751–5.
27. Ferrer-Brechner T. The management of pain associated with malignancy. Semin Anesth. 1985;4:313–22.
28. Schug SA, Zech D, Dorr U. Cancer pain management according to WHO analgesic guidelines. J Symptom Manage. 1994;9:372–82.
29. Ventafridda V, Caraceni A, Gamba A. Field-testing of the WHO guidelines for cancer pain relief: summary report of demonstration projects. In: Proceedings of the second international congress of cancer pain, vol. 16. 1990. p. 451–64.
30. Jacox A, Carr DB, Payne R, Management of cancer pain: clinical practice guideline. No. 9. Rockville: Agency for Health Care Policy and Research 1994 (AHCPR publication no 94–0592).
31. Cherny NI, Portenoy RK. The management of cancer pain. Cancer J Clin. 1994;44: 263–303.
32. Levy MH. Pharmacologic management of cancer pain. Semin Oncol. 1994;21:718–39.
33. Principles of analgesic use in the treatment of acute and cancer pain. American Pain Society; 1992.
34. Twycross R. Pain relief in advanced cancer. London: Churchill Livingstone; 1994.
35. Bonica JJ. History of pain concepts and pain therapy. Mt Sinai J Med. 1991;58(3):191–202.
36. Malmberg AB, Yaksh TL. Hyperalgesia medicated by spinal glutamate and substance P receptor blocked by spinal cyclooxygenase inhibition. Science. 1992;257:1276–9.
37. Willer JC, De Broucker T, Bussel B. Central analgesic effect of ketoprofen in humans: electrophysiological evidence for a supraspinal mechanism in a double-blind and cross-over study. Pain. 1989;38:1–7.
38. Watson AC, Brookes ST, Kirwan JR, Faulkner A. Non-aspirin, non-steroidal anti-inflammatory drugs for osteoarthritis of the knee. Cochrane Database Syst Rev. 2000;(2).

39. Vane JR. Inhibition of prostaglandin synthesis as a mechanism of action for aspirin-like drugs. Nat New Biol. 1971;231:232–5.
40. Simon LS, Lanza FL, Lipsky PT, et al. Efficacy and safety in two placebo-controlled trials in osteoarthritis and rheumatoid arthritis, and studies of gastrointestinal and platelet effects. Arthritis Rheum. 1998;9:1591–602.
41. Stuart MJ, Murphy S, Oski FA, Evans AE, Donaldson MH, Gardner FH. Platelet function in recipients of platelets from donors ingesting aspirin. N Engl J Med. 1972;287:1105–9.
42. Sunshine A. New clinical experience with tramadol. Drugs. 1994;47(Suppl 1):8–18.
43. Wilder-Smith CH, Schmike J, Osterwakder B, Senn HJ. Oral tramadol, a mu-opioid agonist and monoamine reuptake-blocker, and morphine for strong cancer-related pain. Ann Oncol. 1994;5:141–6.
44. Babul N. Efficacy and safety of extended-release, once-daily tramadol in chronic pain: a randomized 12-week clinical trial in osteoarthritis of the knee. J Pain Symptom Manage. 2004;28:497–504.
45. Arbaiza D, Vidal O. Tramadol in the treatment of neuropathic cancer pain. Clin Drug Investig. 2007;27(1):75–83.
46. Eichelbaum M, Evert B. Influence of pharmacogenetics on drug disposition and response. Clin Exp Pharmacol Physiol. 1996;23:983–5.
47. Davis T, Mellar P. Hydrocodone. Opioids for cancer pain. Oxford: Oxford University Press; 2007. p. 59–68.
48. Kirvela M. The pharmacokinetics of oxycodone in uremic patients undergoing renal transplantation. J Clin Anesth. 1996;8:13–8.
49. Bruera E. Randomized, double-blind, cross-over trial comparing safety and efficacy of oral controlled-release oxycodone with controlled-release morphine in patients with cancer pain. J Clin Oncol. 1998;16:3222–9.
50. Heisknen T, Kalso E. Controlled-release oxycodone and morphine in cancer related pain. Pain. 1997;73:37–45.
51. Mucci-LoRosso P. Controlled-release oxycodone compared with controlled-release morphine in the treatment of cancer pain: a randomized, double-blind, parallel-group study. Eur J Pain. 1998;2:239–349.
52. Ananthan S. Identification of opioid ligands possessing mixed micro agonist/delta antagonist activity among pyridomorphinans derived from naloxone, oxymorphone, and hydromorphone. J Med Chem. 2004;47:1400–12.
53. Sloan P, Slatkin N, Ahdieh H. Effectiveness and safety of oral extended-release oxymorphone for the treatment of cancer pain: a pilot study. Support Care Cancer. 2005;13:57–65.
54. Adams MA, Ahdieh H. Single and multiple dose pharmacokinetic and dose proportionality study of oxymorphone immediate release tablets. Drugs R D. 2005;6:91–9.
55. Gutstein HB, Huda A. Goodman and Gilman's the pharmacological basis of therapeutics. 11th ed. McGraw Hill, New York 2006. p. 571.
56. Ahmedzai S, Brooks D. Transdermal fentanyl versus sustained-release oral morphine in cancer pain: preference, efficacy, and quality of life. The TTS-Fentanyl Comparative Trial Group. J Pain Symptom Manage. 1997;13:254–61.
57. Donner B. Long-term treatment of cancer pain with transdermal fentanyl. J Pain Symptom Manage. 1998;15:168–75.
58. Radbruch L. Transdermal fentanyl for the management of cancer pain: a survey of 1005 patients. Palliat Med. 2001;15:309–21.
59. Camps C, Cassinello J, Jara C, et al. Tolerability and effectivity of oral transmucosal fentanyl citrate in the long-term treatment of irruptive pain in oncology patients: ECODIR study. Clin Transl Oncol. 2005;7:205–12.
60. Bulka A. Reduced tolerance to the anti-hyperalgesic effect of methadone in comparison to morphine in a rat model of mononeuropathy. Pain. 2002;95:103–9.
61. Bulka A, Weisenfield-Hallin Z, Xu XJ. Differential antinociception by morphine and methadone in two sub-strains of Sprague-Dawley rats and its potentiation by dextromethorphan. Brain Res. 2002;942:95–100.

62. Davis M, Walsh D. Methadone for relief of cancer pain: a review of pharmacokinetics pharmacodynamics, drug interactions and protocols of administration. Support Care Cancer. 2001;9:73–83.
63. Mercadante S, Casuccio A, Fulfaro F, et al. Switching from morphine to methadone to improve analgesia and tolerability in cancer patients: a prospective study. J Clin Oncol. 2001;19:2898–904.
64. Grochow L. Does intravenous methadone provide longer lasting analgesia than intravenous morphine? A randomized, double-blind study. Pain. 1989;38:151–7.
65. Reddy SF, Fisch M, Bruera E. Oral methadone for cancer pain: no indication of Q-T interval prolongation or torsades de pointes. J Pain Symptom Manage. 2004;28:301–3.
66. Roden M. Drug-induced prolongation of the QT interval. N Engl J Med. 2004; 350:1015–22.
67. Kreek MJ, Gutjahr CL. Drug interactions with methadone. Ann N Y Acad Sci. 1976;281:350–70.
68. Terlinden R, Ossig J, Fliegert F, Lange C, Gohler K. Absorption, metabolism, and excretion of 14C-labeled tapentadol HCl in healthy male subjects. Eur J Drug Metab Pharacokinet. 2007;32:163–9.
69. Hartrick C, Van Hove I, Stegmann JU, Oh C, Upmalis D. Efficacy and tolerability of tapentadol immediate release and oxycodone HCl immediate release in patients awaiting primary joint replacement surgery for end-stage joint disease: a 10-day, phase III, randomized, double-blind, active- and placebo-controlled study. Clin Ther. 2009;31:260–71.
70. Weschules DJ, Bain KT, Reifsnyder J, et al. Toward evidence-based prescribing at end of life: a comparative analysis of sustained-release morphine, oxycodone, and transdermal fentanyl, with pain, constipation, and caregiver interaction outcomes in hospice patients. Pain Med. 2006;7:320–9.
71. Ferrell BR, Griffith H. Cost issues related to pain management: report from the Cancer Pain Panel of the Agency for Health Care Policy and Research. J Pain Symptom Manage. 1994;9:221–34.
72. Kalso E, Vainio A. Morphine and oxycodone hydrochloride in the management of cancer pain. Clin Pharmacol Ther. 1990;47:639–46.
73. Bruera EB, Pereira J, Watanabe S. Systematic opioid therapy for chronic cancer pain: practical guidelines for converting drugs and routes. Cancer. 1996;78:852–7.
74. Acute pain managements in infants, children, and adolescents: operative and medical procedures. In: US Dept of Health and Human Services. Rockville: Agency for Health Care Policy and Research; 1992.
75. Hershey L. Meperidine and central neurotoxicity. Ann Intern Med. 1983;55:425–9.
76. WHO. Cancer pain relief and palliative care. Geneva: WHO; 1996.
77. DuPen A, Shen D, Ersek M. Mechanisms of opioid induced tolerance and hyperesthesia. Pain Manag Nurs. 2007;8(3):113–21.
78. Mercadante S. The role of octreotide in palliative care. J Pain Symptom Manage. 1994;9:406–11.
79. Moulin DE, Iezzi A, Amireh R, Sharpe WK, Boyd D, Merksey H. Randomized trial of oral morphine for chronic non-cancer pain. Lancet. 1996;347:143–7.
80. Bruera E, Brenneis C, Paterson AH, MacDonald RN. Use of methylphenidate as an adjuvant to narcotic analgesics in patients with advanced cancer. J Pain Symptom Manage. 1994;9:3–6.
81. Dahan A. Simultaneous measurement and integrated analysis of analgesia and respiration after an intravenous morphine infusion. Anesthesiology. 2004;101:1201–9.
82. McQuay H. Opioids in pain management. Lancet. 1999;353:2229–32.
83. Portenoy R. Chronic opioid therapy in nonmalignant pain. J Pain Symptom Manage. 1990;5(1 Suppl):S46–62.
84. Sees KL, Clark HW. Opioid use in the treatment of chronic pain: assessment of addiction. J Pain Symptom Manage. 1993;8:257–64.

85. Macaluso C, Weinberg D, Foley K. Opioid abuse and misuse in a cancer pain population. J Pain Symptom Manage. 1998;3:S24.
86. Passik SD, Kirsh KL, McDonald MV, Ahn S, et al. A pilot survey of aberrant drug-taking attitudes and behaviors in samples of cancer and AIDS patients. J Pain Symptom Manage. 2000;19:274–86.
87. Passik SD, Schreiber J, Kirsh KL. A chart review of the ordering of urine toxicology screen in a cancer center: do they influence pain management. J Pain Symptom Manage. 2000;19:44.
88. Schug SA, Zech D, Grond S, et al. A long term survey of morphine in cancer pain patients. J Pain Symptom Manage. 1992;7:259–66.
89. Portenoy RK, Foley KM, Inturrisi CE. The nature of opioid responsiveness and its implications for neuropathic pain: new hypothesis derived from studies of opioid infusions. Pain. 1990;43:273–86.
90. Mizoguchi H, Watanabe C, Yonezawa A, Sakkkurada S. New therapy for neuropathic pain. Int Rev Neurobiol. 2009;85:249–63.
91. McQuay HJ. A systematic review of antidepressants in neuropathic pain. Pain. 1996;68:217–27.
92. Sindrup SH, Jensen TS. Efficacy of pharmacological treatments of neuropathic pain: an update and effect related to mechanism of drug action. Pain. 1999;83:389–400.
93. Jefferies K. Treatment of neuropathic pain. Semin Neurol. 2010;30:425–32.
94. Watson CPN. Antidepressant drugs as adjuvant analgesics. J Pain Symptom Manage. 1994;9:392–405.
95. Potter WZ, Rudorfer MV, Manji H. The pharmacologic treatment of depression. N Engl J Med. 1991;325:633–42.
96. Vanken JH. Elucidation of pathophysiology and treatment of neuropathic pain. Cent Nerv Syst Agents Med Chem. 2012;12:304–14.
97. Backonja M. Gabapentin for the symptomatic treatment of painful neuropathy in patients with diabetes mellitus: a randomized controlled trial. JAMA. 1998;280:1831–6.
98. Bennett MI, Simpson KH. Gabapentin in the treatment of neuropathic pain: a review. Palliat Med. 2004;18:5–11.
99. Rice AS, Maton S. Gabapentin in postherpetic neuralgia: a randomized, double-blind, placebo-controlled study. Pain. 2001;94:215–24.
100. Dworkin RH. Advances in neuropathic pain: diagnosis, mechanisms, and treatment recommendations. Arch Neurol. 2003;60:1523–34.
101. Freynhagen R. Efficacy of pregabalin in neuropathic pain evaluated in a 12-week, randomized, double-blind, multicenter, placebo-controlled trial of flexible- and fixed-dose regimens. Pain. 2005;115:254–63.
102. Ross JR, Goller K, Hardy J, Riley M, Broadley K. Gabapentin is effective in the treatment of cancer-related neuropathic pain: a prospective, open-label study. J Palliat Med. 2005;8(6):1118–26.
103. Caraceni A, Zecca E, Bonezzi C, Arcuri E, YayaTur R, Maltoni M, Visentin M, Gorni G, Martini C, Tirelli W, Barbieri M, De Conno F. Gabapentin for neuropathic cancer pain: a randomized, controlled trial from the Gabapentin Cancer Pain Study Group. J Clin Oncol. 2004;22:2909–17.
104. Gilron I, Bailey JM, Tu D, Holden RR, Weaver DF, Houlden RL. Morphine, gabapentin, or their combination for neuropathic pain. N Engl J Med. 2005;352:1324–34.
105. Dworkin RH, O'Connor AB, Audette J, Baron R, Gourlay GK, Haanpaa ML, Kent JL, Krane EJ, Lebel A, Levy RM, Mackey SC, Mayer J, Miaskowski C, Raja SN, Rice AS, Schmader KE, Stacey B, Stanos S, Treede RD, Turk DC, Walco GA, Wells CD. Recommendations for the pharmacological management of neuropathic pain, an overview and literature update. Mayo Clin Proc. 2010;85(Suppl 3):S3–S14.
106. Lossignol DA, Obiols-Portis M, Body J. Successful use of ketamine for intractable cancer pain. Support Care Cancer. 2005;13:188–93.

107. Attal N, Cruccu G, Bacon R. EFNS Guidelines on the pharmacological treatment of neuro-pathic pain: 2010 revision. Eur J Neurol. 2011;17:1113–23.
108. Ettinger AB, Portenoy RK. The use of corticosteroids in the treatment of symptoms associated with cancer. J Pain Symptom Manage. 1994;3:99–103.
109. Watanabe S, Bruera E. Corticosteroids as adjuvant analgesics. J Pain Symptom Manage. 1994;9:442–5.
110. Jacox A, Carr DB, Payne R. New clinical practice guidelines for the management of pain in patients with cancer. N Engl J Med. 1994;330:651–5.
111. Kerr IG, Sone M, Deangelis C, Iscoe N, MacKenzie R, Schueller T. Continuous narcotic infusion with patient-controlled analgesia for chronic cancer pain in outpatients. Ann Intern Med. 1988;108(4):554–7.
112. Payne R. Role of epidural and intrathecal narcotics and peptides in the management of cancer pain. Med Clin North Am. 1987;71:313–27.
113. Du Pen SL, Williams AR. Management of patients receiving combined epidural morphine and bupivacaine for the treatment of cancer pain. J Pain Symptom Manage. 1992;7:125–7.
114. Glover D, Lipton A, Keller A, et al. Intravenous pamidronate disodium treatment of bone metastases in patients with breast cancer: a dose-seeking study. Cancer. 1994;74:2949–55.
115. Purohit OP, Anthony C, Radstone CR, Owen J, Coleman RE. High-dose intravenous pamidronate for metastatic bone pain. Br J Cancer. 1994;70:554–8.
116. Carlen PL, Wall PD, Nadvorna H, Steinbach T. Phantom limbs and related phenomena in recent traumatic amputations. Neurology. 1978;28:211–7.
117. Raj PP. Practical management of pain. Mosby Year Book: St. Louis; 1992.
118. Wesolowski JA, Lema MJ. Phantom limb pain. Reg Anesth. 1993;18:121–7.
119. Katz J, Melzack R. Pain memories in phantom limbs: review and clinical observations. Pain. 1990;43:319–36.
120. Sherman RA. Stump and phantom limb pain. Neurol Clin. 1989;7:249–64.
121. MacFarlane BV, Wright A, O'Callaghan J, Bensen HA. Chronic neuropathic pain and its control by drugs. Pharmacol Ther. 1997;75:1–19.
122. Wartan SW, Hamann W, Wedley JR, McColl I. Phantom pain and sensation among British veteran amputees. Br J Anaesth. 1997;78:652–9.
123. Postone N. Phantom limb pain: a review. Int J Psychiatry Med. 1987;17:57–70.
124. Roth YF, Sugarbaker PK. Pains and sensations after amputation: character and clinical significance. Arch Phys Med Rehabil. 1980;61:490.
125. Melzack R. Phantom limb pain: Implications for treatment of pathologic pain. Anesthesiology. 1971;35:409–19.
126. Jensen TS, Krebs B, Nielsen J, Rasmussen P. Phantom limb, phantom pain and stump pain in amputees during the first six months following amputation. Pain. 1983;17:243–56.
127. Nikolajsen L, Ilkjaer S, Kroner K, Christensen JH, Jensen TS. The influence of preamputation pain on postamputation stump and phantom pain. Pain. 1997;72:393–405.
128. Smith J, Thompson JM. Phantom limb pain and chemotherapy in pediatric amputees. Mayo Clin Proc. 1995;70:357–64.
129. Knox DJ, McLeod BJ, Goucke CR. Acute phantom limb pain controlled by ketamine. Anaesth Intens Care. 1995;23:620–2.
130. Krane EJ, Heller LB. The prevalence of phantom sensation and pain in pediatric amputees. J Pain Symptom Manage. 1995;10:21–9.
131. Newman P, Fawcett W. Pre-emptive analgesia. Lancet. 1993;342:562.
132. Katz J. Prevention of phantom pain by regional anesthesia. Lancet. 1997;349:519–20.
133. Katz J. Phantom limb pain. Lancet. 1997;350:1338–9.
134. Jahangiri M, Jayatunga AP, Bradley JWP, Dark CH. Prevention of phantom pain after major lower limb amputation by epidural infusion of diamorphine, clonidine and bupivacaine. Ann R Coll Surg Engl. 1994;76:324–6.
135. Pavy TJ, Doyle DL. Prevention of phantom limb pain by infusion of local anaesthetic in the sciatic nerve. Anaesth Intens Care. 1996;24:599–600.

136. Malawer MM, Buch R, Khurana JS, Orth MS, Garvey T, Rice L. Postoperative infusional continuous regional analgesia. A technique for relief of postoperative pain following major extremity surgery. Clin Orthop. 1991;266:227–37.
137. Jaeger H, Maier C. Calcitonin in phantom limb pain: a double-blind study. Pain. 1992;48:21–7.
138. Nikolajsen L, Hansen CL, Nielsen J, Keller J, Arendt-Nielsen L, Jensen TS. The effect of ketamine on phantom pain: a central neuropathic disorder maintained by peripheral input. Pain. 1996;67:69–77.
139. McCormick Z, Chang-Chien G, Marshall B, Huang M, Harden N. Phantom limb pain: a systemic neuroanatomical-based review of pharmacologic treatment. Pain Med. 2014;15:292–305.
140. Varandhan KK, Lobo DN, Ljungqvist O. Enhanced recovery after surgery: the future of improving surgical care. Crit Care Clin. 2010;26(3):527–47.

Rehabilitation for Patients with Bone and Soft Tissue Sarcoma

15

Sanjeev Agarwal, Caitlin Cicone, Paul A. Pipia,
and Aditya V. Maheshwari

15.1 Introduction

Patients with bone and soft tissue sarcoma are susceptible to multiple neurological and musculoskeletal impairments throughout the course of the disease and treatment process, making rehabilitation an essential component of management [1]. Not only are the surgeries complex, requiring the involvement of multiple surgical disciplines, but multi-agent chemotherapy programs are employed along with high-dose radiation treatments, all of which have the potential to result in significant functional impairments and negatively impact quality of life [2]. In addition to the rehabilitative considerations that must be made for all cancer patients, the disease process and treatment course of sarcoma result in unique impairments that require specific attention during rehabilitation. The focus of this section is to review how rehabilitation fits into the treatment model for patients with sarcoma.

15.2 Overview of Cancer Rehabilitation

The overall goal of cancer rehabilitation is to improve or maintain quality of life, function, and independence throughout the course of the disease process [3]. Using a multidisciplinary team approach, cancer rehabilitation aims to increase function, promote community reintegration, assist in psychosocial coping, lower burden of care, and manage comorbid conditions [3]. Cancer rehabilitation ultimately addresses impairments caused by the cancer itself, as well as cancer treatment, in an attempt to lessen the potential disability.

S. Agarwal, M.D. (✉) • C. Cicone, D.O. • P.A. Pipia, M.D. • A.V. Maheshwari, M.D.
Department of Orthopaedic Surgery and Rehabilitation Medicine,
SUNY Downstate Medical Center, Brooklyn, NY, USA
e-mail: Aditya.maheshwari@downstate.edu

© Springer International Publishing Switzerland 2017   295
R.M. Henshaw (ed.), *Sarcoma*, DOI 10.1007/978-3-319-43121-5_15

15.2.1 Phases of Cancer Rehabilitation

Rehabilitation in patients with sarcoma may occur at any or multiple points during the course of the disease process. Cancer rehabilitation in general can be categorized as preventative, restorative, supportive, and palliative [3]. The role of rehabilitation changes depending on where a patient is in this continuum [4].

15.2.1.1 Preventative

While not yet routinely practiced in patients with an extremity sarcoma, general consensus suggests that early intervention by a physiatrist can maximize functional outcome and lower anxiety [5]. Preventative rehabilitation begins before or soon after treatment to stop functional loss or disability from occurring [3]. Rehabilitation that begins prior to cancer therapy has been termed "prehabilitation." [6] During the prehabilitation period, the physiatrist assesses baseline level of function and endurance, preexisting physical deficits, and comorbidities that may impact a patient's tolerance to treatment and overall outcome [6]. If pre-existing deficits are found, management may begin prior to cancer therapy and lead to a smoother transition postoperatively. This phase is especially relevant in patients that are projected to have significant morbidity following treatment, such as the patient with an extremity sarcoma requiring amputation [2]. In this circumstance, prehabilitation allows the physiatrist to familiarize the patient with the implications that are associated with their level of amputation. Referral to a peer support group or a psychiatrist to lessen the psychosocial burden is also appropriate prior to treatment, as there is significant stress associated with loss of a limb [5].

15.2.1.2 Restorative

Restorative therapy occurs if surgery has been curative or the disease process is stable, with the goal of returning the patient to their prior level of function [6]. Early postsurgical rehabilitation for patients with sarcoma will be dictated by multiple factors including immediate postoperative condition, type of surgery, and restrictions on weight bearing and range of motion (ROM) [3]. Rehabilitation extending beyond the immediate postsurgical period is based on the type of surgery performed, amputation, or LSS, as well as any required adjuvant chemotherapy or radiation.

15.2.1.3 Supportive/Palliative

In later stages of sarcoma, or in the case of metastatic disease, rehabilitation continues to play a role in maximizing patient independence, mobility, and comfort [7]. Supportive rehabilitation occurs during progressive disease and disability and focuses on regaining partial independence in daily activities [8]. Palliative rehabilitation aims to maintain comfort, quality of life, and functional independence in those in the terminal phases of cancer [8].

15.2.2 Constitutional Symptoms

Managing cancer-related symptoms during the rehabilitation process is a challenging, but necessary, component of care. Two of the most frequently encountered

Table 15.1 Intervention for cancer-related fatigue in adults

Evaluate for and treat reversible causes of fatigue
Physical activity/exercise
Rehabilitation
Psychoeducation
Meditation, mindfulness-based stress reduction, cognitive behavioral stress management
Cognitive behavioral therapy for fatigue, depression, pain, and sleep
Yoga

Adapted from Berger et al. [10]

symptoms in cancer patients are fatigue and pain [4]. In patients with sarcoma, these symptoms persist even into survivorship, further impacting the rehabilitation process [9].

The overall prevalence of chronic renal failure (CRF) is 70–100%, depending on type and stage of cancer and current anticancer treatments [4, 10]. CRF is not only problematic for patients during the active phase of their disease or treatment but can persist in disease-free survivors [11]. While CRF can be the result of cancer treatment, such as a chemotherapy-induced cascade of biological alterations, or from the cancer itself it is likely multifactorial in nature [10]. If CRF is not addressed during the rehabilitation process, it may prevent successful functional recovery and full participation in therapy [7]. Both pharmacological and non-pharmacological approaches are used to manage cancer-related fatigue, if no reversible sources are identified (Table 15.1).

Cancer-related pain presents another barrier to rehabilitation. The prevalence of pain in patients with sarcoma is about 53%, and the incidence of inadequately treated pain has been reported to be 63% [1]. Even after treatment of sarcoma, pain has been found to persist in some patients, which impacts physical functioning and quality of life [9], and can severely interfere with performing activities of daily living (ADLs) [12]. Cancer patients often experience overlapping pain syndromes that are mostly due to tumor effects, although cancer-related anxiety, depression, or distress can worsen pain [4]. A multimodal approach to pain management is often needed to achieve adequate pain control and should incorporate a combination of agents from multiple analgesic classes, anticancer treatments, interventional techniques, and manual approaches/modalities. Specifics regarding pain management will be discussed in following sections, as well as in Chap. 14.

15.3   Impairments Caused by Sarcoma Treatment

The trend toward combined modality therapy in patients with extremity sarcomas is important from the rehabilitation perspective as surgery, chemotherapy, and radiation all carry the potential to cause functional, neurological, and musculoskeletal impairments. Disease grade and stage, extent of surgical intervention, and side effects from adjuvant therapy all influence the rehabilitation plan and functional outcome [5]. Rehabilitation addresses both the immediate and long-term impairments caused by cancer treatments.

15.3.1 Impairments Caused by Adjuvant Therapy

Antineoplastic agents have the potential to cause significant functional limitations due to the neurotoxicity, cognitive dysfunction, cardiomyopathy, and pulmonary fibrosis that occurs from disruption of normal tissue [4]. Regimens in patients with sarcoma that use platinum and vinca alkaloids are associated with inactivity into survivorship [13, 14]. While chemotherapy-induced peripheral neuropathy is likely to diminish following treatment of extremity sarcomas, mild neurotoxicity, from prior cisplatin exposure, can persist into survivorship [15]. Lastly, chemotherapy may accelerate skin changes from radiation therapy and delay prosthetic fitting [16].

Patients with sarcoma are frequently given radiation at doses that make them susceptible to the negative consequences of the treatment [2]. Radiation fibrosis syndrome (RFS) is a late manifestation of radiation treatment and describes the clinical manifestations of the pathological fibrotic tissue sclerosis that results after radiation treatment due to vascular dysfunction and the abnormal accumulation of thrombin [17]. This subsequent fibrosis occurs to some degree in all muscles and connective tissue in the radiation field, resulting in various consequences [4]. Postradiation, tendons and ligaments become fibrotic, resulting in loss of elasticity, shortening, and contracture, which can then impair function and ROM [17]. In children, functional impairment may result from leg-length discrepancies due to disruption of epiphyseal plates, and scoliosis can occur secondarily [17]. Osteoporosis and osteopenia are common after radiation, which disrupts the integrity of bones and makes patients susceptible to fractures [17]. Effects of radiation can be seen overtime, and, even after radiation therapy is completed, functional status should be assessed regularly.

Patients with bone or soft tissue sarcoma near the axilla or groin are particularly susceptible to developing lymphedema, due to the close proximity to major lymphatic channels and lymph node complexes [18]. Lymphedema is the accumulation of protein-rich lymph fluid in the extracellular spaces and can result either from obstruction of lymphatic channels from radiation or surgical destruction of lymph nodes/vessels [1]. Due to increases in protein concentration, colloid osmotic pressure increases, pulling fluid into the interstitium, causing inflammation, adipose tissue hypertrophy, and fibrosis [1]. Increases in the size and weight of the limb from the soft tissue swelling result in pain, postural dysfunction, impaired mobility, and limited joint movement [19]. Consequently, patients struggle to perform their activities of daily living and have altered body image, psychosocial function, and quality of life [19]. Lymphedema may also lead to skin infections, hyperkeratosis, and papillomatosis [1].

15.3.2 Surgery-Related Impairments

Extent, location, and type of tumor are important factors in determining the primary impairments after surgical intervention. The type of surgery performed on a patient with sarcoma, limb salvage surgery (LSS) vs. amputation, will also cause distinct impairments. Survival and oncologic outcomes are the primary consideration when deciding between surgical approaches; however, function and cosmetic appearance are secondary considerations in the decision [5].

15.3.2.1 Limb Salvage Surgery

LSS is a surgical approach that attempts to avoid amputation but, often, at the expense of damaging many anatomical areas [8]. As a result of the expansive tissue destruction, patients are at risk for a variety of functional complications such as loss of ROM, muscle weakness, poor motor control, leg-length discrepancies, gait impairments, and pain. Site-specific impairments that occur based on anatomical location should be monitored for during the rehabilitation process and are listed below in order of the most commonly effected site.

15.3.2.2 Distal Femur/Knee Joint

The distal femur/knee joint is the most common location for extremity sarcomas [7]. As compared to proximal femur resections, distal femur resection lends to better functional outcomes, as there is a lack of important muscles originating or inserting at this site [20]. While uncommon, peroneal, femoral, and tibialis nerve impairment can occur and negatively impact gait mechanics [7]. Additionally, postoperative patients can develop leg-length discrepancies [7]. Despite these potential functional impairments, with aggressive physical therapy, these patients may be able to walk without a limp [20].

15.3.2.3 Proximal Tibia/Knee Joint

Involvement of this region has a high impact on functional outcome. The patellar tendon inserts on the proximal tibia, and disruption of this attachment can cause weakness in knee extension [20]. Loss of ROM is common in patients undergoing LSS and results in poorer functional outcomes [21]. When loss of ROM occurs at the knee, a crucial component of the gait cycle, patients may compensate by hip hiking or circumduction in order to clear the extremity during swing phase [21]. Alterations in gait mechanics are problematic as they compromise joint and tissue integrity [21]. As with distal femur involvement, peroneal nerve palsy and leg-length discrepancies may occur [7].

15.3.2.4 Shoulder/GHJ/Scapula

Hand dominance is an important factor to consider when evaluating possible functional limitations in patients with a bone or soft tissue sarcoma involving the humerus or gleno-humeral joint (GHJ). If the dominant hand is affected, the patient may have difficulty performing ADLs and completing tasks that require the use of fine motor skills [22]. As opposed to patients who require forequarter amputations, patients who undergo LSS are able to retain their hand function [22]. Despite therapy, however, above shoulder hand activities are generally lost [8]. Patients who undergo intra-articular resection, where the glenoid and deltoid musculature are preserved, may recover some shoulder function (shoulder motion >90°), as opposed to patients undergoing an extra-articular resection in which shoulder function is lost [20]. Additionally, when the proximal humerus and glenohumeral joint is affected, the deltoid muscle and axillary nerve are almost always involved, leading to difficulty with posturing the head, neck, and shoulder [7].

15.3.2.5 Proximal Femur/Hip Joint
Proximal femur resections can lead to significant impairment due to the potential involvement of the hip flexors, extensors, and abductors [20]. Oftentimes, hip abductors are weakened resulting in a Trendelenburg gait [20, 22]. This gait pattern accommodates ipsilateral hip abduction weakness during stance phase but can lead to complications such as low back pain and increased energy expenditure [21]. With hamstring muscle or sciatic nerve compromise, patients develop altered gaits due to knee flexion contractures and ankle instability [20]. Knee dysfunction may also result from quadriceps or femoral nerve destruction, and patients may have difficulty maintaining the stance phase of the gait cycle [20].

15.3.2.6 Pelvis
Pelvic resections can be external or internal hemipelvectomies, the latter being subclassified into Type I (iliac bone), Type II (periacetabular), Type III (ischiopubic), Type IV (en bloc resection of the ilium and sacral ala), or combinations [7]. Impairments in this anatomically complex region differ depending on both surgical technique and anatomical location. Type I resection preserves the hip joint and generally allows for function to be maintained [20]. Sacrifice of the ilium in these patients may result in a leg-length discrepancy, due to the proximal rotation of the remaining portion of the pelvis [20]. In patients undergoing Type II, resections the risk for functional impairment is dependent on the type of reconstruction. Those who undergo no or minimal reconstruction progress slower in terms of mobilization, stability, and weight-bearing ability but have shorter surgical times and fewer complications, compared to those that undergo pelvic reconstruction [20, 23]. Patients with a "flail extremity" may also have slower walking speeds, but their gait cycles are not significantly different than those undergoing more extensive and surgically complicated reconstructions [23]. Type III resections involving loss of the ischium produce an unbalanced and uncomfortable sitting surface [22]. Lastly, pelvic girdle involvement may also cause injury affecting the bladder, bowel, or uterus.

15.3.2.7 Amputation
For the subset of patients with sarcoma that require amputation, disability is largely dictated by level [6]. Functional concerns also differ depending on upper and lower extremity involvement. Considerations regarding handedness, vocation, ADLs, and recreational activities are important factors that play a role in functional outcomes

Table 15.2 Energy expenditure by amputation level

	Increase (%)	% increase above normal 3 METs
Unilateral BKA with prosthesis	9–28	3.3–3.8
Unilateral AKA with prosthesis	40–65%	4.2–5.8
Bilateral BKA with prosthesis	41–100	4.2–6.0
BK plus AKA with prosthesis	75	5.3
Bilateral AKA with prosthesis	> 200	11.4
Unilateral hip disarticulation with prosthesis	82	5.5
Hemipelvectomy with prosthesis	125	6.75

AKA above knee amputation, *BKA* below knee amputation, *MET* metabolic equivalent tasks
Adapted from Tobias and Gillis [6]

for patients undergoing upper extremity amputation [6]. Level of amputation, whether above the elbow or below, plays a large role in determining function, as preservation of the elbow joint generally allows for better outcomes. Furthermore, for patients who undergo a forequarter amputation, the ability to obtain a functional prosthesis is rare, due to the lack of bony/muscular framework on which to suspend the prosthesis [22].

In regard to lower extremity amputation, both the affected and non-affected limb need be assessed, as both will affect ambulation, sitting posture, and standing balance [6]. Pre-existing motor or sensory deficits in the non-amputated limb limit weight bearing, balance, and ambulation [6]. Additionally, the level of amputation, whether proximal or distal, will impact energy expenditure and disability in lower extremity amputations. Normal ambulation requires 3 METs (metabolic equivalent tasks), and this requirement increases after amputation based on level of amputation and whether or not a prosthetic or assistive device is used (Table 15.2). More proximal levels of amputation and lack of an anatomical joint are associated with higher levels of disability and energy expenditure [5]. For example, the majority of individuals who undergo external hemipelvectomy for management of soft tissue sarcoma of the pelvis do not use a prosthetic device due to the increase in energy requirements [24]. Pre-existing cardiopulmonary disease may further limit ambulation with a prosthesis. Lastly, there are psychosocial factors that if left unaddressed can lead to significant disability.

15.4 Rehabilitation Interventions in Patients with Extremity Sarcoma

Despite the need for aggressive rehabilitation in patients with sarcoma, there are few disease-specific approaches. Often, concepts regarding general cancer and musculoskeletal rehabilitation are applied to this patient population [5]. General practices such as early mobilization, gait training, active-assisted range of motion, and isometric exercises are key components in successful rehabilitation following LSS [8].

15.4.1 Scar Tissue Mobilization

Both surgery and radiation therapy destroy the tensile strength of the tissue and result in scar tissue formation that limits ROM and causes pain [7]. Therapeutic techniques aimed at improving ROM and encouraging the tissue to regain its ability to stretch are essential in the rehabilitation of patients with bone and soft tissue tumors, as maintaining ROM correlates with improved functional mobility and QOL [21]. For the postradiation patient, fibrosis will occur to some degree in all tissue within the radiation field. Postradiation, all irradiated muscles must be identified and incorporated into the rehabilitation process, as the absence of ongoing ROM can result in the formation of contractures [4]. Deep friction and stretching exercises can make the scars soften and more flexible [7]. Daily ROM exercises also align scar tissues, which increases overall mobility [6]. Ultrasound, a modality providing deep heat, may improve tissue elasticity if used prior to ROM exercises and fibrous-release techniques [25].

15.4.2 Modalities

Modalities assist in overcoming functional limitations and providing pain relief. Ultrasound, as mentioned previously, can be focused on areas with radiation-induced fibrosis or postsurgical scarring to soften scar tissue [4]. Massage provides therapeutic benefits from its antispasmodic, fibrolytic, and counter-stimulatory effects [4]. Electrical stimulation can be used to decrease muscle spasm, and transcutaneous electrical nerve stimulator (TENS) units can aid in providing pain relief [26]. Desensitization techniques, which produce a tolerance for increasingly intense stimulation, can be used in the management of neuropathic pain, including chemotherapy-induced peripheral neuropathy [25]. Contraindications to modalities, such as massage and ultrasound, arise from fear of spreading cancer both locally and systemically [4]. These precautions should not be disregarded entirely; however, the use of modalities may be of benefit, rather than harm, in certain circumstances [4].

15.4.3 Aerobic Exercise

While not specific to patients with extremity sarcomas, studies consistently suggest that aerobic exercise is safe and lowers symptom burden in patients undergoing cancer treatment and into survivorship [4, 27, 28]. Aerobic exercise potentially combats fatigue, mitigates the impact of high-dose chemotherapy, and improves quality of life [4, 11, 27, 28]. Despite the general consensus regarding improved outcomes with exercise in cancer patients, it has not yet become a routine component in management. As physiatry becomes more involved in the treatment of patients with cancer, physiatrists can integrate physical activity and exercise into practice, a component that may have been overlooked by other members of the team [14, 27].

15.4.4 Lymph Drainage

Complete (or complex) decongestive therapy (CDT) is the current standard of care for managing lymphedema [1]. CDT has been shown to be an effective treatment that also improves quality of life [19]. This is a two-phase, multimodal program that focuses on reduction of fluid, during phase I, and maintaining the reduction, during phase II. The components of CDT include manual lymph drainage (MLD), compression bandages/garments, exercise, and skin care.

During stage I, MLD aims to stimulate the intrinsic contractility of the lymphatic system using a massage technique characterized by a specific stroke duration, orientation, pressure, and sequence [4]. Treatments begin proximally in lymphostatic regions and direct lymph toward functioning lymphotomes [4]. MLD is then followed by compression bandaging, which is a specialized form of bandaging used to achieve gradient compression. Short stretch bandages are applied, with more layers distal than proximal, and are left in place 21–24 h per day during phase I [1]. The bandages exert low pressure in the resting muscle, but as the muscle contracts within the space of the short bandages, interstitial fluid pressure increases [1]. The cycling between high and low pressure creates an internal pump mechanism that encourages lymph to flow along the gradient created by the bandaging. Remedial lymphedema exercises are repetitive movements that produce serial muscle contractions and are used to compress lymph vessels and trigger contraction in lymph vessel walls, so as to further encourage lymph to flow along the established pressure gradient [4].

Once reduction in volume reduction has plateaued, patients enter phase II, a long-term maintenance phase. Compression bandages are used only at night and MLD is performed as needed [4]. Compression garments, such as sleeves or stockings, are worn during the day to maintain the volume reduction and skin integrity, protect the limb from potential trauma, and prevent fibrosis [4]. Additionally, skin care is emphasized in both stages to limit and prevent bacterial/fungal overgrowth and microfissuring. Patients should cleanse and moisturize the skin daily with mineral oil-based soap [4].

15.4.5 Gait Training

There are six determinants of gait that deal with the conservation of energy during normal ambulation: pelvic rotation, pelvic tilt, knee flexion in midstance, foot/ankle motion, knee motion, and lateral pelvic motion [29]. Alterations in biomechanics in any of these components lead to compensatory gait patterns and ultimately increased energy expenditure, muscle fatigue, and pain. As previously discussed, gait impairments are common in patients with extremity sarcomas. During the rehabilitation process, multiple interventions can be employed to address gait dysfunction. Both therapeutic exercises and the use of orthotics/prosthetics can help to optimize alignment and allow for safer ambulation. Therapeutic exercises are typically isometric strengthening exercises, aimed at strengthening the core musculature and the muscles supporting a weak or painful body part [25]. Stabilization and protection of an impaired limb may also be achieved through the use of orthotics, by immobilizing the limb completely or restricting motion at specific joints [25]. For example, patients with peroneal nerve disruption that develop foot drop after a proximal tibia resection may require an ankle-foot orthosis (AFO) to assist with ambulation. For patients with foot drop, the most common AFO is a posterior leaf spring AFO [30]. This is often set in several degrees of dorsiflexion so that the foot clears the ground during swing phase, and also facilitates the ankle going into dorsiflexion after push-off [30]. Subcategories of AFOs exist, such as carbon fiber or plastic fiber, which allow for orthotics to be customized for patient's needs. Carbon fiber AFOs are lighter, assist during toe-off, and may provide a more normal gait pattern; however, patients with spasticity or contractures are not candidates for carbon fiber AFOs as they cannot be molded [1]. For those patients with instability at the knee due to quadriceps or femoral nerve involvement after proximal femur resection, they may require a ground-reactive AFO, which provides a posteriorly directed force at the proximal tibia to encourage knee extension and control knee flexion or a knee-ankle-foot orthosis (KAFO) [20]. If hip flexion and knee extension are not intact, then knee bracing, such as with a KAFO, is needed. Additionally, training with assistive devices and education regarding environmental modifications and energy conservation are also important rehabilitative interventions to address gait impairments. By working with a therapist, patients will learn to recognize which movements are difficult to achieve, whether due to weakness or pain, and develop compensatory strategies to avoid these triggers [25]. Lastly, patients with a lower extremity amputation will need to relearn balance and posturing, even prior to gait training with the prosthesis itself, due to changes in center of balance.

15.4.6 Pain Management

Despite the increased effort to achieve adequate pain control in patients with cancer, pain in patients with sarcoma often remains undertreated or inadequately treated [31]. Quality of life, physical functioning, and psychological features are all negatively impacted by poor pain control [31, 32]. The first step to achieving pain control begins with an adequate pain assessment and goes beyond acquiring a pain rating (i.e., obtain a description of the pain, timing, duration, onset, provoking or palliative features, impact on a patient's life, red flags for abuse of pain medication, etc.). Pain can be categorized as nociceptive or neuropathic. Nociceptive pain is due to pressure on nerves and ongoing tissue damage and is further subdivided into somatic or visceral (distention of a hollow viscus), whereas neuropathic pain is due to direct damage to the nerve and can be either central or peripheral in origin [32]. Determining the etiology of pain in patients with sarcoma may be challenging, as most patients with cancer often experience overlapping pain syndromes due to the interaction between cancer cells, the nervous system, and immune system [32]. Pain

Table 15.3 World Health Organization analgesic ladder for cancer pain management in adults

Pain severity	Analgesic
Mild	Non-opioids such as NSAIDs and/or Tylenol
Mild-moderate	Weak opioid (codeine, tramadol, dihydrocodeine) +/− non-opioid
Moderate-severe	Strong opioid (morphine, methadone, oxycodone, hydromorphone, fentanyl) +/− non-opioid

The oral route of administration is effective and inexpensive and should be tried first when available. Around-the-clock dosing should be given to prevent the onset of pain
Adapted from Smith and Saiki [32]

management can begin once an adequate assessment of a patient's pain has been made. Unique to cancer pain management is the reliance on high-dose opioids, which should be initiated early on in the disease process if needed, rather than withheld until the terminal stages of the disease [1, 4]. For patients with cancer, the World Health Organization (WHO) has developed a severity-based analgesic ladder that provides guidelines on when to initiate non-opioid and opioid medications (Table 15.3).

For mild pain, non-opioid medications, such as acetaminophen and NSAIDs, should be used; for mild to moderate pain, "weak" opioids with or without a non-opioid are used; for moderate to severe pain, strong opioids should be initiated with or without non-opioids [32]. The WHO currently recommends using regularly scheduled dosing of medication to prevent the onset of pain, by taking into consideration the half-life, bioavailability, and duration of action of the analgesic [26]. This around-the-clock scheduling should be supplemented with the option for breakthrough pain medication or rescue doses [32]. While opioids are heavily relied upon for the management of cancer pain and are appropriate for the management of nociceptive pain, opioids do not adequately address all pain syndromes. For neuropathic pain, antidepressants and anticonvulsant medications should be incorporated into treatment regimens, as opioid analgesia does not provide adequate coverage for neuropathic pain [1]. For bone pain, radiotherapy using external beam radiation, and medical management with bisphosphonates, that inhibit osteoclastic bone resorption (the presumed mechanism behind pain from bony metastasis [1]) or Denosumab, a RANKL (receptor activator of nuclear factor kappa-B ligand) inhibitor, have been shown to be beneficial [26]. In some cases, patients experience pain that is refractory to oral medications and may require interventional pain management. Interventional techniques including selective nerve blocks/plexus blocks, neurolysis, and intraspinal devices (i.e., spinal cord stimulators or intrathecal infusion with morphine) should be considered in cases of refractory pain [1, 26]. For example, patients with lower extremity cancer pain or phantom limb pain following an amputation may benefit from a lumbar sympathetic block [32]. Stellate ganglion blocks are indicated for patients with upper extremity, head, or neck pain from phantom limb pain, postradiation pain, postsurgical neuropathy, and neuropathic pain [33].

15.4.7 Site-Specific Considerations Following LSS

Due to the highly complex and individualized nature of LSS, developing a standard-ized rehabilitation regimen is challenging [5]. Basic guidelines for rehabilitation following LSS have been published [7, 8]. Although such protocols have not yet been consistently incorporated into practice, there are site-specific rehabilitation goals and approaches that should be considered. It should be noted that limitations regarding ROM and weight-bearing status will often differ based on surgical technique.

15.4.7.1 Distal Femur/Knee Joint

Physical therapy in these patients aims to achieve knee ROM 0–90° and functional weight bearing [8]. For a distal femur reconstruction, weight-bearing status is typi-cally as tolerated for both cemented and cementless prostheses, if good initial fixa-tion is achieved. For allograft and allograft prosthetic composites, it may be delayed based on the bone-graft interface healing. If wound healing is progressing satisfac-torily, active and active-assisted ROM (AAROM) and strengthening exercises are initiated as soon as possible with the goal of achieving at least 90 degrees of full extension [8].

15.4.7.2 Proximal Tibia/Knee Joint

Rehabilitation focuses on achieving full limb extension without any degree of extension lag, as this may impair ambulation. Although achieving full range of knee flexion at the expense of knee extension is not recommended, many patients may have some residual extension lag [8]. Patients are generally partial weight bearing after surgery [20]. Since the quadriceps mechanism is often reconstructed along with the gastrocnemius flap, knee flexion is initially not allowed, but progressive isometric quadriceps strengthening and ankle ROM exercises may be started early on. Patients are immobilized for 4–6 weeks in a long-leg brace to allow for healing and establishment of a good extensor mechanism [8, 20]. Once the patient is able to do an active straight leg raise (about 4–6 weeks), active knee ROM exercises can begin along with WBAT with a goal to achieve at least 90 degrees of flexion [8]. Additionally, these patients may require management for leg-length discrepancies. This may be treated with up to a 2 cm inch shoe insert; however, if more height is required, then it is necessary to raise the shoe [7].

15.4.7.3 Proximal Humerus/Scapula/GHJ

The goal of rehabilitation in these patients is to have normal hand, wrist, and elbow function, so that feeding and hygiene abilities are preserved, and to achieve shoul-der joint stability [8]. Immobilization of the shoulder generally occurs for 6 weeks after surgery, although pendulum exercises (i.e., Codman I/II exercises) can begin as early as post-op day 10 [8, 20]. Hand and elbow ROM exercises and occupational therapy are encouraged initially, but full elbow flexion should be avoided so flexor muscle attachments are not disrupted [8]. Gradually, full elbow extension is allowed and AAROM at the shoulder may begin when the immobilizer is removed after week 6 [8]. Patients may benefit from a shoulder mold to improve any cosmetic deformity due to the loss of tissue [7].

15.4.7.4 Proximal Femur/Hip Joint

Rehabilitation efforts aim to reestablish abductor strength and prevent hip dislocation [8]. Patients are initially toe-touch weight bearing and generally require hip abduction braces for at least 6 weeks to protect abductor repair and prevent hip dislocation [8]. Initially, knee and ankle exercises are encouraged, as well as abductor muscle strengthening [8]. Patients with instability at the knee from quadriceps or femoral nerve involvement may require an AFO or KAFO [20]. Leg-length discrepancy can also occur and may require a shoe insert for adequate management.

15.4.7.5 Pelvis

With pelvic involvement, the goal is to obtain normal knee and ankle function and have a minimal decrease in hip function [8]. Therapy considerations, including weight-bearing status, are largely variable, based on both anatomic location and surgical technique. In type I and II patients, a hip abduction brace is generally used for 6–8 weeks to protect the abductor muscle repair [8]. Knee and ankle ROM and strengthening exercises can begin initially, but active strengthening of the abductors is avoided until the abduction brace is discontinued [8]. Patients with a type III resection do not typically require an abduction brace and may begin active hip ROM and strengthening as early as post-op week one [8].

15.4.8 Amputation Rehabilitative Care

Rehabilitation for patients with amputation ideally begins preoperatively and prepares patients for the physical and psychological loss. Postoperative rehabilitation is subdivided into pre-prosthetic management and prosthetic training.

During the pre-prosthetic phase, goals include wound healing, controlling edema, suture site desensitization, limb shaping, and addressing functional deficits. Physical and occupational therapy at this time focuses on strength training for ambulation and transfers, stretching to prevent contractures, and reduction of residual limb edema. Shaping the residual limb is essential during this stage, as a poorly shaped limb may lead to skin breakdown or inability to bear weight [5]. Compression therapy with continued wrapping of the residual limb will decrease edema and assist limb shaping [6]. The use of stump shrinkers, however, should be avoided until staples/sutures have been removed. Ambulation with a walker or crutches, as opposed to sitting in a wheelchair, and prone positioning while laying should be encouraged so as to prevent hip or knee flexion contractures [20].

Prosthetic training takes place with the prosthesis itself. In patients with sarcoma that require adjuvant treatment, chemotherapy and radiation may prolong healing or cause edema that will result in delayed prosthesis fitting [6, 16]. Rehabilitation during this stage focuses on donning and doffing the prosthesis, transfers and ambulation with the prosthesis, and increasing dexterity with ADLs (for upper extremity

Table 15.4 United States Medicare K-Levels

K0	Does not have the ability or potential to ambulate or transfer safely with or without assistance; prosthesis does not enhance quality of life
K1	Has the ability or potential to use a prosthesis on level surfaces at a fixed cadence; household ambulator
K2	Has the ability or potential for ambulation with low-level environmental barriers (curbs, stairs, uneven surfaces); community ambulator
K3	Has the ability or potential for ambulation with variable cadence and across most environmental barriers; community ambulator who has vocational, therapeutic, or exercise activity that require prosthetic utilization beyond simple locomotion
K4	Has the ability or potential for ambulation that exceeds basic ambulation skills, exhibiting high impact stress or energy levels; typical of children, active adults, or athletes

K-Levels describe the functional level of patients with prosthetics and ultimately determine the prosthetic components that Medicare will cover

amputations) [6]. Type of prosthesis prescribed for patients is largely impacted by the K-level, or functional level, as outlined in Table 15.4. The knee mechanism of the prosthesis for patients with a transfemoral amputation, and the ankle/foot mechanism of the prosthesis for patients with a transtibial amputation, will be decided by the expected level of activity [6]. Not only does a prosthesis allow for improvement in physical function, but fitting with a prosthesis can help to decrease residual limb and phantom pain and improve quality of life [5].

15.5 Rehabilitation in Sarcoma Survivorship

Today, survival rates following limb salvage surgery for extremity sarcomas are 60–70% [8], but predicting functional outcome still remains challenging [34]. Even after the acute phase of illness, survivors of sarcoma are left to deal with impaired functional status and independence and late effects of treatment [11]. Fatigue, limited physical functioning, and pain are domains that present unique challenges to survivors of sarcoma [9]. While these factors have the potential to negatively impact quality of life, they are also areas where rehabilitative intervention has the potential to make a major impact [9]. Rehabilitation in this patient population is not necessarily short term, and patients may require or benefit from ongoing therapy even into survivorship.

15.6 Rehabilitation in Palliative Care

Even in the case of advanced or metastatic disease, rehabilitation continues to play a role in maintaining function and decreasing symptom burden. Maintaining mobility and independence is essential for many patients throughout the course of their disease process, including the terminal phases. Rehabilitation efforts in such cases can be aimed at educating family members and the patient on mobility, environmental adjustments, appropriate body mechanics/energy conservation, and assistive devices [35]. Physical and occupational therapy also assist in non-pharmacological pain management, relieving symptoms such as dyspnea and edema, and preventing contractures and decubitus ulcers, through low-frequency therapy, repositioning, breathing assistance/decongestive physiotherapy, massage, and heat and relaxation techniques [35]. Many of these techniques can be carried on into very advanced stages of the disease and performed as bedside interventions.

Conclusion

There is a general consensus that early intervention by a physiatrist, even before treatment, will lead to improved functional outcomes in patients with sarcoma [5]. The functional, neurological, and musculoskeletal impairments acquired by patients with sarcoma during the course of the disease and treatment process make it clear that rehabilitation is a necessary component in the multidisciplinary management of these patients. Despite the need for rehabilitation in these patients, much is lacking regarding specific protocol and therapy regimens. General cancer and musculoskeletal rehabilitation principles can be applied to patients with extremity sarcomas; however, additional research and investigation are warranted to address the specific functional limitations and physical impairments that result.

References

1. McMichael B, Wininger YD. Physiatric Approach to Cancer Rehabilitation. UPMC Rehab Grand Rounds. 2015(Winter):7.
2. Siegel GW, Biermann JS, Chugh R, et al. The multidisciplinary management of bone and soft tissue sarcoma: an essential organizational framework. J Multidiscip Healthc. 2015;8: 109–15.
3. Yadav R, Shin KY, Guo Y, Kozen B. Cancer Rehabilitation. In: Yeung S-CJ, Escalante CP, Gagel RF, editors. Medical care of cancer patients. Shelton: People's Medical Publishing House: BC Decker Inc.; 2009. p. 563–9.
4. Cheville AL. Cancer Rehabilitation In: Braddom RL, ed. Physical medicine & rehabilitation. 4th ed. Philadelphia: Saunders Elsevier; 2011:1371–1401.
5. Custodio CM. Barriers to rehabilitation of patients with extremity sarcomas. J Surg Oncol. 2007;95(5):393–9.
6. Tobias K, Gillis T. Rehabilitation of the sarcoma patient-enhancing the recovery and functioning of patients undergoing management for extremity soft tissue sarcomas. J Surg Oncol. 2015;111(5):615–21.
7. Oren R, Zagury A, Katzir O, Kollender Y, Meller I. Principles and Rehabilitation after Limb-sparing Surgery for Cancer. In: Malawer MM, Sugarbaker PH, editors. Musculoskeletal cancer surgery: treatment of sarcomas and allied diseases. Dordrecht: Kluwer Academic; 2001. p. 581–91.
8. Shehadeh A, El Dahleh M, Salem A, et al. Standardization of rehabilitation after limb salvage surgery for sarcomas improves patients' outcome. Hematol Oncol Stem Cell Ther. 2013;6(3–4):105–11.
9. Kwong TN, Furtado S, Gerrand C. What do we know about survivorship after treatment for extremity sarcoma? A systematic review. Eur J Surg Oncol. 2014;40(9):1109–24.

10. Berger AM, Mitchell SA, Jacobsen PB, Pirl WF. Screening, evaluation, and management of cancer-related fatigue: ready for implementation to practice? CA Cancer J Clin. 2015;65(3): 190–211.
11. Eickmeyer SM, Gamble GL, Shahpar S, Do KD. The role and efficacy of exercise in persons with cancer. PM R. 2012;4(11):874–81.
12. Furtado S, Grimer RJ, Cool P, et al. Physical functioning, pain and quality of life after amputation for musculoskeletal tumours: a national survey. Bone Joint J. 2015;97-B(9):1284–90.
13. Wampler MA, Galantino ML, Huang S, et al. Physical activity among adult survivors of childhood lower-extremity sarcoma. J Cancer Surviv. 2012;6(1):45–53.
14. Kimmel GT, Haas BK, Hermanns M. The role of exercise in cancer treatment: bridging the gap. Curr Sports Med Rep. 2014;13(4):246–52.
15. Earl HM, Connolly S, Latoufis C, et al. Long-term neurotoxicity of chemotherapy in adolescents and young adults treated for bone and soft tissue sarcomas. Sarcoma. 1998;2(2): 97–105.
16. So NF, Andrews KL, Anderson K, et al. Prosthetic fitting after rotationplasty of the knee. Am J Phys Med Rehabil. 2014;93(4):328–34.
17. Stubblefield MD. Radiation fibrosis syndrome: neuromuscular and musculoskeletal complications in cancer survivors. PM R. 2011;3(11):1041–54.
18. Black JF. Cancer of the muskuloskeltal system and its rehabilitation. Cancer and rehabilitation 2015. http://emedicine.medscape.com/article/320261-overview - a5. Accessed 18 Oct 2015.
19. Lasinski BB, McKillip Thrift K, Squire D, et al. A systematic review of the evidence for complete decongestive therapy in the treatment of lymphedema from 2004 to 2011. PM R. 2012;4(8):580–601.
20. Konzen B, Cannon CP. Rehabilitation in Orthopedic Oncology. In: Lin PP, Patel S, editors. Bone Sarcoma. Boston: Springer; 2002. p. 215–35.
21. Marchese VG, Spearing E, Callaway L, et al. Relationships among range of motion, functional mobility, and quality of life in children and adolescents after limb-sparing surgery for lower-extremity sarcoma. Pediatr Phys Ther. 2006;18(4):238–44.
22. Gillis T, Yadav R. Rehabilitation of the patient with soft tissue sarcoma. In: Pollock RE, editor. Soft tissue sarcoma. Hamilton: BC Decker Inc; 2002.
23. Carmody Soni EE, Miller BJ, Scarborough MT, Parker Gibbs C. Functional outcomes and gait analysis of patients after periacetabular sarcoma resection with and without ischiofemoral arthrodesis. J Surg Oncol. 2012;106(7):844–9.
24. Schaal Wilson RE. Rehabilitation considerations for a patient with external hemipelvectomy and hemisacrectomy for recurrent soft tissue pelvic sarcoma: a case report. Physiother Theory Pract. 2015;31(6):433–41.
25. Cheville AL, Basford JR. Role of rehabilitation medicine and physical agents in the treatment of cancer-associated pain. J Clin Oncol. 2014;32(16):1691–702.
26. Ripamonti CI, Santini D, Maranzano E, Berti M, Roila F. Management of cancer pain: ESMO clinical practice guidelines. Ann Oncol. 2012;23(Suppl 7):vii139–54.
27. Schmitz KH, Courneya KS, Matthews C, et al. American College of Sports Medicine roundtable on exercise guidelines for cancer survivors. Med Sci Sports Exerc. 2010;42(7):1409–26.
28. Dimeo FC, Tilmann MH, Bertz H, Kanz L, Mertelsmann R, Keul J. Aerobic exercise in the rehabilitation of cancer patients after high dose chemotherapy and autologous peripheral stem cell transplantation. Cancer. 1997;79(9):1717–22.
29. Esquenazi A, Talaty M. Gait analysis: technology and clinical applications. In: Braddom RL, editor. Physical medicine & rehabilitation, vol. 4. Philadelphia: Saunders Elsevier; 2011.
30. Hennessey WJ. Lower limb orthotic devices. In: Braddom RL, editor. Physical medicine and rehabilitation, vol. 4. Philadelphia: Saunders Elsevier; 2011.
31. Kuo PY, Yen JTC, Parker GM, et al. The prevalence of pain in patients attending sarcoma outpatient clinics. Sarcoma. 2011;2011:813483.

32. Smith TJ, Saiki CB. Cancer pain management. Mayo Clin Proc. 90(10):1428–39.
33. Gulati A, Joshi J, Baqai A. An overview of treatment strategies for cancer pain with a focus on interventional strategies and techniques. Pain Manag. 2012;(6):569–80.
34. Kolk S, Cox K, Weerdesteyn V, et al. Can orthopedic oncologists predict functional outcome in patients with sarcoma after limb salvage surgery in the lower limb? A nationwide study. Sarcoma. 2014;2014:436598.
35. Barawid E, Covarrubias N, Tribuzio B, Liao S. The benefits of rehabilitation for palliative care patients. Am J Hosp Palliat Care. 2015;32(1):34–43.

A Multidisciplinary Approach to Physical Therapy for Patients with Sarcomas

16

Kelly O'Mara

16.1 Introduction

In the United States, 900 new cases of bone tumors are diagnosed each year, with approximately 400 of these cases occurring in patients less than 20 years of age. Osteosarcoma accounts for 3.4% of all childhood cancers and 56% of malignant bone tumors in children. Soft-tissue tumors account for 7% of all childhood cancers. Seventy percent of patients diagnosed with osteosarcoma survive greater than five years. Medical and surgical management has progressed to improve these statistics over the past decades. Survivorship is a continuum (acute, transitional, extended, and permanent) (Fig. 16.1). Quality of life and function are crucial to meaningful survivorship. Physical therapists (PT) and occupational therapists (OT) are vital team members for improving quality of life and function in patients diagnosed with sarcomas across the survivorship continuum [1, 2].

16.2 Indications for Rehabilitation

The *International Classification of Functioning, Disability and Health* (ICF; Fig. 16.2) is the standard language of rehabilitation sciences used to describe health and health-related states. This model demonstrates the interactions between health conditions, body functions and structures, activity, participation, and contextual factors (environment and personal). Alteration of health condition is disorder or disease; problems within body functions and structures are impairments; difficulties performing daily tasks are activity (or performance) limitations; and the inabilities to fulfill societal roles are participation restrictions. Environmental factors include

K. O'Mara, PT, DPT, PCS
Children's National Health System, Washington, DC, USA
e-mail: KOmara@childrensnational.org

© Springer International Publishing Switzerland 2017
R.M. Henshaw (ed.), *Sarcoma*, DOI 10.1007/978-3-319-43121-5_16

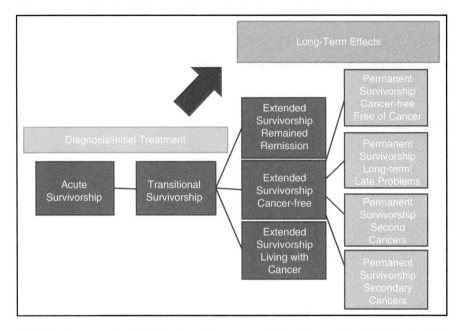

Fig. 16.1 Acute survivorship is the time when a person is being diagnosed and/or in treatment for cancer. Extended survivorship is the time immediately after treatment is completed, usually measured in months. Permanent survivorship is a longer period, often meaning that the passage of time since treatment is measured in years

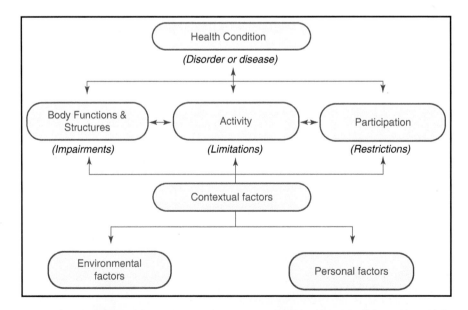

Fig. 16.2 Adapted from The International Classification of Functioning, Disability and Health [3]

the physical, social, and attitudinal environments within a person's life; personal factors include the demographic and psychological components that affect a person's experience [3].

16.2.1 Physical Activity/Performance Limitations

Data regarding survivorship in sarcomas are emerging from the Childhood Cancer Survivor Study (CCSS) that explores long-term survivorship in pediatric cancers. When compared to siblings and leukemia survivors, survivors of musculoskeletal (bone and soft-tissue) tumors have a higher risk of adverse health status, functional impairments, activity limitations, pain, and anxiety [4]. Survivors of brain tumors and bone tumors reported the highest prevalence of physical performance limitations, with one-third of bone cancer survivors reporting physical limitations [5]. A study by Nagarajan et al. [6] explored the population of survivors of lower extremity and pelvic tumors and found 71.8% of survivors report some level of disability, and about a quarter perceive themselves as moderately to severely limited in daily tasks. Despite the secondary physical impairments of rhabdomyosarcoma, only 14.1% of survivors report performance limitations [7, 8].

16.2.2 Participation Restrictions

When compared to matched siblings, survivors of pediatric cancers are more likely to report decreased ability to perform personal care or routine activities (i.e., shopping and housework) [9, 10]. Additionally, survivors are almost six times more likely to have decreased attendance at school or work compared to siblings. In survivors of bone cancers, 11% of survivors reported poor health prevented them from attending school or work, second only to pediatric brain tumor survivors [5].

16.2.3 Impairments

Musculoskeletal tumors, oncological treatments (radiation and chemotherapy), and surgical interventions have primary and secondary effects on body structures and functions: posture, muscle performance, joint mobility, motor function, pain, and range of motion. Impairments may be related to connective tissue dysfunction or localized inflammation post-radiation therapy or surgery, pathological fracture, joint arthroplasty (endoprosthesis), rotationplasty, and/or amputation. These impairments can cause pain and/or decreased quality of gait, locomotion, balance, and upper extremity function. Additionally, survivors of childhood osteosarcoma report adverse health status and pain [2, 11].

Range-of-motion impairments are common after limb sparing surgeries. Tsauo et al. [12] evaluated patients 3 years postwide resection and endoprosthesis placement and found less knee flexion range of motion in the surgical knee ($106.6° \pm 13.0°$) than in nonsurgical lower extremity. Buchner et al. [13] found patients 4 years post-limb-sparing surgery for proximal tibia tumors with medial gastrocnemius flap to have a mean knee flexion range of motion of only 60°. Knee range-of-motion outcomes are less favorable in revision of proximal tibia tumors due to the immobilization required for healing of the knee extensor mechanism.

Strength is negatively affected by disuse/immobilization, surgery, and radiation therapy. During surgical intervention, muscles may be resected, transferred, or denervated, depending on the proximity to the tumor and neurovascular bundle. In addition, chemotherapy causes chronic weakness and fatigue and may require frequent hospitalizations [14].

Gait and functional independence is influenced by strength and range of motion. Decreased knee, hip, and ankle range of motion decreases quality of gait and performance on stairs [15, 16]. In a study by Marchese et al. [17], measurements in knee flexion, hip flexion, and hip extension range of motion correlated with functional outcomes of timed up and down stairs (TUDS), timed up and go (TUG), and 9 minute run-walk distance in patients with lower extremity sarcoma after limb salvage surgery.

Bone health impairments, including osteonecrosis or osteopenia, can occur due to decreased activity and secondary effects of chemotherapy and radiation therapy. These can increase fragility, risk of fractures, and poor healing.

Integumentary system is compromised in survivors of sarcomas due to slowed wound healing secondary to radiation and chemotherapy. Limb edema can arise due to radiation fibrosis and lymphatic dysfunction. Incisions used for biopsies, skin grafts, limb salvage, amputation, and rotationplasty require extra care both for safe healing and for prevention of secondary infection, delayed wound closure, or dehiscence.

Neuromuscular impairments can occur in this population secondary to neurotoxic chemotherapies, radiation, surgical neuropraxia, axonotmesis, or neurotmesis.

Cardiovascular/pulmonary functioning is reduced as a result of acute and chronic injury from chemotherapy, radiotherapy, surgery, and decreased physical activity during diagnosis, treatment, and survivorship.

16.3   Rehabilitation Team Members

Exercise has the potential to reduce these secondary effects and improve physical fitness in pediatric cancer survivors [18] (Table 16.1). The rehabilitation team includes physical therapists, occupational therapists, and physiatrists. The goals of rehabilitation team members are to restore function, minimize impairments, and optimize capacity for activities and participation.

16.3.1 Physical/Occupational Therapists

Physical and occupational therapists are important team members in optimizing treatment outcomes in persons with sarcomas. Physical therapists specialize in movement and function. They assess range of motion, flexibility, strength,

Table 16.1 PT/OT clinical points specific to management of patients with sarcomas

Wound healing: Delayed wound healing with chemotherapy. Care must be taken with progressive range of motion opposing incisions.
Muscles/structures spared, resected, or rerouted: Know what you are and are not strengthening or ranging.
Secondary effects of chemotherapy on overall cardiopulmonary function: Incorporate cardiopulmonary training as appropriate.
Secondary effects of chemotherapy/surgery on neurological system: Screen for neuropathies. Educate on proper supportive shoes or devices.
Secondary effects of chemotherapy/surgery on bone health: Care must be taken with progressive range of motion, weight-bearing, and shearing/contact activities.
Patient/family goals and expectations need to be addressed and readdressed frequently throughout management.
Communication is essential for success: Open communication between oncologists, orthopedic oncologists, social workers, and other physical and occupational therapists.
Be realistic with goal setting.
When in doubt, do no harm. Then seek guidance/knowledge.

functional mobility, gait, integumentary, neuromuscular, and cardiovascular/pulmonary fitness. Occupational therapists specialize in activities of daily living and adaptation. They focus on fine motor and upper extremity function.

16.3.2 Physiatrists (Physical Medicine and Rehabilitation)

Surgery and medical management of sarcomas can have both short- and long-term debilitating effects on patients. Physiatrists specialize in rehabilitation medicine and assist in decision-making regarding intensity and environment of rehabilitation. Some patients may require acute or subacute rehabilitation environments for intensive therapy to safely return to the home environment. Over time, survivors of sarcoma have long-standing secondary effects that can be monitored by physiatrists.

Varying models of rehabilitation teams exist in different hospital systems and centers related to the treatment of survivors of sarcomas. The most common approach is through transdisciplinary care. Within a transdisciplinary model, one discipline—often physical therapy—is responsible for the management and coordination of care regarding function of these patients.

16.4   Points of Entry for Rehabilitation Services

Physical and occupational therapists encounter patients with sarcomas throughout many phases of diagnosis, treatment, and survivorship. Some reasons for referral for physical and/or occupational therapy include decreased functional independence, pain management, risk of fall or injury, difficulty with self-care, bracing or prosthetic management, splinting, and discharge planning.

Table 16.2 Points
of entry for physical and
occupational therapists
during survivorship

- Pre-diagnosis
- Outpatient evaluation and/or treatment
- Outpatient gait training
- Inpatient general medical or orthopedic floors
- Rheumatology, orthopedic, and/or chronic pain clinics
- Diagnosis
- Inpatient admission
- Outpatient solid tumor clinic
- Preoperative
- Chemotherapy admissions
- Postoperative
- Postradiation
- Postsurgical acute stay
- Acute rehabilitation stay
- Outpatient evaluation and/or treatment
- Prosthetic/orthotic fitting and/or training
- Post-lengthening
- Bone marrow transplantation admission
- Long-term follow-up

Physical and occupational therapists may encounter a patient with sarcoma at various points during and prior to diagnosis and survivorship (Table 16.2). In the multidisciplinary team model, physical therapists meet patients and families early in the diagnostic and treatment phases.

16.5 Multidisciplinary Sarcoma Clinic

At Children's National Health System, the majority of patients are seen through the multidisciplinary sarcoma clinic. The team members in this clinic include physical therapists, orthopedic oncologists, pediatric oncologists, radiation oncologists, radiologists, nurse practitioners, physician assistants, residents, fellows, medical students, nurses, and social workers. In addition, consulting services include psychologists, child life specialists, general surgeons, wound care, and nutritionists. External consultation occurs with prosthetics and orthotics specialists.

Face-to-face time and collaboration with other providers allows for patient-centered care. Every clinic visit starts with review of patient cases and discussion regarding scheduled patients. Physical therapists discuss with medical and surgical oncologists the patient's progress, ongoing or new concerns, and radiographic and diagnostic findings. As a team, the physical therapist and orthopedic oncologist evaluate the patient, discuss goal and progress, and provide an updated plan of care to the patient and family. Team members modify the plan of care for rehabilitation intervention based on patient's prognosis, phase of treatment, patient goals, and patient's quality of life. The physical therapist also provides intervention, and relays information to treating therapists.

16.6   Physical Therapy Evaluation

The physical therapy evaluation (Fig. 16.3) includes intake and assessment of history, motivation and understanding, physical examination, and development of a plan.

History intake and assessment helps to understand the patient's current and past status. Important aspects include patient's age, diagnosis, past medical and surgical history, current level of function, interests, limitations, and tolerance to pain. Understanding a patient's prior medical, developmental, surgical, and/or traumatic history helps to establish the patient's current status and impairments. It is important to understand the patient's environment at home and school, including stairs, curbs, bathroom setup, and transportation needs. This information helps to establish what physical/performance and participation limitations a patient may encounter. A physical therapist should evaluate patient and caregiver motivation and understanding in order to establish baseline knowledge. This will provide a framework for education, motivation, and planning. Parent and patient understanding of diagnosis and plan, anticipated outcomes of surgery/radiation, understanding of rehabilitation commitment for optimal outcome, past response to painful experiences (trauma, surgery, change), past response to "hard work" expectations, family dynamics, and relationships should all be considered.

Physical examination is the foundation of the physical therapist evaluation. A thorough examination is critical to measure baseline and subsequent changes throughout the diagnosis and survivorship experience. Physical examination includes integumentary (sensation, vascular integrity, edema, old scars), location of tumor, posture of extremity, range of motion of involved and uninvolved extremities, strength of involved and uninvolved extremities, functional mobility, balance, and gait: assistive devices, weight-bearing status (per orthopedic oncologist), and fitness.

Plan is established with consideration of scheduled systemic control (chemotherapy) and/or local control (surgery/radiation). Physical therapists determine the immediate need for home exercise programs, gait training and assistive devices, weight-bearing status (per orthopedic oncologist), and supportive orthotics (hand/foot splints, knee immobilizers, slings, kinesio tape). They may also connect the patient with a prosthetics, if amputation or rotationplasty is indicated. In addition, the physical therapist determines and plans for future needs that may arise at different phases of medical or surgical intervention and survivorship.

PHYSICAL THERAPY EVALUATION

Tumor Location

Recent Imaging Reviewed by Medical Team

- ☐ X-Ray
- ☐ MRI
- ☐ CT
- ☐ PET
- ☐ Bone Scan

Care Team Rounds Comments

Precautions and Contraindications

- ☐ Weightbearing
- ☐ ROM
- ☐ Strengthening
- ☐ No shearing forces
- ☐ None
- ☐ Other

Access

- ☐ None
- ☐ Port
- ☐ Broviac
- ☐ PICC
- ☐ Peripheral IV

Diagnosis

- ☐ Osteosarcoma
- ☐ Ewing's Sarcoma
- ☐ Desmoid Tumor
- ☐ Synovial Sarcoma
- ☐ Soft Tissue Sarcoma
- ☐ Undifferentiated Sarcoma
- ☐ Osteoid Osteoma
- ☐ Pathological Fracture
- ☐ Undiagnosed
- ☐ Other

Chemotherapy

- ☐ Ifosfamide
- ☐ Doxorubicin
- ☐ Vincristine
- ☐ Cyclophosphamide
- ☐ Actinomycin
- ☐ Etoposide
- ☐ Cisplatin
- ☐ Methotrexate
- ☐ None
- ☐ Other

Surgical History

Procedure	Yes	Date	Comments
Biopsy	☐		
Tumor Resection	☐		
Limb sparing	☐		
Endoprothesis Placement	☐		
Amputation	☐		
Rotationplasty	☐		
Lung Tissue Resection	☐		
Wound Revision	☐		
Central Line Placement	☐		
Central Line Removal	☐		
Other	☐		
Other	☐		

Fig. 16.3 Standardized Physical Therapy patient evaluation form used at Children's National Medical Center. The use of standardized forms allows for rapid collection of reproducible data, which can be easily done electronically, and can facilitate communication with other therapists and providers. This data can be used for research and outcomes analysis

Radiation History

Location	Yes	Type	Dosage	Date	Comments
Tumor	☐				
Lung	☐				
Other	☐				
Other	☐				

Known Late Effects

Subjective (free text)

Current Level of Function

Therapy Services:

☐ None	☐ 1x/week
☐ Outpatient PT	☐ 2x/week
☐ Outpatient OT	☐ 3x/week
☐ Seen by PT during inpatient admissions	☐ 2x/month
☐ Seen by OT during inpatient admissions	☐ 1x/month
	☐ As needed

Equipment:

☐ Knee Immobilizer	☐ Bilateral Crutches
☐ Elbow Immobilizer	☐ Single Left Crutch
☐ Ankle Immobilizer	☐ Single Right Crutch
☐ Cast	☐ Single Point Cane
☐ Hinged Knee Brace	☐ Quad Cane
☐ AFO	☐ Bilateral Loftstrand Crutches
☐ FRC Splint	☐ Single Left Loftstrand Crutch
☐ Hinged Elbow Brace	☐ Single Right Loftstrand Crutch
☐ Ultraflex	☐ Anterior Rolling Walker
☐ Above Knee Prosthesis	☐ Standard Walker
☐ Below Knee Prosthesis	☐ Posterior Walker
☐ Upper Extremity Prosthesis	☐ Rollator
☐ Other	☐ Roll-a-bout
	☐ Other

Fig. 16.3 (continued)

Gait Deviations

SWING	RIGHT	LEFT	COMMENT
Circumduction	☐	☐	
Toe drag	☐	☐	
Hip hike	☐	☐	
Steppage	☐	☐	
Shuffling	☐	☐	

STANCE	RIGHT	LEFT	COMMENT
Foot flat	☐	☐	
Foot slap	☐	☐	
Toe first	☐	☐	
Pronation	☐	☐	
Supination	☐	☐	
In-toeing	☐	☐	
Out-toeing	☐	☐	
Excessive knee flexion	☐	☐	
Buckling	☐	☐	
Genu recurvatum	☐	☐	
Trendelenberg	☐	☐	
Decreased trailing limb	☐	☐	
Decreased weightbearing	☐	☐	
Decreased stance time	☐	☐	
Decreased step length	☐	☐	
Decreased push-off	☐	☐	

Fig. 16.3 (continued)

TRUNK/UPPER EXTREMITY	RIGHT	LEFT	COMMENT
Increased lateral flexion	☐	☐	
Increased forward flexion	☐	☐	
Increased trunk rotation	☐	☐	
Decreased trunk rotation	☐	☐	
Decreased arm swing	☐	☐	
High guard	☐	☐	

Left Upper Extremity

LEFT	WNL	Active	Passive	MMT	Pain	Comments
Shoulder Flexion	☐	#	#	#	☐	
Shoulder Extension	☐	#	#	#	☐	
Shoulder Abduction	☐	#	#	#	☐	
Shoulder External Rotation	☐	#	#	#	☐	
Shoulder Internal Rotation	☐	#	#	#	☐	
Elbow Flexion	☐	#	#	#	☐	
Elbow Extension	☐	#	#	#	☐	
Forearm Supination	☐	#	#	#	☐	
Forearm Pronation	☐	#	#	#	☐	
Wrist Flexion	☐	#	#	#	☐	
Wrist Extension	☐	#	#	#	☐	
Wrist Radial Deviation	☐	#	#	#	☐	
Wrist Ulnar Deviation	☐	#	#	#	☐	

RIGHT Upper Extremity

RIGHT	WNL	Active	Passive	MMT	Pain	Comments
Shoulder Flexion	☐	#	#	#	☐	
Shoulder Extension	☐	#	#	#	☐	
Shoulder Abduction	☐	#	#	#	☐	
Shoulder External Rotation	☐	#	#	#	☐	
Shoulder Internal Rotation	☐	#	#	#	☐	
Elbow Flexion	☐	#	#	#	☐	
Elbow Extension	☐	#	#	#	☐	
Forearm Supination	☐	#	#	#	☐	
Forearm Pronation	☐	#	#	#	☐	
Wrist Flexion	☐	#	#	#	☐	
Wrist Extension	☐	#	#	#	☐	

LEFT Lower Extremity

LEFT	WNL	Active	Passive	MMT	Pain	Comments
Hip Flexion	☐	#	#	#	☐	
Hip Extension	☐	#	#	#	☐	
Hip Abduction	☐	#	#	#	☐	
Hip Adduction	☐	#	#	#	☐	
Hip External Rotation	☐	#	#	#	☐	
Hip Internal Rotation	☐	#	#	#	☐	
Knee Flexion	☐	#	#	#	☐	
Knee Extension	☐	#	#	#	☐	
Ankle Dorsiflexion	☐	#	#	#	☐	
Ankle Plantarflexion	☐	#	#	#	☐	
Ankle Inversion	☐	#	#	#	☐	
Ankle Eversion	☐	#	#	#	☐	

Fig. 16.3 (continued)

RIGHT Lower Extremity

RIGHT	WNL	Active	Passive	MMT	Pain	Comments
Hip Flexion	☐	#	#	#	☐	
Hip Extension	☐	#	#	#	☐	
Hip Abduction	☐	#	#	#	☐	
Hip Adduction	☐	#	#	#	☐	
Hip External Rotation	☐	#	#	#	☐	
Hip Internal Rotation	☐	#	#	#	☐	
Knee Flexion	☐	#	#	#	☐	
Knee Extension	☐	#	#	#	☐	
Ankle Dorsiflexion	☐	#	#	#	☐	
Ankle Plantarflexion	☐	#	#	#	☐	
Ankle Inversion	☐	#	#	#	☐	
Ankle Eversion	☐	#	#	#	☐	

Bony Concerns

	Present	Comment
AvascularNecrosis	☐	
Decreased Bony Density	☐	
Leg Length Discrepancy	☐	
Pathological Fracture	☐	
Stress Fracture	☐	
Other	☐	

Soft Tissue Observations

	Present	Comment
Atrophy	☐	
Edema	☐	
Muscle Asymmetry Left to Right	☐	
Muscle Asymmetry Proximal to Distal	☐	
Incisions/Scars	☐	
Soft Tissue Restrictions	☐	

Neuromuscular System:

Cardiopulmonary System:

Recommendations

☐ HEP
☐ Continue Outpatient PT/OT
☐ Initiate Outpatient PT/OT
☐ Return to Outpatient PT/OT
☐ Follow-up at next scheduled Sarcoma Clinic visit

Fig. 16.3 (continued)

16.7 Physical Therapy Intervention

Physical therapists follow patients during chemotherapy and/or radiation for:

- Individualized conditioning programs
- Strengthening, ROM, cardiovascular/endurance/fitness training
- Reinforcement of active participation and expectations
- Preoperative outpatient consult, as needed, if poor tolerance to chemotherapy regimen

Physical therapists optimize function postsurgically to assist with safe return to the home environment, postsurgical healing/wound management, and pain management. Acute postsurgical physical therapy intervention includes:

- Bed mobility/transfers
- Ambulation with ordered weight-bearing status per orthopedic oncologist
- Assistive device and/or wheelchair prescription and training
- Range of motion as cleared by orthopedic oncologist
- Isometric strengthening, active-assisted range of motion, active range of motion and/or resisted exercise (per orthopedic oncologist)
- Prevention of deep vein thrombosis and impairments in uninvolved extremities
- Edema management
- Sensory assessment and education
- Home exercise program
- Assessment if inpatient acute care rehabilitation is indicated—PM&R
- Planning for outpatient therapies as indicated

Physical therapy intervention continues during inpatient admissions and scheduled outpatient appointments:

- Wound healing/management
- Edema management
- Initiation of ROM/strengthening as cleared by orthopedic oncologist
- Gait training/progression
- Prevention/surveillance of secondary complications
  - Chemotherapy and/or surgically induced neuropathies
  - Neurovascular complications
- Individualized conditioning program
- Cardiovascular/endurance/fitness training
- Reinforcement of active participation and expectations
- Education of therapeutic techniques and progression
- Discontinuation of supportive devices, as appropriate
- Expectations of ROM progression and importance of wound healing
- Progression of isometric, concentric, eccentric, and functional strengthening
- Education of functional ROM goals
- Postamputation desensitization and limb shaping
- Prosthetic preparation, training, and management

16.8   Surgery: Functional Considerations

Local control (surgical and radiation) options are often determined by the location and size of tumor, the involvement of surrounding soft tissue, muscle, and neurovascular structures, as well as the patient and family's expectation and motivation for functional and recreational outcomes. A physical therapist can assist with the plan regarding patient and family expectations of outcomes and can advocate between medical and surgical teams and the patient to assist with optimal selection of surgical techniques. Surgical interventions include:

- Limb salvage
  - Local tumor resection (soft tissue)
  - Wedge resection (bone)
  - Endoprosthesis, allograph, autograph
  - Rotationplasty
- Amputation

When selecting surgical intervention, limb salvage procedures should provide function equal to amputation and survival rates should be no worse [19–21]. Active discussion and decision-making is a team-effort between the patient, family, orthopedic oncologist, oncologist, and physical therapist. Psychological readiness is assessed throughout the planning process through education and discussion of expectations. Physical therapists tailor exercises during the preoperative phase to prepare patients for surgery and specifically to prepare for postoperative success related to planned surgical intervention.

Postoperative considerations and expectations vary with each surgical technique:

- Local tumor resection (soft tissue)
  - Pros: minimal restrictions postoperatively
  - Cons: soft tissue, myofascial, and wound-healing restrictions
- Wedge resection
  - Pros: bone intact, full functional mobility
  - Cons: non-weight bearing until bone fully healed, activity restrictions
- Endoprosthesis, allograft, autograft
  - Pros: intact limb, end-bearing sensation, proprioception, expandable
  - Cons: leg length discrepancies, wound healing, activity restrictions, prolonged use of assistive devices
- Rotationplasty
  - Pros: intact functional joint (knee or hip) with proprioception, full functional mobility with appropriate prosthesis
  - Cons: cosmetics, wound healing, delayed weight bearing with nonunion
- Amputation
  - Pros: functional mobility with appropriate prosthesis based on amputation level, early weight bearing
  - Cons: loss of limb, phantom limb sensation, prolonged use of assistive devices

16.9   Benefits to Multidisciplinary Care

Limited data and standardization of care exist for the rehabilitation management of patients diagnosed with sarcomas [22–24]. Therefore, strong relationships, communication, and collaboration between physical and occupational therapists with medical and surgical oncologists are critical to the safe and effective treatment of this unique population. In a multidisciplinary model, physical therapists are active in the patient's care early on and provide preventative and preparatory guidance (Table 16.3).

Having therapists involved in the early phases of diagnosis and planning assists in effective communication among the team members. Physical therapy sessions require a significant amount of one-on-one time with patients and families, and the well-informed physical therapist can establish stronger bonds and provide realistic approaches and expectations to the patient and families. Physical therapists involved in specialized clinics have increased depth of understanding and knowledge related to the patient's condition and specialized treatment approaches.

Multidisciplinary clinics provide a "one-stop shop" for patients with sarcomas and their families. Because the patient meets with medical, surgical, and rehabilitation specialists in one visit, it prevents the need of juggling multiple appointments within an already busy schedule. Families report satisfaction with the team approach and gain confidence in the collaborative environment.

Table 16.3 Factors influencing patient rehabilitation potential	
	• Location of tumor
	• Size of tumor
	• Involvement of surrounding soft tissue, muscle, and neurovascular structures
	• Radiation and surgical options
	• Medical management
	• Age
	• Patient's general medical condition, fitness, and activity level
	• Family and patient knowledge of disease/treatment options
	• Family and patient expectations
	• Family and patient motivation and psychological acceptance
	• Distance from treatment center
	• Insurance/access
	• Psychosocial issues of patient and family
	• Knowledge and skill of the therapist and prosthetist and/or orthotist

16.10 Patient Case one

16.10.1 Clinical Perspective

The patient is a 15-year-old cheerleader diagnosed with distal femur osteosarcoma. She was followed by physical therapy during inpatient chemotherapy admissions, but surgery was performed at an outside hospital. During surgery, injury occurred to the femoral nerve with a subsequent neuropathic foot. At the outside hospital, the patient was provided with off-the-counter ankle-foot orthosis (AFO) and knee immobilizer postoperatively. Upon discharge from the acute setting, the patient initiated outpatient physical therapy services near her home and presented with anterior knee wound dehiscence requiring revision and delay in chemotherapy regimen. While awaiting healing for resumption of chemotherapy, the patient did not receive physical therapy services, and the previously prescribed AFO no longer fit. Upon return to an inpatient stay, the patient presented with a significant plantarflexion contracture and decreased knee flexion. At this time, the physical therapist and medical team transitioned the patient to the care of outpatient physical therapy services within the multidisciplinary team at treating hospital. The patient was fitted with a custom resting foot splint, and the physical therapist collaborated with a vendor to obtain low-load prolonged-duration bracing for knee flexion and ankle dorsiflexion. The patient received physical therapy treatment 3–5x/week during inpatient chemotherapies and 1x/week outpatient between admissions and after completion of chemotherapy. The patient attends the multidisciplinary clinic to meet with oncologists, orthopedic oncologists, general surgeons, and physical therapists for the management of metastatic disease, and physical therapy intervention and plan are reassessed and modified based on patient and medical goals.

16.10.2 Family Perspective

"It Takes A Village!" My granddaughter was diagnosed with osteosarcoma September 2012. Almost immediately, the process was initiated. The team was identified, the plan established, and the journey began.

My granddaughter's regimen consisted of an aggressive chemotherapy treatment to shrink the tumor on her left femur. Successful shrinkage of the tumor was realized in December 2012. The next phase of the process began—surgery to remove the tumor and femur, then placement of the endoprosthesis. The team guided her successfully through another phase of her treatment.

She then continued on to her next phase of chemotherapy and weekly physical rehabilitative therapy sessions. The physical therapy sessions consisted of rehabilitative work that would allow her to function with her endoprosthesis as close to normal as possible.

We attempted to use a physical therapist closer to our home: however, we missed the team and their collaborative interaction. The trek to Children's every Monday for rehabilitative therapy is well worth it.

Battling cancer is not an easy journey. Remaining positive despite the ongoing obstacles can cause you to become discouraged. It truly helps to have a multidisciplinary team of medical staff at your disposal. So, yes! It truly takes a village!!

16.11 Patient Case two

16.11.1 Clinical Perspective

The patient is an 11-year-old soccer player diagnosed with distal femur osteosarcoma. He initially presented with recent history of knee pain and swelling. He was evaluated by pediatric oncologist with presumed osteosarcoma. The patient presented with difficulty ambulating due to pain; therefore, the oncologist contacted physical therapy who provided education and gait training for joint protection. The patient met with the physical therapist, in addition to the orthopedic oncologist and full multidisciplinary team, a few days later to begin medical and surgical planning. Physical therapists treated patient during chemotherapy admissions providing education regarding the importance of range of motion, strength, and cardiovascular exercise prior to surgery and to prevent secondary complications due to chemotherapy. The patient underwent wide radial resection of distal femur tumor with expandable endoprosthesis placement, and physical therapists provided postoperative care including gait training, isometric knee/hip exercises, and active ankle and foot exercises. Unfortunately, the patient had postoperative delayed wound closure, skin integrity disruptions, and decreased sensation and motor function to foot and ankle. Physical therapists assisted with custom-fabricated resting foot splint and collaborated with wound care nursing to aide in optimizing wound healing. The patient was scheduled for outpatient physical therapy 2x/week and seen 3–5x/week during postoperative chemotherapy admissions for range of motion, strengthening, and progression of functional mobility and gait. The physical therapist coordinated with an orthotist to provide the patient with an orthotic to assist with functional foot dorsiflexion and to provide support during standing and gait activities. Once chemotherapy was completed, physical therapy continued at 2x/week frequency, and the patient will continue to be followed during outpatient multidisciplinary clinic.

16.11.2 Family Perspective

Our second appointment with my son's oncologist was overwhelming. The doctor walked into the room with ten people in tow. He brought his fellow, nurse coordinator, nurse practitioner, two surgeons, another oncologist, physical therapist, child life specialist, social worker, and psychologist. The following week we also met the nutritionist. Aside from the fact that all these people could barely fit into our examining room, I had a hard time processing who they were and why they were there. I remember pulling aside one of the nurses after the appointment and asking why the second oncologist was there. But as the weeks went by, I realized that this was a carefully assembled team, and one that worked well together. I had expected most of the people who directed my son's treatment, such as the oncologist, surgeon, and nurses, and was pleasantly surprised to discover how many people were on board to help with issues as they arose. When my son had difficulty eating, the nutritionist stepped in. When he developed anxiety over so many needles, the psychologist and child life specialist were right there.

The physical therapist emerged as one of the key individuals on the team. My son had osteosarcoma in his right femur, so from his first visit to the clinic, he was having trouble walking. She outfitted him immediately with crutches, then began a pre-surgery program to get him in the best physical shape possible before surgery. Once surgery took place, she helped him figure out how to move safely while his leg was immobilized. PT continued both inpatient and outpatient for the rest of chemotherapy.

As I write this, chemotherapy has ended. 5 days after it ended, my son fell and fractured his arm. Once again, the team approach was invaluable. Nurses and fellows helped arrange orthopedic appointments, and physical therapy helped him figure out how to move safely. Meanwhile, the oncologist is planning for posttreatment scans, the surgeon is preparing us for limb-lengthening procedures, the nutritionist is working with us on transitioning to a healthy diet, and the psychologist is helping my son with the emotional side of restarting school.

The most comforting piece for me as a parent has been knowing that not only are there all of these people to support my son, but they all talk to each other. So when I approached the nutritionist shortly before surgery to discuss my son's weight, she already knew how much he had gained recently and whether or not he had any mouth sores. Similarly, when discussing presurgical concerns with the physical therapist, she knew what the surgeon expected before and after surgery and tailored my son's program to meet that.

Certainly, it hasn't been a panacea. We've been frustrated with everyone at least once. Parents often have an inherent fear of contradicting medical professionals, especially when those same professionals are saving one's child's life! I remember very clearly one afternoon when the nurse coordinator said to me, "You'd tell us if there's something that's not working, right?" Not, "You'd tell me," but, "You'd tell us." As a team, they wanted to do things well, and they wanted to know whether or not their actions were working. And that comment reaffirmed just how effective our multidisciplinary sarcoma team is!

16.12 Barriers to Multidisciplinary Care

Multidisciplinary clinic visits often compliment ongoing or phasic physical or occupational therapy services. Due to space and time constraints, physical therapy intervention within the clinic setting is limited to evaluation, assessment, updating plan of care, and home exercise prescription. The physical therapist serves as a contact person for therapists providing ongoing treatment for these patients.

Additionally, due to the nature of multidisciplinary clinics, physical therapy goals and intervention may not be the top priority at certain phases of diagnosis and treatment. For example, if a patient has new onset or recurrent disease, the family and medical team's focus may be on the establishment or modification of medical, surgical, or radiation plan of care. Physical therapy goals may be secondary or tertiary, but the presence of a physical therapist to recognize the appropriateness of redirection of efforts and focus is important.

Insurance and reimbursement can affect the patient's access to multidisciplinary care. Physical therapists and physicians must advocate for coverage of services. Additionally, in general, multidisciplinary clinics versus individual treatment sessions yield lesser rates of productive, billable time for treating therapists. It is important to recognize the immeasurable benefits to teamwork and collaboration and the cost-effectiveness of decreased unbillable time for communication and planning without the presence of a multidisciplinary environment.

16.13 Challenges without Multidisciplinary Teams

Multidisciplinary clinics are growing throughout the United States and the world, although, the majority of centers currently do not benefit from this model. Due to the decreased number of orthopedic oncology surgical centers compared to cancer centers, physical and occupational therapists often encounter patients at a variety and later stage of treatment. Depending on the center, therapists often do not see patients with sarcomas until after surgical intervention and have reported decreased communication of indications and restrictions for intervention [23].

Oncologists, versus orthopedic oncologists, are often the referring physician for therapy prescription and often have decreased depth of understanding regarding weight-bearing, range of motion, and activity restrictions. Physical and occupational therapists have limitations to safe intervention without clear indications and restrictions. Additionally, the management of sarcomas is not included in entry-level physical or occupational therapy education. Therefore, therapists working with patients at outside facilities are often unfamiliar with the medical and surgical considerations unique to this population. To date, only one article is published related to standardization of rehabilitation after limb salvage surgery [22].

In many pediatric centers, waitlists for outpatient services are significant. Patients that require outpatient therapies may wait excessive periods for a physical or occupational therapy evaluation, and patients may be discharged from therapy due to frequent no shows and cancellations due to chemotherapy and other admissions or appointments. In addition, families may need to travel for healthcare appointments and may have multiple physical therapists and/or occupational therapists at each phase of treatment.

With the lack of interhospital medical record access, therapists have challenges obtaining surgical and follow-up reports from orthopedic oncology, medical oncology, and general surgery physicians. With the increasing demands of productivity within the healthcare system, therapists experience time constraints and therefore decreased ability to contact and communicate with outside providers.

The application of multidisciplinary clinics aids in the growth of understanding of physical and occupational therapists. Through intrahospital, interhospital, and professional organizations, education is improving to increase the knowledge of professionals that may interact with the sarcoma populations [23]. Multidisciplinary care approach to patients with sarcomas should become the standard of care to provide a higher level of quality, consistency, functional, and quality of life outcomes in this uniquely challenging population.

References

1. Geller D, Gorlick R. Osteosarcoma: a review of diagnosis, management, and treatment strategies. Clin Adv Hematol Oncol. 2010;8(10):705–18.
2. Nagarajan R, Kamruzzaman A, Ness K, et al. Twenty year follow-up of survivors of childhood osteosarcoma: a report from the childhood cancer survivor study (CCSS). Cancer. 2011;117(3):625–34.
3. World Health Organization: towards a common language for functioning, disability, and health. http://www.who.int/classifications/icf/icfbeginnersguide.pdf
4. Hudson MM, Mertens AC, Yasui Y, et al. Health status of adult long-term survivors of childhood cancer: a report from the childhood cancer survivor study. JAMA. 2003;290:1583–92.
5. Ness K, Mertens A, Hudson M, Wall M, et al. Limitations on physical performance and daily activities among long-term survivors of childhood cancer. Ann Intern Med. 2005;143: 639–47.
6. Nagarajan R, Clohisy DR, Neglia JP, et al. Function and quality-of-life of survivors of pelvic and lower extremity osteosarcoma and Ewing's sarcoma: the childhood cancer survivor study. Br J Cancer. 2004;91:1858–65.
7. Punyko JA, Gurney JB, Scott Baker K, et al. Physical impairment and social adaptation in adult survivors of childhood and adolescent rhabdomyosarcoma: a report from the childhood cancer survivors study. Psychooncology. 2006;16:26–37.
8. Ness K, Hudson MM, Ginsberg JP, et al. Physical performance limitations in the childhood cancer survivor study cohort. J Clin Oncol. 2009;27:2382–9.
9. Bekkering WP, Vliet Vlieland TP, Koopman HM, et al. Functional ability and physical activity in children and young adults after limbsalvage or ablative surgery for lower extremity bone tumors. J Surg Oncol. 2011;103(3):276–82.
10. Bekkering WP, Vliet Vlieland TP, Koopman HM, et al. Quality of life in young patients after bone tumor surgery around the knee joint and comparison with healthy controls. Pediatr Blood Cancer. 2010;54(5):738–45.
11. Oeffinger KC, Mertens AC, Sklar CA, et al. Chronic health conditions in adult survivors of childhood cancer. N Engl J Med. 2006;355(15):1572–82.
12. Tsauo JY, Li WC, Yung RS. Functional outcomes after endoprosthetic knee reconstruction following resection of osteosarcoma near the knee. Disabil Rehabil. 2006;28(1):61–6.
13. Buchner M, Zeilang F, Bernd L. Medial gastrocnemius muscle flap in limb-sparing surgery of malignant bone tumors of the proximal tibia: mid-term results in 25 patients. Ann Plast Surg. 2003;51:266–72.
14. Gerber LH, Hoffman K, Chaudhry U, et al. Functional outcomes and life satisfaction in long-term survivors of pediatric sarcomas. Arch Phys Med Rehabil. 2006;87(12):1611–17.
15. Norkin CC, Levangie PK. Joint structure and function: a comprehensive analysis. Philadelphia: F.A. Davis Company; 1992.
16. Carty CP, Dickinson IC, Watts MC, Crawford RW, Steadman P. Impairment following limb salvage procedures for bone sarcoma. Knee. 2009;16(5):405–8.

17. Marchese V, Spearing E, Callaway L, Rai S, et al. Relationships among range of motion, functional mobility, and quality of life in children and adolescents after limb-sparing surgery for lower-extremity sarcoma. Pediatr Phys Ther. 2006;18(4):238–44.
18. Tseng-Tien H, Ness K. Exercise interventions in children with cancer: a review. Int J Pediatr. 2011;2011:461512.
19. Pardasaney PK, Sullivan PE, Portney LG, Mankin HJ. Advantage of limb salvage over amputation for proximal lower extremity tumors. Clin Orthop Relat Res. 2006;444:201–8.
20. DiCaprio MR, Friedlaender GE. Malignant bone tumors: limb-sparing versus amputation. J Am Acad Orthop Surg. 2003;11:25–37.
21. Gupta SK, Alassaf N, Harrop AR, Kiefer GN. Principles of rotationplasty. J Am Acad Orthop Surg. 2012;20(10):657–67.
22. Shehadeh A, Dahleh M, Salem A, Sarhan Y, Sultan I, Henshaw R, Aboulafia A. Standardization of rehabilitation after limb salvage surgery for sarcomas improves patients' outcome. Hematol Oncol Stem Cell Ther. 2013;6(3):105–11.
23. O'Mara K, Miale S. Establishing guidelines for safe and effective treatment of pediatric sarcoma survivors: a mission of the pediatric oncology special interest group. Rehabil Oncol. 2016;34:117–9.
24. Corr AM, Liu W, Bischop, et al. Feasibility and functional outcomes of children and adolescents undergoing preoperative chemotherapy prior to limb-sparing procedure or amputation. Rehabil Oncol. 2017;35;38–44.

Howard Rosenthal and Kimberly Haynes

The treatment of bone and soft tissue tumors is a highly specialized field requiring a multidisciplinary team approach. Personnel from a variety of disciplines are needed including medical, nursing, social work, case management, psychology, and rehabilitation. Due to the rarity of the tumor types, and the limited numbers of centers nationwide, even worldwide, this team approach must be able to provide care that is not available through routine or normal medical venues [1]. The lead physician, typically the orthopedic oncologist, must provide leadership and guidance to a group of medical personnel with a varied medical background and practice history. Unlike most other oncologic specialties, whereby the medical oncologist is the team leader, in musculoskeletal oncology, it is most commonly the surgeon who provides that direction and decision-making concerning total care. This total care approach must be delivered in a manner that is understandable to the patient and family, seamless with regard to the physicians, and effective in reference to the disease process. An integral part of the team is the advanced practice providers (APPs), which include advanced practice nurses (APRNs) and physician assistants (PAs) [2]. The APRNs are nurses with an advanced degree such as a master's or doctorate degree in nursing. Nurses with advanced degrees can be a clinical nurse specialist (CNS), nurse practitioner (NP), certified registered nurse anesthetist (CRNA), or nurse-midwife (CNM) depending on the education track followed. This chapter will focus on the roles and responsibilities of the clinical nurse specialists, nurse practitioners, physician assistants, and certified registered nurse anesthetists and describe the treatment and care they provide sarcoma patients. Other personnel experienced in the care and treatment of sarcoma patients include physical therapists, occupational therapists, registered nurses, case managers, social workers, clinical psychologists, athletic trainers, and certified genetic counselors. We will also discuss how the

H. Rosenthal, M.D., F.A.C.S. (✉) • K. Haynes, O.N.C.
University of Kansas Cancer Center, Sarcoma Center, Overland Park, KS, USA
e-mail: hrosenthal@kumc.edu

© Springer International Publishing Switzerland 2017   335
R.M. Henshaw (ed.), *Sarcoma*, DOI 10.1007/978-3-319-43121-5_17

office staff work in conjunction with our providers and make our office run smoothly. We will focus on our experience and successes over a 20-year period as well as provide feedback from patients and primary care physicians and referring other physicians, all that are considered integral parts of the sarcoma team. This feedback has enabled us to create an efficient and streamlined center, providing care to over 3500 patients per year with bone or soft tissue tumors, both benign and malignant.

The treatment and care of the patient with a bone or soft tissue tumor begins well before their arrival at the orthopedic oncologist's office. The presence of a mass or tumor, especially in younger patients, places the patient and his/her family in a very fearful position. The interval duration between the initial visit to the primary referring physician's office, to the time it may take to obtain various radiological scans, and the additional time for ultimate consultation with the orthopedic oncologist contributes to the stress and anxiety regarding the sarcoma diagnosis. That stress extends beyond the patient and direct family. Imagine, for example, the fear, stress, and difficulty from the primary care physician or referring physician standpoint with regard to informing the patient that they are going to be seen by an orthopedic oncologist. Most primary care physicians have known the patient and/or family for quite some time prior to the presentation of the tumor. The patient often presents with nonspecific complaints, possibly aches or pains, many incidentally related to a sports injury, and no other constitutional or laboratory studies to indicate neoplasm. Frequently, a preliminary diagnosis of sports injury or hematoma and other benign nonneoplastic conditions is given initially. Persistence of pain over an extended period of time prompts the patient to return to their primary care physician who may send the patient to the physical therapist for, once again, the diagnosis of sports-related injury. Therefore, once the presence of a mass or persistence of symptoms prompts more in-depth physical examination or radiographic review, weeks to months may have elapsed. The physician's emotional discomfort with his own role in this delay may be perceived by the patient, feeding into the patient's own internal fears. Thus, the treatment for the patient with sarcoma could be said to really start with the treatment of the referring physician. Whereby this may be through educational activities or through emotional and professional support, it must be to the benefit and welfare of the patient. This treatment plan is the responsibility of the entire orthopedic oncology team, from the surgeon to the front office staff, nurses, medical assistants, and even billing personnel. This responsibility and care enhances and may even improve the oncologic outcome of these patients in need.

The rarity of sarcoma poses special problems to medical practitioners as well as to patients and their families. The paucity of medical information, lack of familiarity with the disease, and discomfort of treating cancer patients all play a role in the care of sarcoma patients. Very few sarcoma support groups are available, and it remains one of the few diseases not discussed on television or other media. Many sarcomas occur in the early decades of life, and the additional stresses to the family as well as loss of control of the health of the family also play a role in the care of the patient. The advanced practice providers (APPs) and entire team must work in a uniform fashion, with clearly outlined goals and approaches, individualized to the patient, taking into account all of the above factors [5]. These APPs help navigate the patient through the treatment process. They translate to the patient the role of each of the providers and their treatment recommendations. Advanced practice providers ensure that the patient does in fact follow through with the recommended treatments, procedures, appointments, and myriad tests that are required during the treatment plan. Typically, once the patient presents to the treating orthopedic oncologist, these various procedures and tests move quite promptly, often faster than the patient may have time to absorb the information and necessities presented to them. Fear can become an inhibitor, which can significantly impact treatment. Advanced practice providers help the patient understand the need for consultations with other members of the sarcoma team such as the medical oncologist, radiation oncologist, interventional radiologist, and even geneticists, pathologists, dieticians, and psychologists. The hospital personnel who perform various scheduling of procedures also have an impact on the patient's treatment.

The patient and family members entrust the APRNs and PAs to guide them through the process of care and treatment. Advanced practice providers must be fluent in all aspects of care and be able to educate and delineate to the patient the reasoning behind treatments. Reinforcing the logic of order of treatment plans and the biology of the tumor itself help ensure follow up on a long-term basis. Most APRNs and PAs, who work in conjunction with an orthopedic oncologist, are trained by on-the-job experience or through preceptorship type of practices, serving for long periods of time, with an orthopedic oncologist. Advanced practice providers must be able to communicate with all other members of the team, physicians and therapists, in order to ensure timely and appropriate treatment and to make sure some treatments such as staging studies and surveillance scans are not duplicated or deficient. This active communication serves to improve patient outcomes on the basis that, firstly, appointments, tests, and treatments are not missed due to miscommunication and, secondly, the patient feels as if he/she is a partner in the treatment plan. This integration of care has been shown to improve overall outcomes.

17.1 Historical Aspects of Orthopedic Nursing and Advanced Practice Nursing

Orthopedic nursing can trace its roots to Victorian England, in a village near London, called Baschurch. The specialty's matriarch, Dame Agnes Hunt (December 31, 1866 to July 24, 1948), is generally recognized and accepted as the first orthopedic nurse. As a child, she had developed secondary septic arthritis of the hip following a bout of septicemia. She trained as a nurse at the Royal Alexandria Hospital in Rhyl, a seaside town in Wales, and, soon thereafter, opened a convalescent home for crippled children at the Florence House in Baschurch, England. She espoused the concepts of "open air therapy and happiness," encouraging natural, clean air and nature to assist with the healing of disease. She taught that "no nurse is worth her salt if she has not the joy of life within her and the power of being able to share it with her patients." In 1901, she sought treatment for her own septic arthritis from Sir Robert Jones. She had invited him to the convalescent home which he visited on so many occasions that he built an operating room and introduced the use of diagnostic X-rays in 1907 to be used in the diagnosis and treatment of orthopedic diseases. She devoted her entire nursing career to improving the lives of crippled children and those injured by the ravages of war. She was declared a Dame of the British Empire in 1926, the highest honor that could be awarded to a woman at that time. When asked what were the most important aspects of nursing, she replied, "Common sense, gentleness, and kindliness, and the power to give joy and hope to those who are suffering." Hunt died in 1948 at the age of 81. Her ashes were interred in the parish churchyard at Baschurch, where there is also a plaque inside the church, which reads "Reared in suffering thou shalt know how to solace others' woe. The reward of pain doth lie in the gift of sympathy."

17.1.1 Advanced Practice Providers

Advanced practice providers in the surgical oncology field will typically work alongside the physician, augmenting and ensuring continuity and access to the care required. Specifically, in the orthopedic oncology field, due to the rarity of the disease process itself, the APPs serve many purposes. Due to the educational backgrounds of these providers, they can be used as independent providers seeing new patients and established patients. They can work in the operating room as a first assist and, depending on the practice, can be billed as an assistant surgeon. APPs are educators of patients and staff. They are liaisons, researchers, consultants, expert clinicians, navigators, and leaders [8]. Due to the amount of information a patient receives at the initial visit, the APP will be able to reeducate and reinforce treatment recommendations for the patient throughout the course of therapy, ensure appropriate follow-up on tests and surgeries ordered, and provide education and support for the patient and family members. The APP will communicate with other members of the sarcoma team, including adult and pediatric medical and radiation oncologists, to ensure continuity of care.

The term advanced practice provider is a term used to describe APRNs (NP, CNS, CRNA) and physician assistants (PAs) who work in a clinic setting and/or hospital setting with a physician or group of physicians. Each advanced practice provider brings unique experience to the office practice. APRNs are registered nurses who have completed a master's or doctorate degree in nursing [3]. Doctorate degrees can be a PhD or a DNP (Doctorate of Nursing Practice). APRNs who work in an orthopedic oncology office would be a clinical nurse specialist (CNS) or a nurse practitioner (NP). Neither will have undergone specific class work training in orthopedic oncology but will have been trained on the job. Many will have had prior orthopedic experience and/or oncology experience. There is a difference between a CNS, NP, and PA with respect to their educational classwork and clinical settings.

Historically, the CNS emerged to fill the need for a clinical expert in the hospital setting caring for a specific population of patients. The National Association of Clinical Nurse Specialists website states "The essence of CNS practice is clinical nursing expertise in diagnosis and treatment to prevent, remediate, or alleviate illness and promote health with a defined specialty population-be that specialty broad or narrow, well established, or emerging. The roles of a CNS include expert clinician, consultant (systems and process analysis), educator, researcher, and leader (change agent)."

According to the American Association of Nurse Practitioners website "autonomously and in collaboration with health care professional and other individuals, NP's provide a full range of primary, acute and specialty health care services including: ordering, performing and interpreting diagnostic tests such as lab work and X-rays, diagnose and treat acute and chronic conditions such as diabetes, high blood pressure, infections, and injuries, prescribe medications and other treatments, manage patients overall care, provide counseling and educate patients on disease prevention and positive health and lifestyle choices."

A certified registered nurse anesthetist (CRNA) is also included in the term advanced practice provider. According to the American Association of Nurse Anesthetists (AANA) website "The requirements for becoming a Certified Registered Nurse Anesthetist (CRNA) mainly include having a bachelor's degree in nursing (or other appropriate baccalaureate degree), Registered Nurse licensure, a minimum of 1-year acute care experience (for example, ICU or ER), and the successful completion of both an accredited nurse anesthesia educational program and the national certification examination." Due to some of the surgical techniques and adjuvant treatments that are used during surgery, having an experienced CRNA working with the orthopedic oncologist provides the best and safest care possible. As with an NP, CNS, or PA, a CRNA who works with an orthopedic oncologist during surgery will have learned to care for patients on the job.

Working in conjunction with the surgeon and anesthesiologist, the CRNA must understand how the use of certain bone grafts and bone fillers affect the patient. For example, when bone cement (polymethyl methacrylate) is used to fill the defect in bone where the tumor was removed, the CRNA must be aware of the dangers of cement emboli, exothermic burn reactions, and even odors within the operating room that could cause morbidity to the patient and operating room personnel. Another example is the use of cryosurgery, or the instillation of liquid nitrogen in a tumor cavity. The CRNA needs to be aware of the risk of gas emboli, vascular insult, and even fracture in the patient undergoing cryosurgery. The ability to monitor for gas embolus and then act immediately and appropriately (or even prophylactically) is mandatory.

Communication between the surgeon, anesthesiologist, and CRNA should include directions concerning safety of the patient from a neoplastic standpoint. For example, a tumor located in the forearm might be able to be excised under a Bier block anesthetic. The CRNA must understand that the technique of exsanguination of the extremity prior to instilling the anesthetic agent could potentially spread tumor cells within the vascular tree, potentially resulting in metastatic disease. Therefore, this technique is to be avoided. However, no other specialty including routine orthopedics would a Bier block be contraindicated. Likewise, the prophylactic use of antibiotics is commonly under the purview of the CRNA, and, as important as this is in the limb preservation field, the timing of the administration of the antibiotic may need to be adjusted when infection lies in the differential diagnosis. As one can see, the CRNA must work in collaboration with the surgeon as a team member specific to the type of surgery performed by the orthopedic oncologist.

The American Academy of Physician Assistants states "A physician assistant (or PA) is a nationally certified and state-licensed medical professional. PAs practice medicine on healthcare teams with physicians and other providers. They practice and prescribe medication in all 50 states, the District of Columbia and all U.S. territories, with the exception of Puerto Rico." Physician assistant programs are approximately 26 months, and the course work will include basic sciences, behavioral sciences, and clinical medicine courses including chemistry, biology, microbiology, anatomy, and physiology. Physician assistants can take a medical history, conduct physical exams, diagnose and treat illnesses, order and interpret tests, develop treatment plans, counsel on preventive care, assist in surgery, write prescriptions, and make rounds in hospitals and nursing homes (AAPA website 2015). Over 2000 h of clinical rotations through a variety of settings will complete the training.

The role of advanced practice providers in the orthopedic practice is expanding. A commonly encountered model is a 1:1 ratio of orthopedic surgeons to nurse practitioners. Advanced practice registered nurses (APRNs) and physician assistants (PAs) may practice independently in some states seeing new patients and follow-up patients in the clinic depending on the state's statutes for APRNs and PAs, the nurse practice act for that state, and the patients' insurance. This model would increase patient volumes, reduce weight times, and improve patient satisfaction in a variety of private practice and academic practices. The APP can help overcome patient health education barriers as well as time constraints with regard to scheduling of appointments and surgical procedures. In addition, the use of APPs in the office can significantly diminish phone calls and visits to the emergency room by properly educating patients about symptoms and signs to be monitored. Advanced practice providers function in many roles and are highly important in the care and treatment of patients with sarcoma. Knowledge and skills are mainly obtained by on-the-job training. The benefits of having a knowledgeable APP to the physician and patients is great and can help with patient flow as well as patient and family education, making the patients' experience through a very trying time much easier.

17.1.2 Registered Nurse

The registered nurse is an integral part of the sarcoma team. At least one RN is needed in the office to answer patient phone calls, assist with surgery and radiology scheduling, and assist the physician and APP as needed. Some duties include triaging phone calls, calling results, discussing and answering postoperative care questions, and assisting with surgery scheduling including working with other surgical specialty offices to coordinate a combined surgery. Other duties include filling out FMLA forms and disability paperwork, entering surgery orders, and assisting preanesthesia testing nurses with obtaining cardiac clearances and outside lab work as needed. Ordering radiology testing and even calling for insurance authorizations may be needed. The registered nurse will also have learned about treating sarcomas on the job.

17.1.3 Allied Health Professionals

In our facility, the APRN leads a weekly sarcoma conference with the hospital staff to discuss the upcoming surgery schedule. The attendees include the hospital surgical floor nurse managers, social workers, case managers, operating room personnel, geneticists, and even dieticians. This meeting is a prospective planning meeting discussing the medical, social, emotional, and work-related situations that will impact on the patients' stay in the hospital as well at home when the patient is discharged. All providers who care for sarcoma patients should be knowledgeable about sarcomas and treatment. In much the same fashion that the oncologist's office creates an environment whereby the patient senses expertise and caring, the same goal and motif should be used during every aspect of that patient's care.

By attending this weekly sarcoma conference, nurse managers, social workers, case managers, and operating personnel are aware and prepared for any special needs of the patients and can proactively prepare so the patient can have an optimal surgical, hospital, and discharge experience. Many sarcoma patients undergo very intricate surgical procedures that require significant postoperative restrictions. Therefore, physical and occupational therapists may need extra training to care for these patients. By attending the multidisciplinary weekly meeting, the therapists can prepare for the patients' postoperative needs and can even meet patients before surgery and provide education on crutches, walkers, and other assistive devices that will aid the patient postoperatively. Another way to educate physical and occupational therapists is to invite them to observe during surgery and to shadow the surgeon in clinic. This helps promote a continuum of care for the patient.

Since every sarcoma patient will undergo multiple radiology scans throughout their lifetime, it is important to have radiologists and radiology technicians understand the importance of accurate scanning of these patients. A musculoskeletal radiologist is needed as well as trained radiology technicians. These providers need to know the rationale for the techniques used to scan tumors. The radiology technicians will encounter sarcoma patients frequently and will need education regarding moving and positioning patients pre and postoperatively. They need education regarding the importance of getting an accurate and complete scan of the patient's tumor or surgical site. For example, if a patient has a distal femoral or proximal tibia replacement prosthesis, the technologist must understand the importance of X-raying the entire prosthesis including the tips of the intramedullary stems. When a patient has a tumor around the knee, the technician can explain to the patient that a different type of MRI scan is performed when a patient has a tumor versus a meniscal tear. This knowledge helps the patient and family members feel comfortable that everyone involved in their care is competent.

This communication with all members of the team will certainly improve that care but will also encourage members of the team to be able to explain to the patient that they are aware of that particular patient's situation and that their concerns are being addressed individually. The physicians attend these meetings as well; however it is under the guidance of the APP to organize the plan of care. When all members of the treating team share an understanding of the patient's medical, social, and psychological situation, the ability for that team to deliver tailored care improves. The patient recognizes the team approach to the care and becomes more a part of that team, which also enhances the care as well as the compliance. As a side note, the involvement with the team, including the therapists and case managers, for example, also helps to encourage their personal involvement in each case as well.

An athletic trainer is another allied healthcare provider that may be included in the care of a sarcoma patient. It is not common for the sarcoma patient to require the services of an athletic trainer; however in the young, athletic patient, these services become quite valuable. Specifically, in orthopedics, athletic trainers can expand the scope of practice for the orthopedic sports medicine physician. While historically, the relationship between the physician and athletic trainer took place on the sports field, that relationship is expanding into the physician's office and physical therapist's office as well. Athletic trainers perform histories and physical examinations relative to the musculoskeletal system, evaluate for injuries, and recommend and implement treatment modalities including bracing, therapy, rehabilitation programs, education, and prevention. In the office setting, an athletic trainer can focus on those exercises that might suit a particular patient for a particular sport, both for the prevention of injury and the treatment of injury. In addition, the athletic trainer may work with the patient to enhance their skills at a particular sport by assessing posture, habits, energy expenditure, and other components of the activity.

The athletic trainer industry has already demonstrated significant growth in a very short period of time [9]. In 2006, approximately 34% of certified athletic trainers worked in the healthcare environment with the majority being in hospital settings and in the offices of orthopedic surgeons. According to the Bureau of Labor Statistics, athletic trainer employment is expected to increase by 24% between 2006 and 2016, much faster than the average for other occupations. The scope of practice now includes physical therapy offices, stand-alone offices, and sports teams.

Athletic trainers practice under state statutes, and these rules and regulations do vary by state. They are recognized as healthcare professionals, similar to physical and occupational therapists. They are included in the group of allied healthcare professionals who require licensure in at least 33 states. An additional ten states require abiding by regulations. This increased state regulation and licensure has advanced the professional and publics acceptance of the athletic trainer's role as a qualified healthcare provider. The athletic trainer becomes important in the orthopedic oncology world for a variety of reasons and in numerous situations. As many sarcoma patients and certainly patients with benign bone tumors are young and otherwise healthy, they are commonly involved in various sports activities. Since the treatment that the patient receives for that tumor will require abstention from most sports activities for a period of time, the patient will benefit from the involvement of the athletic trainer in the rehabilitation back to sports. With proper communication with the physician, the AT may initiate some therapies prior to, or even while the patient receives chemotherapy, such that by the end of treatment, the patient may resume those activities. If the surgical reconstruction requires the patient to alter their sports activities, the AT can assist in this fashion as well.

17.2   Phases of Treatment

The Sarcoma Center at the University of Kansas is an independent section within the department of orthopedics as well as the University of Kansas Cancer Center. The facility is an off-campus building within a university medical complex consisting of a medical office building and a hospital with full surgical services, radiology, pathology, and other ancillary services. The campus also houses an administration building and land for expansion. We are very accessible to a multistate region being located on an interstate highway and main thoroughfare. The Sarcoma Center is staffed with one physician whose sole practice is that of orthopedic oncology, a DNP clinical nurse specialist, a registered nurse, medical assistant, two front office employees, a business and practice manager, and a back office employee. In addition, the full staff of the orthopedic department and a sarcoma/breast cancer director maintain various presences within our facility. The accompanying hospital can accommodate all but the most difficult cases that might require ICU coverage.

The hospital was designed specifically for sarcoma surgery and treatment. Prior to treating our first patient, at this new facility, we met with every employee, from the directors to the food service and janitorial staff. In-services were held twice a week for several weeks in order to educate every employee about sarcoma and its treatment. The goal of these in-services was to ensure that any employee that might have contact with our patients would be able to assure that patient that the services rendered to the patient were to be delivered with the specific knowledge that it is tailored to the sarcoma patient. Even the diet that is ordered, the physical therapy they receive, and the cleanliness of the room is tailored specifically for sarcoma patients. It is our belief that in this fashion, while the patient arrives in fear and with lack of knowledge concerning their disease, they are being cared for by a team that is trained specifically in their disease. This gives the patient a better sense of well-being and security, and we believe that this translates into improved care and possibly even better survival. Our operating rooms are staffed with two scrub techs and two circulators for every case, and each is cleansed and sterilized immediately and fully with the closure of every case. Turnover time is less than 15 min. This allows for a very optimized and efficient system to be brought into play.

As mentioned earlier, the initial presentation of the patient with sarcoma actually begins long before the patient arrives at the orthopedic oncologist's office. Many times the patient may suffer an injury such as a fall or an athletic injury, complain of pain, and present to his/her primary care physician's office. During evaluation, various radiographic studies and examinations reveal the presence of a tumor. Given the rarity and concomitant lack of general knowledge concerning sarcomas, there is frequently a delay in the referral process to the orthopedic oncologist. The referring physician must explain to the patient and family the reasoning behind referral to the specialist, not uncommonly located several hundred miles away. In our experience, the patient is frequently not informed as to the possibility that the tumor might be a malignancy. Therefore, when the referring physician calls for the referral, it is prudent upon either the physician or APP in the orthopedic oncologist's office to take the call in a timely manner. This helps expedite the referral process and alleviate the need for the referring physician to order a scan or treatment that may not be necessary or is incorrect. This also provides an opportunity to educate the physician or nurse from the referring office about the unique treatment that sarcomas require and the importance of getting the patient to the orthopedic oncologist before any surgical treatment is rendered.

In our experience, direct communication between the surgeon or APP and the referring physician actually alleviates some of the stresses associated with sarcoma patients. Many times the patient is not aware that the tumor might in fact be a malignancy. The referring physician can inform the patient that he has spoken to the oncologist and that a plan of action and an appointment are already being prepared. In addition, appropriate radiographic studies and other tests can be performed in a timely manner, often prior to the consultation visit.

It is our goal that the time between initial contact and first office visit is within 7 days or less. This allows enough time for all medical records to be received and for the patient to reschedule their activities to allow for a satisfactory consultation and plan development. The APP at this point can also arrange for tests and studies to be scheduled on the same day that the patient arrives. This will impart to the patient a sense of organization, timeliness, and experience when dealing with such a rare disease. The patient and their family, as well as the referring physician, then gain a sense of security that they are being cared for in a facility with experience in sarcoma.

Prior to the patient arriving in the office for their initial appointment, they will have received, by mail, an information packet consisting of information about our Sarcoma Center, directions to the center, lists of items to bring, expectations, and forms that can be filled out ahead of time. There are benefits but also disadvantages to this "preemptive" mailing. The information within the packet provides the patient with educational material that will make the initial visit less frightening. It also allows the patient to fill out forms at his/her leisure rather than while in the waiting room. However, it may also cause fear in some patients. For example, many patients are never told of their presumptive diagnosis. When they receive a mailing discussing cancer, sent by the consulting physician to whom they have not met, many questions and concerns abound. Usually, for most patients, the added information and efficiency are understood and appreciated. In fact, the time saved by not having to fill out forms in the waiting room translates into less waiting time and more face-to-face contact with the surgeon, which is obviously appreciated.

17.2.3 Physician Assistants

Physician assistants require training in accredited programs under the auspices of the Accreditation Review Commission on Education for the Physician Assistant. Most programs are at least 26 months in duration and are associated with medical schools, colleges and universities, and some stand-alone hospitals. The PA education promotes the development of practical skills in clinical problem solving and decision-making [4]. The program consists of classroom and laboratory instruction in basic sciences, medical and behavioral sciences, anatomy, physiology, pharmacology, and clinical diagnosis. Training also requires clinical rotations that may include primary care specialties as well as surgical specialties, psychiatry, and emergency medicine. Prior to being licensed, PAs take a national certifying examination administered by the National Commission on Certification of Physician Assistants. This certifying exam also functions as a de facto licensing exam. All states require passing of this exam as a prerequisite for licensure as a PA. In addition, PAs must complete 100 h of continuing education every 2 years and pass a recertification examination every 6 years.

The scope of practice for the PA is defined by delegation decisions and the scope of practice of the supervising physician, consistent with the PA's education and experience, facility policy, and state laws. Upon graduation the PA may choose specialization, and their scope of practice may then further be defined by the specialty of physician with whom they work [7]. The PA working in the orthopedic oncology specialty will most likely gain most of their postgraduate education from on-the-job training which would be tailored to a specific practice. The PA performs physical examination, checks histories, orders and interprets diagnostic tests, and may prescribe medications and therapies in many states [6]. Like the APRN, the PA may assist in surgery and perform certain surgical procedures outlined by the practices scope. In the hospital setting, the PA conducts rounds, may write orders, take call, and perform admission and discharge work. The physician will most likely define the role of the PA in the orthopedic oncology practice, and their education and involvement will be tailored to that specific practice. This role includes education to the patient and families as well as navigation through the system to ensure timely and appropriate treatment for the patient with sarcoma. The PA must also communicate with the other members of the treatment team and relay relevant information to the patient in a timely manner.

Unlike the APRN who as mentioned above may be employed in a department other than orthopedic surgery, the department of the supervising physician most commonly employs the PA. Therefore, the department may be able to bill for the services rendered by the PA, both in surgical activities and clinical duties. Adherence to Medicare billing procedures is absolutely required in the same fashion as all other employees, residents, and colleagues of the physician. The scope of practice of the PA will be determined and set more precisely by the supervising physician. This allows for a tailored team approach for that specific physician.

References

1. Salsberg E, Grover A. Physician workforce shortages: implications and issues for academic health centers and policymakers. Acad Med. 2006;81(9):782–7.
2. Moote M, Krsek C, Kleinpell R, Todd B. Physician assistant and nurse practitioner utilization in academic medical centers. Am J Med Qual. 2011;26(6):452–60.
3. Mitchell R. Evaluating the clinical preparation of physician assistant versus nurse practitioner students and the characteristics of their preceptors. Internet J Acad Physi Assist. 2003;4(1):1.
4. National Governors Association. NGA paper on the role of physician assistants in health care delivery. J Rural Health. 2014;27(2011):220–9.
5. Jackson D. Physician assistants in orthopedic practices can expand the scope and depth of care. Orthopedics Today. 2009;29(10):18.
6. Larson EH, Coerver DA, Wick KH, Ballweg RA. Physician assistants in orthopedic practice: a national study. J Allied Health. 2011;40(4):174–80.
7. Morgan PA, Shah ND, Kaufman JS, Albanese MA. Impact of physician assistant care on office visit resource use in the United States. Health Serv Res. 2008;43(5 Pt 2):1906–22.
8. Druss BG, Marcus SC, Olfson M, Tanielian T, Pincus HA. Trends in care by non physician clinicians in the United States. N Engl J Med. 2003;348(2):130–7.
9. Overdyk FJ, Harvey SC, Fishman RL, Shippey F. Successful strategies for improving operating room efficiency at academic institutions. Anesth Analg. 1998;86(4):896–906.

Websites

National Association of Clinical Nurse Specialists (NACNS). www.nacns.org.
American Academy of Physician Assistants (AAPA). www.aapa.org.
American Academy of Nurse Practitioners (AANP). www.aanp.org.
America Academy of Nurse Anesthetists (AANA). www.aana.com.
National Athletic Trainers' Association (NATA). www.nata.org.

Psychosocial Issues in Children with Cancer: The Role of Patient Advocacy and Its Impact on Care

18

Victoria A. Sardi-Brown, Mary Jo Kupst, Peter J. Brown, and Lori Wiener

18.1 Introduction

"Your child has cancer." To a family, these four words are excruciating and life altering. Yet, 15,700 families in the United States hear these words each year [1]. Regardless of who you are, no matter what your professional, educational, and cultural backgrounds are, when your child is diagnosed with cancer, it "is not just about the medicine" [2]. The common factors that unite all children and families are the psychological and social concerns, fears, and day-to-day management of the disease. Once parents are told, "your child has cancer," the whole family is affected and forever changed [3–7]. Childhood cancer is as much a psychological disease as it is a physical one in which children and families need help managing the day-to-day isolation, pain, treatment challenges, and the consequences on their daily life. Childhood cancer threatens every aspect of the family's life and the possibility of a future.

This chapter describes psychosocial care, illustrates its critical role in the care of the child with cancer, discusses the importance of a therapeutic alliance with the health-care team, and reviews psychosocial interventions from the time of diagnosis through survivorship, relapse, or end-of-life care. The importance of patient advocacy and its impact on medical care is highlighted, and challenges to achieving optimal

V.A. Sardi-Brown, Ph.D. (✉) • P.J. Brown, M.B.A.
Mattie Miracle Cancer Foundation, Washington, DC, USA
e-mail: vicki@mattiemiracle.com

M.J. Kupst, Ph.D.
Medical College of Wisconsin, Milwaukee, WI, USA

L. Wiener, Ph.D., D.C.S.W.
Psychosocial Support and Research Program, Behavioral Science Core, National Cancer Institute, Bethesda, MD, USA

© Springer International Publishing Switzerland 2017
R.M. Henshaw (ed.), *Sarcoma*, DOI 10.1007/978-3-319-43121-5_18

psychosocial care are discussed. Finally, the collaboration between parent advocates and leading health-care providers that is currently underway to develop and implement national psychosocial standards of care for childhood cancer is described.

It is important to note that the authors of this chapter consist of two parent advocates who lost their only child, Mattie, to osteosarcoma as well as two practicing pediatric psycho-oncologists. Our life circumstances may have brought us together, but it is our great admiration and respect for each other that keep us working together. Throughout the chapter, the unique set of challenges, stressors, and concerns children living with a sarcoma and their families face are illustrated through the experience of Mattie and his parents. Mattie's parents give voice to Mattie's courageous journey.

18.2 Who Was Mattie?

Mattie was born on April 4, 2002, by cesarean section with an Apgar score of 9. Mattie was a precocious child who demonstrated many strengths, such as a sense of humor, observational skills, ability to understand how things worked (at the tender age of 2, he was disassembling and reassembling his Hot Wheel cars with a screwdriver), empathy beyond his years, and a vivacious and veracious need to have fun and convince others to participate in his antics. In July of 2008, when Mattie was 6 years old and attending a tennis camp, he complained of pain in his right arm. When his symptoms got worse, his pediatrician ordered an X-ray, which revealed a mass suggestive of osteosarcoma in Mattie's right humerus. CT, MRI, PET scans and a biopsy confirmed four primary tumor sites: (1) right humerus, (2) left humerus, (3) right femur, and (4) left radius. Mattie's parents were informed that their only child had multifocal synchronous osteosarcoma.

Sixteen days after diagnosis, Mattie began 14 months of treatment including high-dose combination chemotherapy with doxorubicin, cisplatin, methotrexate, ifosfamide, and etoposide. He underwent limb-salvaging resections in two-staged surgical procedures, with custom endoprosthetic reconstruction and autogenous bone grafting. His tumors demonstrated a discordant response to chemotherapy, based on percentage of necrosis: 60% in the right humerus, 80% in the left humerus, 100% in the left radius, and 2% in the right femur. Eleven months after his initial diagnosis, Mattie had another major surgery, a sternotomy, to remove nine metastatic tumors that developed in his lungs. Mifamurtide (L-MTP-PE) was also added to Mattie's treatment.

This only lists the medical procedures Mattie courageously endured. What Mattie's parents and family members observed was his struggle to learn how to cope with the profound functional impact of his surgeries and the change in his daily life thanks to his treatments. He could no longer walk, run, dress, or toilet himself. Within months of his second surgery, Mattie began working with a child psychiatrist who diagnosed him with clinical depression, anxiety, and medical posttraumatic stress disorder. He was started on Celexa and Klonopin to reduce his significant sadness and anxiety.

In August of 2009, only 6 weeks off of chemotherapy, scan results revealed that Mattie's cancer had spread to his lungs and liver. Conversations with Mattie's medical team turned from curative intent to end-of-life care. Mattie's family had to face a parent's worst fear: the reality that their child was dying and the stressful and frightening medical decisions associated with this reality.

18.3 Communicating with Children: History

Given the critical role of psychosocial care in cancer, it is surprising that the subspecialty of psycho-oncology is fairly new. However, prior to the mid-1970s, tremendous stigma surrounded a cancer diagnosis, which was usually fatal. Often, children were not informed of their cancer diagnoses. Over time, as the stigma began to diminish, more open conversations about the name and type of disease, potential side effects, and outcomes were possible. These conversations allowed physicians and other health-care professionals to more fully explore the child's psychosocial well-being and, later, to study children's psychological responses [8].

Important research findings helped change practice as well. Studies found that children who were not provided information about their illness or prognosis understood much more than was originally thought, even when false reassurances were given about their situation [9–11]. Concurrent clinical observations supported the fact that children's anxiety lessened as they found comfort in being able to talk about their own health concerns in a developmentally appropriate manner. The outcome of studies from the 1970s changed the overall practice of pediatric care, emphasizing open communication about cancer between children and their health-care professionals and encouraging parents to dialogue with their children about the disease. The findings illustrated the "enormous strength of children in facing even the most dire news if they can be assured that those around them will answer their questions honestly and not abandon them" [12] (p. 133). Furthermore, this change fueled the inclusion of mental health professionals on childhood cancer treatment teams [9–11].

18.4 What Is Psychosocial Care and Who Provides It?

Psychosocial care can be defined as services and interventions that enable patients, their families, and health-care providers to optimize biomedical health care and to manage the psychological, behavioral, and social aspects of illness and its consequences to promote better health [13]. Specifically, the goal of psychosocial care is to address the effects that cancer and its treatment have on the mental health and emotional well-being of patients, their family members, and their professional caregivers. In addition, provision of psychosocial care has been shown to yield better management of common disease-related symptoms and adverse effects of treatment such as pain and fatigue [14–17]. Research also indicates that distressed emotional states can generate somatic problems, such as sleep difficulties, fatigue, and pain

[18, 19], which can confound the diagnosis and treatment of physical symptoms. Moreover, depression and other psychosocial concerns can affect adherence to treatment regimens by impairing cognition, weakening motivation, and decreasing coping abilities [13].

The American Academy of Pediatrics created guidelines [20] for state-of-the-art care for children and adolescents with cancer. These guidelines delineated the importance of multidisciplinary care in treatment outcomes and recommended that pediatric oncology social workers, pediatric psychologists, and child life specialists work alongside medical staff. Recommendations have been made for families impacted by childhood cancer to also have access to support groups [20, 21]. Other critical disciplines include psychiatry, neuropsychology, nursing, educational specialists, creative arts, chaplaincy, and career and vocational counseling [22]. Though these professional groups are well trained and ethically competent to manage psychosocial issues and concerns, ideally attention to psychosocial issues should not be the sole responsibility or role of just these professionals but rather all providers caring for the child with cancer.

Another critically important component of psychosocial care is palliative care. For many centers, palliative care has been viewed as being synonymous with "end-of-life care," with involvement by subspecialty palliative care teams only when death was imminent [23]. Fortunately, this is changing. Palliative care is now much more holistic, typically comprised of an interdisciplinary approach that includes physicians, nurses, psychosocial clinicians, and others [24] who aim to improve the child's quality of life by alleviating physical, psychosocial, and spiritual suffering of the child and family regardless of disease status [25, 26]. A sarcoma diagnosis is rare in children, and it inherently carries with it medical uncertainty, as well as physical and psychosocial suffering. Therefore, it is appropriate to introduce and include comprehensive palliative care from the time of diagnosis onward [23]. If end-of-life care is needed, the palliative care team will already be in place, with focus transitioning to the child's comfort and family support.

In 2008, psychosocial care received increased attention in the oncology world following the publication by the Institute of Medicine (IOM) entitled *Cancer Care for the Whole Patient: Meeting Psychosocial Health Needs*. The report translated research findings about psychosocial care into practical applications for the purpose of improving the quality of cancer care. Evidence was reported for several effective interventions, including counseling and psychotherapy, pharmacologic support, illness self-management and self-care programs, family and caregiver education, and health promotion interventions [14]. Importantly, the IOM emphasized that optimal care includes the provision of appropriate psychosocial health services [13].

Providing optimal care requires a paradigm shift and an acknowledgment that every patient-health-care professional interaction provides an opportunity to assess the stressors and concerns the patient and their family members are facing, particularly when designing treatment plans. While this should be done for everyone who has cancer and their family, it is especially critical for children. Children who are distressed remember certain procedures with greater negativity, which in turn predicts higher distress with subsequent events [22]. When sufficient information about the child's psychological and social strengths, stressors, and preferences are obtained from the child and the parents, health-care professionals can tailor their specialty services more precisely to the child's needs, thereby averting possible negative or traumatic reactions. Moreover, a therapeutic alliance between the health-care professional and the patient/parent can be formed, which is vital toward pooling resources together toward a common goal [27]. When a therapeutic alliance is established, children and their parents are more likely to feel a part of the treatment team. This is critically important for parents who feel vulnerable and powerless over their child's disease [28]. The following examples illustrate how incorporating psychosocial care into each patient interaction can allow trust to be developed and care to be delivered in a manner that allows children to use their resources to cope more effectively.

During the diagnostic phase of his cancer journey, Mattie underwent countless IV sticks, physical exams, MRI, and CT scans. The pace of these assessments was overwhelming for Mattie, and with each new test, his awareness and knowledge grew that something was very wrong. While at first he handled the tests well, with repeated exams his frustration grew, his tolerance began to decline, and his anxiety rose to the point where even sitting for a brief consultation was impossible. At one point, when entering the CT scanning room, Mattie hid under the scanner in tears. He was absolutely hysterical, refusing to come out from his hiding place. Coaxing by multiple staff members was ineffective. The scheduling window to get his scan done passed, which of course had consequences on the timing of all his other assessments that day. Mattie's response was a sign of fear and trauma. The compounded traumas that Mattie experienced during his first weeks of being diagnosed set the stage for larger issues later in his treatment.

Mattie's parents encouraged his oncologist and treatment team to consider sedating Mattie for all scans, but they were consistently told that PET and CT scans were short and noninvasive and, for safety reasons, it would be better for Mattie to manage without sedation. The team believed that, with staff and family reassurance and some distractions, Mattie could manage the scans without sedation. His parents tried to explain that Mattie had sensory integration issues prior to his cancer diagnosis and that he was highly sensitive to sound, tight spaces, and being confined in any way. They were aware that these neurodevelopmental issues would be key factors in his ability to stay still for the scans. It was not until the head nurse of pediatric sedation and the child life specialist observed the terror Mattie experienced when attempting a CT scan that a new scanning strategy was implemented. If psychosocial information about his sensory issues and coping abilities had been obtained upfront, the additional anxiety, stress, fear, and trauma from having to stay still in the scanner could have potentially been avoided. Unfortunately, this stress carried over into all treatments he perceived as invasive.

The second example occurred while Mattie was undergoing treatment. During morning rounds on the inpatient unit, the attending oncologist found Mattie upset, tired, and feeling ill. When he did not feel well, he tended to emotionally shut down, refusing to cooperate with medical demands, especially when they came from medical personnel he was not familiar with.

The attending oncologist could have left his room and returned when it was a better time. This would have been understandable, as calming Mattie down and reasoning with him was a time-consuming process. Instead, she spent the time figuring out how to relate to Mattie. While in the room, her pager went off. This caught Mattie's attention. He wanted to know more about the pager. The oncologist pulled out her pager, showed it to Mattie, and allowed him to play with it, and they sent messages around the hospital together. A connection was made.

What did this connection accomplish? From a medical standpoint, the oncologist was able to examine Mattie and obtain the medical information she needed in a positive and non-stressful manner. Perhaps more importantly, the beginning of a strong rapport and a trusting therapeutic alliance was formed. Taking the time to understand her patient's fears, behavior, and interests enabled the oncologist to effectively provide Mattie with care. Toward the end of Mattie's life, it was this physician he confided in about his pain. He knew she would take him seriously. If children trust you, they will reveal more to you and also comply more with your medical directions [29].

18.5 Time Points During the Cancer Trajectory for Psychosocial Intervention: Providers' Perspectives

As noted, learning that one's child has cancer is a time of significant distress and family upheaval. Families find themselves confronted with a world where new medical information is being thrust upon them while decisions need to be made about potentially lifesaving treatment options, each of which poses risks for long-term health consequences. The child undergoes many transitions throughout the cancer trajectory from diagnosis to first treatment, intra-treatment transitions (e.g., chemotherapy to surgery, surgery to chemotherapy, radiation to chemotherapy, etc.), resulting in the end of treatment to survivorship, survivorship to relapse, relapse to survivorship, or survivorship to end-of-life care. The following section reviews psychosocial stresses that occur from the point of diagnosis on, with attention provided to the unique needs of youth living with a pediatric solid tumor.

18.5.1 Diagnosis Period

This is a time of tremendous uncertainty. Symptoms that had appeared benign (such as leg pain, a fracture) are worked up to rule out a malignancy. An MRI, CT, or PET scan may be scheduled and blood work obtained while families anxiously await the results. As described in the case with Mattie, children who undergo extensive testing with little psychological preparation can be traumatized by the experience. They can perceive the tests as an assault on their body and feel confused as to why their parents are not protecting them from harm.

When the diagnosis of a sarcoma is given, further testing is required to determine specific histology and to rule out metastatic disease. Parents frantic about their child being diagnosed with cancer may find themselves relieved when the disease appears to be limited to the primary site or even more overwhelmed by news of a less favorable prognosis. While waiting for final results, children perceive their parents' distress, adolescents fear what cancer means in terms of their life expectancy and day-to-day life, and together with the medical team, treatment options are explored. Oncologists should be aware of these dynamics and the enormous stress families are under. This is an important time to engage the help of a mental health professional who can assess the child's understanding, concerns, and ability to adapt to change and the family's strengths and vulnerabilities. When available, the child life specialist can help the child obtain mastery (and therefore be less traumatized) of needle sticks and other invasive and noninvasive tests through medical play, while other professionals, such as a social worker or psychologist, can foster the child's expression of new events and begin to help the family adapt to the changes that will follow. If a line placement is being considered, psychosocial support can be very helpful in introducing the concept of line placement, access, and regular care of dressing changes plus flushing of lines.

Parents also struggle to find the right words to explain cancer and cancer treatments to their child. Mattie's parents worked with his art therapists to find images he would be able to relate to. Since Mattie loved bugs, they created "bone bugs" made out of clay. His disease was conceptualized using a clay bone bug. He visualized the clay bug crawling inside his bones, and when given the option, he grabbed the clay bone bug and smashed it on the floor with his foot to kill it, representing what chemotherapy would be doing inside his body. Other children find it helpful to think of chemotherapy as Pac-Man going through their body, destroying all the cancer cells.

18.5.2 Treatment Considerations

While treatment decisions are being made, the child and family are introduced to new medical and support personnel. The information presented can be quite overwhelming, and the role that each new staff person will have in the child's care can seem similar and be confusing. Providing families written information on the names and roles of the professionals within the team, including psychosocial providers (pictures taken from your institution's website can help enormously) and how they can be contacted begins the process of establishing trust, enhancing a sense of control, and promoting open communication.

The consent process can also be particularly stressful for families. In childhood cancer, families must assimilate a vast amount of information and make decisions in a short period of time. If not all caregivers can be present, audio recording the session allows others to hear the information at a later time. It is important that the patient is included in the consent process along with his or her caregivers and that information is provided using developmentally appropriate language. Families generally have little experience with the difference between standard treatment and clinical trials. In childhood cancer, parents often do not retain the information about the research nature of the protocol, but primarily focus on the specifics of the treatment as well as potential prognosis [30]. They benefit from explanations about experimental questions being asked as part of the recommended therapy. The consent process extends beyond the signing of a document and ideally takes place slowly with multiple opportunities to assess their understanding and answer questions as they occur [31].

18.5.3 Treatment Initiation

The onset of treatment is a particularly stressful time for families. In sarcomas, aggressive surgical options may be considered, especially when the intent is for cure. This includes limb salvage surgeries and, less frequently, amputation. Families benefit from extensive preparation for such surgeries, including opportunities to discuss the multiple consequences of the procedure (expected outcome, functional expectations, pain, disability, deformity, and changes in appearance). Time is needed for the child and family to psychologically prepare for surgery [32].

When available and interested, some children and adolescents can benefit from discussion with other patients who have received similar procedures. As limb salvage surgery does not guarantee postsurgical function at the same level that the child had prior to surgery, expectations need to be clearly spelled out. These include the possibility of surgical complications and the need for future revisions, postsurgical wound healing complicated by adjuvant chemotherapy, and time provided to process the information, ask questions, and obtain support. Staff members who are trained to provide guidance and support at this time are physical and occupational therapists, social workers, child psychologists, and child life specialists [33]. Following surgery, the medical team and psychosocial providers should assess for emotional adjustment, anxiety, depression, family adaptation, and posttraumatic stress-like reactions. The outcome of this assessment can set into place the most appropriate interventions for the child and family.

When a limb-sparing procedure is not possible, amputation can be a very difficult option to accept. Similar to limb sparing, it might be helpful for children and adolescents to discuss the surgery and life after surgery with another amputee, though keep in mind that not all youth are comfortable seeing another person's stump prior to their own surgery. There are books and movies that youth and their parents have found helpful prior to surgery (Table 18.1). Social work, psychology, or recreation therapy may be helpful in preparing for surgery and providing support following amputation. Postsurgery, important concerns and questions pertaining to sexual function, activity, intimacy, and occupational concerns must be addressed and a follow-up plan developed and documented.

Phantom pain can be an issue for which multidisciplinary assistance is needed, including, as noted earlier, the involvement of a palliative care team. In addition to medication (tricyclic antidepressants, anticonvulsants), noninvasive therapies such as acupuncture and biofeedback [34, 35] are often utilized. More invasive options include steroid injection, spinal cord stimulation, or implanted devices. Surgery is done only as a last resort. Physical therapists can be instrumental in providing tools such as mirror therapy and nerve stimulation (TENS), and psychologists have had some success with guided imagery, relaxation techniques, and hypnosis [36–38]. The effectiveness of cognitive behavioral therapy in pediatric pain has been well documented [39, 40], and neuropathic pain syndromes have been reported in a number of case studies [41]. Interestingly, studies have shown little to no difference in quality of life in those who underwent limb salvage as compared to those who

Table 18.1 Psychosocial resources for children and their families with sarcomas

Topic/area	Resources
Books for children	1. *Annie Loses Her Leg but Finds Her Way* by Sandra J. Philipson and Robert Takatch. Chagrin River Publishing Company, 1999
	Annie and her brother Max experience the illness and recovery of their 9-year-old English Springer Spaniel who loses her leg to cancer
	2. *What's Up With Lyndon?* by Dr. Kim Chilman-Blair and John Taddeo. American Cancer Society, 2011. [available in Spanish]
	Childhood osteosarcoma is explained in an informative story that makes the science behind cancer accessible to young readers
Books for teens	1. *Every Child Needs an Angel* by Cosmo Lorusso. iUniverse
	This story narrates Nicole's battle with cancer, her reliance on faith, and her mission to help others and to make a difference. It recounts the unwavering support from friends, neighbors, coworkers, medical staff, and coaches – those who became angels to Nicole in her time of need
	2. *Just Don't Fall: A Hilariously True Story of Cancer, Childhood, Amputation, Romantic Yearning, Truth and Olympic Greatness* by Josh Sundquist. Penguin Group USA, 2010
	At 9 years old, Josh Sundquist was diagnosed with Ewing's sarcoma that eventually claimed his left leg. *Just Don't Fall* is the story of the boy Josh and of the young man he became – an utterly heroic struggle through numerous hospitalizations and worse to become an award-winning skier in the Paralympics and renowned motivational speaker
	3. *A Special Kind of Courage* by Geraldo Rivera. Simon and Schuster, 1976
	True stories of 11 modern youths who have faced various crises, including death, with exemplary courage
	4. *Teenagers: Face to Face with Cancer* by Karen Gravelle and Bertram John. Julian Messner, 1986
	Young people, ranging roughly in age from 13 to 21, speak candidly, recalling the initial shock of their diagnoses, their treatments, and pressures at school. They address how relationships with family, friends, and romantic interests change, reflect on their futures, and discuss how they deal with the possibility of death
	5. *What It Takes: Fighting For My Life and My Love of the Game* by Tom Coughin and Mark Herzlich. ePub, 2013
	Mark Herzlich, a starting linebacker for the New York Giants, was diagnosed with Ewing's sarcoma during his junior year of college. This story is about his fight against the odds to get through treatment and into the NFL

(continued)

Table 18.1 (continued)

Topic/area	Resources
Books for parents/adults	1. *All the Kings Horses, All the Kings Men* by Donna Purves. iUniverse
	All the Kings Horses, All the Kings Men is a moving account of the life of the author's son, previous to and following the discovery of the presence of osteogenic sarcoma
	2. *Childhood Cancer: A Parent's Guide to Solid Tumor Cancers*, 2nd Edition, by Honna Janes-Hodder & Nancy Keene. O'Reilly & Associates, 1999
	Detailed medical information about solid tumor childhood cancers, including neuroblastoma, Wilms tumor, liver tumors, soft tissue sarcomas, and bone sarcomas
	3. *Children with Cancer: A Comprehensive Reference Guide for Parents* by Jeanne Munn Bracken. Oxford University Press, 1986
	A comprehensive road map for families of children diagnosed with various malignancies
	4. *Fighting Chance: Journeys Through Childhood Cancer* by Harry Connolly, Tom Clancy, & Curt I. Civin. Woodholm House Pub, 1998
	This book follows patients, families, and caregivers battling cancer in and out of the hospital. Photographed over the course of 3 years, it includes contributions from best-selling author Tom Clancy and Dr. Curt Civin, director of Johns Hopkins Hospital's Pediatric Oncology Unit. Other insights come from nurses, parents, siblings, and the children themselves
	5. *Fly with a Miracle* by Sheila Belshaw. London: Denor Press. 2001
	Fly with a Miracle describes the details surrounding the pioneering and successful medical treatment in the United Kingdom for bone cancer, through the eyes of a mother and her son (the patient) who is determined to become an airline pilot
	6. *Soul Gifts* by Barbara Gill (2006)
	The author speaks of how we are all connected – "The Human Chain" – and how this connection can be used for peace and prosperity, not by organizing for "the cause" but by living it, one at a time
	7. *What Doctors Cannot Tell You: Clarity, Confidence and Uncertainty in Medicine* by Kevin B. Jones
	What Doctors Cannot Tell You explores the uncertainty that pervades medicine. The patients' stories empower readers to ask questions of their physicians, with a firm belief that healing and hope begin from honesty in those critical conversations
Siblings	1. *Hey, What about Me?: A Personal Journal for Teens Whose Brother or Sister Has Cancer* by Pam Ganz. SuperSibs!, 2003
	2. *When Your Brother Or Sister Gets Cancer* by K. Ballard. Produced in association with Birmingham Children's Hospital Sibling Group and UKCCSG Sibling Project Group, 2004
Survivorship	1. *At Face Value: My Triumph Over A Disfiguring Cancer* by Terry Healey. Cabeat Press, 2006
	The story of Terry Healy who was diagnosed with cancer at age 20 and how he learned to cope with the scars that were left behind
	2. *Very Much Better: A Cancer Memoir of a Boy Who Lived* by Jason Paul Greer. American Cancer Society, LLC, 2011
	The story of Jason, a Ewing's sarcoma cancer survivor

Table 18.1 (continued)

Topic/area	Resources
Grief and loss	1. *Love, Jason* by Doug Anderson. Deep River Books
	The story of a couple's experience during their son's 5-year battle with Ewing's sarcoma and eventual loss
	2. *When The Bough Breaks: Forever After the Death of a Son or Daughter* by Judith R. Bernstein. Andrews McMeel Publishing, 1998
	This book addresses mourning, documenting the process of evolution from initial grief to an altered outlook on life. Excerpts from interviews with 50 parents who lost a child from ages 5 to 45 trace the road from utter devastation to a revised view of life, resulting in a work that is a tribute to resilience and the indomitable human spirit
Helpful websites/ resources	1. *Cancer.net*
	Website: http://www.cancer.net/cancer-types/sarcoma
	This website provides basic information, videos, and links to other resources
	2. *LMSarcoma Direct Research Foundation*
	Phone: 1-888-266-1104
	Website: http://www.lmsdr.org; this website provides specific information and resources for leiomyosarcoma
	3. *Sarcoma Alliance for Research Through Collaboration*
	Phone: 734-930-7600
	Website: http://www.sarctrials.org/
	4. *Sarcoma Foundation of America*
	The website offers patients information and support, informational links, clinical trials, and a public forum
	Website: http://www.curesarcoma.org
	E-mail: info@curesarcoma.org
	Phone: 301.253.8687 Fax: 301.253.8690
	5. *SarcomaHelp.org – The Liddy Shriver Sarcoma Initiative* Phone: 914-762-3251
	Website: http://sarcomahelp.org/
	6. *The Life Raft Group* (supporting the gastrointestinal stromal tumors community)
	Phone: 973–837-9092
	Website: http://www.liferaftgroup.org
Support groups	1. *Synovial Sarcoma Support Group*
	Website: http://www.synovialsarcomasurvivors.org
	2. *The Sarcoma Alliance* (web page has groups for most states in the United States)
	Website: http://sarcomaalliance.org/support-groups/

(continued)

Table 18.1 (continued)

Topic/area	Resources
Financial Services	1. *Aid to Families with Dependent Children (AFDC)*
	A joint federal and state-funded program that offers monthly checks for the care of dependent children who are in financial need because their parent(s) cannot provide them with needed financial support
	Website: http://www.acf.hhs.gov/programs/ofa
	2. *Andre Sobel River of Life Foundation*
	Helps with urgent expenses, allowing single parents to stay at their child's bedside during catastrophic illness. The organization works directly with affiliated children's hospitals
	Website: http://www.andreriveroflife.org
	3. *American Childhood Cancer Organization (formerly Candlelighters)*
	Formed by parents of young cancer patients, has an ombudsman program to assist families and survivors with problems in education, employment, insurance, welfare, or military enlistment. Provides information, local support groups, and specialized information to families and caregivers of children with cancer
	Phone: 855.858.2226
	Website: http://www.acco.org/
	4. *Cancer Care*
	Provides financial assistance to help with some types of costs, including transportation, home care, childcare, and pain medication
	Website: http://www.cancercare.org
	5. *First Hand Foundation*
	Helps children with health-related needs when insurance and other financial resources have been exhausted
	Website: www.firsthandfoundation.org
	E-mail: Firsthandfoundation@cerner.com
	6. *Foundation for Children with Cancer*
	Assists families of children with cancer by providing tangible and direct financial support, such as mortgage payments, insurance premiums, utility bills, or funeral expenses
	Phone: 414.716.6250
	Website: http://www.childrenwithcancer.org
	7. *Insure Kids Now*
	A national campaign to link the nation's uninsured children (0–18) to free and low-cost health insurance
	Phone: 877.Kids.Now (877.543.7669)
	Website: www.insurekidsnow.gov
	8. *Local Department of Human Resources and Social Services*
	Each county's Department of Human Resources (DHR)/Social Services (DSS) has an office or individual to handle requests for emergency assistance. DHR or DSS can assist with rent or monthly payments, moving expenses, utility bills, and financial help toward prescriptions and medical supplies. The phone number of DHR/DSS is in the county government section of one's local telephone directory

Table 18.1 (continued)

Topic/area	Resources
	9. *National Children's Cancer Society (NCCS)*
	Financial and fundraising assistance related to medical treatment, such as lodging and travel. Provides advocacy support, interceding on behalf of children with bills, home care needs, insurance companies, hospitals, and other agencies to negotiate reasonable solutions
	Phone: 314.241.1600
	Website: https://www.thenccs.org/#
	10. *Ruritan Club*
	Local clubs help families pay for medical equipment and supplies, prescription medications, and medical transportation. Listing for local clubs can be found in the business section of a local white pages directory or the national Ruritan office
	Phone: 877.787.8727
	Website: http://www.ruritan.org
	11. State and Local General Assistance Programs
	Designed to provide small amounts of cash assistance to individuals who are not eligible for AFDC or SSI or who are awaiting enrollment in another income subsidy program. Check the county's DHR/DSS to determine if the state or county has a General Assistance Program and where to call or how to apply
Scholarships	1. *Kyle Lee Foundation*
	Awards scholarships to college-bound students who have survived cancer, especially Ewing's sarcoma
	Website: www.kylelee28.com/Kyle
	2. *National Amputation Foundation*
	Awards limited to entering freshmen who have had a major limb amputation and are full-time college or university students
	Phone: 516.887.3600
	Website: http://nationalamputation.org/scholar1.html

underwent amputation, with good adjustment and overall acceptance to amputation by adolescents [42]. In adult populations, limb salvage appears to be more socially acceptable, with lower reported rates of social isolation than in those who had undergone amputation [43, 44]. Clinicians should be astute in asking about perceived social isolation postsurgery and during the child's survivorship phase. Ongoing screening and follow-up are needed to address delayed or previously unidentified psychosocial difficulties.

Chemotherapy is almost always utilized in the treatment of bone sarcomas and many soft tissue sarcomas. Patients are often very concerned about nausea and vomiting as well as hair loss. Consultation with a wig maker prior to all hair loss is preferable as it allows selection of a wig that matches the child's current appearance. Some children are able to donate their own hair prior to it falling out. Others prefer not to wear a wig but opt for hats, scarves, or baldness. Preparation for how the hair starts to fall out is useful as some will choose to avoid the gradual loss by cutting or shaving their hair very short in advance. In addition, following myelosuppressive chemotherapy, patients are encouraged to avoid crowds. This can be most difficult for teens who do not wish to limit social interactions. Furthermore, for adolescent and young adult patients, fertility conversations are necessary prior to induction treatment. Males may delay start of therapy for sperm banking. Some trials exist for ovarian tissue harvest, but for many, chemotherapy cannot be delayed for the necessary hormone treatments.

Radiation is often used at some point during treatment for a sarcoma. Child life specialists, psychologists, or social workers can prepare children for radiation therapy, including what the machines look like and the time required for simulation. Distraction and cognitive behavioral tools can be very effective in reducing anxiety [45, 46]. For those who will require radiation to the brain, neuropsychiatric testing and follow-up assessments should be considered due to the known CNS toxicities. For adolescent males for whom radiation is planned for the testes, sperm banking should be offered and ovarian transposition for ovarian protection considered when radiation is planned for the abdominal/pelvic region [47].

Throughout treatment, physical discomforts and psychosocial stresses persist. Pain, mouth sores, nutritional concerns, diarrhea, or constipation often occurs. As most children are not in the habit of discussing such bodily habits, guidance and support to encourage open disclosure about these important topics can be useful. Psychosocial stresses can persist as well. Poor adherence to medically required care is often a sign of patient or family distress. Routine adherence assessment and monitoring are encouraged. When problems are identified (e.g., doses are missed), a patient or family meeting is needed to understand barriers to compliance and to set clear guidelines and expectations for care. Some centers have found increased monitoring, obtaining the support of additional family members, adjusting medication dose (to address side effects), creating reminder cues, and developing a contract with the adolescent patient that identifies critical elements of care useful.

Other signs of psychosocial stress include increased anxiety, persistent sadness, withdrawal from friends, and difficulty learning to live with reduced physical mobility. Each of these should be a trigger for a consultation with a mental health professional knowledgeable about living with cancer.

18.5.4 Survivorship

Overall, survivors of childhood cancer have been reported to have a high rate of medically significant chronic conditions, particularly those who were treated for a bone sarcoma [48–50]. Chemotherapy and radiation therapy are stressful for youth to undergo, and surgery is often part of the treatment received. Tumor-induced changes in body image, school reentry [51, 52], loss of fertility, and impact on future independence can be especially challenging in the adolescent and young adult population where sarcomas can have their peak occurrence [53, 54]. The Children's Oncology Group [55] has developed comprehensive guidelines for monitoring pediatric cancer survivors. Excellent resources addressing the long-term psychosocial impact of pediatric cancer survivorship are also available. Due to the high rate of obesity in pediatric cancer survivors, physicians actively promoting healthy lifestyles are of utmost importance.

18.5.5 End of Therapy

As exciting as the last cycle of chemotherapy can be, the shift from regular hospital visits, frequent labs, and physical exams to more independence can be anxiety provoking. Parents and children benefit from being prepared for the anxiety that often accompanies scan visits. The psychologist or social worker can introduce the children and family to cognitive and emotionally based behavioral tools that can help reduce anxiety and cope better in the days preceding the scan visits.

Families also benefit greatly from having a transition and survivorship care plan developed by their primary team so that anticipatory guidance can be given. Helping teens learn how to maintain their medical care and advocate for themselves helps make the transition from the pediatric setting to adult oncology care smoother and can lead to better health-care compliance. Many centers now provide patients in their survivorship clinics with survivorship care plans [55, 56] that document the treatments they have had, potential or existing late effects, and a timetable for continued surveillance.

18.5.6 When Cure Is No Longer Possible

The course of sarcoma treatment for some children is characterized by a series of treatment responses and relapses leading to a time when curative options are exhausted. Health-care providers need to respect each family's decisions to stop treatment or to participate in phase I clinical trials, delicately balancing quality of life issues with those related to palliative care, grief, death, and loss. Conversation about the child's and family's goals for care is fundamental to all decisions made. Children, 14 years and older, have been identified as the age group that needs to be routinely included in advance care planning and end-of-life decision-making [57]. Allowing them to be included helps maintain their autonomy in an uncontrollable situation [58]. *Voicing My CHOiCES*, a new adolescent advance care planning guide, can provide the teen with a communication tool to express their opinions about their care and how they wish to be remembered in the future [59–61].

Open discussions that address painful decisions, including home versus hospital care for the dying child, advance directives, autopsy [62], and funeral arrangements, are best held once it is understood that cure is no longer possible. However, the care team needs to respect that families approach a child's pending death differently and therefore the need for access to information about funeral arrangements, autopsies, and other legacy building strategies and materials may vary based on many factors, including the timing of the child's death. Parents appreciate understanding that hope still exists and the important role they play in instilling it within themselves and for their child during the dying process. Hope can be redefined for parents by redirecting their energies toward managing pain and maintaining the highest quality of life possible for their child while striving for a humane and dignified death (the absence of anxiety and pain and the presence of loved ones by their child's side) [31].

It is important to address the emotional needs of parents, siblings, and extended family in the context of families' expectations, unfulfilled dreams, values, and beliefs. As death approaches, families often need assurance that they have done all they could for their child. The health-care team's availability, participation, and investment in caring for the dying child are crucial to and appreciated by all families, even those who appear to be coping well on their own. Spiritual care professionals can be of enormous support for some families during this time.

18.5.7 Bereavement Support

The child's primary medical team (physicians, nurses, social workers, child life specialists, psychologists, and pastoral and other health-care providers who have often developed relationships with the family over a period of months or years) can be an important source of support for bereaved parents and other family members [24]. An abrupt end of contact soon after the child's death can be experienced as abandonment. Although many medical, nursing, and psychosocial providers make an effort to support the bereaved family, there are no existing guidelines and a limited evidence base suggesting timeframes for when staff members should contact the family after the child's death. Clinical practice clearly indicates that hospitals have an obligation to provide some level of bereavement follow-up to the child's family [63–67]. There is also sufficient descriptive evidence to recommend that follow-up calls to assess how the family is managing after a child's death by a member of the medical team who helped care for the child with cancer are helpful and appreciated by the parents [68]. A bereavement assessment is considered essential to the appropriate management of grief-induced emotional distress [69].

Importantly, no qualitative or quantitative data has been found to suggest that a phone call, contact, or conversation can be harmful. In fact, there is data that parents who are not contacted by a member of the team who cared for their child are both "noticed" and "regretted" [70]. Moreover, a minimum period of 13 months of bereavement support is the National Hospice and Palliative Care Association Standard [71]. These facts suggest that the standard of care should consist of at least one meaningful contact between psychosocial staff members and bereaved parents following the death of a child to cancer. The purpose of this call to the child's family is to assess how the family is coping; to let them know they have not been forgotten; to identify families who are at risk for negative physical, psychological, and social sequelae; and to provide resources for community bereavement support [68, 72].

The psychosocial needs and care of patients with pediatric solid tumors and their family members can be particularly challenging at any point along the disease trajectory. Successful treatment requires a comprehensive approach that builds trust and a therapeutic alliance among health-care providers, the patients, and their families. Once this is established, psychosocial support can assist in the treatment-related challenges in a manner that respects the autonomy of the individual and encourages patients to be active participants in their care [56, 73]. While patients can be active participants, to optimize their care, they need and benefit greatly from the advocacy efforts of their families.

18.6   Patient Advocacy and Its Impact on Care

Patient advocacy can be a complex arena to navigate for families whose child has been diagnosed with cancer. Who is the patient's advocate? Does the child have just one advocate? Within the hospital setting, children and their families are introduced to many advocates, most commonly the "patient advocate" or "patient representative." According to the American Hospital Association, "patient advocates are essentially problem solvers. They bridge gaps, ease communication, guide people through bureaucratic mazes, act as liaisons and interpreters and help keep everyone in the system focused on the consumer" [74] (p. 7). These advocates are employed by the hospital, and their goal is to ensure patient satisfaction and the delivery of quality care [75–77]. In addition to advocates within the hospital, families may also have advocates within the community, such as other family members, friends, foundations, and professional organizations who provide essential support for childhood cancer treatment and research and empower the community to join in this fight against cancer.

If you ask parents and family members who the number one advocate for their child with cancer is, the most likely response will be themselves. After all, no one knows the child better, cares, loves, or is as invested in the child as the family. Patient advocacy is defined as "parents speaking and acting on behalf of their child, as an intercessor and champion, to ensure that their child's needs are met" [28]. However, to parents and other family members, hospitals can be intimidating places that have their own culture, use their own language, and have their own hierarchy. Adjusting to all these environmental changes initially can make it difficult for parents and family members to effectively advocate for their child with cancer. Nonetheless, parents and families rise to the occasion under the most dire and stressful circumstances to make complex, life-altering, medical decisions for their children throughout the cancer journey [78, 79].

Parents and families want to be involved in their children's medical care, and this form of advocacy is consistent with family-centered care. The concept of family-centered care arose in the United States in the 1980s as part of the conference of the Surgeon General that was focused on children with special health-care needs [80]. Family-centered care received a legislative mandate in 1986 with passage of US Public Law 99-457 that requires that the whole family be treated as the recipient of services for children with special needs, and with family members deciding ways they want to be involved in decision-making about health and education services for their child [28, 81, 82].

Positive outcomes for both children and their parents have been found when parents play an active role in the health-care process [28, 81, 82]. In fact, parents of children with chronic illness have reported less stress and better emotional well-being when care was rated as more family centered [83]. Specifically, with cancer, parents have been included as coaches and co-therapists in interventions to reduce pain, anxiety, and distress during cancer-related medical procedures such as venipuncture, lumbar puncture, bone marrow aspiration, intramuscular and intravenous injections, and accessing ports. Studies of the efficacy of these interventions indicate that they are successful in reducing child pain, anxiety, and distress [28, 84–88]. The parent advocate influences medical care, and therefore parents must be taken seriously as a valuable member of the medical care team. In fact, parent involvement in medical rounds has been shown to affect medical decision-making in 90% of cases [89]. Therefore, the inclusion of parents in the treatment process is not only beneficial to the child and the family but impacts the overall effectiveness of medical care.

In 2003, Holm et al. conducted a groundbreaking study to explore the ways in which parents participated in their child's medical care [28]. Forty-five parents whose children had completed cancer treatment at least 1 year prior to the study participated. The results found that parents identify themselves as performing the role of an advocate for their child particularly during the diagnosis and treatment phases. However, the disconnect between parents' intimate knowledge of their children and limited knowledge of medical terms and procedures made it difficult for some parents to advocate for their children. Furthermore, given the high regard for medical professionals in our culture, some parents said they did not know whether it was okay to press the medical team, particularly the physicians, when they had questions or concerns because they did not want to be disrespectful. Other parents talked about being intimidated by the environment or by the physicians. Given that parents and family members play a significant role in the treatment team, it is important for physicians to be aware of the fears, insecurities, and other factors that could potentially prevent open communication with these individuals. Ultimately it is the responsibility of parents and family members to ask questions about their child's care, but it is also the responsibility of medical professionals to set the appropriate tone and safe environment to receive such questions.

During the diagnostic phase, parents expressed two main strategies of advocacy such as seeking a medical explanation for their child's symptoms and persisting until a diagnosis is obtained [28]. The research illustrated that parents are keen observers of their children and can identify subtle, yet key, observations that may otherwise be overlooked by the medical community. These observations can impact the timeliness of a cancer diagnosis. When parents bring their children to their pediatrician seeking answers, in most cases the children present with symptoms that are not especially unusual. However, because parents know the nuances of their own child's behavior, they can advocate for their child by insisting that the pediatrician evaluate the symptoms as something beyond the ordinary illness. In some cases, however, families need to be persistent in order to obtain the correct diagnosis. Pediatricians need to respect the role parents play in their child's medical care as well as understand their concerns as it relates to the changes they are observing in their child's health and overall wellness.

During the treatment phase, parents express four main strategies of advocacy [28]. The first strategy is informing. Once children are diagnosed with cancer, most parents develop a veracious appetite to learn everything about their child's cancer. Parents find their own ways of doing this, whether by paper, electronically, or through contacts with friends and family members. The second strategy is deciding upon the course of action for their child's medical treatment. This includes which medical facility to use for treatment, choosing medical team members, deciding on treatment options, whether to participate in clinical trials, and determining when to report changes in symptoms in order to necessitate additional medical care. The third strategy is limiting medical procedures for their child. Examples of a limiting strategy would be when parents refuse to have blood pressure checks taken when the child is sleeping or refusing bedside procedural scans at convenient times for radiology technicians. The final strategy is affirming the child's medical professionals. Relationships often extend throughout treatments and sometimes continue once treatment is over. It is important for health-care professionals to be aware of the strategies associated with patient advocacy, because understanding that such strategies exist will enable professionals to assist families in successfully negotiating through them.

Holm et al.'s advocacy strategies [28] were well operationalized in Mattie's case, particularly the skill of "persisting" as a form of advocacy. When Mattie was 13 months into treatment, his parents persistently advocated to obtain answers as to his constant pain and inability to eat. He was 6 weeks off of chemotherapy, still receiving MTP-PE, an experimental immunotherapy, twice a week. Mattie was weak and participating in an aggressive physical therapy schedule in the hopes of regaining strength and the ability to walk in preparation for returning to school in the fall. However, Mattie refused all food and would not consume even water. He lived on IV fluids only. He kept insisting that he was in pain and that he needed pain medication to manage his symptoms. Mattie's parents received many consults, and the advice ranged from this being a side effect of the chemotherapy, that he was manipulating them for control, or that he was not eating because he was addicted to pain medication. When the symptoms persisted, his parents requested that Mattie undergo new scans, despite only being 6 weeks from completing a very aggressive course of chemotherapy. The team agreed and CT results confirmed that Mattie's cancer had metastasized to his liver and lungs. This scenario illustrates that childhood cancer does not always follow any set scientific pathway or checklist and therefore it is vital to listen to the insights from the patient. There should also be some caution used about assigning blame to parents regarding their child's behavior (in this case with regard to the manipulation of food and pain medication) before ruling out other medical explanations for symptoms. Such pronouncements to parents can have devastating and long-lasting consequences.

Another advocacy strategy that parents find helpful is the "informing strategy." This can be implemented by maintaining a webpage, updating Facebook or a Caring Bridge page, or, as in the case of Mattie's parents, creating a blog. Mattie's mother (Victoria Sardi-Brown) still maintains the blog today though the focus of her writing has shifted from helping Mattie battle osteosarcoma to the aftermath of losing an only child. Though "informing" is typically thought of as acquiring as much information about cancer as possible, health-care professionals should be aware of the positive benefits families may receive from informing friends, family, and their care communities about their child's cancer journey and their experiences.

The second form of advocacy during the treatment phase [28] is the "deciding strategy." Following a cancer diagnosis, most parents know very little about childhood cancer. They express shock and feel overwhelmed when presented with a variety of treatment options for their child. Many of the options may entail care at a center that is geographically distanced from the family's home. Mattie's parents were presented with a treatment option at one major comprehensive cancer center that involved high-dose chemotherapy and limb-salvaging surgery with Repiphysis technology. They found the whole notion of surgery daunting and felt the need to consult with another major cancer institution for a second opinion before consenting to surgery. To their dismay, they found that these cancer institutions recommended two very different treatment plans. In fact, the recommendation presented to Mattie's parents at the second cancer institution was to move directly to end-of-life care, since they felt Mattie had no chance of survival.

Parents consult medical professionals for help making decisions regarding their child's cancer care. They are under tremendous stress when asked to understand medical facts, clinical research, and what seems to be a whole new set of language skills. Contrary recommendations are not only confusing, but induce feelings of confusion and helplessness. Health-care professionals need to be aware of these stressors on families and provide the necessary support to make decisions during such critical times. The Mattie Miracle Cancer Foundation [2] points out that childhood cancer care "is not just about the medicine," a point illustrated by how the two institutions looked at Mattie's case differently. One focused on the sheer medical probability of successfully surviving cancer, whereas the second was willing to fight his cancer aggressively so that he could have as much time with his family as possible. These are subtle differences that have an enormous and empowering impact on the family. Parents respond best to having options presented that take into account evidence-based data along with parental priorities, the child's psychosocial needs and abilities, and short- and long-term consequences. Treatment choices should always be within the hands of the parents as they are the ones who have to live with the long-term consequences of these decisions. Once a decision is made, the team should support the parents' choice. What may appear to be an innocent comment by a health-care professional may not be perceived that way by a parent. Furthermore, such comments may be remembered many years later by parents. Similarly, health-care professionals should acknowledge that the patient/family/physician fit is crucial for effective cancer care. While rare, physicians and their pediatric families should confront a poor fit head on, and when resolution attempts are not effective, changes to care team members should be recommended in order to impact optimal care.

The last advocacy strategy Holm et al. highlighted in the treatment phase was "affirming" [28]. The relationships that parents establish with medical professionals extend throughout treatment and sometimes continue after treatment is over. The treatment protocol that Mattie and his parents endured was extremely grueling, resulting in Mattie spending most of the 14 months of treatment within a hospital setting, with very few days at home. Mattie even elected to die at the hospital. He selected that option because, by that point, the hospital was his second home. Other than Mattie's parents, he had no other family geographically close by; effectively, hospital personnel had become his extended family. On the day that Mattie died, hospital personnel who were part of Mattie's care team came to visit him and his parents to pay their respects and say their final farewell. In essence there was an impromptu memorial service in Mattie's room with 20 people sitting around him in a circle, sharing stories, reflections, and supporting Mattie's parents and each other through this loss. Mattie's parents remain close to several members of Mattie's care team, and it is through these continued connections and relationships that they feel they are further able to keep Mattie's presence and memory alive. The lesson learned for optimal care is that there is a great deal clinicians can gain from the lived experiences of patients and their families who have received your medical and psychosocial services. Families are usually eager to share their insights and feedback with health-care professionals and are most grateful for the care provided to their child.

Advocating for one's child is part of the expected role of being a parent. What sets parents of children with cancer apart from those with normal developmental issues is that they face life and death situations, make difficult decisions, and observe their child endure painful and frightening treatments. The very nature of cancer and its uncertain prognosis contributes to a chronic sense of vulnerability and powerlessness. Actively advocating for their child's needs appears to be one important way parents are able to restore a sense of control and protect their child as well as cope with their own grief and uncertainty [28]. Parents want the medical team to ask them about their child, above and beyond their medical needs. Parents bring the expertise of being vigilant, knowing their child best, and noticing and responding to subtle changes in their child that are important from the time of diagnosis and throughout treatment. Developing a therapeutic alliance, based on active collaboration and mutual respect, is a fundamental key to childhood cancer care.

18.7 The Need for National Psychosocial Standards of Care

Given the growing recognition that psychosocial care is an important component of comprehensive care for people diagnosed with cancer [13], there is a demand for accountability and outcome-driven, cost-effective models for this care. Psychosocial clinicians are being challenged to standardize their approach and evaluate the efficacy of their clinical efforts [90, 91]. There are potential barriers that can prevent high-quality care from being provided consistently across sites. Table 18.2 identifies specific problems that can become barriers to care and suggests interventional strategies for programs to consider in order to reduce obstacles to care.

Table 18.2 Barriers and recommendations to achieve optimal psychosocial care

Problem	Barrier	Recommendation
Financial and system constraints	Pediatric cancer centers have varying amounts of resources and funding which can limit the depth and breadth of psychosocial services	• Provide psychosocial staff with opportunities to network with staff at comprehensive centers; attend relevant meetings
		• Efforts to obtain funding for positions from local foundations
Access to psychosocial services	Billing structures and mental health carve-outs limit who can be seen in many centers	• Administration efforts to include staff in panels
		• Educate staff to advocate with insurance companies
		• Letters of medical necessity
		• Obtain local funding to cover uninsured costs
Access to resources	Health-care team lacks information about existing resources and how to access them	• Designate knowledgeable psychosocial staff to present information, algorithms to access information
Conflict and confusion in medical situations	Differing goals of medical team and family	• Early meetings with team and family to discuss goals
		• Continued check-in with family through treatment
Problems in communication	Lack of time, differing schedules, avoidance, lack of understanding of the skill sets of interdisciplinary team members	• Regular care conferences
		• Psychosocial staff can facilitate communication in meetings with medical team
Problems in staff expertise in pediatric psychosocial issues	Lack of training and experience in understanding family dynamics and belief systems as well as coping with the stresses of diagnosis, treatment, and end of life	• Ensure hiring of appropriate staff
		• Provide opportunities for relevant training through coursework, conferences, in-services

In 2012, adult psychosocial researchers formulated standards addressing the psychosocial component of adult cancer care and issued clinical practice guidelines [92]. They also developed and implemented measurable indicators for the quality of psychosocial care in oncology settings. Recent standards for the psychosocial care of children with cancer and their family members have been published [93]. Though the methods utilized in the development of standards of psychosocial care for adult cancer patients may be useful to the process of developing childhood cancer standards, the specific elements are most likely to differ significantly [91, 93].

18.8   The Impetus Behind the Development of National Childhood Cancer Psychosocial Standards of Care

The devastation of losing a child to cancer is both unimaginable and indescribable for parents. Such a death symbolizes a reversal of the natural order of life, and it erases the dreams and hopes that parents have for their child and for themselves [94]. Parents may continue to grieve long after the death of their child [95, 96]. Such chronic grief has been associated with many psychological (e.g., depression, anxiety) and somatic symptoms (e.g., loss of appetite, sleep disturbances, fatigue), including increased mortality risk [94, 96–98].

After the death of a child, many parents are left with a changed attitude about their employment. They may find that work is no longer rewarding and that their priorities in life are quite different. Instead, they are compelled to be involved in more meaningful activities that will build a legacy for their deceased child [94], such as the creation of a cancer foundation. Many nonprofit childhood cancer foundations across the United States have been started as the direct result of a child's cancer diagnosis or death. Foundation work is a heartfelt, passionate labor of love in which parents dedicate their time and energy to memorialize their child, to help other children and families battle cancer, and to find a way to reengage back into a world which no longer includes their child.

In November of 2009, 2 months after the Browns lost Mattie, they created the Mattie Miracle Cancer Foundation, a 501(c)(3) tax-exempt public charity. Mattie Miracle, based in Washington DC, is dedicated to addressing the psychosocial needs of children and families living with childhood cancer as well as educating healthcare providers on the impact of such a diagnosis on children and their families. The Foundation enhances awareness, advocacy, and access to psychosocial support on both the local and national level. Locally, Mattie Miracle funds a child life specialist position and offers a pediatric nursing support group and free snack carts to inpatient pediatric families at hospitals in Washington DC and Baltimore, MD.

The Browns' cancer experience has inspired them to voice a vision for pediatric psychosocial standards of care, in which every child and family should have access to an optimal level of critical psychosocial services, regardless of where a child is treated. After Mattie's death, they began advocating on Capitol Hill. Though staffers were supportive of the concerns addressed, the number one question posed at each visit was "what are the evidenced-based practices for psychosocial care and treatment for children with cancer and their families?" Mattie Miracle did not have answers to this question, but felt compelled and motivated to find them. In 2011, Mattie Miracle had the opportunity to connect with Brett Thompson, a lobbyist and now partner at Banner Public Affairs. Brett worked with the Foundation on a pro bono basis and convinced the cofounders that they should take a risk and hold the first ever Childhood Cancer Psychosocial Symposium at the Capitol Hill Visitor's Center. The goal of this event was to provide the community and lawmakers with access to cutting-edge psychosocial research and clinical practice delivered by a panel of psychosocial oncology experts (Anne Kazak, PhD, Scientific Chair of the

Symposium; Robert B. Noll, PhD; Andrea Farkas Patenaude, PhD; Ken Tercyak, PhD; and Lori Wiener, PhD), along with insights from parents whose children battled cancer. The Symposium was filled to capacity with registrants representing 12 different states from across the country. Attendees included nurses, social workers, professional counselors, child life specialists, art therapists, occupational therapists, psychologists, medical doctors, congressional staffers, and childhood cancer advocates. Mattie Miracle wanted to capitalize on the momentum from the Symposium on Capitol Hill and consulted with Dr. Lori Wiener and Dr. Anne Kazak on next steps. They encouraged Mattie Miracle to think more broadly and to sponsor a psychosocial think tank where leaders in the field could brainstorm the creation of Standards of Care for Childhood Cancer. The American Psychosocial Oncology Society, a national organization dedicated to psychosocial aspects of cancer care, invited Mattie Miracle to host the think tank at their 2013 annual conference in Huntington Beach, CA. It was at this think tank that the Psychosocial Standards of Care Project for Childhood Cancer was born.

18.9 The Psychosocial Standards of Care Project for Childhood Cancer

Extensive preparation work by the Mattie Miracle psychosocial core team of experts was done to launch the first think tank, whose long-term goal was the development of evidence-and consensus-based, comprehensive, implementable twenty-first-century pediatric psycho-oncology standards of care. The first step was a synthesis of existing attempts to standardize the clinical practice in pediatric psycho-oncology. Wiener et al. [91] reviewed literature from 1980 to 2013 to identify existing guidelines, consensus-based reports, and standards for psychosocial care of children with cancer and their families. Twenty-seven publications about psychosocial care met the inclusion criteria, consisting of (1) articles describing standards, guidelines, or consensus-driven reports in the field of pediatric psycho-oncology with an explicit focus on pediatric or adolescent oncology patients published in a peer-reviewed journal in English between 1980 and 2013 or (2) psychosocial cancer care standards which did not exclude pediatric oncology patients. Despite persistent calls by a number of international childhood cancer oncology and psycho-oncology professional organizations about the urgency to address the psychosocial needs of children with cancer, none of these articles were sufficiently up-to-date, comprehensive, specific enough, or evidence or consensus based to serve as a current standard for psychosocial care of children with cancer and their families.

In addition to the literature review, think tank participants and their colleagues completed an online survey exploring the perceived needs of children with cancer and their families in all settings where a child with cancer could be treated. This data was qualitatively analyzed and presented at the think tank. A major goal of the think tank was to obtain consensus on what the "essential" elements for psychosocial care should be. An "essential" element, as developed by Livestrong [99], is defined as having a positive impact on morbidity, mortality, and/or quality of life, can be implemented across a variety of care settings, is supported by an evidence base, and has been agreed upon through consensus of the provider community. Recognizing varying resources and data to support the provision of each recommended standard, elements were identified as "essential" (to be provided to all children with cancer), a "high need element" (all settings should provide direct access or referral to this element of care when possible), or a "strive element" (all settings should strive to provide direct access or referral to this element of care).

During the think tank, participants reached consensus on essential elements for the care of children with cancer, and, as a result, four working groups (Screening and Assessment, Child and Family Psychotherapeutic Interventions, Staff and Documentation, School Issues (social and neurocognitive)) were formed. The working groups consisted of 22 psychologists, three psychiatrists, five social workers, one nurse, two oncologists, and five parents from the United States, Canada, and the Netherlands. The working groups were represented by several professional groups: American Psychosocial Oncology Society (APOS); International Psychosocial Oncology Society (IPOS); Society of Pediatric Oncology (SIOP); Children's Oncology Group (COG); National Association of Pediatric Social Work (APOSW); American Psychological Association, Division 54 (APA); Oncology Nursing (APHON); and American Association of Child Psychiatry (AACAP).

Following this groundbreaking think tank, working groups held monthly conference calls, led by a core think tank group leader. Each group reviewed the clinical literature to ensure, when possible, that standards generated were evidence based. A consensus-based approach was used to determine whether enough evidence was available for the element to remain essential. To systematically guide the process among the work groups, the Appraisal Guidelines for Research and Evaluation [100] was followed. The groups conducted further evaluations of their work by sending supporting data and a rating form to pediatric oncologists, pediatric psycho-oncologists, or other applicable health-care providers (such as child life specialists, educational specialists, oncology nurses, etc.) for feedback.

A second psychosocial think tank was sponsored by the Mattie Miracle Cancer Foundation and held at the 2014 American Psychosocial Oncology Society Conference in Tampa, FL. Small working groups reviewed the created standards, evidence summaries, and rating forms and conducted additional reviews of specific portions of the standards generated by a different working group. In addition to achieving consensus on the recommendations, think tank participants were asked to rate whether each recommendation should continue to be considered an essential element, a high need element, or a strive element.

The standards were consolidated and further revision, literature appraisal, and GRADE [101] analysis for each standard element by working group members were performed. The standards were evaluated for quality and rigor and vetting from outside organizations and individuals. As a result, 15 evidence-based "Psychosocial Standards of Care for Children with Cancer and Their Families" were published in a special supplemental issue of *Pediatric Blood & Cancer* [93]. This 3-year-long, international project involved 85 health-care professionals from 44 institutions across the United States, Canada, and the Netherlands. The project resulted in the largest and most comprehensive compilation of psychosocial standards to date in which 1217 journal articles were reviewed and appraised for rigor. These historic evidence-based standards define what children with cancer and their families must receive to effectively support their psychosocial needs from the time of diagnosis, through survivorship or end-of-life and bereavement care. The standards have been endorsed by 14 professional organizations: (1) American Academy of Child and Adolescent Psychiatry (AACAP), (2) American Childhood Cancer Organization (ACCO), (3) American Psychosocial Oncology Society (APOS), (4) Association of Pediatric Hematology/Oncology Educational Specialists (APHOES), (5) Association of Pediatric Hematology/Oncology Nurses (APHON), (6) Association of Pediatric Oncology Social Workers (APOSW), (7) American Society of Pediatric Hematology/Oncology (ASPHO), (8) B+ Foundation, (9) Canadian Association of Psychosocial Oncology (CAPO), (10) Cancer Support Community (CSC), (11) Children's Cause for Cancer Advocacy (CCCA), (12) Children's Oncology Group (COG), (13) National Children's Cancer Society (NCCS), and (14) Society of Pediatric Psychology (SPP; Division 54 of the American Psychological Association). The standards' authors and the Mattie Miracle Cancer Foundation are committed to creating, disseminating, and implementing a twenty-first-century, widely applicable blueprint to support universally available psychosocial services [91, 93].

Conclusion

This chapter reviewed the trajectory of sarcoma care from a psychosocial perspective. The importance of strengthening the alliance among the provider, patient, and the family was emphasized as the key to improving both the cancer experience and the outcomes of a childhood cancer diagnosis. Examples were provided to illustrate how a comprehensive alliance of professionals, patients, and families is needed in order for psychosocial care to be effective and meaningful. All health-care practitioners, regardless of their profession, need to be aware that psychosocial elements are just as important as the medical care and service that they deliver. Finally, psychosocial care must be a standard part of all cancer care. With the development and implementation of Childhood Cancer Psychosocial Standards of Care, the health-care industry will help lessen the potentially devastating psychological, social, and emotional impact that such a diagnosis can have on children and their families and help improve coping and adaptation for the entire family system.

References

1. CureSearch for Children's Cancer. Childhood cancer statistics. 2014. http://www.curesearch.org/Childhood-Cancer-Statistics/
2. Mattie Miracle Cancer Foundation. 2014. https://www.mattiemiracle.com/
3. Alderfer M, Kazak AE. Family issues when a child is on treatment for cancer. In: Brown RT, editor. Comprehensive handbook of childhood cancer and sickle cell disease. New York: Oxford; 2006. p. 53–75.
4. Cohen MS. Families coping with childhood chronic illness: a research review. Fam Syst Health. 1999;17:149–64.
5. Overholser JC, Fritz GK. The impact of childhood cancer on the family. J Psychosoc Oncol. 1990;8:71–85.

6. Varni JW, Katz ER, Colegrove R, Dolgin M. Family functioning predictors of adjustment in children with newly diagnosed cancer: a prospective analysis. J Child Psychol Psychiatry. 1996;37:321–8.
7. Wallander JL, Varni JW, Babani L, Banis HT, Wilcox KT. Family resources as resistance factors for psychological maladjustment in chronically ill and handicapped children. In: Roberts MC, Wallander JC, editors. Family issues in pediatric psychology. Hillsdale: Lawrence Erlbaum Associates; 1992. p. 129–45.
8. Holland J. History of psycho-oncology: overcoming attitudinal and conceptual barriers. Psychosom Med. 2002;64:206–21.
9. Patenaude AF, Kupst MJ. Psychosocial functioning in pediatric cancer. J Pediatr Psychol. 2005;30(1):9–27.
10. Spinetta JJ. The dying child's awareness of death. Psychol Bull. 1974;81:256–60.
11. Waechter EH. Death anxiety in children with fatal illness. Unpublished doctoral dissertation. Stanford University, Palo Alto, California.
12. Patenaude AF, Kupst MJ. SIOP education book. International Society of Paediatric Oncology (pp. 133–137). 2010. http://www.siop-online.org/sites/default/files/SIOP%20Education%20 Book%202010.pdf
13. Institute of Medicine of the National Academies. Cancer care for the whole patient: meeting psychosocial health needs. Washington, DC: National Academies Press; 2008.
14. Jacobsen PB, Holland JC, Steensma DP. Caring for the whole patient: the science of psychosocial care. J Clin Oncol. 2012;30(11):1151–3.
15. Jaaniste T, Hayes B, von Baeyer CL. Providing children with information about forthcoming medical procedures: a review and synthesis. Clin Psychol Sci Pract. 2007;14:124–43.
16. Kazak A. Evidence-based interventions for survivors of childhood cancer and their families. J Pediatr Psychol. 2005;30(1):29–39.
17. Powers S. Empirically supported treatments in pediatric psychology: procedure-related pain. J Pediatr Psychol. 1999;24:131–45.
18. American Psychiatric Association (APA). Diagnostic and statistical manual of mental disorders, text revision (DSM-IV-TR). 4th ed. Washington, DC: APA; 2000.
19. Spitzer RL, Kroenke K, Linzer M, Hahn SR, Williams JB, deGruy FV, Brody D, Davies M. Health-related quality of life in primary care patients with mental disorders. Results from the PRIME-MD 1000 study. JAMA. 1995;274(19):1511–7.
20. American Academy of Pediatrics. Guidelines for the pediatric cancer center and the role of such centers in diagnosis and treatment. Pediatrics. 1997;99:139–40.
21. Kazak A. Comprehensive care for children with cancer and their families: a social ecological framework guiding research, practice, and policy. Child Serv. 2001;4(4):217–33.
22. Askins MA, Moore BD. Psychosocial support of the pediatric cancer patient: lessons learned over the past 50 years. Curr Oncol Rep. 2008;10:469–76.
23. Rosenberg AR, Wolfe J. Palliative care for adolescents and young adults with cancer. Clin Oncol Adolesc Young Adults. 2013;3:41–8.
24. Institute of Medicine of the National Academies. When children die: improving palliative and end-of-life care for children and their families. 2003. http://iom.edu/Reports/2002/When-Children-Die-Improving-Palliative-and-End-of-Life-Care-for-Children-and-Their-Families.aspx
25. Waldman E, Wolfe J. Palliative care for children with cancer. Nat Rev Clin Oncol. 2013; 10(2):100–7.
26. Wein S, Pery S, Zer A. Role of palliative care in adolescent and young adult oncology. J Clin Oncol. 2010;28(32):4819–24.
27. Masera G, Spinetta JJ, Jankovic M, Ablin AR, Buchwall I, Van Dongen-Melman J, Eden T, Epelman C, Green DM, Kosmidis HV, Yoheved S, Martins AG, Mor W, Oppenheim D, Petrilli AS, Schuler D, Topf R, Wilbur JR, Chesler MA. Guidelines for a therapeutic alliance between families and staff: a report of the SIOP working committee on psychosocial issues in pediatric oncology. Med Pediatr Oncol. 1998;30:183–6.
28. Holm KE, Patterson JM, Gurney JG. Parental involvement and family-centered care in the diagnostic and treatment phases of childhood cancer: results from a qualitative study. J Pediatr Oncol Nurs. 2003;20(6):301–13.

29. Goold SD, Lipkin M. The doctor-patient relationship. J Gen Intern Med. 1999;14(Suppl 1):S26–33.
30. Kupst MJ, Patenaude AF, Walco GA, Sterling C. Clinical trials in pediatric cancer: parental perceptions on informed consent. J Pediatr Hematol Oncol. 2003;25:787–90.
31. Wiener L, Alderfer M, Pao M. Psychiatric and psychosocial support for child and family. In: Pizzo PA, Poplack DG, editors. Principles and practice of pediatric oncology. 7th ed. Philadelphia: Lippincott; 2015. p. 1124–40.
32. Kusch M, Labouvie H, Ladisch V, Fleischhack G, Bode U. Structuring psychosocial care in pediatric oncology. Patient Educ Couns. 2000;40(3):231–45.
33. Robert RS, Ottaviani G, Huh WW, Palla S, Jaffe N. Psychosocial and functional outcomes in long-term survivors of osteosarcoma: a comparison of limb-salvage surgery and amputation. Pediatr Blood Cancer. 2010;54(7):990–9.
34. Bradbrook D. Acupuncture treatment of phantom limb pain and phantom limb sensation in amputees. Acupunct Med. 2004;22(2):93–7.
35. Prakash S, Golwala P. Phantom headache: pain-memory-emotion hypothesis for chronic daily headache? J Headache Pain. 2011;12(3):281–6.
36. Cassileth R, Keefe FJ. Integrative and behavioral approaches to the treatment of cancer-related neuropathic pain. Oncologist. 2010;15(Suppl):19–23.
37. MacIver K, Lloyd DM, Kelly S, Roberts N, Nurmikko T. Phantom limb pain, cortical reorganization and the therapeutic effect of mental imagery. Brain. 2008;131(8):2181–91.
38. Ramachandran VS, Brang D, McGeoch PD. Size reduction using mirror visual feedback (MVF) reduces phantom pain. Neurocase. 2009;15(5):357–60.
39. Chambless DL, Ollendick T, Thomas H. Empirically-supported psychological interventions: controversies and evidence. Annu Rev Psychol. 2001;52:685–716.
40. Palermo TM. Cognitive-behavioral therapy for chronic pain in children and adolescents. Oxford: New York; 2012.
41. Wetering EJ, Lemmens KM, Nieboer AP, Huijsman R. Cognitive and behavioral interventions for the management of chronic neuropathic pain in adults—a systematic review. Eur J Pain. 2010;14(7):670–81.
42. Nagarajan R, Neglia JP, Clohisy DR, Robison LL. Limb salvage and amputation in survivors of pediatric lower extremity bone tumors: what are the long-term implications? J Clin Oncol. 2002;20:4493–501.
43. Harris IE, Leff AR, Gitelis S, Simon MA. Function after amputation, arthrodesis, or arthroplasty for tumors about the knee. J Bone Joint Surg Am. 1990;72:1477–85.
44. Postma A, Kingma A, De Ruiter JH, Schraffordt Koops H, Veth RP, Goëken LN, Kamps WA. Quality of life in bone tumor patients comparing limb salvage and amputation of the lower extremity. J Surg Oncol. 1992;51:47–51.
45. Pao M, Wiener L. Anxiety and depression. In: Wolfe J, Hinds P, Sourkes B, editors. Textbook of interdisciplinary pediatric palliative care. Philadelphia: Elsevier; 2011. p. 229–38.
46. Wiener L, Pao M. Comprehensive and family-centered psychosocial care in pediatric oncology: integration of clinical practice and research. In: Kreitler S, Ben-Arush MW, Martin A, editors. Pediatric oncology: psychosocial aspects and clinical interventions. 2nd ed. West Sussex: Wiley; 2012. p. 7–17.
47. Martin JR, Kodaman P, Oktay K, Taylor HS. Ovarian cryopreservation with transposition of a contralateral ovary: a combined approach for fertility preservation in women receiving pelvic radiation. Fertil Steril. 2007;87(1):189 e5–7.
48. Ginsberg JP, Goodman P, Leisenring W, Ness KK, Meyers PA, Wolden SL, Smith SM, Stovall M, Hammond S, Robison LL, Oeffinger KC. Long term survivors of childhood Ewing sarcoma: a report from the Childhood Cancer Survivorship Study. J Natl Cancer Inst. 2010;102:1272–83.
49. Hudson MN, Jones KE, Mulrooney DA, Avedian R, Donaldson S, Popat R, West DW, Fisher P, Leisenring W, Stovall M, Robison LL, Ness KK. Change in health status of pediatric upper

and lower extremity sarcoma: a report from the Children's Cancer Survivorship Study. Arch Phys Med Rehabil. 2013;94:1062–73.

50. Wiener L, Battles H, Bernstein D, Long L, Derdak J, Mackall CL, Mansky P. Persistent psychological distress in long-term survivors of pediatric sarcoma: the experience at a single institution. Psychooncology. 2006;15(10):898–910.

51. Koopman HM, Koetsier JA, Taminiau AHM, Hijnen KE, Bresters D, Egeler RM. Health related quality of life and coping strategies of children after treatment of a malignant bone tumor: a five year follow up study. Pediatr Blood Cancer. 2005;45(5):694–9.

52. Van Riel CAHP, Meijer-van den Bergh EEM, Kemps HLM, Feuth T, Schreuder HWB, Hoogerbrugge PM, Groot IJM, Mavinkurve-Groothuis AM. Self-perception and quality of life in adolescents during treatment for a primary malignant bone tumour. Eur J Oncol Nurs. 2014;18(3):267–72.

53. Fritz GK, Williams JR, Amylon M. After treatment ends: psychosocial sequelae in pediatric cancer survivors. Am J Orthopsychiatry. 1988;58:552–61.

54. Merchant M, Wright M. Sarcomas and other solid tumors. In: Wiener L, Pao M, Kazak AE, Kupst MJ, Patenaude AF, editors. Quick reference for pediatric oncology clinicians: the psychiatric and psychological dimensions of cancer symptom management. Charlottesville, VA: Oxford University Press; 2015.

55. Children's Oncology Group. Long-term follow-up guidelines for survivors of childhood, adolescent, and young adult cancers. Version 3.0, Appendix 1, Arcadia, CA; 2008.

56. Horowitz ME, Fordis M, Krause S, McKellar J, Poplack DG. Passport for care: implementing the survivorship care plan. J Oncol Pract. 2009;5(3):110–2.

57. Weir RF, Peters C. Affirming the decision adolescents make about life and death. Hastings Cent Rep. 1997;27:29–40.

58. Wicks L, Mitchell A. The adolescent cancer experience. Loss of control and benefit finding. Eur J Cancer Care (Engl). 2010;19(6):778–85.

59. Wiener L, Zadeh S, Battles H, Baird K, Ballard E, Osherow J, Pao M. Allowing adolescents and young adults to plan their end-of-life care. Pediatrics. 2012;130(5):897–905.

60. Wiener L, Zadeh S, Wexler L, Pao M. When silence is not golden: engaging adolescents and young adults in discussions around end-of-life care choices. Pediatr Blood Cancer. 2013;60(5):715–8.

61. Zadeh S, Pao M, Wiener L. Opening end-of-life discussions: how to introduce voicing my CHOiCES™, an Advance Care Planning Guide for Adolescents and Young Adults. Palliative and supportive care, E-published ahead of print; 2014.

62. Wiener L, Sweeney C, Baird K, Merchant MS, Warren KE, Corner GW, Roberts KE, Lichtenthal WG. What do parents want to know when considering autopsy for their child with cancer? J Pediatr Hematol Oncol. 2014;36(6):464–70.

63. deCinque N, Monterosso L, Dadd G, Sidhu R, Lucas R. Bereavement support for families following the death of a child from cancer: practice characteristics of Australian and New Zealand Paediatric Oncology Units. J Paediatr Child Health. 2004;40:131–5.

64. Heiney S, Wells L, Ruffin J. A memorial service for families of children who died from cancer and blood disorders. J Pediatr Oncol Nurs. 1996;13:72–9.

65. Johnson L, Rincon B, Gover C, Rexin D. The development of a comprehensive bereavement program to assist families experiencing pediatric loss. J Pediatr Nurs. 1993;8:142–6.

66. Neidig J, Dalgas-Pelish P. Parental grieving and perceptions regarding health care professionals' interventions. Issues Compr Pediatr Nurs. 1991;14:179–91.

67. Whittam EH. Terminal care of the dying child. Cancer. 1993;71:3450–2462.

68. Davies B, Limbo R, Jin J. Grief and bereavement in pediatric palliative care. In: Ferrell BR, Coyle N, editors. Oxford textbook of palliative nursing. 3rd ed. New York: Oxford University Press. p. 1081–97).

69. Kissane DW. Bereavement. In: Doyle D, Hanks G, Cherny N, Calman K, editors. Oxford textbook of palliative medicine. Oxford: Oxford University Press; 2004. p. 1137–51.

70. Macdonald ME, Liben S, Carnevale FA, Rennick JE, Wolf SL, Meloche D, Cohen SR. Parental perspectives on hospital staff members' acts of kindness and commemoration after a child's death. Pediatrics. 2005;116(4):884–90.
71. National Hospice and Palliative Care Association. Standard, bereavement care and services, BCS 1. Defined Bereavement Program; 2000.
72. Wolfe J, Hinds PS, Sourkes BM. Textbook of interdisciplinary pediatric palliative care. Philadelphia: Elsevier; 2011.
73. Kurt BA, Armstrong GT, Cash DK, Krasin MJ, Morris EB, Spunt SL, Robison LL, Hudson MM. Primary care management of the childhood cancer survivor. J Pediatr. 2008; 152(4):458–66.
74. American Hospital Association (AHA). In the name of the patient. Chicago: American Hospital Association; 2002.
75. Goehring K. New tools to measure patient satisfaction. Health Care Exec. 2001;15:71–2.
76. Martin DR, Tipton BK. Patient advocacy in the USA: key communication role functions. Nurs Health Sci. 2007;9:185–91.
77. Ross J. Keeping the focus on satisfaction. Health Care Exec. 2001;16:62–3.
78. Kupst MJ, Schulman JL. Long-term coping with pediatric leukemia: a six-year follow-up study. J Pediatr Psychol. 1988;13(1):7–22.
79. Kupst MJ, Natta MB, Richardson CC, Schulman JL, Lavigne JV, Das L. Family coping with pediatric leukemia: ten years after treatment. J Pediatr Psychol. 1995;20(5):601–17.
80. U.S. Department of Health and Human Services (Division of Maternal and Child Health). Surgeon general's report: children with special health care needs (DHHS Publication No. HRS/D/MC 87–2). Washington, DC: Government Printing Office; 1987.
81. Rosenbaum P, King S, Law M, King G, Evans J. Family-centered service: a conceptual framework and research review. Phys Occup Ther Pediatr. 1998;18:1–20.
82. Woodside JM, Rosenbaum PL, King SM, King GA. Family-centered service: developing and validating a self-assessment tool for pediatric service providers. Child Health Care. 2001;30:237–52.
83. King SM, Rosenbaum PL, King GA. Parents' perceptions of caregiving: development and validation of a measure of processes. Dev Med Child Neurol. 1996;38:757–72.
84. Barrera M. Brief clinical report: procedural pain and anxiety management with mother and sibling as co-therapists. J Pediatr Psychol. 2000;25:117–21.
85. Broome ME, Rehwaldt M, Fogg L. Relationships between cognitive behavioral techniques, temperament, observed distress, and pain reports in children and adolescents during lumbar puncture. J Pediatr Nurs. 1998;13:48–54.
86. Manne SL, Redd WH, Jacobsen PB, Gorfinkle K, Schorr O, Rapkin B. Behavioral intervention to reduce child and parent distress during venipuncture. J Consult Clin Psychol. 1990;58:565–72.
87. Powers SW, Blount RL, Bachanas PJ, Cotter MW, Swan SC. Helping preschool leukemia patients and their parents cope during injections. J Pediatr Psychol. 1993;18:681–95.
88. Smith JT, Barabasz A, Barabasz M. Comparison of hypnosis and distraction in severely ill children undergoing painful medical procedures. J Couns Psychol. 1996;43:187–95.
89. Rosen, P., Stenger, E., Bochkoris, M., Hannon, M., J., & Kwoh, C. K. (2009). Family-centered multidisciplinary rounds enhance the team approach in pediatrics. Pediatrics, 123, 4, e603-e608.
90. Noll RB, Patel SK, Embry L, Hardy KK, Pelletier W, Annett RD, Patenaude A, Lown EA, Sands SA, Barakat LP. Children's Oncology Group's 2013 Blueprint for research: behavioral science. Pediatr Blood Cancer. 2013;60:1048–54.
91. Wiener L, Viola A, Koretski J, Perper ED, Patenaude AF. Pediatric psycho-oncology care: standards, guidelines, and consensus reports. Psychooncology. 2014;24(2):204–11. doi:10.1002/pon.3589.
92. Jacobsen PB, Wagner LI. A new quality standard: the integration of psychosocial care into routine cancer care. J Clin Oncol. 2012;30(11):1154–9.

93. Wiener L, Kazak AE, Noll R, Patenaude AF, Kupst MJ. Standards for the psychosocial care of children with cancer and their families. Pediatr Blood Cancer. 2015;62(S5):425.
94. Alam R, Barrera M, D'Agostino N, Nicholas DB, Schneiderman G. Bereavement experiences of mothers and fathers over time after the death of a child due to cancer. Death Stud. 2012;36(1):1–22.
95. Kreichbergs U, Valdimarsdottir U, Onelov E, Henter JI, Steineck G. Talking about death with children who have severe malignant disease. N Engl J Med. 2004;351:1175–86.
96. Wing DG, Clance PR, Burge-Callaway K, Armistead L. Understanding gender differences in bereavement following the death of an infant: implications for treatment. Psychotherapy. 2001;38:60–73.
97. Li J, Precht DH, Mortensen PB, Olsen J. Mortality in parents after death of a child in Denmark: a nationwide follow-up study. Lancet. 2003;361:363–7.
98. Znoj HJ, Keller D. Mourning parents: considering safeguards and their relationship to health. Death Stud. 2002;26:545–65.
99. Rechis R, Beckjord EB, Arvey SR, Reynolds KA, McGoldrick D. The essential elements of survivorship care: a livestrong brief. 2011. Retrived from http://www.livestrong.org/pdfs/3-0/EssentialElementsBrief
100. AGREE Collaboration. Development and validation of an international appraisal instrument for assessing the quality of clinical practice guidelines: the AGREE project. Qual Saf Health Care. 2003;12:18–23.
101. Guyatt GH, Oxman AD, Vist GE, Kunz R, Falck-Ytter Y, Alonso-Coello P, Schünemann HJ. GRADE: an emerging consensus on rating quality of evidence and strength of recommendations. BMJ. 2008;336:924–6.

Treatment Effects and Long-Term Management of Sarcoma Patients and Survivors

19

Luca Szalontay and Aziza Shad

19.1 Introduction

The diagnosis of cancer in children and adolescents is a life-altering event for them as well as their families. In 2014, an estimated 15,780 new cases of cancer were diagnosed among children and adolescents aged birth to 19 years in the USA [1]. The 5-year survival rate of children diagnosed with cancer before the age of 15 years is approximately 83%, and according to data from 2013, it results in an estimated 420,000 survivors of childhood cancer in the USA [2]. Solid tumors make up about 55–62% of all pediatric tumors, with brain tumors being the most common (26%), followed by neuroblastoma (8%), soft tissue sarcomas (7%), bone tumors (4%), and kidney tumors (4%) [3].

Sarcomas originate primarily from the elements of the mesodermal embryonic layer. Staging to determine the extent of the disease is crucial for determining therapy and prognosis. Current treatment consists of three modalities: surgery, chemotherapy, and radiation. A complete surgical resection is ideal, but often is not possible owing to tumor invasion of the surrounding structures; hence, the initial surgery may only be a biopsy or debulking at best. A second surgery (usually preceded by neo-adjuvant chemotherapy) aims to resect the tumor completely with a fair margin of healthy tissue around the tumor. Following surgery, more chemotherapy is given

L. Szalontay, M.D. (✉)
Division of Hematology, Oncology and Stem Cell Transplantation, Department of Pediatrics, Morgan Stanley Children's Hospital of New York, Columbia University Medical Center, New York, NY, USA
e-mail: ashad@lifebridgehealth.org

A. Shad, M.D.
The Herman & Walter Samuelson Children's Hospital at Sinai, Baltimore, MD, USA

Georgetown University School of Medicine, Washington, DC, USA

© Springer International Publishing Switzerland 2017
R.M. Henshaw (ed.), *Sarcoma*, DOI 10.1007/978-3-319-43121-5_19

and the patient is monitored closely for recurrent disease and physical function [4]. In some cases, following biopsy and induction chemotherapy, radiation is used as the second modality of treatment.

Over the last several decades, due to advances in treatment protocols and supportive care, survival rates have improved tremendously, and as a result, almost 80% of children treated for cancer will be long-term survivors. However, it has also become clear that this cure has come at a price. It has been proven that survivors are at risk for a number of chronic or late-occurring health problems caused by their cancer or its treatment, often referred to as "late effects of therapy," which can affect the physical, cognitive, and psychosocial health of the survivors. Reports from the Childhood Cancer Survivorship Study (CCSS) estimate that almost 75% of all survivors will develop at least one chronic health problem, more than 40% will suffer from a severe life-threatening or disabling condition, and one third will have multiple health problems [5]. Long-term follow-up programs and services are essential in order to address the unique needs of this ever-growing population.

Below is a discussion of the causes and follow-up of late effects of therapy specific to patients with sarcomas. The recommendations for screening and follow-up have been taken from the Children's Oncology Group (COG) Long-Term Follow-Up (LTFU) Guidelines [6].

19.2 Late Effects by Systems

19.2.1 Anthracycline Cardiotoxicity

Anthracyclines are antibiotic drugs with effective antitumor cytotoxic activity, and they are extensively used in the chemotherapy of various sarcomas [7]. The main mechanism of their activity involves the inhibition of topoisomerase IIα, an enzyme, which relaxes supercoiled DNA, allowing DNA replication and transcription. Interfering with DNA synthesis and RNA transcription in cancer cells induces cell cycle blocks at the G1 or G2 phases causing arrest in mitosis and cell death.

The clinical manifestations of anthracycline-induced cardiotoxicity have been categorized into an acute form, which shows symptoms within 24 h of the anthracycline intravenous infusion, and a late-onset chronic progressive form, characterized by left ventricular systolic dysfunction, that can remain subclinical for many years. These cardiotoxic effects are dose dependent and cumulative, and the cumulative dose is the most important cardiotoxic risk factor.

There are three main hypotheses on the molecular mechanisms through which anthracyclines induce cellular degenerative changes in the myocardiocytes [8]. One of those theories is the oxidative stress hypothesis: anthracyclines enter the cell through passive diffusion, and anthracycline-induced reactive oxygen species are produced by the intracellular redox metabolism of the drug. Oxidative stress induces nitric oxide synthase, and nitric oxide can inactivate key enzymes of the heart muscle, including myofibrillar creatine kinase. The second concept is the topoisomerase IIβ hypothesis, which suggests that the formation of a ternary complex consisting of an anthracycline, DNA, and topoisomerase IIβ triggers DNA damage in the form of double-strand breaks in the DNA and activates the p53 pathway, which induces apoptosis, ultrastructural and functional mitochondrial defects, and fibrosis leading to decreased left ventricular ejection fraction and increased left ventricular end-systolic and end-diastolic volumes. The third hypothesis is the alcoholic metabolite hypothesis, which proposes that the C-13 hydroxy metabolite of doxorubicin, referred to as doxorubicinol, accumulates within membranous compartments acting as low-clearance storage sites and is more potent in interfering with the iron homeostasis of the cardiomyocyte resulting in alterations in the redox, energetic, and ionic balance of the cells. This can also explain why anthracyclines can induce a lifelong risk of cardiotoxicity.

There are several mechanisms that can explain myocyte destruction. Generation of free oxygen radicals leads to lipid peroxidation of membranes, causing vacuolation, which is irreversible, and repair is only possible via replacement of the myocytes by fibrous tissue. Another possible mechanism of cardiotoxicity is cardiac cell death by apoptosis. Because of the limited regenerative capacity of the heart, the number of cardiomyocytes decreases, which results in ventricular remodeling. In vivo experimental evidence suggests that doxorubicin-induced cardiomyopathy might be mediated by the loss of cardiac stem cells [9].

There are several factors, which make cardiomyocytes more susceptible to injury [10]. Mitochondria are one of the key mediators of anthracycline-induced cardiotoxicity, and their abundance in cardiomyocytes could make the heart muscle more vulnerable to injury. Additionally, cardiomyocytes have low concentrations of free radical scavengers, such as catalase and glutathione peroxidase, and therefore they are more sensitive to ROS (Reactive Oxygen Species) injury. Cardiolipin, found in the inner mitochondrial membrane, has a high affinity to anthracyclines. Binding to this specific phospholipid molecule inhibits the respiratory chain and interacts with mitochondrial DNA.

Clinical manifestations of anthracycline-induced cardiotoxicity can present at various time periods. Acute cardiotoxicity, when patients become symptomatic, occurs within 1 week of treatment, documented in less than 1% of the cases, and is usually self-limiting [11]. Early-onset cardiotoxicity (symptoms presenting within 1 year of treatment) includes electrophysiological changes, left ventricular dysfunction, decreased exercise capacity, and clinical heart failure. Late-onset cardiotoxicity may present with acute cardiomyopathy or progression of left ventricular dysfunction. Diagnostic markers include cardiac troponin T, N-terminal pro-brain natriuretic peptide, and C-reactive protein [12].

The cardiac toxicity of doxorubicin may be attributable in part to genetic variations in drug targets or genetic differences in drug disposition, such as in biotransformation enzymes and drug transporters [13].

It has been recently demonstrated that anthracycline treatment induces a specific cardiac iron overload, which is independent of systemic iron load, and the cardiotoxic effects of doxorubicin develop from mitochondrial iron accumulation [14, 15]. Certain genotypes of the HFE gene were associated with higher cardiac iron levels further increasing the cardiac iron load caused by doxorubicin therapy [14, 16]. Since heterozygosity for HFE mutations has a high prevalence in the western countries, these results suggest that HFE genotyping could become a useful strategy for identifying patients with a higher risk of anthracycline-related cardiac damage.

Anthracyclines induce a cardiac remodeling pattern characterized by interstitial or patched fibrosis. It has been recently revealed that NADPH oxidase polymorphism rs4673 protects against focal myocardial necrosis, whereas rs1883112 is strongly associated with cardiac fibrosis [17]. These findings may lead to better individualized strategies for early detection and prevention of anthracycline cardiotoxicity.

To identify genetic markers predictive of anthracycline-induced cardiotoxicity in children, Visscher et al. conducted a genetic study of 220 key genes involved in absorption, distribution, metabolism, elimination, and toxicity of medications and found single nucleotide polymorphisms (SNPs) in several genes that are significantly associated with cardiotoxicity following anthracycline treatment [18].

There have been different approaches to prevent anthracycline-related cardiotoxicity. One of them is to modify treatment protocols to achieve the best outcome with the least amount of exposure to the toxic drug. Limiting the total cumulative anthracycline dose to 300 mg/m^2 resulted in fewer cases with severe left ventricular dysfunction; however, it has become clear that there is no safe dose of anthracyclines [19]. Randomized trials comparing continuous infusion with bolus infusion found that it decreased acute onset cardiotoxicity in adults, but showed no significant difference in cardiac outcomes in children with high-risk ALL [20, 21]. Epirubicin and idarubicin are structural analogs of doxorubicin and daunorubicin, respectively, and were designed to reduce cardiotoxicity. Liposomal anthracyclines have a more favorable oncological and a safer cardiovascular profile than conventional anthracyclines [22].

Several agents have been tested to determine whether they can protect the heart against anthracycline-related cardiotoxicity. Dexrazoxane is an iron-chelating agent, which prevents the formation of iron-anthracycline complexes. The combination of dexrazoxane and doxorubicin resulted in less cardiac damage in children than that caused by doxorubicin alone [23]. Amifostine reduces chemotherapeutic drug damage in normal tissue. It is less cardioprotective than dexrazoxane; it scavenges free radicals, but it does not reduce their production [24].

Animal studies provide novel mechanistic insight into the pathogenesis of anthracycline toxicity. It has recently become known that gene therapy with soluble Fas, an inhibitor of Fas/Fas ligand interaction, in mice prevents the progression of doxorubicin-induced acute cardiotoxicity, accompanying attenuation of the cardiomyocyte degeneration, inflammation, and oxidative damage caused by Fas signaling [25]. Carvedilol has been shown to offer some cardioprotection from its antioxidant activity, and it reduced anthracycline-induced cardiomyopathy when tested on rats [26]. Probucol is an antioxidant and lipid-lowering agent, and studies in rats showed that pretreatment with probucol negates the toxic impact of doxorubicin therapy on cardiomyocytes [27]. Sildenafil, a phosphodiesterase inhibitor, could also protect against anthracycline-induced cardiotoxicity when given to mice treated with doxorubicin [28]. Li et al. used murine models to investigate the effects of erythropoietin (EPO) and reported that the administration of EPO prior to the appearance of the cardiac dysfunction resulted in less left ventricular dilatation and dysfunction [29]. Animal studies have also demonstrated that phosphodiesterase 5 inhibitors have powerful protective effect against doxorubicin cardiotoxicity through the cGMP signaling pathway [30]. Coenzyme Q, L-carnitine, and glutathione are supplements with antioxidant activity protecting the heart against anthracycline-induced lipid peroxidation [31–33].

19.2.1.1 Recommended Screening

Currently, there is no consistently used, precise definition of anthracycline-induced cardiotoxicity. It can manifest as either clinical or subclinical heart failure. The American Heart Association's class I recommendation for children receiving anthracycline treatment is serial monitoring of both the left and the right ventricular functions by echocardiography starting at diagnosis and then periodically throughout treatment (Table 19.1a, b) [6, 34]. Exercise stress testing may detect asymptomatic cardiac dysfunction in patients treated with anthracyclines or mediastinal radiation, but its application in monitoring cardiac function of childhood survivors is uncertain. Although these patients may have adequate cardiac function at rest, they may decompensate if cardiac demands are increased [35, 36]. Results closely correspond with prognosis in patients with congestive heart failure.

Biomarkers may help identify patients undergoing treatment who are at high risk for cardiotoxicity. Cardiac troponin I (cTnI) assays are the best-studied biomarkers, and monitoring cTnI levels may provide information regarding the development of cardiac toxicity before left ventricular dysfunction becomes apparent on echocardiography or via clinical symptoms. It might also allow for earlier realization of the degree of cardiac damage occurring during treatment, creating the opportunity for more timely modulation of therapy [37]. When the contribution of modifiable risk factors on the development of major cardiac events was investigated among adult survivors of childhood cancer, it was found that hypertension could potentiate therapy-related risk in this patient population [38].

It has been challenging to manage patients with heart failure secondary to anthracycline toxicity. ACE inhibitors have been shown to improve left ventricular mass, dimension, and fractional shortening [39]. Beta-blockers reverse the intrinsic mechanisms of myocardial dysfunction and remodeling mediated by the adrenergic pathway [40]. Growth hormone concentrations are found to be low in survivors treated with anthracycline and cranial irradiation. GH acts indirectly on the heart through IGF-1 to maintain adequate left ventricular mass. Replacement therapy increases left ventricular mass during anthracycline therapy, but cannot provide long-term gain preventing cardiomyopathy [41]. Cardiac transplantation remains the last resort for patients in whom cardiomyopathy develops after anthracycline therapy; their survival rates are almost the same as those after transplant for other indications.

Table 19.1 (**a**) End-treatment follow-up echocardiogram schedule to monitor cardiac late effects after treatment with anthracyclines per COG survivorship guidelines [6]; (**b**) calculating total anthracycline dose

a

Age at treatment	Chest radiation	Anthracycline dose	Recommended schedule
< 1 year old	yes	any	annually
	no	< 200 mg/m^2	every 2 years
		≥ 200 mg/m^2	annually
1-4 years old	yes	any	annually
	no	< 100 mg/m^2	every 5 years
		≥ 100 to < 300 mg/m^2	every 2 years
		> 300 mg/m^2	annually
> 5 years old	yes	< 300 mg/m^2	every 2 years
		≥ 300 mg/m^2	annually
	no	< 200 mg/m^2	every 5 years
		≥ 200 to < 300 mg/m^2	every 2 years
		> 300 mg/m^2	annually
any age with decrease in serial function			annually

b

Anthracycline drug	Equivalent factor
Adriamycin	x 1.0
Mitoxantrone	x 2.5
Daunomycin	x 0.75
Idarubicin	x 3.0

19.2.2 Bone Disease

Patients with cancer have an increased incidence of bone disease. Malignant tumors can not only form osteolytic or osteoblastic bone metastases, but the treatment to eliminate the tumor can also result in bone loss leading to osteoporosis and fractures.

Measuring bone mineral density (BMD) in children and adolescents has its challenges [42], since it varies on the basis of height and stage of puberty, which may not even correlate with age in a chronically ill child. Dual-radiograph absorptiometry (DXA) has traditionally been used to determine BMD, and height age (the age at which 50% of normal children would be the patient's current height) is often used to get a more accurate measurement and fracture risk. Quantitative computed tomography (QCT) provides direct and more precise volumetric measurement; however it is not currently universally available and involves increased radiation doses. A newer technique is directed at peripheral anatomic sites, but this has to be validated and standardized in the pediatric population.

Steroids have an effect on bone metabolism in multiple ways including: decreasing osteoblast activity, increasing bone resorption, interfering with the growth hormone/IGF-1 axis, reducing muscle strength, and disturbing calcium homeostasis at the level of the kidney and gut [43]. Methotrexate's cytotoxic effect on osteoblasts results in reduced bone volume and formation of new bone [44]. Alkylating agents can cause gonadal dysfunction that can impact BMD when deficiencies of ovarian and testicular hormones develop. Estrogens play an important role in achieving and maintaining peak bone mass, while androgens help in periosteal apposition, adding to the biochemical strength of the bone [45]. Radiation to the neuroendocrine axis can lead to growth hormone deficiency and hypogonadism.

Osteonecrosis is a condition where there is cellular death of bone components due to interruption of the blood supply. It is a relatively rare condition in the general population, but shows increased incidence among children with cancer. Overall estimates for the incidence have ranged from 1 to 9% [46], and the cumulative incidence was found to increase with time for many years after treatment. The necrosis occurs at one or more bone sites, usually at weight-bearing joints, resulting in pain and loss of mobility. The most common sites are the hips (72%), followed by the shoulders (24%) and the knees (21%) [47]. Bone sarcoma survivors are among patients with the greatest risk. Older age at diagnosis, shorter elapsed time, exposure to dexamethasone, and gonadal and non-gonadal radiotherapy were independently associated with osteonecrosis.

19.2.2.1 Recommended Screening

The latest COG-LTFU Guidelines recommend a baseline evaluation of BMD by DXA or QCT at entry into long-term follow-up for survivors treated with agents that predispose to BMD deficits or with medical conditions associated with BMD deficits.

Treatment of BMD deficits in children includes increasing weight-bearing exercise, optimizing nutritional intake of calcium and vitamin D, nutrient supplementation, and treatment of underlying conditions that may exacerbate BMD [48, 49].

Counseling cancer survivors on healthy lifestyle choices is also a crucial part of treatment. Cancer survivors with significantly decreased BMD may benefit from endocrinology consultation. Treatment options such as calcitonin and bisphosphonates are currently reserved for patients with recurrent fractures or those who are on clinical trials.

19.2.3 Rehabilitation After Limb-Sparing Surgery

Until around 1970, amputation was the treatment choice for primary high-grade malignant bone and soft tissue tumors of the limb. The management of these tumors has changed dramatically since that time, and today about 85% of these patients undergo limb-sparing surgery. This means that instead of amputating part of or the entire limb, the surgical team reconstructs the bony and soft tissue defects using custom or modular endoprostheses, allografts, or composite materials [50]. The goal is to preserve the patient's physical, psychological, social, occupational, creative, and economical function to the highest possible level in conjunction with malignant disease and treatment.

Limb-sparing surgery can result in survival rates and disease-free periods that equal those achieved with amputation [51]. Limb-sparing surgery offers better psychological functioning and an intact body image, but is more complex and associated with more morbidity, including infection, pain, and other postoperative complications. Limb-sparing surgery is an extensive procedure, and it deliberately damages many anatomic areas potentially causing several problems such as bone and joint, muscle, skin, nerve, vascular, and lymphatic system damages, scars, and infections. Therefore, rehabilitation is performed by a multidisciplinary team, which includes an orthopedic oncologist, nurses, social workers, dietitians, physiotherapists, occupational therapists, and orthopedic technicians.

Children who undergo limb-sparing surgery may need to be hospitalized repeatedly for lengthening procedures which prolongs rehabilitation and causes repeated cycles of functional regression. Complications following endo-prosthetic reconstruction fall into two main categories: mechanical (breakage/fracture of the implant, instability due to wear) and biological (infection, aseptic loosening, wound/soft tissue breakdowns). A recent retrospective study including 232 patients who underwent endo-prosthetic reconstruction for malignant and aggressive bone tumors between 1980 and 2002 found that the overall incidence of complications was 41% [52]. Mechanical complications were the most common cause of implant failure, which occurred in 21% of the patients. Data have also shown that modular implants were much less likely to fail than custom implants. Infection was the most common complication seen in this study and was also the most common cause of loss of limb; 51% of infections resulted in eventual amputation. The limb salvage rate for all patients was 90% after 20 years, demonstrating that many complications were successfully managed, particularly in the absence of an infection.

Many children experience psychological problems during the course of the disease and the surgical management of the tumor [53]. Young children feel frustrated by being isolated from their environment; there are losses of opportunity for play, feelings of inadequacy due to impaired mobility, and problems at school. The issues affecting teenagers are often related to their body image. They also have problems in identifying with their peer group.

19.2.4 Gonadal Damage and Fertility

Chemotherapy and radiotherapy can both have a deleterious effect on the gonads. Consideration of fertility preservation is a quality of life issue, and discussion of potential fertility problems at the time of diagnosis provides the patients and their families with the reassurance that the oncology team believes in a future when these issues become important.

19.2.4.1 Male Fertility

Reduced fertility is common among adult survivors of cancer who received some form of chemotherapy, testicular radiation, or experienced damage to the hypothalamus or pituitary glands [54]. We often see sterilization, but at the same time preservation of Leydig function, as testicular hormonal production is more resistant to treatment-induced damage and is independent of the presence of spermatogonia.

If chemotherapeutic agents do not kill stem spermatogonia, spermatogenesis recovers within 12 weeks after cessation of therapy [55]. Spermatogenesis can be impaired by agents that alkylate or cross-link DNA, like cyclophosphamide, ifosfamide, or cisplatin. The cumulative dose of a cytotoxic agent determines the duration and magnitude of impaired spermatogenesis [56, 57]. The Childhood Cancer Survivor Study reported that survivors aged 15–44 years were less likely to sire a pregnancy than siblings [58]. Whether the prepubertal testis is less sensitive than the postpubertal testis to chemotherapy is not known. Although the prepubertal testis does not show complete spermatogenesis, there is evidence that cytotoxic treatment given to prepubertal boys affects their fertility. COG suggests that having a prepubertal status at diagnosis is not protective against germ cell toxicity of alkylating agents [59].

Testicular germ cells are very sensitive to radiation and germinal cell depletion is dose dependent. Differentiating cells are damaged by doses as low as 1 Gy, which reduce the number of spermatogonia and spermatocytes [60]. A single testicular dose of radiation exceeding 4–6 Gy can result in permanent azoospermia. Fractionated irradiation of the testes can be even more harmful; with doses of more than 2 Gy, aspermia may be permanent [61]. Gonadotropin deficiency can develop when the hypothalamus and pituitary gland are damaged by surgery, tumors, or cranial radiation. The severity varies from subclinical to severe, when it can diminish the levels of circulating sex hormones.

19.2.4.2 Recommended Screening for Males

Assessment of male reproductive function starts from the assessment of pubertal development. For survivors exposed to alkylating agents or radiation before the onset of puberty, the COG-LTFU Guidelines recommend annual assessment of pubertal development until sexual maturity using Tanner staging and measurement of testicular volume. Semen analysis is the initial investigation of fertility potential. It provides information about the functional status of the germinal epithelium, epididymis, and accessory sex glands. Hormonal evaluation should include the measurements of serum FSH, LH, and testosterone levels. Testicular volume change can also be an indicator of decreased fertility. Approximately 85% of the testicular mass consists of germinal tissue, so a reduced germinal mass is associated with reduced testicular size and soft consistency.

Patients with hypogonadotropic hypogonadism usually require therapy with gonadotropin-releasing hormone and human menopausal gonadotropin to induce spermatogenesis [62]. Cryopreservation of sperm before cancer therapy is a successful method for fertility preservation in postpubertal individuals. Recent advances in assisted reproductive technology can allow men to father successful pregnancies [63]. Fertility preservation for prepubertal boys continues to be a challenge because their spermarche has not started yet. Harvesting spermatogonial stem cells from preserved testicular tissue for in vitro maturation might be an option in the future [64]. Men with oligospermia can achieve fatherhood using in vitro fertilization or intracytoplasmic sperm injection [65].

19.2.4.3 Female Fertility

Loss of ovarian function after chemotherapy that includes an alkylating agent, procarbazine, or ovarian irradiation can result in both sterilization and loss of hormonal production, because ovarian hormonal production is closely related to the presence of ova and maturation of the primary follicle [66]. Survivors who lose ovarian function during or shortly after the completion of cancer therapy are classified as having acute ovarian failure (AOF). It includes patient who reported never menstruating or who had ceased having menses within 5 years after their cancer diagnosis. According to the CCSS data, only a relatively small number, about 6% of childhood cancer survivors, developed AOF. They were older at cancer diagnosis, more likely to have received abdominal or pelvic radiotherapy, or more likely to have been diagnosed with Hodgkin's lymphoma. Previous data indicate that radiation affects the ovaries in a dose-dependent fashion [67]. Doses in a range of 10–30 Gy cause AOF in the majority of patients treated during childhood and adolescent [68].

Some survivors who retain ovarian function after the completion of cancer treatment and experience menopause at younger than 40 years of age are classified as having "premature menopause." It leads to the early and often unexpected loss of reproductive potential as well as the cessation of ovarian sex hormone production. These women are at risk for developing various adverse health outcomes, including osteoporosis, death from cardiovascular disease, and psychosexual dysfunction, just to name a few. The risk factors for premature menopause are older age, exposure to increasing doses of radiation to the ovaries, or increasing alkylating agent score (based on the number of alkylating agent and their cumulative dose).

The offspring of women whose treatment included pelvic irradiation are more likely to be premature, have a low birth weight, and be small for gestational age [69]. Prior treatment with doxorubicin or daunorubicin increased the risk of low birth weight, which was independent from pelvic irradiation. The risk of miscarriage was increased among women whose treatment included high-dose cranial or cranio-spinal irradiation.

The intense radiotherapy and chemotherapy received by cancer survivors are known to cause somatic mutations in humans and germ line mutations in animals [70]. Preliminary results of the evaluation of self-reported genetic and congenital diseases among offspring of survivors and offspring of sibling controls were reassuring that cancer treatment using modern protocols does not carry a large risk of genetic disease in offspring conceived after treatment [71].

19.2.4.4 Recommended Screening for Females

As per COG-LTFU Guidelines, hormonal studies including FSH, LH, estradiol, and anti-Mullerian hormone should be done annually or more frequently if needed in pubertal and postpubertal females.

A number of strategies to protect the ovaries and preserve fertility during cancer therapy have been attempted with limited success. The gamete pool in females is fixed at birth and collection is technically more difficult. Collection of mature oocytes for fertilization and subsequent cryopreservation for young sexually mature females with partners has the most success. Cryopreservation of oocytes is an alternative option [72].

19.2.5 Renal Adverse Effects

Nephrotoxicity is a known side effect of certain childhood cancer therapies, resulting in a decline in glomerular filtration rate (GFR), deterioration of tubular function, development of albuminuria/proteinuria, or renovascular hypertension during or after treatment [73]. Potentially nephrotoxic agents include ifosfamide, the platinum compounds, cisplatin and carboplatin, and methotrexate, all of which are used in the treatment of solid tumors [73, 74]. Abdominal and total body irradiation may also cause radiation nephropathy [75].

Ifosfamide can have serious adverse effects on the kidney despite concurrent use of the uroprotectant mesna. The most common manifestation is proximal tubular dysfunction and less often decreased GFR [76, 77]. A reduction in GFR occurs in 25% of patients treated with high-dose ifosfamide [78], and approximately 30% of children develop a persistent tubulopathy, some of them with a clinically significant

Fanconi syndrome [79]. In most of the cases, tubular dysfunction is asymptomatic, but growth failure and rickets are serious sequelae of this disorder if untreated. Several risk factors have been recognized for chronic ifosfamide-induced nephrotoxicity, the most important being the cumulative dose but also including age less than 3 years, concurrent or previous platinum therapy, renal irradiation, unilateral nephrectomy, or hydronephrosis [80–82].

Kidney damage is the major dose-limiting side effect of cisplatin. Most children treated with cisplatin will have some acute renal loss with an average of 8% decrease in GFR per 100 mg/m^2 dose received [83]. The decline in GFR directly correlates with peak serum or urine platinum concentrations and infusion rates [84]. A magnesium-wasting tubulopathy occurs in almost every patient treated with cisplatin. Magnesium supplementation is often needed and can cause hypocalcemia and/or hypokalemia. The outlook for long-term recovery or stability of renal function is generally favorable, but magnesium wasting tends to be long-lasting [85].

Carboplatin is a cisplatin analog, but it is less nephrotoxic than cisplatin, since it is not transformed into toxic metabolites by renal tubule cells. On the other hand, the risk of renal insufficiency and tubulopathies is higher with the combination therapy of carboplatin and ifosfamide than with cisplatin and ifosfamide [86].

High-dose methotrexate (MTX) therapy is associated with acute renal dysfunction with an overall incidence rate of 1.8% [87], and it results in delayed elimination of the drug and its metabolite. Toxicity is due to the precipitation of the drug within the renal tubular lumen. MTX-related nephrotoxicity appears to be entirely reversible, with a medium recovery time of 16 days [87]. Irradiation of the kidney occurs when the primary tumor is located near the kidney. Radiation nephritis or radiation nephropathy usually presents after a latent period of 3–12 months and manifests by hypertension, proteinuria, renal insufficiency, and anemia [88]. Doses greater than 20 Gy result in significant nephropathy [89].

19.2.5.1   Recommended Screening

Assessment of childhood cancer survivors for late renal sequelae should be part of every checkup [73]. Baseline screening recommendations for asymptomatic survivors of potentially nephrotoxic therapy include blood pressure measurement; serum electrolytes including calcium, magnesium, and phosphorus; BUN/creatinine; and urinalysis. After the baseline evaluation, annual follow-up includes blood pressure measurement and urinalysis. Currently, the definition of hypertension is a blood pressure level at or above the 95th percentile. Proteinuria is first detected by urinary dipstick, which primarily detects albumin. Persistent proteinuria warrants referral to a nephrologist. Abnormal GFR is most often detected by elevated serum creatinine concentrations. Patients at risk for renal late effects should be counseled to avoid lifestyles that put them at risk for renal injury such as tobacco use, excessive alcohol consumption, dehydration, and NSAID use.

19.2.6 Secondary Malignancies

Childhood cancer survivors are at risk for development of subsequent malignant neoplasms. This risk is approximately tenfold greater than the general population and an important health-related concern [90]. Secondary malignancies are the leading cause of treatment-related mortality in long-term childhood cancer survivors. The cumulative incidence of all subsequent neoplasms after 30 years following diagnosis was 20.5% and was higher in patients who received radiation therapy [91]. For many second malignancies, the incidence continues to increase with longer follow-up, with no plateau of risk over time. Underlying genetic susceptibility, such as mutation of the retinoblastoma or p53 gene (i.e., Li-Fraumeni syndrome), also plays an important role. Therapy-associated leukemia has a shorter latency, typically less than 10 years from the primary cancer diagnosis [92], and has a well-defined association with alkylating agents and topoisomerase II inhibitor chemotherapy.

Radiotherapy is a double-edged sword. Solid malignancies include breast, thyroid, skin, and brain cancer, and there is a strong association with radiation exposure with a latency that exceeds 10 years [92]. Additionally, Henderson et al. found an increased number of gastrointestinal cancers in childhood cancer survivors as compared to general population, with 87% of those patients having received radiotherapy for treatment of the primary cancer [93]. The goal of radiation treatment planning should be to keep the normal tissue exposures to a minimum, and every effort should be made to minimize the influence of factors that could potentially increase the risk of secondary malignancies, including lower total dose or a nonradiation approach whenever evidence supports the benefit without compromising tumor cure [94].

Childhood cancer survivors have an increased risk of secondary sarcomas [95]. Exposure to therapeutic radiotherapy for the primary cancer is the most significant risk factor observed in secondary sarcoma development, and this risk showed sharp increase with the radiation dose of 50 Gy or more. Anthracycline chemotherapy is also associated with secondary sarcomas. Those who survived Hodgkin's lymphoma or sarcoma were more likely to develop a secondary sarcoma compared to other types of cancer. Schwartz et al. showed that the increase in the risk of bone sarcoma is well described by a linear function of the radiation dose received by the bones [96].

19.2.6.1 Recommended Screening
Annual follow-up with recommended screening as per COG-LTFU Guidelines is suggested.

19.2.7 Neuropathy and Hearing Loss

Chemotherapy-induced peripheral neuropathy is a common and potentially dose-limiting side effect of many chemotherapy drugs [97]. It primarily affects sensory nerves, which allow perception of touch, pain, temperature, position, and vibration, and several pathobiologic mechanisms have been discovered. Platinum compounds irreversibly bind to DNA inducing apoptosis of primary sensory neurons [98]. Antitubulins, such as vincristine, bind to microtubules, which interrupt axonal transport, target the soma of sensory neurons as well as the nerve axons, and induce neuronal death [99].

Cisplatin is widely used in the treatment of bone sarcomas, and it produces a well-recognized neurotoxicity. Factors that influence the degree of toxicity are total cumulative dose, the dose of individual injection, the schedule of drug delivery, renal function, and previous neurological damage from other conditions [100]. Earl et al. conducted a study examining 36 patients treated for bone and soft tissue sarcomas and found that 44% had a significant reduction in deep tendon reflexes; 55% had raised vibration perception threshold, which was the most sensitive single test in the assessment of neuropathy; and 35% had abnormal nerve conduction studies [101].

Management of neuropathic pain includes systemic and topical medications, such as NSAIDs, opioids, tricyclic antidepressants, gabapentin and pregabalin, topical lidocaine and capsaicin, as well as non-pharmacological options like applying heat or ice at the affected area, physical therapy, massage therapy, or in severe cases transcutaneous electrical nerve stimulation and spinal cord stimulation.

Children treated for malignancies may be at risk for early- or delayed-onset hearing loss that can affect learning, communication, school performance, social interaction, and overall quality of life [102]. Survivors at particular risk include those treated with platinum compounds, but this risk is modified by the variability of the individual's susceptibility to cisplatin ototoxicity [103]. The mechanism of platinum cochlear toxicity is through interference with signal transduction from the organ of Corti in the cochlea. The sites of the damage are the outer hair cells, the spiral ganglion, and the stria vascularis, and it results in hearing loss involving the speech frequencies (500–2000 Hz). Several factors determine the risk of hearing loss besides the individual's susceptibility, including younger age, higher cumulative doses of chemotherapy, CNS tumors, and concomitant CNS radiation [102].

19.2.7.1 Recommended Screening

All childhood cancer survivors exposed to ototoxic therapy should undergo a yearly audiological evaluation. Upon entry into long-term follow-up, evaluation should consist of air conduction study, bone conduction study, tympanometry, and speech audiometry in survivors at risk for hearing loss [104]. Change in hearing sensitivity following ototoxic therapy should be evaluated relative to pretreatment measures [105].

The general principles managing hearing loss include appropriate referrals to an audiologist and otolaryngologist and implementation of hearing device and other adaptive strategies when indicated. Evaluation by language and speech therapists should also be obtained. Avoidance of loud noise and ototoxic medications, such as aminoglycoside antibiotics and diuretics, are also recommended.

19.2.8 Post-Traumatic Stress Disorder

Childhood cancer can be a devastating experience that places patients at an increased risk for disruption in psychological functioning [106]. The fourth edition of the Diagnostic and Statistical Manual for Mental Disorders (DSM-IV) in 1994 expanded the possible list of A1 stressors for post-traumatic stress disorder (PTSD) to include a "diagnosis of a life-threatening illness." Since this modification, many studies have investigated the incidence of PTSD among patients with cancer diagnosed at childhood. Researchers found that the incidence of the full PTSD syndrome was relatively low in this population [107], so they shifted their attention onto subclinical levels of post-traumatic stress symptomatology (PTSS), identifying specific factors associated with trauma response in this population which became the focus of their research.

There are several risk factors that may increase the risk of poor adaptation for children. Female patients appear to be more vulnerable [108], and the age of the child and the family's socioeconomic status can also influence the child's ability to adapt to the negative experience [109]. There is evidence that suggests a higher incidence of PTSS among children on active treatment and those who recently received the diagnosis [110]. Children with a previously diagnosed mental disorder have greater risk for stress-related mental disorder [111]. Severity of parental PTSS in response to the child's illness is a well-studied risk factor which is a significant correlate of child PTSS [112]. History of stressful life events in the child's life is also a critical factor regarding adaptation to childhood cancer.

The impact of these events on a developing personality is significant, and they have been linked to behavior issues, worsened physical health, and maladjustment at home and school [113]. Epidemiologic research has shown that individuals with PTSD tend to report a history of multiple potentially traumatic events rather than an isolated experience [114]. It can support a "multiple hit hypothesis" for traumatized children, for whom cancer either being the hit that precipitates the stress reaction or representing one of the several hits that together increase the risk of poor adaptation.

Stress or trauma-related symptoms such as heightened arousability, intrusive thoughts, and avoidant behavior have been frequently reported among children undergoing treatment for cancer [115]. PTSD among survivors is also associated with lower income, unemployment, single status, and intense treatment [116].

19.2.8.1 Recommended Screening

Given the potential benefit of interventions for those with prior psychopathology, that children are less likely to verbalize emotional problems, and the detrimental implications of undiagnosed mental disorders, the follow-up visits for the survivors should incorporate assessment for mental disorders, especially stress-related mental problems.

19.2.9 Sleep Disorders

The prevalence of sleep problems in children in the general population is estimated to be up to 30% [117]. Sleep problems are more prevalent in children and adolescents with chronic medical, neurodevelopmental, and social conditions [118]. There are several factors contributing to sleep disruption, and they can be a direct result of brain injury or an indirect result of chemotherapy. Stress on the child and the family resulting from a life-threatening disease can exacerbate sleep disorders.

A Childhood Cancer Survivorship Study examined the prevalence of, and risk factors for, fatigue and sleep disturbance among adult survivors of childhood cancer [119]. It showed that 19% of survivors were in the most fatigued range, 16.7% reported disrupted sleep, and 14% complained of excessive daytime sleepiness. A retrospective study was done among children with cancer, who were referred to a pediatric sleep clinic [120]. Excessive daytime sleepiness was the most common problem, followed by sleep-disordered breathing, such as obstructive sleep apnea, and insomnia.

When assessing survivors of childhood cancer for sleep problems, a detailed history is crucial. Subjective evaluation of sleep disorders is based on a sleep diary, use of validated scales for quantifying sleepiness, and sleep questionnaires. Objective measures include multiple sleep latency test, maintenance of wakefulness test, and nocturnal polysomnography.

Treatment of excessive daytime sleepiness is usually based on the cause [121]. Insufficient or inadequate sleep and disorders of arousal are treated with a behavioral approach and creating a safe sleeping environment. Obstructive sleep apnea requires weight reduction, tonsillectomy, or nasal CPAP. Treatment for delayed sleep phase syndrome often involves light therapy, appropriate sleep hygiene, and melatonin. To improve wakefulness physicians often prescribe methylphenidate, amphetamine, or modafinil.

Recently, several prospective interventional trials and analyses have been initiated to better understand sleep dysfunction in patients with childhood cancer and to provide information, which will inform future pharmacologic interventions, thereby improving patient quality of life.

19.2.9.1 Recommended Screening

A detailed history of sleep patterns should be included in the annual LTFU of all cancer survivors.

19.2.10 Resilience, Posttraumatic Growth, and Positive Sequelae

With increasing cognitive maturity, adolescent and young adult survivors may experience positive benefits or perceived positive impact as a result of their cancer experience [122]. Parents and siblings are also likely to experience positive benefits. These include enhanced coping abilities and motivation in various life domains. Posttraumatic growth is defined as the process of applying positive interpretations and finding meaning in a traumatic event. Self-awareness of inner resources and available social support may facilitate positive changes related to self-concept, relationships, and life philosophy. Survivors are more likely than siblings to report perceived positive impact. Predictors include malignancy or relapse, older age at diagnosis, and fewer years since diagnosis.

19.2.11 Employment Status After Childhood Cancer

The health and behavioral consequences of cancer may significantly affect long-term vocational and employment opportunities. Although not all studies have demonstrated deficits in employment, many report employment difficulties in adult childhood cancer survivors, with survivors being nearly twice as likely to be unemployed compared to healthy controls [123].

Survivors of bone and soft tissue sarcomas such as Ewing's sarcoma are less likely to be employed full time compared to sibling controls due to physical limitations that can restrict activity and job performance. Adult survivors of certain sarcomas, including rhabdomyosarcoma, are significantly more likely to report physical impairment characterized by one or more chronic health conditions, cancer-related pain, performance limitations of routine activities, and health-related inability to work, compared to sibling controls. Individuals treated with amputation have been shown to exhibit significant deficits in education, employment, and insurance access compared to sibling controls [124].

19.2.11.1 Recommended Screening
A detailed employment history and consultation/intervention by social work and rehabilitation specialists is important at the LTFU annual visits.

19.2.12 Insurance Status After Childhood Cancer

In the USA, where health insurance is provided largely through employers, restricted employment opportunities affect healthcare access. In the past, long-term childhood cancer survivors were significantly less likely to have health insurance, have more difficulty obtaining insurance due to restrictive policies excluding preexisting medical conditions, and more likely to be denied health insurance because of their cancer history [125].

There has been significant improvement in recent years in the disparity of insurance access between childhood cancer survivors and sibling or population controls due to legislation prohibiting employment discrimination and facilitating insurance access and portability. With the introduction of the Affordable Care Act in 2010, it is expected that more childhood cancer survivors will retain or have access to health insurance, either through long-term coverage under parental health insurance policies or the ability to purchase affordable state or federal health insurance plans.

Given that a substantial body of evidence confirms that childhood cancer may negatively affect vocational and employment opportunities and insurance access, providers should be aware of legislation that facilitates survivor employment and insurance access.

19.2.12.1 Recommended Screening

A detailed health insurance history and intervention by social work is important at the LTFU annual visits.

19.2.13 Healthcare Behaviors

Risk-based care incorporates the previous cancer, cancer therapy, genetic predispositions, lifestyle behaviors, age, and comorbid health conditions. Quality care for cancer survivorship has been defined as "a risk based approach to health care and a systematic plan for life-long screening, surveillance and prevention." Childhood cancer survivors continue to demonstrate significant lack of knowledge and misperceptions about their cancer diagnosis, treatment, and cancer-related health risks following completion of therapy; therefore, healthcare providers must focus on health maintenance and promotion along with surveillance for the early identification of late effects. With many pediatric cancer survivors continuing to engage in high-risk-taking behaviors at a rate similar to their peers, it falls on the clinicians to educate youths to focus on modifiable risk factors (diet, exercise, smoking, drinking alcohol) and to undergo routine surveillance. Potentially, a healthy lifestyle can help minimize the negative physical and psychological effects of cancer and its treatment.

It is important to develop an individual risk profile, which contains cancer diagnosis and treatment, complications during treatment, complications after treatment, family history, current problems and medications, physical examination and findings, laboratory test results and scan to date, health maintenance and screening behaviors, psychosocial health, and neurocognitive function status.

19.2.13.1 Recommended Screening

Educating young adult survivors of childhood cancer on the importance of modifiable risk factors and prevention cannot be overemphasized. Topics, which should be included, are eating a balanced diet, exercising regularly, smoking cessation, limiting alcohol intake, sun protection, minimizing environmental or industrial exposures, safe sex practices, and health maintenance. Secondary prevention of cancer is just as important as primary prevention. It involves breast self-examination and mammography for girls, testicular self-examination and PSA blood test for boys, regular skin examination, eye examination, colonoscopy, DEXA scan, regular dental checkup, and other case-specific screening and laboratory tests [126–128].

19.3 Models of Long-Term Follow-Up Care [129]

There are a variety of models for delivering care to survivors. The model best suited for an institution depends in large part on the population of survivors served and the resources available in the facility. From a different perspective, the best model may vary from patient to patient, those with the most complex treatment history requiring the most specialized level of care. But no matter what model is chosen, all survivors need education about their health risks and ongoing screening for potential late effects that may occur as they age.

19.3.1 Cancer Center Models

19.3.1.1 Primary Oncology Care

Patients continue to see their treating oncologist in the oncology clinic. This model is often the most comfortable for the patient, who has developed a relationship and a level of trust with the physician, nurses, and ancillary staff; the focus may remain on disease surveillance rather than the potential for late effects.

19.3.1.2 Specialized Long-Term Follow-Up Clinic

This is probably the most common model. It involves transitioning the patient from the primary oncologist to a specialized long-term follow-up team within the same cancer center, usually when the patient has been off therapy for at least 2 years. It provides expertise in the long-term effects of therapy and has a health promotion/wellness focus. It is designed to examine and evaluate the patient as well as to provide risk-based screening and recommendations and education about potential late effects (Tables. 19.2, 19.3, and 19.4). The team can provide support for transitioning the patient to adult-focused care, while others can follow patients for life. Patients follow up with a community healthcare provider for routine healthcare needs.

Table 19.2 End-treatment follow-up exams to monitor late effects in Ewing's sarcoma per COG survivorship guidelines [6]

Exam	Frequency
History and physical exam	1st - 4th year: every 3 months 5th year: every 6 months
Blood tests	1st - 4th year: every 3 months 5th year: every 6 months
Chest and extremity X-ray	1st - 4th year: every 3 months 5th year: every 6 months
CT/MRI chest and tumor site	end of treatment and if clinically indicated
Cardiac evaluation (EKG, echocardiogram)	end of treatment and then at 1-5 years depending on anthracycline dose received
Functional evaluation	1 year off treatment, then at 2.5 and 5 years
Fertility evaluation	1 year off treatment, then as needed

Table 19.3 End-treatment follow-up exams to monitor late effects in osteosarcoma per COG survivorship guidelines [6]

Exam	Frequency
History and physical exam	1st year: every 2-3 months 2nd year: every 3-4 months 3rd-4th year: every 6 months 5th-10th year: every 12 months
Blood tests	1st-2nd year: every 6 weeks-3 months 3rd-4th year: every 2-4 months 5th-10th year: every 6 months
Chest and extremity X-ray	1st year: every 3 months 2nd-3rd year: every 6 months 4th-10th year: every 12 months
CT/MRI chest and tumor site	every 4-6 months for the first 3 years, or as indicated
Cardiac evaluation (EKG, echocardiogram)	end of treatment and then at 1-5 years depending on anthracycline dose received
Hearing test	end of treatment, 2.5 years or as indicated
Functional evaluation	1 year off treatment, then at 2.5 and 5 years
Fertility evaluation	1 year off treatment, then as needed

19.3.1.3 Formalized Transition Programs

Many pediatric institutions have upper age limit for care, recognizing that the needs of older survivors can be better served in an adult-focused healthcare environment. These clinics are stuffed by pediatric and adult oncologists, family practitioners, internists, and nurse practitioners, who are experts in the care of pediatric cancer survivors. Multidisciplinary referrals to other subspecialties are made on an as-needed basis, often to an established network of adult providers.

19.3.1.4 Adult Oncology-Directed Care

Another option for transitioning young adult patients is to refer them to an adult oncologist for long-term follow-up. However, once minimal risk for disease recurrence has been identified, care is frequently transitioned to a primary care provider.

Table 19.4 End-treatment follow-up exams to monitor late effects in rhabdomyosarcoma/soft tissue sarcoma per COG survivorship guidelines [6]

Exam	Frequency
History and physical exam	1st year: every 3 months 2nd-3rd year: every 4 months 4th year: every 6 months 5th-10th year: every 12 months
Blood tests	1st year: every 3 months 2nd-3rd year: every 4 months 4th year: every 6 months 5th-10th year: every 12 months
Urinalysis	1st year: every 3-6 months 2nd year: every 6 months 3rd-10th year: every 12 months
CT/MRI of primary tumor	1st year: every 3 months 2nd year: every 4 months 3rd-4th year: every 6 months
Chest x-ray	1st year: every 3 months 2nd year: every 4 months 3rd-4th year: every 6 months
Other specific testing	based on site of the primary tumor

19.3.2 Community-Based Models

19.3.2.1 Shared Care

This has been defined as a joint partnership between a specialist and a primary care provider in the planned delivery of care for a particular patient. This model has been used safely and successfully in improving patient outcomes with various chronic illnesses. It offers a practical solution for meeting the complex needs of cancer survivors. In reality, however, it has not been yet embraced as the norm for survivorship care. The barriers of implementing this model are lack of knowledge and experience of the primary care physician on complex oncological problems and treatment protocols, the lack of time needed to provide a comprehensive preventive and chronic disease care, and the lack of continual communication and the clear delineation of roles between the oncologist and the primary care physician [130].

19.3.3 Need-Based Models

In the UK, models based on intensity of treatment are being explored to guide decisions about type and frequency of long-term follow-up for pediatric cancer survivors. Three levels of care have been proposed [131], and patients are followed either via telephone every 1–2 years, by primary care physician or nurse practitioner every 1–2 years, or by a specialized late-effect clinic.

19.4 Transition of Care

To optimize the health and quality of life of childhood cancer survivors, it is important to develop a systematic care that continues beyond the childhood years. There are two key phases in the management of a cancer patient: transition to long-term follow-up and transition to adult healthcare.

19.4.1 Transition to Long-Term Follow-Up

Following completion of cancer treatment, patients enter an initial phase of follow-up care, which focuses on surveillance for disease recurrence. Later it should transition to survivorship-focused care, where the emphasis is placed on risk-based screening and health promotion.

At the end of therapy, all treating oncologists should provide survivors with a clinical summary that details cancer treatment exposures, potential cancer treatment-related health risks, and recommendations for health screening and risk-reducing behaviors. The summary should include date of diagnosis, cancer histology and stage, specific treatment modalities, and cumulative chemotherapy dose and radiation treatment volumes and doses [119].

19.4.2 Transition to Adult Healthcare

This occurs when the survivor moves from pediatric long-term follow-up care to adult-oriented healthcare. In this adult setting, the patients assume primary responsibility for their own care.

19.5 Summary

Advances in the treatment of childhood sarcoma have resulted in increasing numbers of survivors. Numerous studies have demonstrated that survivors of childhood cancer are likely to present with adverse health-related consequences of their treatment, and they can develop side effects any time later in life.

Current treatment protocols for childhood cancer are designed to minimize late effects without compromising survival, but further research is crucial to improve the quality of life for current and future survivors. Current strategies are focusing on eliminating or reducing exposures to specific chemotherapies with known late toxicities, identifying individuals with increased susceptibility for specific treatment-associated late effects, and improving care for individuals, who developed treatment-related side effects.

The care of the child diagnosed with cancer does not end with the completion of therapy. We need to make sure that this vulnerable population continues to get access to best practices to detect and manage late effects, which will significantly improve their quality of life, which should be our ultimate goal.

References

1. Ward E, DeSantis C, Robbins A, Kohler B, Jemal A. Childhood and adolescent cancer statistics. CA Cancer J Clin. 2014;64:83–103.
2. Armstrong GT, Chen Y, Yasui Y, Leisenring W, Gibson TM, Mertens AC, Stovall M, Oeffinger KC, Bhatia S, Krull KR, Nathan PC, Neglia JP, Green DM, Hudson MM, Robinson LL. Reduction in late mortality among 5-year survivors of childhood cancer. NEJM. 2016;374: 833–42.
3. http://www.cancer.org/cancer/cancerinchildren/detailedguide/cancer-in-children-types-of--childhood-cancers. Accessed 10 Jul 2016.
4. Kline NE, Sevier N. Solid tumors in children. J Pediatr Nurs. 2003;18:96–102.
5. Oeffinger KC, Mertens AC, Sklar CA, et al. Chronic health conditions and in adult survivors of childhood cancer. N Engl J Med. 2006;355:1572–82.
6. http://www.survivorshipguidelines.org/pdf/LTFUGuidelines_40.pdf.
7. Eschenhagen T, Force T, Ewer MS, de Keulenaer GW, Suter TM, Anker SD, et al. Cardiovascular side effects of cancer therapies: a position statement from the Heart Failure Association of the European Society of Cardiology. Eur J Heart Fail. 2011;13:1–10.
8. Corradi F, Paolini L, De Caterina R. Ranolazine in the prevention of anthracycline cardiotoxicity. Pharmacol Res. 2014;79:88–102.
9. Rosa GM, Gigli L, Tagliasacchi MI, Di Iorio C, Carbone F, Nencioni A, Montecucco F, Brunelli C. Update on cardiotoxicity of anti-cancer treatments. Eur J Clin Investig. 2016;46:264–84.
10. Lipshultz SE, Karnik R, Sambatakos P, Franco VI, Ross SW, Miller TL. Anthracycline-related cardiotoxicity in childhood cancer survivors. Curr Opin Cardiol. 2014;29:103–12.
11. Diamond M, Franco V. Preventing and treating anthracycline-related cardiotoxicity in survivors of childhood cancer. Curr Cancer Ther Rev. 2012;8:141–51.
12. Lipshultz SE, Miller TL, Scully RE, et al. Changes in cardiac biomarkers during doxorubicin treatment of pediatric patients with high-risk acute lymphoblastic leukemia: associations with long-term echocardiographic outcomes. J Clin Oncol. 2012;30:1042–9.

13. Jungsuwadee P, Zhao T, Stolarczyk EI, Paumi CM, Butterfield DA, St. Clair DK, Vore M. The G671V variant of MRP1/ABCC1 links doxorubicin-induced acute cardiac toxicity to disposition of the glutathione conjugate of 4-hydroxy-2-trans-nonenal. Pharmacogenet Genomics. 2012;22:273–84.
14. Cascales A, Sanchez-Vega B, Navarro N, Pastor-Quirante F, Corral J, Vicente V, Ayala de la Pena F. Clinical and genetic determinants of anthracycline-induced cardiac iron accumulation. Int J Cardiol. 2012;154:282–6.
15. Ichikawa Y, Ghanefar M, Bayeva M, Wu R, Khechaduri A, Naga Prasad SV, Mutharasan RK, Naik TJ, Ardehali H. Cardiotoxicity of doxorubicin is mediated through mitochondrial iron accumulation. J Clin Invest. 2014;124:617–30.
16. Lipshultz SE, Lipsitz SR, Kutok JL, Miller TL, Colan SD, Neuberg DS, et al. Impact of hemochromatosis gene mutations on cardiac status in doxorubicin-treated survivors of childhood high-risk leukemia. Cancer. 2013;119:3555–62.
17. Cascales A, Pastor-Quirante F, Sanchez-Vega B, Luengo-Gil G, Corral J, Ortuno-Pacheco G, Vicente V, de la Pena FA. Association of anthracycline-related cardiac histological lesions with NADPH oxidase functional polymorphisms. Oncologist. 2013;18:446–53.
18. Visscher H, Ross CJ, Rassekh SR, Barhdadi A, Dube MP, Al-Saloos H, et al. Pharmacogenomic prediction of anthracycline-induced cardiotoxicity in children. J Clin Oncol. 2012;30:1422–8.
19. Nysom K, Holm K, Lipsitz SR, et al. Relationship between cumulative anthracycline dose and late cardiotoxicity in childhood acute lymphoblastic leukemia. J Clinic Oncol. 1998;16:545–50.
20. Legha SS, Benjamin RS, Mackay B, et al. Reduction of doxorubicin cardiotoxicity by prolonged continuous intravenous infusion. Ann Intern Med. 1982;96:133–9.
21. Lipshultz SE, Giantris AL, Lipsitz SR, et al. Doxorubicin administration by continuous infusion is not cardioprotective: the Dana-Farber 91-01 Acute Lymphoblastic Leukemia protocol. J Clinic Oncol. 2002;20:1677–82.
22. Gabizon AA, Lyass O, Berry GJ, Wildgust M. Cardiac safety of pegylated liposomal doxorubicin (Doxil/Caelyx) demonstrated by endomyocardial biopsy in patients with advanced malignancies. Cancer Investig. 2004;22:663–9.
23. Lipshultz SE, Rifai N, Dalton VM, et al. The effect of dexrazoxane on myocardial injury in doxorubicin-treated children with acute lymphoblastic leukemia. N Engl J Med. 2004;351:145–53.
24. Herman EH, Zhang J, Chadwick DP, Ferrans VJ. Comparison of the protective effects of amifostine and dexrazoxane against the toxicity of doxorubicin in spontaneously hypertensive rats. Cancer Chemother Pharmacol. 2000;45:329–34.
25. Miyata S, Takemura G, Kosai K, Takahashi T, Esaki M, Li L, et al. Anti-Fas gene therapy prevents doxorubicin-induced acute cardiotoxicity through mechanisms independent of apoptosis. Am J Pathol. 2010;176:687–98.
26. Spallarossa P, Garibaldi S, Altieri P, et al. Carvedilol prevents doxorubicin-induced free radical release and apoptosis in cardiomyocytes in vitro. J Mol Cell Cardiol. 2004;37:837–46.
27. Siveski-Iliskovic N, Hill M, Chow DA, Singhal PK. Probucol protects against doxorubicin cardiomyopathy without interfering with its antitumor effect. Circulation. 1995;91:10–5.
28. Fischer PW, Salloum F, Das A, Hyder H, Kukreja RC. Phosphodiesterase-5 inhibition with sildenafil attenuates cardiomyocyte apoptosis and left ventricular dysfunction in a chronic model of doxorubicin cardiotoxicity. Circulation. 2005;111:1601–10.
29. Li L, Takemura G, Li Y, et al. Preventive effect of erythropoietin on cardiac dysfunction in doxorubicin-induced cardiomyopathy. Circulation. 2006;113:535–43.
30. Jin Z, Zhang J, Zhi H, Hong B, Zhang S, Guo H, Li L. Beneficial effects of tadalafil on left ventricular dysfunction in doxorubicin-induced cardiomyopathy. J Cardiol. 2013;62:110–6.
31. Iarussi D, Auricchio U, Agretto A, Murano A, Giuliano M, Casale F, Indolfi P, Iacono A. Protective effect of coenzyme Q10 on anthracyclines cardiotoxicity: control study in children with acute lymphoblastic leukemia and non-Hodgkin lymphoma. Mol Asp Med. 1994;15(Suppl):s207–12.

32. Wouters KA, Kremer LC, Miller TL, Herman EH, Lipshultz SE. Protecting against anthracycline-induced myocardial damage: a review of the most promising strategies. Br J Haematol. 2005;131:561–78.
33. Arrick BA, Nathan CF, Griffith OW, Cohn ZA. Glutathione depletion sensitizes tumor cells to oxidative cytolysis. J Biol Chem. 1982;257:1231–7.
34. Barry E, Alvarez JA, Scully RE, Miller TL, Lipshultz SE. Anthracycline-induced cardiotoxicity: course, pathophysiology, prevention and management. Expert Opin Pharmacother. 2007;8:1039–58.
35. Schwartz CL, Hobbie WL, Truesdell S, Constine LC, Clark EB. Corrected QT interval prolongation in anthracycline-treated survivors of childhood cancer. J Clin Oncol. 1993;11:1906–10.
36. Harake D, Franco VI, Henkel JM, Miller TL, Lipshultz SE. Cardiotoxicity in childhood cancer survivors: strategies for prevention and management. Futur Cardiol. 2012;8:647–70.
37. Christenson ES, James T, Agrawal V, Park BH. Use of biomarkers for the assessment of chemotherapy-induced cardiac toxicity. Clin Biochem. 2015;48:223–35.
38. Armstrong GT, Oeffinger KC, Chen Y, Kawashima T, Yasui Y, Leisenring W, et al. Modifiable risk factors and major cardiac events among adult survivors of childhood cancer. J Clin Oncol. 2013;31:3673–80.
39. Lipshultz SE, Lipsitz SR, Sallan SE, et al. Long-term enalapril therapy for left ventricular dysfunction in doxorubicin-treated survivors of childhood cancer. J Clin Oncol. 2002;20:4517–22.
40. Bristow MR. Mechanism of action of beta-blocking agents in heart failure. Am J Cardiol. 1997;80:26–40.
41. Lipshultz SE, Vlach SA, Lipsitz SR, et al. Cardiac changes associated with growth hormone therapy among children treated with anthracyclines. Pediatrics. 2005;115:1613–22.
42. Wasilewski-Masker K, Kaste SC, Hudson MM, Esiashvili N, Mattano LA, Meacham LR. Bone mineral density deficits in survivors of childhood cancer: long-term follow-up guidelines and review of the literature. Pediatrics. 2008;121:705–13.
43. Hochberg Z. Mechanisms of steroid impairment of growth. Horm Res. 2002;58:33–8.
44. Davies JH, Evans BA, Jenney ME, Gregory JW. Skeletal morbidity in childhood acute lymphoblastic leukemia. Clin Endocrinol. 2005;63:1–9.
45. Syed F, Khosla S. Mechanisms of sex steroid effects on bone. Biochem Biophys Res Commun. 2005;328:688–96.
46. Burger B, Beier R, Zimmermann M, et al. Osteonecrosis: a treatment related toxicity in childhood acute lymphoblastic leukemia (ALL)—experiences from trial ALL-BFM 95. Pediatr Blood Cancer. 2005;44:220–5.
47. Kadan-Lottick NS, Dinu I, Wasilewski-Masker K, et al. Osteonecrosis in adult survivors of childhood cancer. A report from the childhood cancer survivor study. J Clin Oncol. 2008;26:3038–45.
48. Mays D, Gerfen E, Mosher RB, Shad AT, Tercyak KP. Validation of a milk consumption stage of change algorithm among adolescent survivors of childhood cancer. J Nutr Educ Behav. 2012;44:464–8.
49. Mays D, Black JD, Mosher RB, Heinly A, Shad AT, Tercyak KP. Efficacy of the Survivor Health and Resilience Education (SHARE) program to improve bone health behaviors among adolescent survivors of childhood cancer. Ann Behav Med. 2011;42:91–8.
50. Lampert MH, Sugarbaker PH. Rehabilitation of patients with extremity sarcoma. In: Sugarbaker PH, Malawer MM, editors. Musculoskeletal surgery for cancer. New York: Thieme; 1992. p. 55–73.
51. Lewis MM. Musculoskeletal oncology: a multidisciplinary approach. In: Ragnarsson KT, editor. Rehabilitation of patients with physical disabilities caused by tumors of the musculoskeletal system. Philadelphia: WB Saunders; 1992. p. 429–48.
52. Shehadeh A, Noveau J, Malawer M, Henshaw R. Late complications and survival of endoprosthetic reconstruction after resection of bone tumors. Clin Orthop Relat Res. 2010;468:2885–95.

53. Frieden RA, Ryniker D, Kenan S, et al. Assessment of patient function after limb-sparing surgery. Arch Phys Med Rehabil. 1993;74:38–43.
54. Lee SH, Shin CH. Reduced male fertility in childhood cancer survivors. Ann Pediatr Endocrinol Metab. 2013;18:168–72.
55. Meistrich ML, Wilson G, Mathur K, Fuller LM, Rodriguez MA, McLaughlin P, et al. Rapid recovery of spermatogenesis after mitoxantrone, vincristine, vinblastine, and prednisone chemotherapy for Hodgkin's disease. J Clin Oncol. 1997;15:3488–95.
56. Buchanan JD, Fairley KF, Barrie JU. Return of spermatogenesis after stopping cyclophosphamide therapy. Lancet. 1975;2:156–7.
57. Hansen PV, Trykker H, Helkjoer PE, Andersen J. Testicular function in patients with testicular cancer treated with orchiectomy alone or orchiectomy plus cisplatin-based chemotherapy. J Natl Cancer Inst. 1989;81:1246–50.
58. Green DM, Kawashima T, Stovall M, Leisenring W, Sklar CA, Mertens AC, et al. Fertility of male survivors of childhood cancer: a report from the Childhood Cancer Survival Study. J Clin Oncol. 2010;28:332–9.
59. Kenney LB, Cohen LE, Shnorhavorian M, Metzger ML, Lockart B, Hijiya N, et al. Male reproductive health after childhood, adolescent and young adult cancers: a report from the Children's Oncology Group. J Clin Oncol. 2012;30:3408–16.
60. Rowley MJ, Leach DR, Warner GA, Heller CG. Effect of graded doses of ionizing radiation on the human testis. Radiat Res. 1974;59:665–78.
61. Ash P. The influence of radiation on fertility in man. Br J Radiol. 1980;53:271–8.
62. Han TS, Bouloux PM. What is the optimal therapy for young males with hypogonadotropic hypogonadism? Clin Endocrinol. 2010;17:21–30.
63. Neal MS, Nagel K, Duckworth J, Bissessar H, Fischer MA, Portwine C, et al. Effectiveness of sperm banking in adolescents and young adults with cancer: a regional experience. Cancer. 2007;110:1125–9.
64. Wyns C, Curaba M, Vanabelle B, Van Langendonckt A, Donnez J. Options for fertility preservation in prepubertal boys. Hum Reprod Update. 2010;16:312–28.
65. Schwarzer JU, Fiedler K, v Hertwig I, Krusmann G, Wurfel W, Schleyer M, et al. Sperm retrieval procedures and intracytoplasmic spermatozoa injection with epididymal and testicular sperms. Urol Int. 2003;70:119–23.
66. Green DM, Sklar CA, Boice JD, Mulvihill JJ, Whitton JA, Stovall M, Yasui Y. Ovarian failure and reproductive outcomes after childhood cancer treatment: results from the Childhood Cancer Survivor Study. J Clin Oncol. 2009;27:2374–81.
67. Wallace WH, Thomson AB, Saran F, et al. Predicting age of ovarian failure after radiation to a field that includes the ovaries. J Radiat Oncol Biol Phys. 2005;62:738–44.
68. Sklar C. Reproductive physiology and treatment-related loss of sex hormone production. Med Pediatr Oncol. 1999;32:2–8.
69. Green DM, Whitton JA, Stovall M, et al. Pregnancy outcome of female survivors of childhood cancer: a report form the Childhood Cancer Survivor Study. Am J Obstet Gynecol. 2002;187:1070–80.
70. Boice JDJ, Tawn EJ, Winther JF, et al. Genetic effects of radiotherapy for childhood cancer. Health Phys. 2003;85:65–80.
71. Mulvihill JJ, Munro H, Whitton JA et al. Genetic disease in offspring of survivors of childhood and adolescent cancer. Presented at the annual meeting of the American Society of Human Genetics, October 23–27, 2007, San Diego, CA (abstr 2002).
72. Wallace WH, Thomson AB. Preservation of fertility in children treated for cancer. Arch Dis Child. 2003;88:493–6.
73. Jones DP, Spunt SL, Green D, Springate JE. Renal late effects in patients treated for cancer in childhood: a report from the Children's Oncology Group. Pediatr Blood Cancer. 2008;51:724–31.
74. Rossi R, Pleyer J, Schafers P, Kuhn N, Kleta R, Deufel T, et al. Development of ifosfamide-induced nephrotoxicity: prospective follow-up in 75 patients. Med Pediar Oncol. 1999;32:177–82.

75. Breitz H. Clinical aspect of radiation nephropathy. Cancer Biother Radiopharm. 2004;19:359–62.
76. Loebstein R, Atanackovic G, Bishai R, et al. Risk factors for long-term outcome of ifosfamide-induced nephrotoxicity in children. J Clin Pharmacol. 1999;39:454–61.
77. Stohr W, Paulides M, Bielack S, et al. Ifosfamide-induced nephrotoxicity in 593 sarcoma patients: a report from the Late Effects Surveillance System. Pediatr Blood Cancer. 2007;48:447–52.
78. Berrak SG, Pearson M, Bielack S, et al. High-dose ifosfamide in relapsed pediatric osteosarcoma: therapeutic effects and renal toxicity. Pediatr Blood Cancer. 2005;44:215–9.
79. Suarez A, McDowell H, Niaudet P, et al. Long-term follow-up of ifosfamide renal toxicity in children treated for malignant mesenchymal tumors: an International Society of Pediatric Oncology report. J Clin Oncol. 1991;9:2177–82.
80. Fels LM, Bokemeyer C, van Rhee J, et al. Evaluation of late nephrotoxicity in long-term survivors of Hodgkin's disease. Oncology. 1996;53:73–8.
81. Marina NM, Poquette CA, Cain AM, et al. Comparative renal tubular toxicity of chemotherapy regimens including ifosfamide in patients with newly diagnosed sarcomas. J Pediatr Hematol Oncol. 2000;22:112–8.
82. Raney B, Ensign LG, Foreman J, et al. Renal toxicity of ifosfamide in pilot regimens of the intergroup rhabdomyosarcoma study for patients with gross residual tumor. Am J Pediatr Hematol Oncol. 1994;16:286–95.
83. Erdlenbruch B, Nier M, Kern W, et al. Pharmacokinetics of cisplatin and relation to nephrotoxicity in paediatric patients. Eur J Clin Pharmacol. 2001;57:393–402.
84. Skinner R, Pearson AD, English MW, et al. Cisplatin dose rate as a risk factor for nephrotoxicity in children. Br J Cancer. 1998;77:1677–82.
85. Ariceta G, Rodriguez-Soriano J, Vallo A, et al. Acute and chronic effects of cisplatin therapy on renal magnesium homeostasis. Med Pediatr Oncol. 1997;28:35–40.
86. Hartmann JT, Fels LM, Franzke A, et al. Comparative study of the acute nephrotoxicity from standard dose cisplatin +/− ifosfamide and high-dose chemotherapy with carboplatin and ifosfamide. Anticancer Res. 2000;20:3767–73.
87. Widemann BC, Balis FM, Kempf-Bielack B, et al. High-dose methotrexate-induced nephrotoxicity in patients with osteosarcoma. Cancer. 2004;100:2222–32.
88. Cohen EP, Robbins ME. Radiation nephropathy. Semin Nephrol. 2003;23:486–99.
89. Rossi R, Kleta R, Ehrlich JH. Renal involvement in children with malignancies. Pediatr Nephrol. 1999;13:153–62.
90. Neglia JP, Friedman DL, Yasui Y, et al. Second malignant neoplasms in five-year survivors of childhood cancer: childhood cancer survivor study. J Natl Cancer Inst. 2001;93:618–29.
91. Friedman DL, Whitton J, Leisenring W, Mertens AC, Hammond S, Stovall M, Donaldson SS, Meadows AT, Robinson LL, Neglia JP. Subsequent neoplasms in 5-year survivors of childhood cancer: the Childhood Cancer Survivor Study. J Natl Cancer Inst. 2010;102:1083–95.
92. Bahtia S, Sklar C. Second cancers in survivors of childhood cancer. Nat Rev Cancer. 2002;2:124–32.
93. Henderson T, Oeffinger K, Whitton J, Leisenring W, Neglia J, Meadows A, et al. Secondary gastrointestinal cancer in childhood cancer survivors a cohort study. Ann Intern Med. 2012;156:757–66.
94. Kumar S. Second malignant neoplasms following radiotherapy. Int J Environ Res Public Health. 2012;9:4744–59.
95. Henderson TO, Rajaraman P, Stovall M, Constine LS, Olive A, Smith SA, et al. Risk factors associated with secondary sarcomas in childhood cancer survivors: a report from the Childhood Cancer Survivor Study. Int J Radiat Oncol Biol Phys. 2012;84:224–30.
96. Schwartz B, Benadjaoud MA, Cléro E, Haddy N, El-Fayech C, Guibout C, et al. Risk of second bone sarcoma following childhood cancer: role of radiation therapy treatment. Radiat Environ Biophys. 2014;53:381–90.
97. Han Y, Smith MT. Pathobiology of cancer chemotherapy-induced peripheral neuropathy (CIPN). Front Pharmacol. 2013;4:art156.

98. Velasco R, Bruna J. Chemotherapy induced peripheral neuropathy: an unresolved issue. Neurologia. 2010;25:116–31.
99. Bennett GJ. Pathophysiology and animal models of cancer-related painful peripheral neuropathy. Oncologist. 2010;15:9–12.
100. Cersosimo RJ. Cisplatin neurotoxicity. Cancer Treat Rev. 1989;6:195–211.
101. Earl HM, Connolly S, Latoufis C, Eagle K, Ash CM, Fowler C, Souhami RL. Long-term neurotoxicity of chemotherapy in adolescents and young adults treated for bone and soft tissue sarcomas. Sarcoma. 1998;2:97–105.
102. Grewal S, Merchant T, Reymond R, McInerney M, Hodge C, Shearer P. Auditory late effects of childhood cancer therapy: a report from the Children's Oncology Group. Pediatrics. 2010;125:938–50.
103. Dolan ME, Newbold KG, Nagasubramanian R, et al. Heritability and linkage of analysis of sensitivity to cisplatin-induced cytotoxicity. Cancer Res. 2004;64:4353–6.
104. Association AS-L-H. Guidelines for the audiologic management of individuals receiving cochleotoxic drug therapy. ASHA. 1994;35:11–9.
105. Nagy JL, Adelstein DJ, Newman CW, Rybicki LA, Rice TW, Lavertu P. Cisplatin ototoxicity: the importance of baseline audiometry. Am J Clin Oncol. 1999;22:305–8.
106. Currier JM, Jobe-Shields LE, Phipps S. Stressful life events and posttraumatic stress symptoms in children with cancer. J Trauma Stress. 2009;22:28–35.
107. Kazak AE. Posttraumatic distress in childhood cancer survivors and their parents. Med Pediatr Oncol. 1998;S1:60–8.
108. Stuber M, Kazak AE, Meeske K, Barakat L, Guthrie D, Garnier H, et al. Predictors of posttraumatic stress symptoms in childhood cancer survivors. Pediatrics. 1997;100:958–64.
109. Landolt MA, Vollrath M, Ribi K, Gnehm HE, Sennhauser FH. Incidence and association of child and parental posttraumatic stress symptoms in pediatric patients. J Child Psychol Psychiatry. 2003;44:1199–207.
110. Phipps S, Long A, Hudson M, Rai SN. Symptoms of post-traumatic stress in children with cancer and their parents: effects of informant and time from diagnosis. Pediatr Blood Cancer. 2005;45:952–9.
111. Schrag NM, McKeown RE, Jackson KL, Cuffe SP, Neuberg RW. Stress-related mental disorders in childhood cancer survivors. Pediatr Blood Cancer. 2008;50:98–103.
112. Barakat LP, Kazak AE, Gallagher PR, Meeske K, Stuber M. Posttraumatic stress symptoms and stressful life events predict the long-term adjustment of survivors of childhood cancer and their mothers. J Clin Psychol Med Settings. 1997;22:843–59.
113. Hodges WF, London J, Crolwell JB. Stress in parents and late elementary age children in divorced and intact families and child adjustment. J Divorce Remarriage. 1990;14:63–79.
114. Gerhardt CA, Yopp JM, Leininger L, Valerius KS, Correll J, Vannatta K, Noll RB. Brief report: post-traumatic stress during emerging adulthood in survivors of pediatric cancer. J Pediatr Psychol. 2007;32:1018–23.
115. Nir Y. Post-traumatic stress disorder in children with cancer. In: Eth S, Pynoos R, editors. Posttraumatic stress disorder in children. Washington: American Psychiatric Press; 1985. p. 123–32.
116. Meeske KA, Patel SK, Palmer SN, Nelson MB, Parow AM. Factors associated with health related quality of life in pediatric cancer survivors. Pediatr Blood Cancer. 2007;49:298–305.
117. Archbold KH, Pituch KJ, Panahi P, et al. Symptoms of sleep disturbances among children at two general pediatric clinics. J Pediatr. 2002;140:97–102.
118. Owens J. Classification and epidemiology of childhood sleep disorders. Prim Care. 2008;35:533–46.
119. Mulrooney DA, Ness KK, Neglia JP, et al. Fatigue and sleep disturbance in adult survivors of childhood cancer: a report from the childhood cancer survivor study (CCSS). Sleep. 2008;31:271–81.
120. Rosen G, Brand SR. Sleep in children with cancer: case review of 70 children evaluated in a comprehensive pediatric sleep center. Support Care Cancer. 2011;19:985–94.

121. Kaleyias J, Manley P, Kothare SV. Sleep disorders in children with cancer. Semin Pediatr Neurol. 2012;19:25–34.
122. Zebrack BJ, Stuber ML, Meeske KA, et al. Perceived positive impact of cancer among long-term survivors of childhood cancer: a report from the childhood cancer survivor study. Psychooncology. 2012;21:630–9.
123. Kirchhoff AC, Krull KR, Ness KK, et al. Occupational outcomes of adult childhood cancer survivors: a report from the childhood cancer survivor study. Cancer. 2011;117:3033–44.
124. Kirchhoff AC, Leisenring W, Krull KR, et al. Unemployment among adult survivors of childhood cancer: a report from the childhood cancer survivor study. Med Care. 2010;48:1015–25.
125. Park ER, Kirchhoff AC, Zallen JP, et al. Childhood Cancer Survivor Study participants' perceptions and knowledge of health insurance coverage: implications for the Affordable Care Act. J Cancer Surviv. 2012;6:251–9.
126. Schwartz L, Rowland J, Shad A. Pediatric cancer survivors: moving beyond cure. Pediatric psycho-oncology: a quick reference on the psychosocial dimensions of cancer symptom management. 2nd ed. Oxford: Oxford University Press; 2015.
127. Tercyak KP, Donze JR, Prahlad S, Mosher RB, Shad AT. Multiple behavioral risk factors among adolescent survivors of childhood cancer in the Survivor Health and Resilience Education (SHARE) program. Pediatr Blood Cancer. 2006;47:825–30.
128. Tercyak KP, Donze JR, Prahlad S, Mosher RB, Shad AT. Identifying, recruiting, and enrolling adolescent survivors of childhood cancer into a randomized controlled trial of health promotion: preliminary experiences in the Survivor Health and Resilience Education (SHARE) program. J Pediatr Psychol. 2006;31:252–61.
129. Landier W, CureSearch COG. Establishing and enhancing services for childhood cancer survivors: long-term follow-up program resource guide. Available from: http://www.survivor-shipguidelines.org/pdf/LTFUResourceGuide.pdf
130. Shad A, Myers SN, Hennessy K. Late effects in cancer survivors: "The shared care model". Curr Oncol Rep. 2012;14:182–90.
131. Eiser C, Absolom K, Greenfield D, et al. Follow-up after childhood cancer: evaluation of a three-level model. Eur J Cancer. 2006;42:3186–90.

Follow-Up/Late Effects Clinics

20

Allison B. Spitzer and Aditya V. Maheshwari

20.1 Introduction

Integral to the multidisciplinary model of care for the treatment of bone and soft tissue sarcomas is maintaining long-term follow-up for patients [1]. In general, during the past five decades, long-term survival into adulthood is expected for greater than 80% of children with pediatric malignancies who have access to contemporary cancer therapies [1, 2]. With the increasing use of modern interventional therapies, survival rates for patients living with sarcoma have increased markedly over the past few decades. Specifically, Jacobs et al. [3] demonstrated that 5-year overall survival rates for soft tissue sarcoma increased from 28% from 1991 to 1996 to 62% from 2004 to 2010 ($p < 0.0001$) and that radiation therapy was an independent prognostic indicator of survival.

While the therapies responsible for increased survival rate are certainly to be lauded, these therapies can also result in adverse long-term health outcomes, which are collectively referred to as "late effects" [4]. Because late effects manifest themselves months to years after the patient in question has completed their cancer treatment, they can be associated with their own array of costly treatments, screening tests, and social and psychological issues. Perhaps as expected, the prevalence of these late effects increases as the time from cancer diagnosis and treatment increases [5].

The importance of and need for high-quality late effect clinics for cancer survivors and specifically for sarcoma survivors, as will be discussed in this chapter, have increased proportionately with prolonged patient survival. Using these late effects clinics to identify clinical and treatment characteristics of patients with the greatest morbidity and mortality may help to develop a global set of risk assessment tools as well as counseling and health screening recommendations for long-term sarcoma survivors around the world [6].

A.B. Spitzer, M.D. • A.V. Maheshwari, M.D. (✉)
Department of Orthopaedic Surgery and Rehabilitation Medicine, SUNY Downstate Medical Center, Brooklyn, NY, USA
e-mail: Aditya.maheshwari@downstate.edu

© Springer International Publishing Switzerland 2017
R.M. Henshaw (ed.), *Sarcoma*, DOI 10.1007/978-3-319-43121-5_20

20.2   Overview of Late Effects

Late effects encompass a number of broad domains, which include growth and development, organ function, reproductive capacity and offspring health, secondary carcinogenesis, and psychosocial sequelae of disease. Aksnes et al. [7] studied the health status at long-term follow-up for patients with "extremity bone sarcoma" (EBS) and found that over a median follow-up period of 12 years (range 6–22 years), 33% of EBS survivors had ototoxicity, 13% had reduced renal function, and that EBS survivors were statistically more likely than age- and gender-matched controls to have heart disease ($p = 0.001$), hypertension ($p = 0.03$), thyroid disease ($p = 0.04$), more diarrhea ($p = 0.02$), palpitations ($p = 0.01$), and shortness of breath ($p = 0.01$). The authors concluded that since EBS survivors had relatively poorer health status than the control group, long-term follow-up was mandatory. Similarly, Paulides et al. studied a cohort of 67 patients with Ewing's sarcoma (with a median follow-up of 3.5 years) and found that 10.4% of these patients developed nephrotoxicity, 8.9% cardiotoxicity, and 34.3% all other toxicities; there was no difference between the short- and long-term rates of these toxicities, leading the authors to conclude that Ewing's sarcoma has an overall relatively poor prognosis compared with other sarcomas and that appropriate short- and long-term follow-up is essential for survivors of Ewing's sarcoma [8].

Although late effects can be somewhat anticipated based on therapeutic exposures, individual risk and disease manifestation can be influenced by a multitude of factors related to the tumor, to the treatment, and to the host. Tumor-related factors can include tumor location, effect on local tissue, tumor-induced organ dysfunction, and mechanical effect. Treatment-related factors include dose and target organ size during radiation therapy; agent, intensity, cumulative dose, and schedule of chemotherapy; surgical technique and site; use of a combined modality therapy; and management of chronic graft-versus-host disease. Host-related factors can include gender, genetics, prior health state, developmental status, age at diagnosis, time elapsed from diagnosis or therapy, individual capacity for tissue healing, normal organ function, and socioeconomic status. These late effects occur in adults who are childhood cancer survivors, whether from sarcoma or other malignant origin, and must be addressed with effective long-term follow-up [9].

In the Childhood Cancer Survivor Study (CCSS) [10], the investigators demonstrated that morbidity and mortality in childhood cancer survivors increased after the fourth decade of life (Fig. 20.1). Specifically, the incidence of a self-reported debilitating health condition was 53.6% among survivors compared with 19.8% in a sibling control group. Also, among survivors who were 35 years old (and had not previously experienced a disabling or life-threatening health condition), 25.9% experienced a new grade 3 (severe or disabling) to grade 5 (life-threatening or fatal) health condition within 10 years, compared to 6% of healthy siblings [10]. Such debilitating or life-endangering health conditions can result in significant functional impairment of survivors. Female survivors in particular demonstrated a steeper age-dependent diminished health status compared with male survivors.

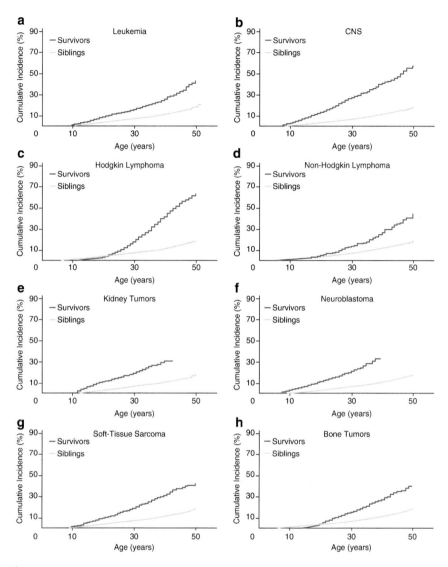

Fig. 20.1 Cumulative incidence of chronic health conditions for severe, disabling, life-threatening, or fatal health conditions by primary childhood cancer diagnosis: (**a**) leukemia, (**b**) central nervous system tumors, (**c**) Hodgkin lymphoma, (**d**) non-Hodgkin lymphoma, (**e**) kidney tumors, (**f**) neuroblastoma, (**g**) soft tissue sarcoma, and (**h**) bone tumors (Reproduced with permission [10])

20.3   Overview of Sarcoma Prognosis

Relapsed primary cancer is the most frequent cause of mortality among survivors of childhood cancer, followed by cause-specific mortality from subsequent primary cancers and cardiac and pulmonary toxicity [11]. More specifically, bone and soft tissue sarcomas are an extremely heterogeneous set of tumors with variable behavior and prognoses. Choong et al. [12] described the long-term follow-up (mean of 44 months) of 20 patients with nonmetastatic, low-grade, central osteosarcoma, all of which arose in the lower limb and presented with a primary symptom of pain. Five- and 10-year survival with wide surgical margins was 90% and 85%, respectively. Berlanga et al. [13] described a 51% and 45% overall survival rate for high-grade osteosarcoma at 5 and 10 years, respectively. Kinsella et al. [14] also found relatively poor survival rates (51% and 39% overall survival at 5 and 10 years, respectively) in a cohort of 107 patients with Ewing's sarcoma of the bone, in which metastatic disease at presentation, age greater than 25, elevated lactate dehydrogenase, and central primary tumor in localized disease patients were associated with decreased disease-free survival and overall survival and where a majority of the patients relapsed within 5 years of presentation and a minority relapsed within 5–15 years. These varied prognoses among patients with tumors in the sarcoma family serve to emphasize the importance of consistent long-term follow-up for all sarcoma survivors and may help guide diagnosis-specific guidelines for sarcoma follow-up.

With improved survival and an increasing number of middle-aged childhood sarcoma survivors, it becomes important to investigate the late effects of these tumors and their treatments, which range from radical surgical excision to chemotherapy to radiation therapy depending on the type of tumor. For example, the British Childhood Cancer Survivor Study described long-term adverse outcomes in a large cohort of 664 childhood bone sarcoma survivors. Although the authors found that after 25 years of follow-up, the overall mortality risk was comparable to the general population, mortality within the first 25 years of follow-up was 12.7× greater than the general population; survivors were four times more likely to develop a subsequent neoplasm and had overall poorer health status and exhibited increased healthcare usage [9].

Generally, all childhood and young adult cancer survivors have greater hospital-related morbidity compared with age- and gender-matched controls, and late effects from childhood or young adult cancer treatment contribute markedly to these patients' morbidity [6, 15, 16]. Other studies have found that 60% to upward of 90% of childhood sarcoma survivors develop one or more chronic health conditions and that 20–80% of survivors experience severe, sometimes life-threatening, complications during adulthood [17, 18]. In spite of higher all-around morbidity, overall mortality for all childhood and young adult cancers has decreased over time due to improved therapeutic efficacy, awareness of late effects (including subsequent cancers), and how to prevent or treat them. Significantly, there has been a resultant reduction in deaths from primary cancer. With increasingly widespread implementation of therapeutic protocols and effective multidisciplinary long-term follow-up into adulthood, late morbidity and mortality can be further curbed, and we may be able to better ascertain how individual tumors and therapeutic interventions affect long-term mortality.

20.4   Multidisciplinary Long-Term Follow-Up Clinics

While many patients diagnosed with sarcoma may be "cured" of their disease and live cancer-free lives, a significant number of these patients are at risk of developing serious chronic medical conditions with age that are related to their sarcoma treatment. It is very important for childhood and young adult sarcoma survivors to have an appropriate transition from the pediatric to the adult health-care setting. The long-term outcomes, livelihood, and well-being of these patients depend on access to appropriate resources, including multidisciplinary late effects clinics, which have been described as the "optimal model" to facilitate coordination between the patient's cancer center oncology team and community physician specialists who will manage the patient's health care longitudinally [19].

The continued development of special multidisciplinary long-term follow-up clinics is critical. For example, one of the limitations of the current system is limited ability of childhood cancer survivors to access appropriate risk-based care. For example, Casillas et al. [20] found that survivors without access to health insurance were less likely to report cancer-related visits or cancer center visits (RR 0.83; 95% CI) and that uninsured survivors had lower levels of care utilization overall compared with privately insured survivors. Further, Kirchhoff et al. [21] found that certain survivor subgroups such as younger survivors aged 20–29 years, females, nonwhites, and survivors self-reporting poorer health faced more cost barriers to appropriate follow-up care, which may put them at greater risk of succumbing to the late effects of their disease. In addition, Nathan et al. [22] found that survivors at the highest risk of colon, breast, or skin cancer had very low surveillance, which emphasizes the need for education about appropriate surveillance and risk of new malignancies for both childhood cancer survivors and physicians. They also found that 31.5% of survivors reported receiving survivor-focused care, that is, care focusing on their previous cancer, while 17.8% also received advice about risk reduction or ordering of screening tests; overall, approximately 88.8% of survivors received some form of medical care. In sum, there is a clear discrepancy between the care childhood cancer survivors should receive and the care they are getting, and increasing the creation and utilization of multidisciplinary late effects clinics specifically for sarcoma survivors will help to eradicate this discrepancy.

One of the essential services provided to patients by such multidisciplinary clinics is the coordination of an individualized survivor's care plan in order to record and monitor the therapeutic interventions the patient has previously received (and their associated health risks), individualized health screening recommendations, and education about risk modification through lifestyle choices. These clinics can streamline the care model, through efforts to pair patients with two or more specialists in the same appointment, thereby increasing efficient use of patient and provider time and potentially increasing the rate of patient follow-up. For example, a patient may see both a medical oncologist specializing in the treatment of sarcoma and a cardiologist specializing in the treatment of heart problems caused by cancer treatment in the same appointment. In addition, renal, endocrinology, physical medicine and rehabilitation, and psychiatry specialists are also available through these clinics to help manage conditions in these patients that are most commonly seen in sarcoma survivors [23].

The primary focus of these clinics is on early detection and surveillance, since chronic conditions that typically occur at a later age in the general population, such as cardiac disease, can occur at a much younger age in sarcoma survivor patients, even as young as 30 years old, and occur in nearly one-third of soft tissue sarcoma survivors after treatment [24]. Other common chronic conditions in sarcoma survivors (occurring as soon as 2 years after treatment) include type 2 diabetes, hypertension, dyslipidemia, renal failure, mental health problems, recurrence of sarcoma, and new malignancies. These conditions are often treatable with early detection and intervention through established medical techniques. The occurrence of these conditions at young ages demonstrates the need for multidisciplinary late effects clinics, as primary care providers may not have the clinical experience to look for heart disease or renal failure in a 30-year-old patient, regardless of previous treatments received. Of note, some clinics may only accept patients who have been out of therapy for 2 or more years, or adult patients only, in order to encourage short-term follow-up with the patient's surgical team or in pediatric hospitals with the appropriate pediatric oncological resources.

In addition, while these clinics are invaluable for helping sarcoma survivors receive the highest quality of care, such clinics may also serve as research recruitment sites where the effectiveness of new interventions intended to improve survival and quality of life in sarcoma survivors can be tested on a relatively wide scale.

Beyond assisting sarcoma patients with coordinating care and developing new treatment strategies, such clinics may also provide patients with another equally valuable but perhaps unquantifiable resource: that of human solidarity and friendship. Attending such clinics and interacting with other individuals with similar health backgrounds may help sarcoma survivors meet other individuals with similar medical histories and treatment experiences and, thereby, foster acquaintances among those with similar struggles, as well as successes, associated with a diagnosis of sarcoma and its long-term sequelae. An individual patient may experience enrichment of their mental health status (often plagued by the depression and anxiety associated with a cancer diagnosis) through exposure to, and contact with, a population of similar individuals. Finally, it is possible that the course of an individual patient's disease may be altered through such clinics, by helping providers more easily to identify successful (or ineffective) treatment trends for late effects on a large scale and by helping patients to share successful late effect treatment information. Patient-driven interactions can potentially identify particular treatment options in their early stages, before a given therapy has become widely adopted and thoroughly substantiated in the literature.

Unfortunately, lack of health insurance still seems to be an important concern for survivors of childhood cancer because of health issues, unemployment, and other societal factors. Access to, and retention of, health insurance for childhood cancer survivors has improved with the passing of recent legislation such as the Health Insurance Portability and Accountability Act, although further studies are required to clarify the durability and limitations of such legislation [25].

20.5 Follow-Up Intervals

Currently, there are no published data outlining specific universal and widely acceptable policies for follow-up of surgically treated patients. However, it has been shown that clear protocols for sarcoma survivor follow-up can improve both the consistency and availability of long-term care [26]. Follow-up strategy for soft tissue sarcoma should be tailored to the individual risk of recurrence and based on the most efficient means of surveillance [24]. Early detection of resectable local or metastatic (especially to the lungs) recurrent disease can help prolong patient survival, as can new advances in sarcoma treatment. Also, given that 40–60% of patients with soft tissue sarcoma experience relapse, with the majority occurring within the first 5 years after primary treatment (about 80% of metastases to the lung and almost 70% local recurrences occur in the first 2–3 years), close surveillance during the first 2–3 years after treatment is essential [24]. Generally, high-risk patients are more likely to relapse within the first 2–3 years, while lower-risk patients may relapse later and less frequently.

There is currently a wide spectrum of surveillance strategies, which can vary widely from provider to provider. Rutkowski et al. [24] advocate for a somewhat conservative approach, focusing on the most effective (rather than the most sophisticated) forms of surveillance, including a careful history, physical exam (including scrutiny of postoperative scars at the primary tumor site), and chest X-ray or chest computed tomography (CT) [depending on provider preference] to screen for lung metastases in asymptomatic patients. This is justified by the authors given that lung metastases are the most frequent location of disease recurrence in patients with soft tissue sarcoma of the extremity and that multiple patient series have demonstrated that radical excision of resectable lung metastases afforded overall longer survival compared with patients with inoperable disease [27, 28]. Rutkowski et al. also recommend that patients with soft tissue sarcomas that are retroperitoneal or intraperitoneal (such as gastrointestinal stromal tumor) in location may also benefit from contrast-enhanced computed tomography of the abdomen and pelvis during follow-up. Importantly, the risk assessment (based on tumor grade, size, and site) can help to determine the frequency of each patient's routine follow-up intervals. For example, certain rare subtypes of soft tissue sarcoma tend to spread consistently to specific geographic locations, such as the lymph nodes for rhabdomyosarcoma, epithelioid sarcoma, clear cell sarcoma and synovial sarcoma, and intra-abdominally for myxoid liposarcoma.

With respect to recommended follow-up intervals, the European Society for Medical Oncology (ESMO) [29, 30] published a set of clinical guidelines for soft tissue sarcoma follow-up, describing the following follow-up intervals for high-grade surgically treated soft tissue sarcomas: every 3–4 months with clinical exam and chest X-ray or chest CT for intermediate-/high-grade surgically treated soft tissue sarcoma patients during the first 2–3 years after surgery, every 6 months until the 5th year after surgery, and annually after the 5-year mark with primarily clinical follow-up. For low-grade sarcoma patients, they recommend follow-up every 4–6 months with slightly less frequent chest X-rays or chest CTs with clinical exam for the first 3–5 years, then annually [30].

In addition, Alberta Health Services in Canada [31] put out another set of recommended clinical practice guidelines for soft tissue sarcoma follow-up surveillance in 2014, with the following recommendations: clinical exam and chest X-ray or chest CT every 6 months in the first 2 years and annually for 5 years after surgical resection for low-risk/low-grade sarcomas and exam and chest X-ray every 4 months for 2 years after surgical resection, then every 6 months for the 3rd year, and every 6–12 months for years 4–5 for high-risk/moderate- or high-grade sarcoma. The authors also recommended baseline post-resection imaging at least 3 months after surgery in patients felt to be at higher risk of recurrence or who had unreliable local tissues on physical examination, and that routine use of computed tomography for pulmonary imaging was not recommended unless enhanced imaging sensitivity was required due to clinical suspicion for local recurrence. However, neither these guidelines nor the ESMO guidelines include recommendations for bone sarcomas, and while evidence-based literature is referenced, the Alberta authors admit that their recommendations, like other guidelines before them, are primarily based on expert consensus rather than evidence-based literature. The authors cite the relatively rare occurrence of soft tissue sarcomas compared with other cancers as a potential cause for the dearth of high-quality evidence available to help guide follow-up strategies. The Children's Oncology Group (COG) [32] also provides a comprehensive set of guidelines titled "Long-Term Follow-Up Guidelines for Survivors of Childhood, Adolescent and Young Adult Cancer" (COG LTFU), which provides recommended guidelines for health-care professionals caring for asymptomatic survivors presenting for routine exposure-based medical follow-up and is intended to help standardize the care of childhood cancer survivors [33].

Combination of imaging techniques, such as positron-emission tomography with fluorine-18-fluorodeoxyglucose (18-FDG-PET) and CT, can provide both anatomical and functional data, and there is a growing body of evidence demonstrating the effectiveness of PET-CT and other newer imaging methods for the detection and staging of tumors, assessing treatment response, follow-up, and surveillance [34]. These new modalities also have the potential to decrease both the sample sizes required for, and duration of, clinical trials by providing an early indication of therapeutic response that is well correlated with clinical outcomes, such as time to tumor progression or overall survival.

20.6   Cost of Follow-Up

It is important to note that although MRI may be most sensitive to detect local relapse and CT most sensitive to detect lung metastases, it has not been clinically proven that use of these advanced imaging modalities improves clinical outcomes compared to simple clinical assessment (physical examination) of the primary site and interval chest X-rays. Further, Fleming et al. [35] found that performing a chest CT added minimal clinical benefit for surveillance when there was a low risk of pulmonary metastasis. There is a need for clinical trials to identify the optimal strategy for sarcoma surveillance that will balance enhanced survival, quality of life, cost, and willingness of society to contribute resources. Obstacles to the completion of such trials include the rarity of extremity soft tissue sarcoma, the cost of conducting a clinical trial, and the willingness of cancer survivors to participate.

There is currently a wide disparity in the cost of sarcoma surveillance methods, despite surveillance guidelines issued by prominent national and international organizations such as the National Comprehensive Cancer Network. Specifically, Goel et al. [36] conducted a literature search of all published extremity soft tissue sarcoma 5-year surveillance strategies from 1982 to 2003 using Medicare-allowed charges as a proxy. They identified 54 strategies for follow-up in 34 published studies. Total Medicare-allowed charges in year 2003 US dollars ranged from $485 for follow-up of low-grade sarcoma to $21,235 for follow-up of high-grade sarcoma, a 42.8-fold cost differential with an average of $ 6401. Of note, clinical examination and chest X-ray were the two most commonly utilized screening modalities, again emphasizing the need for clinical trials to ascertain whether these modalities are not only the least costly but also the most cost-effective form of sarcoma surveillance screening. Given the marked disparities in cost for different surveillance methods, it is clear that cost is an important factor that needs to be addressed and standardized in future sarcoma surveillance guidelines.

20.7   Future Directions

There is significant potential for future studies and a demonstrated need for the publication of universal clinical practice guidelines for the treatment and surveillance of patients with extremity bone-based and soft tissue sarcomas that account for the individual characteristics and expected prognosis of each patient and tumor. In order to help lay the groundwork for such a study, Gerrand et al. [29] conducted a survey of current practice in the United Kingdom, which confirmed that clinicians in the United Kingdom vary follow-up recommendations according to the patient's perceived risk of relapse, which respondents associated with surgical margin status, histological grade and size and depth, tumor diagnosis, site, and patient age, all findings supported by peer-reviewed literature. There was significant variation in current practice with respect to the types of imaging studies used for follow-up (e.g., chest X-ray versus computed tomography of the chest) and the frequency and cost of follow-up. Of note, the findings of the UK survey are similar to a survey conducted by the American Society of Surgical Oncology by Sakata et al. [31]

Given the significant variation in physician approach to surveillance, Damery et al. [26] surveyed 132 patients and found that patients generally preferred follow-up appointments consisting of physical examination and chest X-ray in a secondary care location rather than the primary care setting. It is important to incorporate patient preferences into clinical surveillance strategies in order to maximize both patient follow-up and satisfaction.

Variation in management and cost reflected in these current practice surveys emphasizes the current absence of high-quality evidence supporting any one follow-up strategy and clearly suggests there is a role for future higher-level studies to determine the optimal follow-up strategy for each individual sarcoma survivor patient. Factors such as the economic cost of follow-up, psychological impact to the patient, and the prognostic effect of more intensive versus less intensive follow-up algorithms should all be further elucidated in these randomized studies and reflected in subsequent evidence-based clinical practice guidelines.

Conclusions

There is a clear, demonstrated need for a *universal* set of *evidence-based* clinical guidelines for both soft tissue and bone sarcomas in order to best streamline care and in order to clarify the standard of follow-up care for sarcoma survivors. Interestingly, the recommendation that these late effects clinics be "multidisciplinary" appears currently to be the only universally recognized clinical practice guideline. Future guidelines should ideally be evidence based, should reflect the findings of existing literature regarding the impact of specific tumor and individual characteristics on prognosis and treatment of late effects including but not limited to recurrence, and should also reflect previously unaddressed questions such as the effect of patient health insurance on the care received. In summary, there has been significant therapeutic progress in the treatment of certain types of sarcomas in the past century, which is reflected by the increased number of sarcoma survivors in need of long-term clinical follow-up. To this end, we must continue to find ways to fund the expansion of multidisciplinary late effect sarcoma clinics where patients and providers can effectively coordinate their long-term follow-up care for the diverse and sometimes unexpected late effects known to be associated with sarcoma treatment.

In addition, there is a demonstrable need for future high-powered, higher-level studies regarding the optimal follow-up algorithm that will maximize the efficacy of the increasing numbers of multidisciplinary late effect clinics. Importantly, these late effects clinics are poised to serve as recruitment centers for high-quality randomized, controlled clinical trials that would help provide the best evidence for follow-up protocols for sarcoma survivors, further highlighting their integral role in the future enhanced treatment of sarcoma survivors.

References

1. Lin PP, Patel S. Bone sarcoma. New York: Springer; 2013.
2. Hudson MM, Oeffinger KC, Jones K, Brinkman TM, Krull KR, Mulrooney DA, et al. Age-dependent changes in health status in the childhood cancer survivor cohort. J Clin Oncol. 2015;33(5):479–91.
3. Jacobs AJ, Michels R, Stein J, Levin AS. Improvement in overall survival from extremity soft tissue sarcoma over twenty years. Sarcoma. 2015;2015:279601.
4. Late Effects of Treatment for Childhood Cancer—for health professionals (PDQ®) 2015 [cited 27 Dec 2015]. http://www.cancer.gov/types/childhood-cancers/late-effects-hp-pdq. Accessed 22 Nov 2015.
5. Mols F, Helfenrath KA, Vingerhoets AJ, Coebergh JW, van de Poll-Franse LV. Increased health care utilization among long-term cancer survivors compared to the average Dutch population: a population-based study. Int J Cancer. 2007;121(4):871–7.
6. Rebholz CE, Reulen RC, Toogood AA, Frobisher C, Lancashire ER, Winter DL, et al. Health care use of long-term survivors of childhood cancer: the British Childhood Cancer Survivor Study. J Clin Oncol. 2011;29(31):4181–8.
7. Aksnes LH, Bauer HC, Dahl AA, Fossa SD, Hjorth L, Jebsen N, Lernedal H, Hall KS. Health status at long-term follow-up in patients treated for extremity localized Ewing Sarcoma or osteosarcoma: a Scandinavian sarcoma group study. Pediatr Blood Cancer. 2009;53(1):84–9.
8. Paulides M, Dorr HG, Stohr W, Bielack S, Koscielniak E, Klingebiel T, et al. Thyroid function in paediatric and young adult patients after sarcoma therapy: a report from the Late Effects Surveillance System. Clin Endocrinol. 2007;66(5):727–31.
9. Fidler MM, Frobisher C, Guha J, Wong K, Kelly J, Winter DL, et al. Long-term adverse outcomes in survivors of childhood bone sarcoma: the British Childhood Cancer Survivor Study. Br J Cancer. 2015;112(12):1857–65.
10. Armstrong GT, Kawashima T, Leisenring W, Stratton K, Stovall M, Hudson MM, Sklar CA, Robison LL, Oeffinger KC. Aging and risk of severe, disabling, life-threatening, and fatal events in the childhood cancer survivor study. J Clin Oncol. 2014;32(12):1218–27.
11. Reulen RC, Winter DL, Frobisher C, Lancashire ER, Stiller CA, Jenney ME, Skinner R, Stevens MC, Hawkins MM, British Childhood Cancer Survivor Study Steering Group. Long-term cause-specific mortality among survivors of childhood cancer. JAMA. 2010;304(2):172–9.
12. Choong PF, Pritchard DJ, Rock MG, Sim FH, McLeod RA, Unni KK. Low grade central osteogenic sarcoma. A long-term follow up of 20 patients. Clin Orthop Relat Res. 1996;322:198–206.
13. Berlanga P, Canete A, Diaz R, Salom M, Baixauli F, Gomez J, Llavador M, Castel V. Presentation and long-term outcome of high-grade osteosarcoma: a single-institution experience. J Pediatr Hematol Oncol. 2015;37(5):e272–7.
14. Kinsella TJ, Miser JS, Waller B, Venzon D, Glatstein E, Weaver-McClure L, Horowitz ME. Long-term follow-up of Ewing's sarcoma of bone treated with combined modality therapy. Int J Radiat Oncol Biol Phys. 1991;20(3):389–95.
15. Zhang Y, Lorenzi MF, Goddard K, Spinelli JJ, Gotay C, McBride ML. Late morbidity leading to hospitalization among 5-year survivors of young adult cancer: a report of the childhood, adolescent and young adult cancer survivors research program. Int J Cancer. 2014;134(5):1174–82.

16. Lorenzi MF, Xie L, Rogers PC, Pritchard S, Goddard K, McBride ML. Hospital-related morbidity among childhood cancer survivors in British Columbia, Canada: report of the Childhood, Adolescent, Young Adult Cancer Survivors (CAYACS) program. Int J Cancer. 2011;128(7):1624–31.
17. Hudson MM, Ness KK, Gurney JG, Mulrooney DA, Chemaitilly W, Krull KR, et al. Clinical ascertainment of health outcomes among adults treated for childhood cancer. JAMA. 2013;309(22):2371–81.
18. Geenen MM, Cardous-Ubbink MC, Kremer LC, van den Bos C, van der Pal HJ, Heinen RC, et al. Medical assessment of adverse health outcomes in long-term survivors of childhood cancer. JAMA. 2007;297(24):2705–15.
19. Oeffinger KC, McCabe MS. Models for delivering survivorship care. J Clin Oncol. 2006;24(32):5117–24.
20. Casillas J, Castellino SM, Hudson MM, Mertens AC, Lima IS, Liu Q, Zeltzer LK, Yasui Y, Robison LL, Oeffinger KC. Impact of insurance type on survivor-focused and general preventive health care utilization in adult survivors of childhood cancer: the Childhood Cancer Survivor Study (CCSS). Cancer. 2011;117(9):1966–75.
21. Kirchhoff AC, Lyles CR, Fluchel M, Wright J, Leisenring W. Limitations in health care access and utilization among long-term survivors of adolescent and young adult cancer. Cancer. 2012;118(23):5964–72.
22. Nathan PC, Greenberg ML, Ness KK, Hudson MM, Mertens AC, Mahoney MC, et al. Medical care in long-term survivors of childhood cancer: a report from the childhood cancer survivor study. J Clin Oncol. 2008;26(27):4401–9.
23. Crom DB, Lensing SY, Rai SN, Snider MA, Cash DK, Hudson MM. Marriage, employment, and health insurance in adult survivors of childhood cancer. J Cancer Surviv. 2007;1(3):237–45.
24. Rutkowski P, Lugowska I. Follow-up in soft tissue sarcomas. Memo. 2014;7(2):92–6.
25. Warner EL, Park ER, Stroup A, Kinney AY, Kirchhoff AC. Childhood cancer survivors' familiarity with and opinions of the Patient Protection and Affordable Care Act. J Oncol Pract. 2013;9(5):246–50.
26. Damery S, Biswas M, Billingham L, Barton P, Al-Janabi H, Grimer R. Patient preferences for clinical follow-up after primary treatment for soft tissue sarcoma: a cross-sectional survey and discrete choice experiment. Eur J Surg Oncol. 2014;40(12):1655–61.
27. Patel SR, Zagars GK, Pisters PW. The follow-up of adult soft-tissue sarcomas. Semin Oncol. 2003;30(3):413–6.
28. van Geel AN, Pastorino U, Jauch KW, Judson IR, van Coevorden F, Buesa JM, Nielsen OS, Boudinet A, Tursz T, Schmitz PI. Surgical treatment of lung metastases: the European organization for research and treatment of cancer-soft tissue and bone sarcoma group study of 255 patients. Cancer. 1996;77(4):675–82.
29. Gerrand CH, Billingham LJ, Woll PJ, Grimer RJ. Follow up after primary treatment of soft tissue sarcoma: a survey of current practice in the United Kingdom. Sarcoma. 2007;2007:34128.
30. Casali PG, Jost L, Sleijfer S, Verweij J, Blay JY, Group EGW. Soft tissue sarcomas: ESMO clinical recommendations for diagnosis, treatment and follow-up. Ann Oncol. 2009;20(Suppl 4):132–6.
31. Sakata K, Johnson FE, Beitler AL, Kraybill WG, Virgo KS. Extremity soft tissue sarcoma patient follow-up: tumor grade and size affect surveillance strategies after potentially curative surgery. Int J Oncol. 2003;22(6):1335–43.
32. Landier W, Bhatia S, Eshelman DA, Forte KJ, Sweeney T, Hester AL, et al. Development of risk-based guidelines for pediatric cancer survivors: the children's oncology group long-term follow-up guidelines from the children's oncology group late effects committee and nursing discipline. J Clin Oncol. 2004;22(24):4979–90.

33. National Comprehensive Cancer Network Soft Tissue Sarcoma Guidelines [12 Jan 2015]. http://www.nccn.org/professionals/physician_gls/pdf/sarcoma.pdf. Accessed 2 Dec 2015.
34. Scott M, Schuetze SM, Laurence H, Baker LH, Benjamin RS, Canettac R. Selection of response criteria for clinical trials of sarcoma treatment. Oncologist. 2008;13(Suppl 2):32–40.
35. Fleming JB, Cantor SB, Varma DG, Holst D, Feig BW, Hunt KK, Patel SR, Benjamin RS, Pollock RE, Pisters PW. Utility of chest computed tomography for staging in patients with T1 extremity soft tissue sarcomas. Cancer. 2001;92(4):863–8.
36. Goel A, Christy ME, Virgo KS, Kraybill WG, Johnson FE. Costs of follow-up after potentially curative treatment for extremity soft-tissue sarcoma. Int J Oncol. 2004;25(2):429–35.

Clinical Trials for Sarcomas

21

Neel Pancholi, Eish Maheshwari, Julio Jauregui, and Aditya V. Maheshwari

21.1 Introduction

Clinical trials provide the best way for clinicians and researchers alike to discover the optimal medical strategy, treatment, or device for patients [1]. Additionally, clinical trials allow for a determination on treatment safety and efficacy in humans. Clinical trials provide the highest level of evidence available for health-care decision-making. In progression from medical idea to implementation in clinical practice, the clinical trial is one of the final stages of a long and rigorous research process. Clinical trials start with small groups of patients to determine if a new approach causes any harm, and once that hurdle is cleared, the next stage is to determine the risks and benefits of the new approach [2]. A recommendation is made if the new approach, device, or treatment option improves patient outcomes, provides no benefit, or causes harm [1]. A discussion will be provided on what clinical trials are, how they work, their risks and benefits, and their importance in medicine. Furthermore, a survey of significant clinical trials in the study of various sarcomas will be provided.

21.2 What Are Clinical Trials/How Do They Work

When a clinical trial is first proposed, a protocol is created which details how the trial will work [2]. The principal investigator (PI) prepares the protocol for the clinical trial outlining what will be done during the study and why. It is important that every center that participates in the trial uses the same protocol for reproducibility. The protocol establishes study parameters including: a number of patients

N. Pancholi, M.D. • J. Jauregui, M.D. • A.V. Maheshwari, M.D. (✉)
Department of Orthopaedic Surgery and Rehabilitation Medicine, SUNY Downstate Medical Center, Brooklyn, NY, USA
e-mail: Aditya.maheshwari@downstate.edu

E. Maheshwari
Department of Orthopaedic Surgery and Rehabilitation Medicine, SUNY Downstate Medical Center, Brooklyn, NY, USA

© Springer International Publishing Switzerland 2017
R.M. Henshaw (ed.), *Sarcoma*, DOI 10.1007/978-3-319-43121-5_21

that will participate, patient eligibility, treatment(s) or interventions received, frequency of treatment, the type of data that will be collected, and detailed information on the treatment plan. Avoiding bias in a clinical trial is paramount, and researchers help achieve this by using strategies of randomization and blinding. The study group and comparison group in a clinical trial are assigned patients by chance (randomization) rather than by choice, which establishes statistically relevant groups. Blinding is achieved when patients are not informed if they will be in the treatment or control group. Double blinding is achieved when the investigator is also blinded from whether the patient is receiving the experimental or control treatment. These techniques significantly decrease the potential for bias influencing outcomes, improving the statistical power and credibility of the clinical trial.

In addition to the PI, sponsors and the institutional review board (IRB) are the two other key groups involved in clinical trials. The sponsor serves as an overseer of the trial. Sponsors are commonly pharmaceutical or device companies that indicate a clinical trial for one of their products. Furthermore, government agencies such as the National Institutes of Health (NIH); the National Heart, Lung, and Blood Institute (NHLBI); and the United States (US) Departments of Defense and Veterans Affairs sponsor clinical trials. Private companies such as universities and nonprofit organizations may also sponsor clinical trials [1]. Some companies and groups sponsor clinical trials that test the safety of products, such as medicines, and how well they work. The US Food and Drug Administration (FDA) oversees these clinical trials. The NIH may partner with these companies or groups to help sponsor some trials. Sponsors select qualified investigators, monitor the investigation, provide investigators with information they need, and ensure that all parts of the study adhere to general investigational plans and protocols. The sponsor is responsible for all operational aspects of the study.

The IRB is a regulatory group whose primary goal is the protection of the rights and welfare of human subjects. The IRB is a body designated by an institution to review, approve the initiation of, and conduct periodic review on studies involving human subjects. Responsibilities of the IRB include conducting initial and periodic review of research to ensure the safety of human subjects, establish adequate informed consent for participants, and approve any changes to the initial protocol [3]. In addition to the IRB, there are other notable regulatory bodies for patient protection in clinical trials. The Office of Human Rights Protections provides guidance and oversight to the IRB by offering advice and developing educational programs for research-related issues. The Data Safety Monitoring Board is comprised of research and study topic expert and is required to review all NIH phase 3 clinical trials for their safety profiles and identify and resolve any unforeseen risks to patients. The Food and Drug Administration provides further protection for study participants by reviewing applications for drugs or medical devices before any human testing is done [1].

21.3   Historical Perspectives

James Lind is considered the first physician to have conducted a controlled clinical trial in the modern era [4]. In 1747, as a surgeon on board his ship the HMS Salisbury, he sought to investigate scurvy's response to various diets. He took 12 of his men who suffered from scurvy and assigned two of them to six different diets. His results were remarkable in that the group given oranges and lemons were effectively cured of scurvy. Although the results were clear, Lind hesitated to recommend citrus for sailors, as oranges/lemons were expensive at the time. Not until 50 years later did the British Navy make citrus a compulsory part of its diet, dramatically decreasing scurvy and providing substantial clinical benefit. In 1946 the first randomized controlled trial was conducted by Sir Bradford Hill using streptomycin to treat pulmonary tuberculosis [4]. His landmark clinical trial established randomization as superior to alternation in order to better conceal the allocation schedule. Randomization is now the standard in clinical trials [5].

In 1947 the Nuremberg Code was developed, outlining ten basic statements for the protection of human participants in clinical trials (Appendix) [6]. Today clinical trials are widely accepted in the medical community as the best method for obtaining data for health-care decision-making and include stringent measures to avoid bias and ensure human subject safety.

21.4   Types of Trials

The NIH organizes clinical trials into six different categories: treatment trials which test experimental treatments, natural history trials which provide information on how diseases progress, prevention trials which look for better ways to prevent disease, diagnostic trials which are conducted to find better tests or procedures for diagnosing a particular disease, screening trials which test the best way to detect certain diseases, and quality of life trials which explore ways to improve comfort and quality of life for individuals with chronic illness [7]. While these types of trials each investigate different aspects of care, all are integral to improving patient care.

Furthermore, clinical trials are divided into four phases (Table 21.1) [8]. Prior to any testing on humans, there are preclinical trials, frequently performed with relevant and suitable animal models. After preclinical trials have shown some efficacious results, phase 1 trials are conducted with a limited number of human volunteers. Phase 1 trials are generally done on healthy people where a treatment is tested to verify that there are no adverse or toxic effects. Phase 2 trials are then performed with a small group of actual patients to demonstrate effect of treatment. After a treatment has shown some clinical benefit, phase 3 trials are performed on a large scale with multiple patients in multiple centers to determine efficacy. After regulated trials with many built-in safeguards to protect study participants have risks. It is critical that study participants be thoroughly educated on the known specific risks and benefits of a given trial. Patients must also be informed that unforeseen effects may occur and what strategies are in place to detect and minimize such effects. A goal of each clinical trial should be to improve public and patient literacy making patients and their families into informed decision-makers [1].

21.6   Importance of Clinical Trials

Clinical trials are a key research tool for establishing that new treatments or strategies are both safe and effective in addressing an illness in a specific population. Clinical trials show us what works and what doesn't work in medicine and health care by answering two important questions: does the treatment work in humans and is the treatment safe [10]? Furthermore, these trials can inform health-care decision-makers and allow for allocation of resources to treatments that work best. In the next section, we will review some of the landmark studies in sarcoma which have changed how we treat patients and outline the importance of clinical trials.

21.7   Examples of Clinical Trials in Sarcoma

In contrast to the commonly occurring carcinomas, there are relatively fewer clinical trials in sarcoma due to the low incidence of sarcoma in the population. As a result, there are few universally accepted recommendations for the treatment of sarcoma. Multicenter trials have been useful in studying rare tumors and thus serve as a useful application in sarcomas. Some examples of clinical trials in sarcoma are discussed below.

In most cases of soft tissue sarcomas, a multimodal approach to treatment including surgery, radiation therapy, and chemotherapy is used [11]. However, there are no universal guidelines. In a landmark randomized trial, patients with extremity soft tissue sarcomas (STS) were randomized to receive limb-sparing surgery plus postoperative radiation therapy vs. limb amputation [12]. All patients received doxorubicin-based chemotherapy. Although local recurrence was higher in the limb-sparing group, the overall survival was identical between the two groups. Therefore, for patients with a limb-sparing option, multimodality therapy with local resection and radiation therapy is preferable, and amputation for extremity STS is rarely performed these days.

However, the role of adjuvant chemotherapy in soft tissue sarcoma remains controversial. Several randomized but underpowered clinical trials with doxorubicin have been unable to show consistent beneficial results. As with much of clinical research in sarcoma, the absence of large, randomized trials limits interpretation of such data. To overcome this, a meta-analysis [13] of all randomized trials performed by the *Sarcoma Meta-analysis Collaboration*, doxorubicin-based adjuvant therapy for soft tissue sarcomas, showed that chemotherapy statistically improves the time

18. Coens C, van der Graaf WT, Blay JY, Chawla SP, Judson I, Sanfilippo R, Manson SC, Hodge RA, Marreaud S, Prins JB, Lugowska I, Litière S, Bottomley A. Health-related quality-of-life results from PALETTE: a randomized, double-blind, phase 3 trial of pazopanib versus placebo in patients with soft tissue sarcoma whose disease has progressed during or after prior chemotherapy—a European Organization for Research and Treatment of Cancer Soft Tissue and Bone Sarcoma Group Global Network Study (EORTC 62072). Cancer 2015;121:2933–41.
19. Demetri GD, Chawla SP, von Mehren M, Ritch P, Baker LH, Blay JY, Hande KR, Keohan ML, Samuels BL, Schuetze S, Lebedinsky C, Elsayed YA, Izquierdo MA, Gómez J, Park YC, Le Cesne A. Efficacy and safety of trabectedin in patients with advanced or metastatic liposarcoma or leiomyosarcoma after failure of prior anthracyclines and ifosfamide: results of a randomized phase II study of two different schedules. J Clin Oncol. 2009;27:4188–96.
20. Kawai A, Araki N, Sugiura H, Ueda T, Yonemoto T, Takahashi M, Morioka H, Hiraga H, Hiruma T, Kunisada T, Matsumine A, Tanase T, Hasegawa T, Takahashi S. Trabectedin monotherapy after standard chemotherapy versus best supportive care in patients with advanced, translocation-related sarcoma: a randomised, open-label, phase 2 study. Lancet Oncol. 2015;16:406–16.
21. Eilber FC, Eilber FR, Eckardt J, Rosen G, Riedel E, Maki RG, Brennan MF, Singer S. The impact of chemotherapy on the survival of patients with high-grade primary extremity liposarcoma. Ann Surg. 2004;240:686–97.
22. Eilber FC, Brennan MF, Eilber FR, Eckardt JJ, Grobmyer SR, Riedel E, Forscher C, Maki RG, Singer S. Chemotherapy is associated with improved survival in adult patients with primary extremity synovial sarcoma. Ann Surg. 2007;246:105–13.

Novel Therapies and Future Directions in Treatment of Musculoskeletal Sarcomas

Ratesh Khillan, Mohan Preet, Tanya DiFrancesco, Uchechi Uzoegwu, Osman Ali, and Aditya V. Maheshwari

22.1 Introduction

Musculoskeletal sarcomas (MSS) of the extremities are a heterogeneous group of neoplasms arising from cells of mesenchymal origin. Optimal patient care of MSS is best provided by a multidisciplinary team (consisting of radiology, medical and surgical oncology, radiation medicine, pathology, and psychosocial experts) with experience dealing with these types of tumors. The mainstay of treatment is limb salvage/function-preserving surgery with neoadjuvant or adjuvant radiation. Although response to aggressive chemotherapy has been documented using doxorubicin, ifosfamide, and dacarbazine, proof of efficacy in improving long-term survival is still controversial [1]. Moreover, the prognosis of these patients has plateaued over the last several years with the abovementioned conventional treatment modalities [2]. This has fueled research into the distinct molecular mechanisms of tumorigenesis and disease progression for various sarcoma subtypes.

The prognosis of patients with extremity MSS is often associated with histological diagnoses [3]. In recent times, our molecular and genetic understanding of the different histologies of MSS has rapidly advanced [4]. Not only useful for

R. Khillan, M.D. (✉) • M. Preet, M.D.
Hematology and Oncology, Brooklyn Cancer Care, Medical PC, Brooklyn, NY 11203, USA

Department of Orthopaedics Surgery and Rehabilitation Medicine, SUNY Downstate Medical Center, 450 Clarkson Ave, Box 30, Brooklyn, NY 11203, USA
e-mail: brooklyncancercare@gmail.com

T. DiFrancesco, M.D. • U. Uzoegwu, M.D. • O. Ali, M.D.
Hematology and Oncology, Brooklyn Cancer Care, Medical PC, Brooklyn, NY 11203, USA

A.V. Maheshwari, M.D.
Department of Orthopaedics Surgery and Rehabilitation, State University of New York (SUNY) Downstate Medical Center, 450 Clarkson Ave, Box 30, Brooklyn, NY 11203, USA
e-mail: Aditya.maheshwari@downstate.edu

© Springer International Publishing Switzerland 2017
R.M. Henshaw (ed.), *Sarcoma*, DOI 10.1007/978-3-319-43121-5_22

prognostic classifications, this information can provide insight for more specific therapeutic targeted options. Currently, gastrointestinal stromal tumors (GIST) are the prototype of targeted molecular therapy for sarcoma, with imatinib targeting the c-Kit (CD 117) and PDGFRα receptors [5]. Thus, newer modalities and regimens, in combination with newer targeted therapies, have become the area of interest for these tumors.

22.2 Specific Targeted Pathways by Sarcoma Subtype

Soft tissue sarcomas harbor very specific mutations, which vary considerably depending on their specific histology. This section will discuss these mutations and their targeting by promising novel therapies (Table 22.1). Most of these treatments are still in their early phase of development.

22.2.1 Liposarcomas

Well-differentiated liposarcomas (WDLPS) and dedifferentiated liposarcomas (DDLPS) have amplifications of chromosomal region 12q13-15 [6]. Various

Table 22.1 Soft tissue sarcoma subtypes with specific mutations and potential targeted therapies (adapted with permission from Frith et al. [4])

Soft tissue sarcoma type	Mutation/target	Targeted therapy
Well-differentiated/dedifferentiated liposarcoma	Amplification of MDM2	MDM 2 inhibitors
Solitary fibrous tumor	Translocation of NAB2-STAT6	TKIs
Wild-type GIST	SDH dysfunction/HIF-1 pathway	HIF-1 pathway inhibitor (mTOR inhibitor, Hsp90 inhibitor, histone deacetylase inhibitors)
Angiosarcoma	Angiopoeitin-TIE pathway	Angiopoeitin inhibitor (AMG 386)
Synovial sarcoma	BCL-2 overexpression	BCL-2 inhibitors (e.g., ABT-263, ABT-737)
Malignant peripheral nerve sheath tumor	Constitutive expression of Ras	Dual mTOR/AKT inhibitor (e.g., PI-103 or XL765)
Alveolar rhabdomyosarcoma	Amplification of CDK4	CDK4 inhibitor (e.g., PD0332991)
Ewing's sarcoma family of tumors	IGF1R	IGF1R inhibitors (ganitumumab, cixutumumab)
Most sarcomas	Argininosuccinate synthase 1 deficiency	ADI-PEG20

oncogenes are found including, but not limited to, MDM2, CDK4, and HMGA2 [7]. MDM2 amplification is seen in majority of WDLPS/DDLPS, making it a key feature of this cancer [8]. MDM2 encodes a negative regulator of the tumor suppressorgene tumor protein 53 (p53). There are several small molecules that have been identified to inhibit MDM2-p53 interaction. Nutilin is the most studied of the MDM2 inhibitors. It has an imidazoline structure and acts by binding to MDM2, resulting in unbound active p53. In vitro studies using cell lines with wild-type and mutant p53 have clearly shown that only cells with wild-type p53 are sensitive to these compounds [9]. A neoadjuvant trial using RG7112 (Roche, Nutley, NJ) in WDLPS and DDLPS demonstrated p53 upregulation and reactivation, with one partial response and 14 patients with stable disease [9]. There are additional MDM2 antagonists that are available for human use. For example, MI219 (Ascenta Therapeutics, Malvern, PA) has a spiro-oxindole structure that binds to MDM2, inhibiting p53 binding and allowing for p53 activation in tumor cell lines with wild-type p53 [10]. MDM2 antagonists are promising drugs for the treatment of sarcomas, but resistance to these agents has already been observed. Further clinical trials are needed to check efficacy and potential side effects of these agents.

22.2.2 Solitary Fibrous Tumors

Solitary fibrous tumors are mostly benign, CD34-positive fibroblastic cells. They have translocations NAB2 and STAT6 on chromosome 12q14, but are transcribed in the opposite direction. Before the translocations of NAB2 and STAT6 were discovered, a group of patients with metastatic PDGFRβ-positive solitary fibrous tumors were treated with sunitinib (a tyrosine kinase inhibitor). Six of these patients showed partial response and one patient responded with stable disease [11]. Developments in molecular genetic medicine studying tyrosine kinase inhibitors and Janus kinase-2 (JAK2), targeting FGF and PDGFR, will allow for future treatment of solitary fibrous tumors.

22.2.3 Malignant Peripheral Nerve Sheath Tumors

New evidence in molecular science shows that nerve sheath tumors have mutations in the (mTOR) pathway [12]. Rapamycin, a fungicidal agent, binds to and inhibits the (mTOR) complex. Rapamycin derivative was able to prove cytostatic activity in sarcoma patients [13, 14]. Blocking mTOR signaling with rapamycin results in an increase in phospho-AKT. Preclinical studies have been done to evaluate the effect of RAD001 (an oral rapamycin derivate) (Novartis, Basel, Switzerland). RAD001 was able to induce a 50 % growth reduction in four of five cell lines, although it failed to induce apoptosis, making RAD001 a cytostatic therapy for sporadic and NF1-derived MPNST cells. Additionally, in vivo models using mice with MPNST xenografts treated with RAD001 had a significant decrease in tumor growth in 76 % of mice [12, 15].

22.2.4 Angiosarcomas

Angiosarcomas are an aggressive subset of soft tissue sarcomas comprised of malignant endothelial cells of a vascular or lymphatic origin. As a tumor of vascular origin, there is potential for anti-angiogenic therapy. However, a recently published study on bevacizumab (Genentech, San Francisco, CA) demonstrated very low activity of bevacizumab in this sarcoma [16]. Data suggest that the angiopoietin-TIE2 pathway could be a promising target for the pharmacologic blockade of angiopoietin 2. Blocking this pathway leads to decreased endothelial cell proliferation and blocked VEGF-induced neovascularization in rat corneal models consistent with an anti-angiogenic mechanism [17].

22.2.5 Synovial Sarcomas

Ninety-five percent of synovial sarcomas are characterized by a chromosomal translocation t(X;18)(p11.2;q11.2) resulting in a fusion protein comprised of the SS18 gene (also known as SYT) and the SSX gene (SSX1, SSX2, or rarely SSX4) [18, 19]. Compared to other sarcomas, synovial sarcomas have a high level of B-cell lymphoma 2 protein (Bcl2) [20]. Bcl2 inhibitors have the potential to be used in synovial sarcomas either bypassing the MCL-1 pathway or through SS18-SSX fusion oncogene inhibiting BCL2A1.

22.2.6 Alveolar Rhabdomyosarcomas

Alveolar rhabdomyosarcomas (RMS), primarily tumors of children, are rarer and more aggressive than embryonal rhabdomyosarcomas [21, 22]. The chromosomal translocation t(2;13)(q35;q14) is a characteristic of this tumor. It causes an oncogenic fusion of the transcription factor for PAX3 with the potent transcriptional activation domain of FOX01, which is thought to halt normal muscle differentiation by several mechanisms, including suppression of MyoD [23] and the activation of cyclin D1/cyclin-dependent kinase 4 (CDK4) complexes [24]. CDK4 directly phosphorylates PAX3-FOX01 at Ser430 which enhances PAX3-FOX01 transcriptional activity [25, 26]. Currently, phase I clinical trials are underway studying compounds PD0332991, P276-00, and LY2835219 for the treatment of alveolar RMS. PD0332991 (Pfizer, New York, NY) is an oral pyridopyrimidine-derived CDK inhibitor with a high specificity for CDK4 and CDK6. P276-00 (Piramal Enterprise Limited, Mumbai, India) is a flavone inhibiting both CDK4-D1 and CDK1-B. LY2835219 (Lilly, Indianapolis, IN) is an oral small molecule inhibitor of a potent oral inhibitor of the cyclin-dependent kinases 4 and 6 (CDK4/6) with broad in vivo antitumor activity [27].

22.2.7 Alveolar Soft Part Sarcomas

Surgical treatment is the gold standard of alveolar soft part sarcoma (ASPS) treatment. However, recent data shows that sunitinib is clinically active in the metastatic setting [28]. ASPS has a translocation between the ASPS locus and TFE3, t(Xp11:17q25). The fusion protein, driving cMET expression [29], arises by using the ASPS promoter to drive the transcription factor TFE3 [31]. With sunitinib (Phizer, New York, NY) inhibiting RET-driven cMET, the development of direct cMET inhibitors offers promise for this rare disease [30].

22.2.8 Ewing's Family of Tumors

The most common translocations in Ewing's family of tumors (EFT) involve the EWS and FLI1 genes [t(11;22)(q24;q12)] [31]. The EWS-FLI1 translocation upregulates IGF-1 levels and increases dependence on IGF1R-mediated signaling. Prognosis for patients with relapsed disease still remains poor. Recently, two major phase II trials reported modest efficacy for patients with relapsed EFT. In 38 patients, Tap et al. [31] used a fully humanized monoclonal antibody, ganitumumab; 22 had EFT and 16 had desmoplastic small round cell tumors. Two patients had an objective response, one remaining on treatment for almost 1 year. An additional four patients with stable disease for more than 24 weeks resulted in a clinical benefit rate of 17%. Pharmacodynamic measures of IGF1R treatment, including serum IGF1 levels, were consistent with IGF1R inhibition. Major side effects included cytopenia and hyperglycemia in a minority of patients and one patient with a grade 3 transient ischemic attack. The second study, a multicenter, open-label phase II trial, combined IGF1R inhibitor cixutumumab and mTOR inhibitor temsirolimus in bone and soft tissue sarcomas [32]. Patients were stratified by IGF1R expression, and the primary endpoint was a 12-week PFS rate greater than 40%. In the IGF1R-positive bone sarcoma cohort, 6 patients (11%) had an objective response and 19 patients (35%) were progression-free at 12 weeks (90% confidence interval 24–47%), meeting the primary endpoint. While tissue samples obtained from the patients during treatment showed adequate target inhibition downstream of IGF1R and mTOR, these decreases were unable to correspond to clinical outcomes [12].

Single enantiomer of YK-4-279 demonstrates specificity in targeting the oncogene EWS-FLI1. Enantiospecific effects are also established in cytotoxicity assays and caspase assays, where up to a log-fold difference is seen between (S)-YK-4-279 and the racemic YK-4-279 [33].

Another study revealed that substitution of electron-donating groups at the para-position on the phenyl ring was the most favorable for inhibition of EWS-FLI1 by analogs of 2. Compound 9u (with a dimethylamino substitution) was the most active inhibitor with GI50 = 0.26 ± 0.1 μM. Further, a correlation of growth inhibition (EWS-FLI1expressing TC32 cells) and the luciferase reporter activity was established ($R(2) = 0.84$) [34].

Recently, another in vivo study highlights the efficacy of YK-4-279 to treat EWS-FLI1expressing neoplasms and support its therapeutic potential for patients with Ewing's sarcoma and other ETS-driven malignancies [35].

22.2.9 Chondrosarcoma

Mutations in isocitrate dehydrogenases 1 and 2 (IDH1 and IDH2) have been found to be a common occurrence in several central and periosteal cartilage tumors [36]. More specifically, IDH1 R132 and IDH2 R172 mutations, identified by Amary et al., comprise approximately 56% of these mutations. Observations that patients with hereditary Maffucci and Ollier syndromes express these mutations in enchondromas suggest that the mutations occur early in tumorgenesis [36]. Studies suggest that chondrosarcomas with mutant IDH grow due to hypermethylation of key regulatory genes as well as an accumulation of (D-2-hydroxyglutarate) D2HG, a rare oncometabolite [36]. This understanding has broadened the scope for evaluation of new treatments including therapeutic trials of demethylating agents such as 5-azacitadine. Currently, oral inhibitors of IDH1 (AG-120) and ID2 (AG-221) are in preclinical development and phase 1 trials, respectively. IDH-specific inhibitors for chondrosarcomas are being tested as well [36].

22.3 Immunotherapy

New understanding of the immune system has led to the development of novel therapies against cancer. Immunotherapy involves targeting cancer cells with the patient's own immune cells (Fig. 22.1). Immunotherapy includes agents such as interleukins and interferons, use of vaccines to promote immune responses, and adoptive cell transfer therapy. Tables 22.2 and 22.3 show some of the clinical trials involving innate and adaptive immunity against musculoskeletal sarcomas.

22.3.1 Cytokine Therapies

The immune system is regulated by proteins called cytokines. Clinically significant cytokines in the treatment of sarcomas are interleukin-2 (IL-2) and interferons (IFNs) [37]. IL-2 works by activation and expansion of CD4 and CD8 T cells [38]. Rosenberg et al. produced a tumor regression model involving recombinant

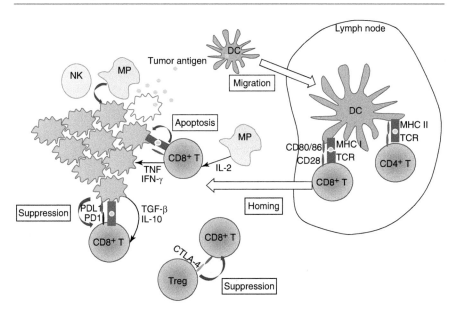

Fig. 22.1 An overview of tumor immunology. Tumor cells are initially attacked by the innate immune system. DCs capture tumor antigens at the tumor site and migrate to the tumor-draining lymph nodes. DCs present the tumor antigen to T cells within the lymph node. Antigen-specific CD4 and CD8 T cells are stimulated by DCs. After stimulation, T cells differentiate into effector cells and activate at the tumor site. Effector CD8 T cells kill tumor cells, although their function is regulated by the immune checkpoint mechanism. *NK* natural killer cell, *MP* macrophage, *DC* dendritic cell (reproduced with permission from Uehara et al. [2])

IL-2 injection for murine melanoma and sarcomas [39]. Due to IL-2 success in metastatic melanoma, it was used in bone and soft tissue sarcomas [40, 41]. Schwinger et al. reported response with high-dose IL-2 therapy in two patients with Ewing's sarcoma and four patients with metastatic osteosarcoma. These patients were heavily pretreated with chemotherapy and radiation and had multiple surgeries. There were two complete responses in two patients of osteosarcoma. High-dose IL-2 treatment is associated with fatigue, anorexia, diarrhea, nausea, vomiting, and high-grade fever; some deaths were also reported with IL-2 therapy [42].

IFN-therapy has shown improved patient survival when used as adjuvant therapy [43, 44]. The COSS-80 study investigated the effectiveness of using adjuvant chemotherapy with IFN [45]. The 30-month disease-free survival rate of the IFN arm was 77% and that of non-IFN arm 73%, although this difference was not statistically significant. The EURAMOS-1 study, a recent study in Europe, investigated the efficacy of the use of adjuvant chemotherapy with pegylated IFN-2b [46]. These studies infer that conventional chemotherapy with IFN improves the prognosis of bone and soft tissue sarcomas.

Table 22.2 Clinical trials stimulating innate immunity against musculoskeletal sarcomas (reproduced with permission from Uehara et al. [2])

Agent	Number of patients	Diagnosis	Treatment	Follow-up	Clinical result
IL-2 [12]	6	Osteosarcoma, Ewing's sarcoma	$6-12 \times 10^6$ IU/m^2 for 5 days by every 3 weeks	7–71 months	Complete response (CR): 5
					Progressive disease (PD): 5
IFNs [16]	3	Osteosarcoma	$2.5-5 \times 10^6$ IU/mL twice or thrice weekly	6–8 months	CR: 2
					PD: 1
IFN-α2 [17]	20	Osteosarcoma, fibrosarcoma, chondrosarcoma, and malignant fibrous histiocytoma	5×10^7 IU/m^2 thrice weekly	1–3 months	Partial response (PR): 3
INF-α [18]	89	Osteosarcoma	Cohort 1 (70 patients); 3×10^6 IU daily for a month	10 years	Metastatic-free survival: 39%
			Cohort 2 (19 patients); 3×10^6 IU for 3–5 years		Sarcoma-specific survival: 43%
INF-β [19]	158	Osteosarcoma (COSS-80)	1×10^5 IU/kg for 22 weeks	30 months	Disease-free survival
					+IFN: 77%
					−IFN: 74%
Pegylated INF-α2b [20]	715	Osteosarcoma (EURAMOS-1)	Methotrexate, adriamycin, and cisplatin (MAP) ± IFN (0.5–1.0 µg/kg/week) for 2 years	Median follow-up 3.1 years	Event-free survival
					+IFN: 77:%
					−IFN: 74% (N.S.)
L-MTP-PE [21]	662	Osteosarcoma (INT 0133)	MAP + L-MTP-PE, MAP + ifosfamide, MAP + ifosfamide + L-MTP-PE	6 years	Overall survival
					+L-MTP-PE: 78%
					−L-MTP-PE: 70%
					Event-free survival
					No significant difference

Table 22.3 Clinical trials stimulating adaptive immunity against musculoskeletal soft tissue sarcomas (reproduced with permission from Uehara et al. [2])

Agent	Number of patients	Diagnosis	Treatment	Immune response	Clinical result
Autologous tumor cells [22]	23	Sarcoma	Total 1.0×10^7 cells	Delayed-type hypersensitivity (DTH) positive: 8 patients	Median survival DTH responder: 16.6 months Non-responder: 8.2 months
Tumor translocation breakpoint-specific peptide-pulsed DCs [23]	52	Ewing's sarcoma, rhabdomyosarcoma	Total 4.2–143.0×10^6 cells	39% with immune response to the translocation breakpoint, 25% with response to E7 specific	Overall survival Vaccination: 43% Control: 31%
Tumor-specific synthetic peptides or tumor lysates pulsed DCs [24]	5	Ewing's sarcoma, synovial sarcoma, neuroblastoma	2–15×10^6 pulsed DCs injected 6–8 times	DTH positive: 1 patient	CR:1 (77 months) PD: 4 (2–27 months)
A 9-mer peptide from SYT-SSX fusion site [25]	21	Synovial sarcoma	0.1 or 10 mg peptide ± adjuvant 6 times at 14-day interval	Tetramer positive CD8: 7 patients	Stable disease (SD): 1/9 peptide alone 6/12 vaccine with adjuvant
Anti-CTLA-4 antibody [26]	6	Synovial sarcoma (expressed NY-ESO-1)	Ipilimumab 3 mg/kg every 3 weeks for 3 cycles	DTH: all patients negative	Time to progression 0.47–2.1 months (median 1.85) overall survival time 0.77–19.7 months (median 8.75)
T-cell receptor (TCR)-transduced T cells (NY-ESO-1 specific) [27]	6	Synovial sarcoma (expressed NY-ESO-1)	TCR-transduced T cells + 720,000 IU/kg of IL-2	Tetramer positive CD8: 5 patients	PR: 4 PD: 2

22.3.2 Mifamurtide

A new agent, mifamurtide (Takeda, Cambridge, MA), liposomal muramyl tripeptide phosphatidylethanolamine (L-MTP-PE), is a synthetic analog of a muramyl dipeptide (MDP) [47]. NOD2, the intracellular pattern recognition molecule, recognizes MDP and enriches NF-κB signaling [48]. Thus, when NOD2 detects L-MTP-PE, it stimulates production of IL-1β, IL-6, and TNF-α by activating NF-κB signaling in monocytes and macrophages [49, 50]. In 1993, 662 patients with osteosarcoma took part in an intergroup study 0133 (INT 0133) determining the efficacy of supplementing basic adjuvant chemotherapy (cisplatin, doxorubicin, and high-dose methotrexate (MAP)) with ifosfamide (IFO) and L-MTP-PE. Study participants were randomly assigned treatment with MAP alone, MAP + IFO, MAP + L-MTPPE, and MAP + IFO + L-MTP-PE. The addition of L-MTP-PE to chemotherapy was found to improve the 6-year overall survival rate from 70 to 78% ($P = 0.03$). The hazard ratio for overall survival with the addition of MTP was 0.71 (95% CI: 0.52–0.96) [51]. Consequently, L-MTP-PE combined with chemotherapy received approval for the treatment of osteosarcoma in Europe, although it has not been approved by the FDA for use in the United States [50].

22.3.3 Vaccine Therapy Against Soft Tissue Sarcomas

Stimulating the immune system with cancer vaccines to target and eliminate sarcomas has been studied in various clinical trials. In combination with GM-CSF, IL-2, or other co-stimulatory adjuvants to enhance the immune response, vaccines can target whole cells, proteins, lysates, and peptides [52, 53]. Antigen-presenting cells present the vaccines as antigen epitopes on MHC molecules and tumor antigen-specific T cells are then activated.

Autologous sarcoma cell lysates which are a cell lysate derived from sarcoma cells with potential immunostimulatory and antineoplastic activities can be used as a vaccine in patients with sarcomas. In a clinical trial, patients who became positive for delayed-type hypersensitivity (DTH) had median survival of 8 months longer than patients who were DTH negative. Also, the size of the tumor decreased [54].

Autologous dendritic cells (DC), pulsed ex vivo with tumor cell lysate, can also stimulate host immunity [55]. This has been used as adjuvant therapy for chemotherapy; one patient had complete remission and five patients with stable disease [56].

Tumor-specific or overexpressed peptides are possible for therapeutic targets for antigen-specific immunotherapy [56–58]. In a study, patients are given nine-mer peptide with or without incomplete Freund's adjuvant (IFA), which is a solution of antigen emulsified in mineral oil and used as an immunopotentiator (booster) and IFN. In patients who received the vaccination, the disease was stabilized as compared to patients who did not receive the vaccine [57].

22.3.4 Adoptive Cell Transfer

Adoptive cell transfer therapy involves the transfer of antigen-specific T cells obtained from the patient [59]. Harvested T cells are expanded ex vivo and transferred back to the patient. Tumor-reactive CD8 T cells secrete very high levels of cytokines, IFN, TNF, and IL-2 [60]. A small study examined six patients with synovial sarcoma or metastatic melanomas expressing NY-ESO-1. To initiate tumor lysis, T cell receptor (TCR) gene-modified T cells redirected toward NY-ESO-1 were produced [60]. In the study, two patients with melanoma showed complete regression, and one patient with synovial sarcoma has stable disease for 18 months. Some types of adoptive cell transfer therapies are ongoing for patients with sarcomas, including autologous DC transport therapy for soft tissue sarcomas (NCT01347034) and hematopoietic cell transplantation and natural killer cell transport therapies for Ewing's sarcomas and rhabdomyosarcomas (NCT02100891) [2].

22.3.5 Immune Checkpoint Blockade

Immune checkpoint blockade has the potential to further anticancer immunology through interference and downregulation of normal inhibitory pathways that modulate self-tolerance and the duration and amplitude of immune responses. Promoting antitumor immunity, ipilimumab, a fully human monoclonal antibody (IgG1), blocks CTLA-4 [61]. In patients with metastatic melanomas receiving ipilimumab, overall survival improved from 6.4 months to 10.0 months [62]. In a phase II study, six patients with advanced synovial sarcoma treated with ipilimumab showed a survival time ranging from 0.77 to 19.7 months (median: 8.75 months). In each patient, posttreatment immunological responses were different, and three patients had an enhanced titer of CT24 (an uncharacterized CTA). Even though all sarcomas expressed NY-ESO-1, no remarkable change was shown in the NY-ESO-1 titer [60]. Nivolumab, a human monoclonal anti-PD-1 antibody, has shown effectiveness in several types of cancers including melanoma, prostate cancer, NSCLC, renal cell carcinoma, and colorectal cancer [63, 64]. Reported clinical outcomes of nivolumab therapies include a cumulative response rate of 18% in patients with NSCLC, 28% in patients with melanoma, and 27% in patients with renal cell carcinoma [65]. Eighty-six patients with advanced melanoma participated in a phase I trial combining both agents nivolumab and ipilimumab. Fifty-three percent of patients experienced grade 3 or 4 adverse effects related to the therapy, as compared with previous rates of 20% among patients treated with ipilimumab monotherapy at a dose of 3 mg/kg. Nine out of 17 patients who received the maximum doses associated with an acceptable level of adverse events (cohort 2, with nivolumab at a dose of 1 mg/kg and ipilimumab at a dose of 3 mg/kg) had an objective response [66]. While ipilimumab and nivolumab have been found effective in certain types of tumors, further research is needed to determine the effectiveness of these immune checkpoint blockade agents for bone and soft tissue sarcomas.

22.4   Miscellaneous Novel Agents

In this section, we will discuss other novel therapies used in the treatment of musculoskeletal sarcomas in clinical practice. Some are not approved in the United States (USA) but are being used in Europe and other countries. After getting data from those countries, these agents will potentially be approved in the USA. We will discuss specific types of sarcomas treated by these novel agents, their mechanism of action, and side effect profile.

22.4.1 Pegylated Arginine Deiminase (ADI-PEG20)

Argininosuccinate synthetase 1 (ASS1) is an integral enzyme in the urea cycle. It is responsible for the combination of the amino acids citrulline and aspartate to form argininosuccinic acid which is later used to form urea [67]. Recent studies have shown that more than 88% of sarcomas, signifying 45 subtypes, have a loss of ASS1 expression [68]. This finding is highly suggestive that these soft tissue tumors may be responsive to the elimination of arginine. Selective arginine depletion with enzymes such as pegylated arginine deiminase (ADI-PEG20) (Polaris Group, San Diego, CA) may prove beneficial and should be exploited as a promising and effective anticancer therapy.

22.4.2 Pazopanib (Votrient)

Pazopanib is a multi-tyrosine kinase inhibitor of vascular endothelial growth factor receptor (VEGFR 1, 2, and 3), platelet-derived growth factor receptor (PDGFR-A and PDGFR-B), and v-kit Hardy-Zuckerman 4 feline sarcoma viral oncogene homolog (c-kit). This agent has demonstrated activity in phase II studies in non-adipocytic sarcomas [69]. Pazopanib is currently indicated for use in advanced soft tissue sarcomas in patients who have received prior chemotherapy.

22.4.3 Regorafenib (Stivarga, BAY 73-4506)

Regorafenib is an oral multi-tyrosine kinase inhibitor of VEGFRs 2 and 3, RET, Kit, PDGFR, and Raf kinases. It is being used for the treatment of GIST in patients who fail to respond to imatinib and sunitinib [70].

22.4.4 Trabectedin (ET-743, Yondelis)

Trabectedin is a novel marine antineoplastic alkaloid with unique mechanism of action. It binds to the minor groove of DNA at the N2 position of guanine, particularly at CGG sequences, and interferes with transcription-coupled nucleotide excision repair, thereby inducing a lethal DNA strand break. This drug has activity against myxoid MSS [71]. This drug is approved in Europe for the treatment of advanced soft tissue sarcomas in patients who have failed anthracyclines and ifosfamide and was approved by the FDA in 2015 for patients with advanced or unresectable liposarcoma and leiomyosarcoma.

22.4.5 Ridaforolimus (AP23573; MK-8669)

Ridaforolimus is a mTOR inhibitor. This medication failed to get FDA approval after studies in soft tissue and bone sarcomas demonstrated a 3-week survival advantage [72].

22.4.6 Palifosfamide (Z10-201)

Palifosfamide is a tris formulation of functional active metabolite of ifosfamide isophosphoramide mustard. It has been studied in combination with doxorubicin, but has shown no survival advantage [73].

22.5   Electroporation

New research is exploring the use of electroporation therapy (EPT), which uses electrical currents to increase cell wall permeability to cytotoxic drugs [74]. One chemotherapy agent used with EPT is bleomycin, a cytotoxic agent that inhibits DNA synthesis by breaking the double strands of DNA. Bleomycin does not cross cell membranes, but in concert with EPT creating transient pores in cell membranes, bleomycin is able to act. Clinical studies show that EPT combined with bleomycin shows response in cutaneous malignancies such as squamous cell carcinomas, basal cell carcinomas, and melanomas [75, 76]. Some of the side effects of EPT are feelings of unpleasantness due to muscle or nerve-related spasms.

22.6   Conclusion and Future Directions

Recent breakthroughs in growth signaling pathways, metabolic reprogramming, and immune therapy have opened the potential for targeted treatment for many sarcomas (Fig. 22.2). It is through an improved fundamental understanding of sarcoma biology that clinical trials based on molecular targets are being developed. These trials form the foundation for further improvements in our ability to care for patients with these tumors and may offer clinical insights into a wide range of other tumors.

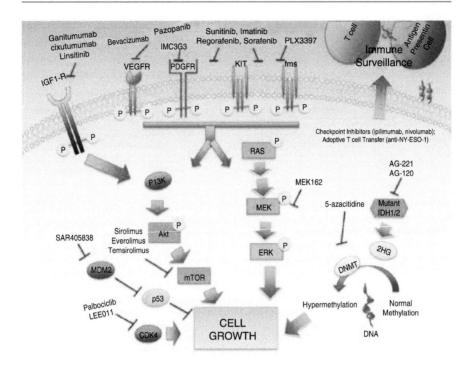

Fig. 22.2 A schematic diagram showing selected signaling, epigenetic, and immune targets used in sarcoma therapy or under clinical development. *IGF1R* insulin growth factor-1 receptor, *VEGFR* vascular endothelial growth factor receptor, *PDGFR* platelet-derived growth factor receptor, *2PG* 2-hydroxyglutarate, *DNMT* DNA methyltransferase (reproduced with permission from Shoustary et al. [27])

Although most of these agents are in very early phases of clinical trials and are not the standard of care, targeted therapy is a significant step in a new and hopefully right direction. With time, these treatments will improve and translate into significant clinical responses. As our knowledge of these targets advances, we will have more effective, personalized therapy and less toxic treatment options for these highly aggressive chemoresistant tumors.

References

1. Kraybill WG, Harris J, Spiro IJ, Ettinger DS, DeLaney TF, Blum RH, Lucas DR, Harmon DC, Letson GD, Eisenberg B. Phase II study of neoadjuvant chemotherapy and radiation therapy in the management of high-risk, high-grade, soft tissue sarcomas of the extremities and body wall: Radiation Therapy Oncology Group Trial 9514. J Clin Oncol. 2006; 24(4):619–25.
2. Uehara T, Fujiwara T, Takeda K, Kunisada T, Ozaki T, Udono H. Immunotherapy for bone and soft tissue sarcomas. Biomed Res Int. 2015;2015:820813. doi:10.1155/2015/820813.
3. Italiano A, Le Cesne A, Mendiboure J, Blay JY, Piperno-Neumann S, Chevreau C, Delcambre C, Penel N, Terrier P, Ranchere-Vince D, Lae M, Le Guellec S, Michels JJ, Robin YM,

Bellera C, Bonvalot S. Prognostic factors and impact of adjuvant treatments on local and metastatic relapse of soft-tissue sarcoma patients in the competing risks setting. Cancer. 2014;120(21):3361–9.

4. Frith AE, Hirbe AC, Van Tine BA. Novel pathways and molecular targets for the treatment of sarcoma. Curr Oncol Rep. 2013;15(4):378–85.

5. Rajendra R, Pollack SM, Jones RL. Management of gastrointestinal stromal tumors. Future Oncol. 2013;9:193–206.

6. Rieker RJ, Weitz J, Lehner B, Egerer G, Mueller A, Kasper B, Schirmacher P, Joos S, Mechtersheimer G. Genomic profiling reveals subsets of dedifferentiated liposarcoma to follow separate molecular pathways. Virchows Arch. 2010;456:277–85.

7. Jemal A, Siegel R, Xu J, Ward E. Cancer statistics, 2010. CA Cancer J Clin. 2010;60:277–300.

8. Jones B, Komarnitsky P, Miller GT, Amedio J, Wallner BP. Anticancer activity of stabilized palifosfamide in vivo: schedule effects, oral bioavailability, and enhanced activity with docetaxel and doxorubicin. Anticancer Drugs. 2012;23:173–84.

9. Kindblom LG. Lipomatous tumors-how we have reached our present views, what controversies remain and why we still face diagnostic problems: a tribute to Dr Franz Enzinger. Adv Anat Pathol. 2006;13:279–85.

10. Jones RL, Fisher C, Al-Muderis O, Judson IR. Differential sensitivity of liposarcoma subtypes to chemotherapy. Eur J Cancer. 2005;41:2853–60.

11. Pedeutour F, Forus A, Coindre JM, Berner JM, Nicolo G, Michiels JF, Terrier P, Ranchere-Vince D, Collin F, Myklebost O, Turc-Carel C. Structure of the supernumerary ring and giant rod chromosomes in adipose tissue tumors. Genes Chromosomes Cancer. 1999;24:30–41.

12. Hay N, Sonenberg N. Upstream and downstream of mTOR. Genes Dev. 2004;18:1926–45.

13. Vignot S, Faivre S, Aguirre D, Raymond E. mTOR-targeted therapy of cancer with rapamycin derivatives. Ann Oncol. 2005;16(4):525–37.

14. Meric-Bernstam F, Mills GB. Mammalian target of rapamycin. Semin Oncol. 2004;31(6 Suppl 16):10–7.

15. Johannessen CM, Reczek EE, James MF, et al. The NF1 tumor suppressor critically regulates TSC2 and mTOR. Proc Natl Acad Sci U S A. 2005;102:8573–8.

16. Angulnik M, Yarber JL, Okuno SH, et al. An open-label, multicenter, phase II study of bevacizumab for the treatment of angiosarcoma and epithelioid hemangioendotheliomas. Ann Oncol. 2013;24(1):3148–53.

17. Dei Tos AP, Piccinin S, Doglioni C, Vukosavljevic T, Mentzel T, Boiocchi M, Fletcher CD. Coordinated expression and amplification of the MDM2, CDK4, and HMGI-C genes in atypical lipomatous tumors. J Pathol. 2000;190:531–6.

18. Nagao K, Ito H, Yoshida H. Chromosomal translocation t(X;18) in human synovial sarcomas analyzed by fluorescence in situ hybridization using paraffin-embedded tissue. Am J Pathol. 1996;148:601–9.

19. Jones KB, Su L, Jin H, Lenz C, Randall RL, Underhill TM., Nielsen TO, Sharma S, Capecchi MR. SS18-SSX2 and the mitochondrial apoptosis pathway in mouse and human synovial sarcomas. Oncogene. 2013;32(18):2365–71, 2375.e1–5. doi: 10.1038/onc.2012.247.

20. Hirakawa N, Naka T, Yamamoto I, Fukuda T, Tsuneyoshi M. Overexpression of bcl-2 protein in synovial sarcoma: a comparative study of other soft tissue spindle cell sarcomas and an additional analysis by fluorescence in situ hybridization. Hum Pathol. 1996;27:1060–5.

21. Marshall AD, Grosveld GC. Alveolar rhabdomyosarcoma—the molecular drivers of PAX3/7-FOXO1-induced tumorigenesis. Skelet Muscle 2012;2:25.

22. Seitz G, Dantonello TM, Int-Veen C, Blumenstock G, Godzinski J, Klingebiel T, Schuck A, Leuschner I, Koscielniak E, Fuchs J. Survival following disease recurrence of primary localized alveolar rhabdomyosarcoma. Pediatr Blood Cancer. 2013;60(3):1267–73.

23. Calhabeu F, Hayashi S, Morgan JE, Relaix F, Zammit PS. Alveolar rhabdomyosarcoma-associated proteins PAX3/FOXO1A and PAX7/FOXO1A suppress the transcriptional activity of MyoD-target genes in muscle stem cells. Oncogene. 2013;32:651–62.

24. Charytonowicz E, Matushansky I, Doménech JD, Castillo-Martín M, Ladanyi M, Cordon-Cardo C, Ziman M. PAX7-FKHR fusion gene inhibits myogenic differentiation via NFkappaB upregulation. Clin Transl Oncol. 2012;14:197–206.
25. Liu L, Wu J, Ong S, Chen T. Cyclin-dependent kinase 4 phosphorylates and positively regulates PAX3-FOX01 in human alveolar rhabdomyosarcoma cells. PLoS One. 2013;8:e58193.
26. Sorensen PH, Lynch JC, Qualman SJ, Tirabosco R, Lim JF, Maurer HM, Bridge JA, Crist WM, Triche TJ, Barr FG. PAX3-FKHR and PAX7-FKHR gene fusions are prognostic indicators in alveolar rhabdomyosarcoma: a report from the children's oncology group. J Clin Oncol. 2002;20:2672–9.
27. Gelbert LM, Cai S, Lin X, Sanchez-Martinez C, Del Prado M, Lallena MJ, Torres R, Ajamie RT, Wishart GN, Flack RS, Neubauer BL, Young J, Chan EM, Iversen P, Cronier D, Kreklau E, de Dios A. A potent oral inhibitor of the cyclin-dependent kinases 4 and 6 (CDK4/6) with broad in vivo antitumor activity [abstract B233]. Mol Cancer Ther. 2011.
28. Stacchiotti S, Tamborini E, Marrari A, Brich S, Rota SA, Orsenigo M, Crippa F, Morosi C, Gronchi A, Pierotti MA, Casali PG, Pilotti S. Response to sunitinib malate in advanced alveolar soft part sarcoma. Clin Cancer Res. 2009;15:1096–104.
29. Tsuda M, Davis IJ, Argani P, Shukla N, McGill GG, Nagai M, Saito T, Laé M, Fisher DE, Ladanyi M. TFE3 fusions activate MET signaling by transcriptional up-regulation, defining another class of tumors as candidates for therapeutic MET inhibition. Cancer Res. 2007;67:919–29.
30. Ladanyi M, Lui MY, Antonescu CR, Krause-Boehm A, Meindl A, Argani P, Healey JH, Ueda T, Yoshikawa H, Meloni-Ehrig A, Sorensen PH, Mertens F, Mandahl N, van den Berghe H, Sciot R, Dal Cin P, Bridge J. The der(17)t(X;17)(p11;q25) of human alveolar soft part sarcoma fuses the TFE3 transcription factor gene to ASPL, a novel gene at 17q25. Oncogene. 2001;20:48–57.
31. Tap WD, Demetri G, Barnette P, Desai J, Kavan P, Tozer R, Benedetto PW, Friberg G, Deng H, McCaffery I, Leitch I, Badola S, Chang S, Zhu M, Tolcher A. Phase II study of ganitumab, a fully human anti-type-1 insulin-like growth factor receptor antibody, in patients with metastatic Ewing family tumors or desmoplastic small round cell tumors. J Clin Oncol. 2012;30:1849–56.
32. Schwartz GK, Tap WD, Qin LX, Livingston MB, Undevia SD, Chmielowski B, Agulnik M, Schuetze SM, Reed DR, Okuno SH, Ludwig JA, Keedy V, Rietschel P, Kraft AS, Adkins D, Van Tine BA, Brockstein B, Yim V, Bitas C, Abdullah A, Antonescu CR, Condy M, Dickson MA, Vasudeva SD, Ho AL, Doyle LA, Chen HX, Maki RG. Cixutumumab and temsirolimus for patients with bone and soft-tissue sarcoma: a multicentre, open-label, phase 2 trial. Lancet Oncol. 2013;14:371–82.
33. Barber-Rotenberg JS, Selvanathan SP, Kong Y, Erkizan HV, Snyder TM, Hong SP, Kobs CL, South NL, Summer S, Monroe PJ, Chruszcz M, Dobrev V, Tosso PN, Scher LJ, Minor W, Brown ML, Metallo SJ, Üren A, Toretsky JA. Single enantiomer of YK-4-279 demonstrates specificity in targeting the oncogene EWS-FLI1. Oncotarget. 2012;3(2):172–82.
34. Tosso PN, Kong Y, Scher L, Cummins R, Schneider J, Rahim S, Holman KT, Toretsky J, Wang K, Üren A, Brown ML. Synthesis and structure-activity relationship studies of small molecule disruptors of EWS-FLI1 interactions in Ewing's sarcoma. J Med Chem. 2014;57(24):10290–303. doi:10.1021/jm501372p.
35. Minas TZ, Han J, Javaheri T, Hong SH, Schlederer M, Saygideǧer-Kont Y, Çelik H, Mueller KM, Temel I, Özdemirli M, Kovar H, Erkizan HV, Toretsky J, Kenner L, Moriggl R, Üren A. YK-4-279 effectively antagonizes EWS-FLI1 induced leukemia in a transgenic mouse model. Oncotarget. 2015;6(35):37678–94. doi:10.18632/oncotarget.5520.
36. Amary MF, Bacsi K, Maggiani F, et al. IDH1 and IDH2 mutations are frequent events in central chondrosarcoma and central and periosteal chondromas but not in other mesenchymal tumours. J Pathol. 2011;224:334–43.
37. Lee S, Margolin K. Cytokines in cancer immunotherapy. Cancer. 2011;3(4):3856–93.

38. Shaw JP, Utz PJ, Durand DB, Toole JJ, Emmel EA, Crabtree GR. Indentication of a putative regulator of early T cell activation genes. Science. 1988;241(4862):202–5.
39. Rosenberg SA, Mule JJ, Spiess PJ, Reichert CM, Schwarz SL. Regression of established pulmonary metastases and subcutaneous tumor mediated by the systemic administration of high-dose recombinant interleukin 2. J Exp Med. 1985;161(5):1169–88.
40. Lotze MT, Chang AE, Seipp CA, Simpson C, Vetto JT, Rosenberg SA. High-dose recombinant interleukin 2 in the treatment of patients with disseminated cancer. Responses, treatment-related morbidity, and histologic findings. J Am Med Assoc. 1986:256(22):3117–24.
41. Atkins MB, Lotze MT, Dutcher JP, Fisher RI, Weiss G, Margolin K, Abrams J, Sznol M, Parkinson D, Hawkins M, Paradise C, Kunkel L, Rosenberg SA. High-dose recombinant interleukin 2 therapy for patients with metastatic melanoma: analysis of 270 patients treated between 1985 and 1993. J Clin Oncol. 1999;17(7):2105–16.
42. Schwinger W, Klass V, Benesch M, Lackner H, Dornbusch HJ, Sovinz P, Moser A, Schwantzer G, Urban C. Feasibility of high-dose interleukin-2 in heavily pretreated pediatric cancer patients. Ann Oncol. 2005;16(7):1199–206.
43. Schwartz RN, Stover L, Dutcher J. Managing toxicities of high-dose interleukin-2. Oncology. 2002;16(11):11–20.
44. Schwartzentruber DJ. Guidelines for the safe administration of high-dose interleukin-2. J Immunother. 2001;24(4):287–93.
45. Winkler K, Beron G, Kotz R, Salzer-Kuntschik M, Beck J, Beck W, Brandeis W, Ebell W, Erttmann R, Göbel U. Neoadjuvant chemotherapy for osteogenic sarcoma: results of a cooperative German/Austrian study. J Clin Oncol. 1984;2(6):617–24.
46. Bielack SS, Smeland S, Whelan JS, Marina N, Jovic G, Hook JM, Krailo MD, Gebhardt M, Pápai Z, Meyer J, Nadel H, Randall RL, Deffenbaugh C, Nagarajan R, Brennan B, Letson GD, Teot LA, Goorin A, Baumhoer D, Kager L, Werner M, Lau CC, Sundby Hall K, Gelderblom H, Meyers P, Gorlick R, Windhager R, Helmke K, Eriksson M, Hoogerbrugge PM, Schomberg P, Tunn PU, Kühne T, Jürgens H, van den Berg H, Böhling T, Picton S, Renard M, Reichardt P, Gerss J, Butterfass-Bahloul T, Morris C, Hogendoorn PC, Seddon B, Calaminus G, Michelagnoli M, Dhooge C, Sydes MR, Bernstein M, EURAMOS-1 investigators. MAP plus maintenance pegylated interferon alpha-2b (MAPIfn) versus MAP alone in patients with resectable high-grade osteosarcoma and good histologic response to preoperative MAP: rst results of the EURAMOS-1 good response randomization. J Clin Oncol. 2013;31(18).
47. Kager L, Potschger U, Bielack S. Review of mifamurtide in the treatment of patients with osteosarcoma. Ther Clin Risk Manag. 2010;6:279–86.
48. Anderson PM, Tomaras M, McConnell K. Mifamurtide in osteosarcoma—a practical review. Drugs Today. 2010;46(5):327–37.
49. Geddes K, Magalhaes JG, Girardin SE. Unleashing the therapeutic potential of NOD-like receptors. Nat Rev Drug Discov. 2009;8(6):465–79.
50. Frampton JE, Anderson PM, Chou AJ. Mifamurtide: a review of its use in the treatment of osteosarcoma. Pediatr Drugs. 2010;12(3):141–53.
51. Meyers PA, Schwartz CL, Krailo MD, Healey JH, Bernstein ML, Betcher D, Ferguson WS, Gebhardt MC, Goorin AM, Harris M, Kleinerman E, Link MP, Nadel H, Nieder M, Siegal GP, Weiner MA, Wells RJ, Womer RB, Grier HE, Children's Oncology Group. Osteosarcoma: the addition of muramyl tripeptide to chemotherapy improves overall survival—a report from the children's oncology group. J Clin Oncol. 2008;26(4):633–8.
52. Harrison C. Vaccines: nanorings boost vaccine adjuvant effects. Nat Rev Drug Discov. 2014;13(7):496.
53. Finkelstein SE, Fishman M, Conley AP, Gabrilovich D, Antonia S, Chiappori A. Cellular immunotherapy for so tissue sarcomas. Immunotherapy. 2012;4(3):283–90.
54. Dillman R, Barth N, Selvan S, Beutel L, de Leon C, DePriest C, Peterson C, Nayak S. Phase I/II trial of autologous tumor cell line-derived vaccines for recurrent or metastatic sarcomas. Cancer Biother Radiopharm. 2004;19(5):581–8.

55. Celluzzi CM, Mayordomo JI, Storkus WJ, Lotze MT, Falo Jr LD. Peptide-pulsed dendritic cells induce antigenspecific, CTL-mediated protective tumor immunity. J Exp Med. 1996;183(1):283–7.

56. Geiger JD, Hutchinson RJ, Hohenkirk LF. Vaccination of pediatric solid tumor patients with tumor lysate-pulsed dendritic cells can expand specific T cells and mediate tumor regression. Cancer Res. 2001;61(23):8513–9.

57. Gnjatic S, Nishikawa H, Jungbluth AA. NY-ESO-1: review of an immunogenic tumor antigen. Adv Cancer Res. 2006;95:1–30.

58. Kawaguchi S, Tsukahara T, Ida K. SYT-SSX breakpoint peptide vaccines in patients with synovial sarcoma: a study from the Japanese Musculoskeletal Oncology Group. Cancer Sci. 2012;103(9):1625–30.

59. Dudley ME, Rosenberg SA. Adoptive-cell-transfer therapy for the treatment of patients with cancer. Nat Rev Cancer. 2003;3(9):666–75.

60. Robbins PF, Morgan RA, Feldman SA. Tumor regression in patients with metastatic synovial cell sarcoma and melanoma using genetically engineered lymphocytes reactive with NY-ESO-1. J Clin Oncol. 2011;29(7):917–24.

61. Weber J. Review: anti-CTLA-4 antibody ipilimumab: case studies of clinical response and immune-related adverse events. Oncologist. 2007;12(7):864–72.

62. Hodi FS, O'Day SJ, McDermott DF. Improved survival with ipilimumab in patients with metastatic melanoma. N Engl J Med. 2010;363(8):711–23.

63. Wiater K, Switaj T, Mackiewicz J, Kalinka-Warzocha E, Wojtukiewicz M, Szambora P, Falkowski S, Rogowski W, Mackiewicz A, Rutkowski P. Efficacy and safety of ipilimumab therapy in patients with metastatic melanoma: a retrospective multicenter analysis. Contemp Oncol. 2013;17(3):257–62.

64. Deeks ED. Nivolumab: a review of its use in patients with malignant melanoma. Drugs. 2014;74(11):1233–9.

65. Topalian SL, Hodi FS, Brahmer JR, Gettinger SN, Smith DC, McDermott DF, Powderly JD, Carvajal RD, Sosman JA, Atkins MB, Leming PD, Spigel DR, Antonia SJ, Horn L, Drake CG, Pardoll DM, Chen L, Sharfman WH, Anders RA, Taube JM, McMiller TL, Xu H, Korman AJ, Jure-Kunkel M, Agrawal S, McDonald D, Kollia GD, Gupta A, Wigginton JM, Sznol M. Safety, activity, and immune correlates of anti-PD-1 antibody in cancer. N Engl J Med. 2012;366(26):2443–54.

66. Wolchok JD, Kluger H, Callahanetal MK. Nivolumab plus Ipilimumab in advanced melanoma. N Engl J Med. 2013;369(2):122–33.

67. Shoushtari AN, Van Tine BA, Schwartz GK. Novel treatment targets in sarcoma: more than just the GIST. Am Soc Clin Oncol Educ Book. 2014:e488–95.

68. Kobayashi E, Masuda M, Nakayama R, Ichikawa H, Satow R, Shitashige M, Honda K, Yamaguchi U, Shoji A, Tochigi N, Morioka H, Toyama Y, Hirohashi S, Kawai A, Yamada T. Reduced argininosuccinate synthetase is a predictive biomarker for the development of pulmonary metastasis in patients with osteosarcoma. Mol Cancer Ther. 2010;9:535–44.

69. van der Graaf WT, Blay JY, Chawla SP, Kim DW, Bui-Nguyen B, Casali PG, Schöffski P, Aglietta M, Staddon AP, Beppu Y, Le Cesne A, Gelderblom H, Judson IR, Araki N, Ouali M, Marreaud S, Hodge R, Dewji MR, Coens C, Demetri GD, Fletcher CD, Dei Tos AP, Hohenberger P. Pazopanib for metastatic soft-tissue sarcoma (PALETTE): a randomized, double-blind, placebo-controlled phase 3 trial. Lancet. 2012;379(9829):1879–86.

70. George S, Wang Q, Heinrich MC, Corless CL, Zhu M, Butrynski JE, Morgan JA, Wagner AJ, Choy E, Tap WD, Yap JT, Van den Abbeele AD, Manola JB, Solomon SM, Fletcher JA, von Mehren M, Demetri GD. Efficacy and safety of regorafenib in patients with metastatic and/or unresectable GI stromal tumor after failure of imatinib and sunitinib: a multicenter phase II trial. J Clin Oncol. 2012;30(19):2401–7.

71. Grosso F, Jones RL, Demetri GD, Judson IR, Blay JY, Le Cesne A, Sanfilippo R, Casieri P, Collini P, Dileo P, Spreafico C, Stacchiotti S, Tamborini E, Tercero JC, Jimeno J, D'Incalci M,

Gronchi A, Fletcher JA, Pilotti S, Casali PG. Efficacy of trabectedin (ecteinascidin-743) in advanced pretreated myxoid liposarcomas: a retrospective study. Lancet Oncol. 2007;8(7):595–602.

72. Demetri GD, Chawla SP, Ray-Coquard I, Le Cesne A, Staddon AP, Milhem MM, Penel N, Riedel RF, Bui-Nguyen B, Cranmer LD, Reichardt P, Bompas E, Alcindor T, Rushing D, Song Y, Lee RM, Ebbinghaus S, Eid JE, Loewy JW, Haluska FG, Dodion PF, Blay JY. Results of an international randomized phase III trial of the mammalian target of rapamycin inhibitor rida-forolimus versus placebo to control metastatic sarcomas in patients after benefit from prior chemotherapy. J Clin Oncol. 2013;31(19):2485–92.

73. Ryan CW. PICASSO 3: a phase 3 international randomized double-blind, placebo-controlled study of doxorubicin plus palifosfamide vs dox plus placebo for patients in first-line for meta-static soft tissue sarcoma. Abstract 3802, ESMO 2013;49.

74. de Bree R, Tijink BM, van Groeningen CJ, Leemans CR. Electroporation therapy in soft tissue sarcoma: a potentially effective novel treatment. Sarcoma. 2006;2006:85234.

75. Rols M-P, Bachaud J-M, Giraud P, Chevreau C, Roche H, Teissie J. Electrochemotherapy of cutaneous metastases in malignant melanoma. Melanoma Res. 2000;10(5):468–74.

76. Rodrıguez-Cuevas S, Barroso-Bravo S, Almanza-Estrada J, Cristobal-Martınez L, Gonzalez-Rodrıguez E. Electrochemotherapy in primary and metastatic skin tumors: phase II trial using intralesional bleomycin. Arch Med Res. 2001;32(4):273–6.

Part II

International Approaches to the Multidisciplinary Care of Sarcoma Patients

Multidisciplinary Approach to Treatment: An Australian Perspective

23

Susan J. Neuhaus and David M. Thomas

23.1 Introduction

Optimal treatment for sarcoma requires knowledge of a large, continually changing body of literature that contains significant contributions from multiple specialties. The rarity of sarcoma and its subtypes makes it challenging to determine optimal treatment strategies. Multidisciplinary input, including specialist pathology and radiology expertise, is essential to providing best clinical practice outcomes. However, there are significant gaps in the evidence base used to underpin clinical decision making for patients with sarcoma and significant geographic and institutional treatment disparities.

Each of these challenges is amplified in the Australian setting. Australia has a publicly funded universal health-care system (Medicare). Medicare funds affordable primary health-care treatment for all Australian citizens and permanent residents and provides free treatment in all public hospitals. The programme is nominally funded by an income tax surcharge known as the *Medicare levy*, currently set at 1.5%. Exemptions apply to low-income earners, with different thresholds applying to singles, families, seniors and pensioners. Individuals may choose to purchase privately funded health care through insurance or self-payment systems or utilize a mixture of privately and publicly funded services.

To date, there is no published data reporting the incidence of sarcoma in Australia. However, data from the National Cancer Registry at the Australian Institute of Health and Welfare suggests a crude incidence rate of 4.6/100,000,

S.J. Neuhaus, MD, MBBS, PhD, FRACS (✉)
Department of Surgery, University of Adelaide, Adelaide, SA, Australia
e-mail: susanneuhaus@apsa.com.au

D.M. Thomas, MD, MBBS, PhD, FRACP
Faculty of Medicine, Cancer Division, St Vincent's Clinical School, Garvan Institute of Medical Research, The Kinghorn Cancer Centre, East Melbourne, Australia

© Springer International Publishing Switzerland 2017
R.M. Henshaw (ed.), *Sarcoma*, DOI 10.1007/978-3-319-43121-5_23

which is comparable to published data from Europe (RARECARE studies) and the USA (SEER database). This suggests that there are approximately 850 new cases of sarcoma per year in Australia [1], although these numbers omit sarcomas misclassified into topologic cancer groups (e.g. breast angiosarcoma and uterine leiomyosarcomas). In general, accurate and consistent pathological diagnosis is an issue for population-level mapping of the true incidence of connective tissue tumours.

There is marked geographic disparity in sarcoma management across Australia. For example, the probability of radiotherapy as a primary (pre-surgical) modality in Australia is largely determined by centre-based preferences and access to sarcoma specialist centres. Similarly, availability and involvement of paediatric oncology expertise in treating patients in the Adult and Young Adolescent (AYA) age range (15–30 years) varies by referral centre, co-location of paediatric and adult treatment centres and/or local networks. In addition, the mixture of private and public health funding models in Australia and national approval processes and funding for drugs have implications for Australian practice guidelines. For example, trabectedin is approved and reimbursed for the treatment of sarcomas in Europe, but not Australia.

This chapter will discuss some of the challenges, obstacles and barriers to good multidisciplinary care for sarcoma patients in Australasia and provide an insight into new and innovative ways they are being addressed.

23.2   Multidisciplinary Care in Australia: The Framework

A multidisciplinary care approach to patients with cancer is well established in Australia and accepted as 'best practice' [2]. Based largely on the model of multidisciplinary care for women with breast or ovarian cancer [3], a number of common national principles have been adopted and underpin multidisciplinary care for all cancers:

- A *team approach*, involving core disciplines integral to the provision of good care, with input from other specialties as required
- *Communication* among team members regarding treatment planning
- Access to the *full range of diagnostic services and approved therapies* for all patients, regardless of geographical remoteness or size of institution
- Provision of care in accord with *nationally agreed standards*
- *Involvement of patients* in decisions about their care

At the national and strategic level, multidisciplinary cancer care has been promoted in national and state cancer plans and frameworks [4–7].

National, state and regional networks have been established and promote exchange of knowledge and expertise between centres to support the implementation of multidisciplinary cancer care. A comprehensive strategy to support multidisciplinary care for cancer treatment planning in regional and country areas, including resources to support increased use of telemedicine, has also been developed in most regions. This enables centres with smaller caseloads, or those that are geographically isolated, to link into larger or specialized centres and expertise, often on a 'case-by-case' basis. In addition, teleconferencing and videoconferencing facilities are frequently used to ensure that all core disciplines are represented at meetings.

Government initiatives have also supported the implementation of multidisciplinary cancer care in Australia through incentive funding. In 2006, new Medicare Benefits Schedule (MBS) item numbers to support attendance by specialists at multidisciplinary treatment planning meetings were introduced. This provides a mechanism for individual 'per patient' reimbursement for clinicians leading a case discussion and for pathology and radiology review.

Further national education and promotion strategies undertaken over the last decade have helped target health services, at national and state levels to emphasize the Principles of Multidisciplinary Care [3], and specifically highlight the importance of:

- Core membership of a cancer type-specific multidisciplinary team (MDT)
- Resource and workforce planning
- Links to the full therapeutic range of services
- Processes for MDT data collection and review
- Communication with GPs and continuity of care
- Patient consent
- Patient involvement in treatment planning

In most centres, specific health service-level protocols exist defining the principles and procedures for provision of multidisciplinary cancer care [8].

23.3 Sarcoma Centres in Australia: A History of the Sarcoma MDT

In January 2008, the Australasian Sarcoma Study Group (ASSG) was formed [9]. Its primary focus was to improve the outcomes for sarcomas and related tumours in the Australian community through research and development. Given the aggressive nature and rarity of sarcoma, and the vast geographic distances in Australia, it was recognized that a collaborative approach was needed to fight the disease. One of the key strategies adopted was to use multidisciplinary teams in the clinical environment to create a network of clinicians, allied health workers, nurses and researchers within Australia and, internationally, all of whom share the common goal of finding solutions to treat sarcoma.

From 2009, with funding from Cancer Australia, the University of Melbourne became the administering institution for the group through Cancer Australia's 'Support for Cancer Clinical Research Program' [10]. Under this programme, the Australian Government provides funding to build Australia's capacity to conduct cancer clinical research. The ASSG is 1 of 13 Multisite Collaborative National Cancer Clinical Trials Groups supported under the programme. Groups were established to help reduce the impact of cancer in the community through facilitating coordination of and collaboration between all stakeholders, including people affected through cancer, health professionals, researchers, cancer societies and government agencies. The group has grown significantly in a short period in both membership and achievement, with work focusing on three areas: research, engagement and organizational capacity.

To establish an infrastructure framework for collaboration between multidisciplinary teams, an audit of existing sarcoma treatment centres within Australia was undertaken in 2009. An online survey of 15 centres was designed, primarily to compile a register of sarcoma treatment centres of excellence and to determine the services offered at those sites. A secondary purpose was to gain knowledge about infrastructure and the capability of sites to conduct sarcoma research [11].

At all 15 sites, either a medical (80%) or paediatric oncologist (47%) was part of the sarcoma team. Similarly, all sites reported employing the range of allied health personnel—social workers, psychologists, physiotherapists, occupational therapists and nutritionists. Twelve sites (80%) offered the services of a clinical nurse consultant or coordinator. All sites provided access to palliative care, pathology and haematology services. Other services available included podiatry and education, with the latter being for the paediatric and adolescent populations.

Regarding diagnostic services, all sites offered MRI scanning, with 73% offering FDG-PET and 93% intervention radiology; only the Peter MacCallum Cancer Centre reported offering alternative scanning devices such as fluorinated azomycin arabinoside (FAZA), fluorinated L-thymine (FLT) and fluorinated misonidazol (F-MISO).

Prince of Wales Hospital in New South Wales and Sir Charles Gardiner Hospital in Western Australia treat both adult and paediatric patients. All sites treated outpatients and inpatients, with the exception of the Adelaide Cancer Centre. It is noteworthy that the Adelaide Cancer Centre is a specialist outpatient centre, whereas all other sites are multi-facility hospitals.

It should also be noted that each of the participating centres is located in state capital cities (Fig. 23.1). This reflects the geographic distribution of the Australian population and availability of specialist health resources [12]. The majority (64.0%) of the Australian population reside in one of the eight capital cities. In fact, the five largest cities in the country (Sydney, Melbourne, Brisbane, Perth and Adelaide) account for 60.9% of the country's population [13]. Although major regional health facilities exist outside of capital cities, they are rarely able to provide the full suite of tertiary-level care. For example, access to external beam radiotherapy, PET scanners and often MRI scans is usually limited to capital cities (Fig. 23.2). This has significant implications for the 36% of Australians that live in rural or remote regions of the country.

Fig. 23.1 Multidisciplinary sarcoma teams in Australia (by state)

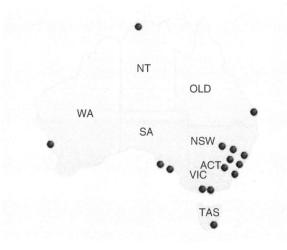

	n	%
Disciplines		
Clinical nurse consultant	12	80
Haematology	15	100
Medical oncology	12	80
Nutrition and dietetics	15	100
Occupational therapy	15	100
Paediatric oncology	7	47
Palliative care	15	100
Pathology	15	100
Physiotherapy	15	100
Psychology	15	100
Radiation oncology	14	93
Social work	15	100
Surgical oncology	14	93
Other services	7	47
Diagnostic Services		
FDG-PET	11	73
Interventional radiology	14	93
MRI	15	100
Other PET tracers	1	7
Age Range		
Adolescent Young Adult (AYA)	13	87
Adult	10	67
Paediatric	8	53
Ambulatory Care		
Home based	13	87
In-patients	14	93
Out-patients	15	100

	n (%)
Discipline	
Clinical nurse consultant	12 (80)
Haematology	15 (100)
Medical oncology	12 (80)
Nutrition and dietetics	15 (100)
Occupational therapy	15 (100)
Paediatriconcology	7 (47)
Palliative care	15 (100)
Pathology	15 (100)
Physiotherapy	15 (100)
Psychology	15 (100)
Radiation oncology	14 (93)
Social work	15 (100)
Surgical oncology	14 (93)
Other services	7 (47)
Diagnostic Services	
FDG-PET	11 (73)
Interventional radiology	14 (93)
MRI	15 (100)
Other PET tracers	1 (7)
Age Range	
Adolescent Young Adult	13 (87)
Adult	10 (67)
Paediatric	8 (53)
Ambulatory Care	
Home based	13 (87)
In-patients	14 (93)
Out patients	15 (100)

Fig. 23.2 Summary of the distributions for disciplines, diagnostics services, age range and ambulatory care

All 15 sites held multidisciplinary team meetings and of these, 8 (53%) were held on a weekly basis. Of the remaining sites, three (20%) held meetings monthly and four (26%) met as required.

All sites reported involvement in hospital run clinical trials. Moreover, all sites expressed willingness to participate in multicentre trials and provided at least one specialist contact to receive inquiries about clinical research. Eight percent ($n = 12$) of sites reported recording sarcoma-specific clinical data, whilst 73% ($n = 11$) collected sarcoma biospecimens.

One of the key outcomes of the ASSG has been the ability to register sarcoma treatment centres of excellence and to create a networked clinical sarcoma community.

The ASSG strongly supports and advocates for multidisciplinary sarcoma care. A critical component of these recommendations is that all patients with sarcoma should be treated at centres with appropriate expertise and relevant multidisciplinary teams. Key recommendations are based on the National Institute for Health and Clinical Excellence Guidance on Cancer Services [14], but, as these recommendations are based on the different populations and health-care systems in the USA and UK, the ASSG have modified them for the Australian setting [15]:

1. All patients with a confirmed diagnosis of bone or soft tissue sarcoma (except children with certain soft tissue sarcomas) should have their care supervised by or in conjunction with a sarcoma multidisciplinary team.
2. A soft tissue and bone sarcoma MDT should meet minimum criteria for caseload. In the UK this is specified as at least 100 new patients with soft tissue sarcoma per year or at least 25 new patients with bone sarcoma per year. Given the difference in population and the size of the landscape, these figures must be modified for the Australian setting.
3. The sarcoma MDT should include:
   (a) A specialist sarcoma pathologist and/or radiologist who is able to review each patient's pathology and radiology.
   (b) A surgeon who is a member of a sarcoma MDT or a surgeon with tumour site-specific or age-appropriate skills, in consultation with the sarcoma MDT.
   (c) Medical and radiation oncology expertise. Chemotherapy and radiotherapy should be carried out by appropriate specialists as recommended by a sarcoma MDT.
   (d) Dedicated ancillary supportive care, which includes nursing, physiotherapy and occupational therapy, age-appropriate psychosocial support and palliative care.
   (e) Access to relevant clinical trials.
4. All sarcoma MDTs should participate in national audit, data collection and training.
5. Patients with functional disabilities as a consequence of their sarcoma should have timely access to appropriate support and rehabilitation services.

The recommendations for centralisation of care for paediatric sarcomas (osteosarcoma, Ewing sarcoma/primitive neuroectodermal tumour, rhabdomyosarcoma) are particularly important, owing to the rarity of these cancers, the lack of a large evidence base for treatment, the complexity and intensity of the treatment regimens and the high mortality from these cancer types [16]. As a consequence, the ASSG strongly recommends that all patients with paediatric sarcomas under the age of 16 years be treated at a paediatric cancer centre and that older patients be treated at a specialist sarcoma centre. For other sarcoma types, the recommendation is that a specialist sarcoma multidisciplinary team assesses patients even if subsequent treatment is carried out elsewhere.

23.4 What Does It Mean in Practice? A Case Example

In 2008, a state-based sarcoma multidisciplinary meeting was established at the Royal Adelaide Hospital. The MDT draws cases from the South Australian population (1.65 million) and the adjacent Northern Territory (population 223,000), encompassing a geographic area of over 2.3 million square km. In addition, although Northern Territory is sparsely populated, approximately 32% of the population are indigenous, many of whom live in isolated and remote communities. Sarcoma incidence in indigenous populations is not known. Prior to 2013, external beam radiotherapy was not available in the Northern Territory. PET scanning remains available only in Adelaide, a distance of over 3000 km.

The SA/NT Adult and AYA Sarcoma Multidisciplinary Team Meeting was set up under nationally accepted guidelines [17]. Meetings were held fortnightly (initially monthly) with videoconferencing facilities to enable other state and interstate hospitals and clinicians to dial in. The key members attending the meeting were surgical oncologists (sarcoma surgeon, plastic surgeon), radiation and medical oncologists (Adult and AYA), radiologist, pathologist, sarcoma data manager, sarcoma research staff and social worker. Attendance records were documented at each meeting. Presence of the referring clinician/representative was mandatory.

An audit of the Adult and AYA sarcoma MDT in SA was conducted in 2012 using an established Multidisciplinary Meeting Tool 4, developed by the Victorian Department of Human Services (DHS) to measure the team's performance against the guidelines and protocols [18].

The number of cases referred to the SA/NT Adult and AYA Sarcoma Multidisciplinary Team Meeting and the breakdown of these cases is illustrated in Fig. 23.3. The purpose of the meeting was to discuss all newly diagnosed cases of sarcoma in SA/NT and those requiring review. Patients were discussed at varying stages of their management, with 60% representing new cases and 40% review. There was no additional educational component to the meetings. Clinical summaries of the recommendations were provided to all treating clinicians and the primary care physician of the patient, in addition to inclusion in the case file. Since inception of the MDT process, engagement with the clinical sarcoma community has continued to broaden, with increased participation of clinical and allied health-care workers (Fig. 23.4).

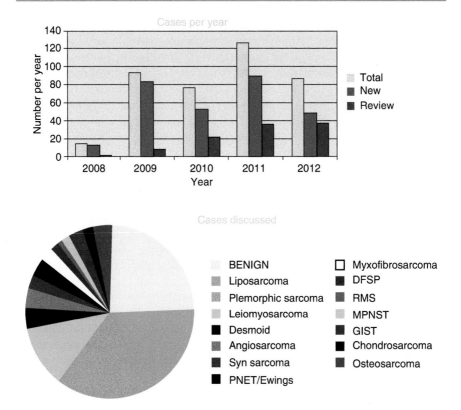

Fig. 23.3 Number of cases per year (2008–2012) presented to the SA/NT Adult and AYA Sarcoma Multidisciplinary Team and breakdown by subtype

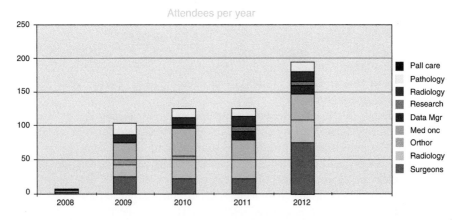

Fig. 23.4 Attendance at SA/NT SARCOMA MDT (2008–2012) by number and discipline

The benefits of increased MDT participation are well recognized [19]. There is sound evidence to support the following conclusions:

- Specialist review of diagnostic imaging in patients with suspected sarcoma reduces clinical error rates and delay in diagnosis.
- The histopathological diagnosis of sarcoma is often changed on review by an expert pathologist. This includes the diagnosis of sarcoma, sarcoma subtype and tumour grade.
- Treatment guided by a sarcoma-specific multidisciplinary team results in better overall survival, improved disease-free survival, reduced risk of amputation, better conformity to clinical practice guidelines and greater use of preoperative imaging and biopsy.
- Participation in clinical trials correlates with improved survival rates for patients with sarcoma.

Whilst metrics to demonstrate these outcomes in the South Australian/Northern Territory scenario above are not available, anecdotal evidence of their benefits has been manifested particularly in increased referral patterns and increased involvement in clinical trials. Two notable patterns of change include an increase in the number of indigenous patients presented for MDT discussion and the number of patients considered for preoperative radiotherapy.

23.5   National Cooperation: A Federated Sarcoma Database

Good quality multidisciplinary care requires accurate and relevant data collection and analysis. A major project for the ASSG, as part of its mandate to improve national sarcoma outcomes, was to establish a national sarcoma clinical database.

A collaborative effort between three major sarcoma centres (Victoria, New South Wales and the Australian Capital Territory) and the ASSG resulted in the development of a minimum sarcoma data set. In 2009, a federated database, based on the BioGrid system [20] and using the sarcoma minimum data set, was built, tested and began being populated in Victoria at the Peter MacCallum Cancer Centre (national data on 3200 patients has since been recorded) and was selected to allow clinicians to collect a comprehensive data set relating to the diagnosis, treatment and follow-up of patients diagnosed with sarcoma.

The governance of the data set is provided by BioGrid Australia. BioGrid Australia has obtained approval from 23 Human Research Ethics Committees for the federated data linkage processes at 39 sites across the Australian Capital Territory (ACT), New South Wales (NSW), Queensland (QLD), South Australia (SA), Tasmania (TAS), Victoria (VIC) and Western Australia (WA). The data set is available to each contributing centre, for research, evaluation and quality control purposes.

In a nation characterized by a small sarcoma patient population and marked geographic disparity, collaboration, cooperation and innovation remain the key to developing and maintaining a research capability.

23.8   Practice Guidelines for the Australian Environment

One example of this innovation is the recent development of Wiki-based Clinical Practice Guidelines for the Management of Adult Onset Sarcoma [22]. The sarcoma guidelines project was a collaborative project between the ASSG and Cancer Council Australia (CCA). Utilizing a modified media-Wiki website platform, it has enabled development of evidence-based (as opposed to existing consensus-based) guidelines to be developed and tailored to the Australian environment [23]. The purpose of these guidelines was not restrictive, but focused on the clinical questions that were most relevant to different disciplines. The selected questions reflected the gaps in knowledge that impacted most on daily management decisions.

As an ab initio set of guidelines, the scope was initially broad. The key areas were then refined to include:

- Diagnosis
- Multidisciplinary treatment
- Chemotherapy (systemic therapies)
- Radiotherapy
- Surgery
- Follow-up

For reasons of pragmatism and resource, the scope of the first iteration was restricted to adult onset bone and soft tissue sarcoma. Gastrointestinal stromal tumours (GIST), Kaposi's sarcoma and aggressive (desmoid) fibromatosis were excluded. Childhood, adolescent (AYA) and gynaecological sarcomas are priorities for the next iteration of the guidelines.

Increasingly, multidisciplinary care acknowledges the central role of consumers in care delivery and optimization. Whilst historically clinical practice guidelines in Australia have been accompanied by separate written consumer guidelines, a decision was made not to do this. Instead, leveraging the technology platform afforded by Wiki-based guidelines, available 'online' consumer resources from within Australia and elsewhere were integrated as 'linked pages' and embedded within the guidelines.

Other external linkages were also embedded, including links to the ASSG, geographic sarcoma expertise ('Find a Sarcoma Specialist') and linkages to available clinical trial sites, such as the NHMRC Australian and New Zealand Clinical Trials Registry (www.anzctr.org.au) and sites presenting detailed clinical treatment protocols such as eviQ (www.eviq.org.au).

The release of these guidelines has had important benefits for the Australian sarcoma community. It has started a conversation about the evidence basis that underpins clinical management, identified key areas where evidence gaps exist and identified key research priorities. In addition, the process brought together key clinical thought leaders and identified areas of marked variance in clinical practice.

The guidelines were released nationally on 15 November 2013 and can be accessed at: www.wiki.cancer.org.au/Australia/Guidelines:sarcoma. The guidelines highlight the importance of early referral to multidisciplinary centres that specialize in treating sarcoma. The importance of the multidisciplinary team in initial assessment, diagnosis and making decisions about treatment is strongly endorsed. A multidisciplinary approach (involving pathologists, radiologists, surgeons, radiation therapists, medical oncologists with experience in sarcoma) or within reference networks sharing expertise and treating a high number of patients annually is preferred. Caseload and experience is associated with improved rates of function limb preservation, lower rates of local recurrence, good rates of overall survival and improved quality of life. The guidelines also support and encourage enrollment of sarcoma patients into clinical trials.

The Australian Clinical Practice Guidelines for the Management of Adult Onset Sarcoma are the first step towards more standardized care for patients with sarcoma across the nation and provide a framework to educate the community about referral pathways and develop more formal communications between sarcoma centres and clinicians, particularly in relation to current trials and access.

The use of existing and emerging technology platforms, such as Internet-based guidelines and Web-based education resources, offers a cost-effective way of engaging with health providers and consumers who may not otherwise have been able to access these opportunities. Further, such a platform provides an accessible up-to-date platform for dissemination of current evidence in a rapidly changing landscape, as well as a national and regional resource for multidisciplinary sarcoma teams, individual clinicians and consumers.

In addition, education modules can be linked to key stakeholder groups such as radiology, pathology, primary care providers and surgical colleges and societies [24]. Such Web-based education resources are not only cost effective, but can be stratified by level of expertise (e.g. medical student vs. specialist) and by resource availability.

From release in November 2013 to May 15, 2014, the guidelines received 3475 page views with 1344 visits and an average of 2.6 pages per visit. Of these 52% of visits were from Australia, 8.9% the USA, 6% the UK, 6% India, 2% Singapore, 1.9% Germany and the remaining 25.3% from 39 additional countries. Engagement from the breadth of the sarcoma community, both in Australia and internationally, via comments and submissions of new evidence is actively encouraged.

23.9   What Does It Mean for Our Region?

Australia is situated within a region that is rapidly expanding in population terms. The Asia-Pacific region accounts for more than four billion people and is arguably the most rapidly developing region globally [25]. It is also a region characterized by great diversity, both in ethnographic and economic terms. The per person gross domestic product for Asia-Pacific countries ranges from $US 1700 in Burma to $US 62,400 in Singapore (Australia is $US 43,000). Little is known about variations in incidence of sarcoma within the region, but standardized mortality rates and other outcome measures suggest that expectations and outcomes for sarcoma are likely to be similarly varied, and guidelines that may be appropriate in one country may be quite unrealistic in another. The concept of resource stratified guidelines within the Asia-Pacific region has been addressed by the *Lancet Oncology,* which included specific guidelines for sarcoma [26].

In a regional and global sense, this poses challenges for equity of sarcoma care. Expectations vary; there are significant economic and social and resource disparities that impact on provision of sarcoma management. However, to make progress, these borders need to be crossed. Expanded collaborative approaches, development of research infrastructure, interoperability of clinical data management platforms and facilitated research collaboration between nations in our region offer the opportunity to develop powerful data sets and address clinical questions that could not be addressed by any one nation alone.

Conclusions

Advances in multidisciplinary sarcoma care in Australia over the last decade have resulted in significant changes in sarcoma management. Formalized multidisciplinary meetings at sarcoma-specific centres have created new awareness of the need for specialist multidisciplinary input at all stages of diagnosis, treatment and follow-up.

As these processes have become embedded as 'best standard of care', new opportunities to establish and maintain a national sarcoma research capability have arisen. These include development of a national clinical sarcoma database, sarcoma biospecimen registers and expanded opportunities for clinical trial participation both nationally and internationally. In addition, new technology platforms have enabled the sarcoma community to address areas of evidence-based practice and identified new opportunities to engage more effectively with the broader sarcoma community, both nationally and across the Asia-Pacific region.

Acknowledgements Australasian Sarcoma Study Group
Cancer Council Australia
Dr. Raghu Gowda and Ms. Sonya Stephens for their assistance and provision of data from the SA/NT MDT.

References

1. Potter JA, Woods R, Bessen T, Farshid G, Roder D, Neuhaus SJ. Incidence and reconstructive demand of sarcoma in Australia: first national data analysis. In: Royal Australasian College of Surgeons Annual Scientific Congress, Singapore May 2014. Abstract 21859.
2. Ruhstaller T, Roe T, Thurlimann B, Nicoll JJ. The multi-disciplinary meeting: an indispensable aid to communication between different specialities. Eur J Cancer. 2006;42:2459–62.

3. Zorbas H, Barraclough B, Rainbird K, et al. Multidisciplinary care for women with breast cancer in the Australian context: what does it mean? Med J Aust. 2003;179(10):528–31.
4. NSW Cancer Plan 2011–15 Cancer Institute NSW, Sydney, November 2010. www.cancerinstitute.org.au/publications Accessed 30 June 2014.
5. The Cancer Council South Australia and South Australian Department of Health. Statewide cancer control plan 2011-2015. 2011 Government of South Australia, Adelaide. http://wwwsa-healthsagovau/wps/wcm/connect/public+content/sa+health+internet/clinical+resources/clinical+topics/cancer+and+oncology/state-wide+cancer+control+plan+2011+2015. Accessed 30 June 2014.
6. Metropolitan Health and Aged Care Services Division. Achieving best practice cancer care—a guide for implementing multidisciplinary care. Victorian Government Department of Human Services, Melbourne, Victoria. 2007. http://wwwgicscomau/resources/multidisciplinarypolicy0702pdf. Accessed 30 June 2014.
7. Department of Health, Western Australia. WA Cancer Plan 2012-2017. Perth: WA Cancer & Palliative Care Network, Department of Health, Western Australia. 2011. http://wwwhealthnetworkshealthwagovau/cancer/docs/12196_WA_Cancer_PLANpdf. Accessed 30 June 2014.
8. Sidhom MA, Poulsen MG. Multidisciplinary care in oncology: medicolegal implications of group decisions. Lancet Oncol. 2006;7:951–4.
9. Thomas D, Whyte S, Choong PFM. Australian Sarcoma Study Group: development and outlook. Cancer Forum. 2009;33(1):25–8.
10. Cancer Australia [monograph on the internet]. Support for clinical trials. http://www.cancer-australia.gov.au/cancer-australia/research-and-clinical-trials/support-clinical-trials. Accessed 30 June 2014.
11. White S, Gatenby S. Sarcoma capability audit: a register of centres of excellence. Cancer Forum 2010 Reports. http://wwwcancerforumorgau/issues/2010/july/reports/sarcoma_capability_audithtm#1. Accessed 30 June 2014.
12. Australian Bureau of Statistics. Australian demographic statistics. December 2013. http://www.abs.gov.au/ausstats/abs@.nsf/mf/3101.0. Accessed 30 June 2014.
13. Population centralization. The Australian Way. http://blog.rpdata.com/2012/04/population-centralizationthe-australian-way/. Accessed 2 Jun 2014.
14. National Institute for Health and Clinical Excellence, 2006. Improving outcomes for people with sarcoma. NICE guidance on cancer services. http://wwwniceorguk/guidance/CSGSARCOMA. Accessed 30 June 2014.
15. Why multi-disciplinary care is important in sarcomas. Australasian Sarcoma Study Group. http://www.australiansarcomagroup.org/multi-disciplinary-care.html. Accessed 30 June 2014.
16. Bleyer A, Montello M, Budd T, Saxman S. National survival trends of young adults with sarcoma: lack of progress is associated with lack of clinical trial participation. Cancer. 2005;103:1891–7.
17. Metropolitan Health and Aged Care Services Division. Achieving best practice cancer care—a guide for implementing multidisciplinary care. Melbourne, Victoria: Victorian Government Department of Human Services; 2007.
18. Cancer Co ordination Unit. Multidisciplinary Meeting Toolkit. Melbourne, Victoria: Victorian Department of Human Services; 2006.
19. Ruhstaller T, Roe H, Thürlimann B, Nicoll JJ. The multidisciplinary meeting: an indispensable aid to communication between different specialities. Eur J Cancer. 2006;42(15):2459–62.
20. Biogrid Australia (Internet). Homepage. http://www.biogrid.org.au/wps/portal. Accessed 30 June 2014.
21. Clark MA, Fisher C, Judson I, Thomas JM. Soft-tissue sarcomas in adults. N Engl J Med. 2005;353:701–11.
22. Cancer Clinical Practice Guidelines. Management of adult onset sarcoma 2013. http://www.wiki.cancer.org.au/australia/Guidelines:Sarcoma. Accessed 30 June 2014.
23. Olver I, Von Dinklage J. It is time for clinical guidelines to enter the digital age. Med J Aust. 2013;199(9):569–70.

24. Kerfoot BP, Kearney MC, Connelly D, Ritchey ML. Interactive spaced education to assess and improve knowledge of clinical practice guidelines: a randomized controlled trial. Ann Surg. 2009;249:744–9.
25. Central Intelligence Agency. The World Factbook. March 2014. https://www.cia.gov/library/publications/the-world-factbook/rankorder/2004rank.html. Accessed 2 June 2014.
26. Lewin J, Puri A, Quek R, Wood D, Alcasabas A, Ngan R, Thomas DM. A consensus statement on resource-stratified management of sarcoma in the Asia-Pacific region. Lancet Oncol. 2013;14:e562–70.

Multidisciplinary Musculoskeletal Oncology Care in Scotland: A Virtual Clinic

24

P.S. Young, D.T. Wallace, M. Halai, H. Findlay, and A. Mahendra

24.1 Demographics and Geography

Early diagnosis and treatment by appropriate specialists is the cornerstone of sarcoma management, and delay or inappropriate intervention can have significant ramifications for patients' morbidity and mortality [1]. Sarcoma services in Scotland are challenged by population distribution and geography. Scotland has a population of around 5.3 million, growing by around 0.5% per annum [2]. Around 70% of the population live within the central belt, an area between the two largest cities with Glasgow in the west and Edinburgh to the east; however, the remaining population is scattered over 79,000 km^2 of what is highly varied and often adverse geography. The incidence of sarcoma in this population is around 180 new cases per annum [3].

The National Health Service (NHS) delivers health care across Scotland which is free at the point of access. The NHS is primarily funded through central taxation which is accountable to the Scottish Government. However, due to the varying geography and health demographics of Scotland, the NHS services are further subdivided into 14 Health Boards, which are responsible for delivering care within their

P.S. Young, B.M.B.S., F.R.C.S. (Tr. & Orth.)
Glasgow Royal Infirmary, Glasgow, Scotland, UK

Scottish Sarcoma Research Group, University of Glasgow, Glasgow, Scotland, UK

D.T. Wallace, M.B.Ch.B., M.R.C.S. (Ed.)
Golden Jubilee National Hospital, Glasgow Royal Infirmary, Glasgow, Scotland, UK

M. Halai, M.B.Ch.B., F.R.C.S. (Tr. & Orth.) • H. Findlay, RGN, ONC, MSc.
Glasgow Royal Infirmary, Glasgow, Scotland, UK

A. Mahendra, M.B.Ch.B., F.R.C.S. (Tr. & Orth.) (✉)
Scottish Sarcoma Managed Clinical Network, Glasgow Royal Infirmary,
Glasgow, Scotland, UK
e-mail: ashish.mahendra@ggc.scot.nhs.uk

© Springer International Publishing Switzerland 2017
R.M. Henshaw (ed.), *Sarcoma*, DOI 10.1007/978-3-319-43121-5_24

local region. Each Health Board has funds allocated from their annual budget to fund tertiary sarcoma services according to a number of factors, such as population. Tertiary sarcoma services are delivered within the three largest cities, Glasgow, Edinburgh and Aberdeen and are co-ordinated nationally through the Scottish Sarcoma Network (SSN). Guidance for all health services within the United Kingdom is provided by the National Institute of Clinical Excellence (NICE) which states that all patients with a confirmed bone or soft tissue sarcoma should have their care supervised or in conjunction with a sarcoma multidisciplinary team (MDT) and that the sarcoma MDT should manage the care of at least 50 new patients with bone sarcoma and 100 new patients with soft tissue sarcoma per year [4]. These are broadly similar to sarcoma guidelines worldwide [5, 6]. The SSN thus provides co-ordinated sarcoma care with a single multidisciplinary team making clinical decisions for all patients with a confirmed sarcoma diagnosis within Scotland. Specific surgical and oncological care is then provided within one of the three primary centres. Furthermore, due to the volume of referrals of patients with a suspected sarcoma, each of the three centres acts as a hub within its own region and co-ordinates subsequent investigations for these patients.

Specific to the West of Scotland (Glasgow) sarcoma service, this catchment area covers around half of the population of Scotland (around 2.5 million), and adult tertiary referrals are received from secondary care centres within Greater Glasgow & Clyde Health Board (46%), secondary care centres from distant health boards (42%) and local primary care practitioners (12%).

24.2   Service History and Redesign

Historically Scotland's geography and demographics meant suspected soft tissue, and osseous tumours were often referred for investigation by primary or secondary care practitioners prior to tertiary referral. This may have led to potential diagnostic delay, unnecessary invasive investigations and/or surgical intervention without prior biopsy, factors well recognised to be associated with delay in diagnosis and poorer patient outcome [1]. Furthermore, of those patients referred to the tertiary centre, a significant number would be required to travel long distances for multiple outpatient consultations. In recent years, however, it has become widely accepted that investigations and management of soft tissue and osseous tumours should be performed in specialist sarcoma centres. This has led to increasing demand on these services given the high ratio of benign to malignant lesions (reportedly as high as 100:1 [7]) and the high incidence of suspected sarcoma compared to the relatively low incidence of actual sarcoma. In the West of Scotland, referrals to the musculoskeletal (MSK) multidisciplinary oncology team typically include soft tissue and bony lesions suspected to be neoplastic.

In 2010, due to increasing demand on the West of Scotland MSK oncology service, a virtual referral clinic was designed and implemented. This aims to utilise modern electronic technology and a centralised multidisciplinary team to provide rapid advice and diagnosis for efficient patient care avoiding unnecessary clinic appointments and a streamlined service to optimise timely investigations for those patients.

24.3   West of Scotland Musculoskeletal (MSK) Oncology Virtual Clinic

The service accepts referrals for adult patients by phone, letter or more commonly by e-mail to the MSK oncology team. At present this service does not cover paediatric referrals (under 16 years of age), which are directly referred to the paediatric musculoskeletal oncologist via a more traditional pathway. E-mails are monitored daily by the lead clinician and the MSK clinical nurse specialist. Immediate advice can be given with regard to baseline imaging as required, including x-rays, CT, MRI, NM bone scan and blood tests. To allow patients to be discussed at the weekly MSK Radiology Meeting, referrers are expected to provide key information including: patient demographics, referrer's contact details, comprehensive clinical information and up-to-date imaging. Patients referred without this baseline information or without the possibility of timely investigation are appointed on an urgent basis to the next clinic to avoid any delay in making a diagnosis.

The MSK Radiology Meeting runs weekly with key personnel comprising a consultant orthopaedic oncologist, MSK consultant radiologist and the orthopaedic oncology clinical nurse specialist. Patient's referrals are discussed with particular scrutiny given to radiological investigations. Patient imaging is available on the Scotland wide digital national archiving system which allows access to all digital imagery from all NHS radiology departments across the country.

Following discussion, a decision is made for each patient (Fig. 24.1); if sufficient clinical information is available for an accurate diagnosis to be made, the patient is either discharged back to referring team with advice or the patient is given the next clinic appointment to apprise them of the diagnosis and discuss treatment options including surgery. Where insufficient clinical information is available to make the diagnosis, the patient may be referred for biopsy (either open or under radiological guidance) or a request for specific urgent radiological investigation is made. Upon referring the patient for radiological guided biopsy, the recommended biopsy

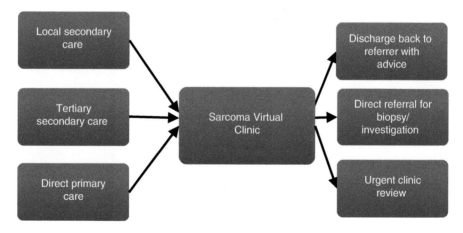

Fig. 24.1 MSK oncology virtual clinic referral management pathway

tract is identified by the surgical team in concert with the specialist radiologist, electronically marked on the available imaging, and saved for use by the interventional radiologist at the time of biopsy. This helps to reduce morbidity associated with inappropriately placed biopsy tracts. Patients requiring biopsy are contacted by telephone after the meeting by the orthopaedic oncology clinical nurse specialist to explain the rationale for biopsy and the timescale for pathology results being available. Contact information is shared and the patient is encouraged to call back with any questions or issues. A formal letter is dictated and sent back to the referring provider the same day, detailing the outcome of the MSK virtual clinic. All patients' journey information is recorded on a secure audit system to allow robust evaluation of the service.

24.4   Service Review

Following inception, we audited all patients seen at the MSK virtual clinic between January 2010 and September 2012. One thousand and twenty-seven patients were referred during that time, of which 12% were from local primary care practitioners (GPs), 46% were from local secondary care institutions (hospitals) within our Health Board and 42% were from secondary care outwith our Health Board. Only 25.5% of the referred patients were given an urgent clinic appointment for further assessment or to discuss surgical intervention, while 45.8% were directly appointed for biopsy prior to clinic review, and 30.3% were discharged immediately back to the referring clinician (Table 24.1). The diagnosis, made either radiologically or histologically when appropriate, was also recorded (Table 24.2).

Table 24.1 Final patient outcome from audit of MSK oncology virtual clinic between January 2010 and September 2012

Final outcome		
Discharged after further investigations	160	15.6%
Discharged after MSK oncology discussion	311	30.3%
Discharged after surgery	2	0.2%
Routine follow-up	135	13.14%
Surgery	379	37%
Deceased	36	3.50%
Total	1027	

Table 24.2 Diagnostic spread of benign and malignant lesions referred to MSK oncology virtual clinic between January 2010 and September 2012

Bone tumour benign	182	17.7%
Bone tumour malignant	74	7.20%
Metastases	88	8.56%
Other (benign)	380	37.0%
Soft tissue sarcoma	71	6.91%
Soft tissue tumour (benign)	227	22.1%
Total	1027	

24.5   Impact of Service Change

Following the implementation of the virtual multidisciplinary team (MDT) meeting for MSK oncology referrals, we have noted a significant improvement in the service overall. All patients who are referred with detailed clinical history and availability of radiological imaging are discussed within 1 week of referral and provided with an agreed upon management plan. Three-quarters of these patients did not subsequently require an initial subspecialty clinic appointment. For over one-quarter of patients, this meant specialist review within 1 week with continued care by their own physician and reassurance regarding their lesion. This reduces patient anxiety and eliminates the need for potentially long distance travel to a clinic appointment for reassurance only.

Almost half the patients referred are directly scheduled to undergo image guided biopsy, performed by the MSK Interventional Radiologist with biopsy tract agreed at the virtual clinic, and the image saved onto the digital archiving system. Patients are scheduled directly to the new patient clinic once final histology results become available and have been discussed at the weekly sarcoma MDT meeting to decide management plan, normally within 2–3 weeks. Streamlining of this service eliminates unnecessary clinic appointments, leads to rapid histological diagnosis and enables swift surgical or oncological intervention if required or reassurance in the majority of cases. Furthermore, planning the biopsy tract in conjunction with the surgical team avoids morbidity associated with inappropriately placed biopsy tracts. This is compared to the previous system where the patient might expect to wait 2–3 weeks for an urgent initial appointment and then subsequent referral for biopsy or further imaging, which might then require expert review by our specialist radiologists. For one-quarter of patients, their clinical journey is not altered by the virtual clinic review; however, their available radiology will have already undergone specialist review.

From the surgeon's perspective, we have seen a drastic reduction in clinic pressures as three quarters of patients require either one less appointment or no appointment. Furthermore, both referring clinician and patient satisfaction with the service is high. Service satisfaction audit completed in 2015 showed referrer satisfaction overall 63% very satisfied, 30% satisfied and 7% fairly satisfied; particular notes were made regarding good accessibility and communication. Patient satisfaction as assessed by the EORTC QLQ-C36 (quality of life) questionnaire showed 95% patients very satisfied with the referral and assessment service. Furthermore, the virtual MSK clinic pathway allows for ease of audit, patient tracking and accountability.

Conclusion

Multidisciplinary sarcoma care is funded and provided in Scotland by a national service and delivered in three main cities. This is challenged by the geography and wide population distribution of the country. Historically, patients would often be investigated and treated in secondary care settings prior to tertiary referral. It has been well established that specific cancer patient pathways can accelerate diagnosis and improve patient management [8]. However, in order to improve patient care and streamline provision of services in the West of Scotland, we have developed a tertiary multidisciplinary virtual MSK oncology clinic. This allows all secondary care clinicians' rapid access to advice and provides patients with efficient, expert review followed by reassurance or referral for histological investigation where appropriate, thereby reducing the need for long-distance travel for patients to unnecessary clinics as well as reducing time to diagnosis and appropriate treatment.

References

1. Johnson GD, Smith G, Dramis A, Grimer RJ. Delays in referral of soft tissue sarcomas. Sarcoma. 2008;2008:378574. doi:10.1155/2008/378574.
2. The Registrar General's annual review of demographic trends. 157th ed. 2012. http://www.gro-scotland.gov.uk/files2/stats/annual-review-2011/rgar-2011.pdf
3. Sarcoma v1.0 2014. Information services division, NHS national services.
4. Referral guidelines for suspected cancer. NICE guideline 27.
5. Guidance on cancer services. Improving outcomes for people with sarcoma. The manual. NICE guidelines.
6. Hooper G. Sarcoma services in New Zealand. N Z Med J. 2011;201:5–6.
7. Hogendoorn PCW. Bone sarcomas: ESMO Clinical Practice Guidelines for diagnosis, treatment and follow-up. Ann Oncol. 2010;21(Suppl 5):v204–13.
8. Dyrop HB, Safwat A, Vedsted P, Maretty-Nielsen K, Hansen BH, Jørgensen PH, Badd-Hansen T, Bünger C, Keller J. Cancer patient pathways shortens waiting times and accelerates the diagnostic process of suspected sarcoma patients in Denmark. Health Policy. 2013;113:110–7.

Limb Salvage in India

25

Shah Alam Khan, Venkatesan S. Kumar,
and Rishi Ram Poudel

25.1 Introduction

In the last couple of decades, the management of musculoskeletal sarcomas has seen a sea change. Limb salvage is now the standard of care for limb sarcomas. Despite high volumes of limb salvage surgery for limb sarcomas, the components of limb salvage surgery are constantly on scrutiny. With advances in chemotherapy, there has been a significant improvement in the survival rates, but still bone sarcomas have the poorest survival rates among pediatric cancers [1]. Limb salvage surgery is an interactive, coordinated sequence of events, which leads to local control of malignancy and restoration of important functions of the affected limb. Thus, limb salvage would include biopsy, disease staging (local and systemic), chemotherapy protocols, surgical procedures, and finally regular follow-up. The aim is to achieve an acceptable oncologic, functional and cosmetic result. Such an exhaustive exercise is therefore possible only through a committed multidisciplinary team.

In developing countries like India, malignant bone and soft tissue tumors occur in huge numbers. The shear population of a billion plus people predisposes to high numbers of sarcoma patients at any given time. In the absence of definitive population-based data on bone sarcomas, the magnitude of occurrence of malignant bone sarcomas in countries like India can be anyone's guess. The general orthopedic surgeons see a large part of these bone tumors. With few centers doing specialized limb salvage surgery, amputation is still the commonest surgery done for malignant bone tumors in the developing world.

S.A. Khan, M.D. (✉)
Department of Orthopaedics, All India Institute of Medical Sciences,
Ansari Nagar, New Delhi, India
e-mail: shahalamkhan70@gmail.com

V.S. Kumar, M.D. • R.R. Poudel, M.D.
All India Institute of Medical Sciences, Ansari Nagar, New Delhi, India

© Springer International Publishing Switzerland 2017
R.M. Henshaw (ed.), *Sarcoma*, DOI 10.1007/978-3-319-43121-5_25

Load of Bone Tumors in India: As mentioned above, the absence of a standardized database in India makes it difficult to estimate the absolute numbers of bone sarcomas being treated in the country. Significant underreporting and poorly reported diagnoses in peripheral setups make the picture even gloomier. Rathi et al. (2007) reported bone tumors to form 7.66% of all pediatric malignancies from a medical college (tertiary health-care setup) in New Delhi [2]. The figure appears to have a significant referral bias. In 2011, Jignasa, from the western Indian state of Gujarat, reported that bone tumors formed 2.32% of all the different pediatric malignancies in a cohort of 2150 malignancies (of which 2% were pediatric malignancies) [3]. In a cohort of 117 patients of bone tumors reported from South India, the authors concluded that primary benign bone tumors significantly outnumber the malignant one, but 35% of all primary malignant bone tumors were osteosarcomas [4]. The Indian Council of Medical Research (ICMR) started the National Cancer Registry Programme (NCRP) in December 1981 [5]. Despite a presence of more than 30 years, the registry has poor reporting of bone sarcomas. In conclusion, absence of a formal databank on malignant bone tumors in India leads to underreporting and "mis-reporting" of these patients. Lack of coordination in information sharing and nonavailability of specialized centers dealing with musculoskeletal tumors in the developing world add to the problems of doing a successful limb salvage surgery.

25.2 Special Challenges in Tumor Surgery

In India a host of challenges make limb salvage surgery a difficult task. The factors, which make this surgery difficult to perform, are as follows:

1. *Delayed diagnosis*: In the developing world, a large number of bone tumors present very late. The delayed diagnosis has both social and medical causes with patient's illiteracy and ignorance playing an important part in seeking advice at an advanced stage. Such high volume tumors are difficult to manage surgically (Fig. 25.1). The delay in diagnosis is also attributable to an ill functioning peripheral health-care setup, which is commonly encountered in countries like India.
2. *Availability of alternative systems of medicine*: Poverty is known to invent its own systems of cure. In India, alternative forms of medicine such as *Ayurveda*, *Siddha*, and homeopathy are popular, and a large section of the society seeks help from these systems especially for bone and joint ailments [6]. The initial treatment is usually taken from the village osteopath and referral to a primary health-care facility is delayed. In the wake of ignorance of disease, even those patients who are already under the care of an allopathic system tend to take advice from other systems of medicines. This causes delayed diagnosis, irrational use of medicines, and undue delay in surgery leading to either primary amputations or a poor outcome of limb salvage surgery in malignant bone tumors.
3. *Poor availability of resources*: Availability of resources is an important factor to consider before attempting limb salvage. Universal insurance coverage is not mandatory in India. As a result, many families face difficulty in meeting the huge economic burden imposed by the cost of chemotherapeutic drugs and

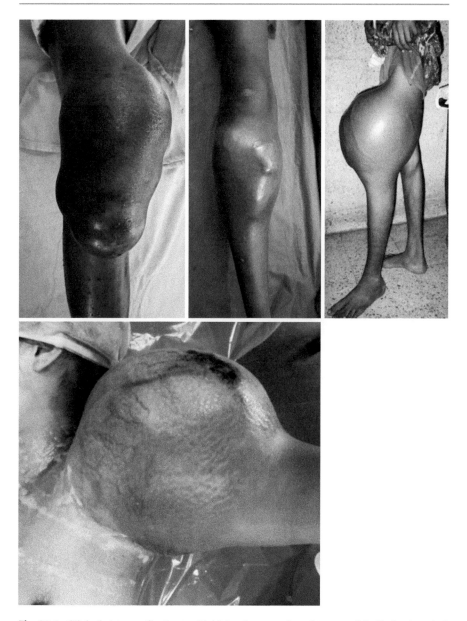

Fig. 25.1 Clinical pictures of patients with high volume, neglected tumors of the limbs. A typical sight in the developing world

surgery. Limb salvage in bone tumors is an implant-dependent procedure. With poor economic resources, majority of surgeons are forced to choose low cost, indigenous implants for limb salvage, thereby jeopardizing the salvage surgery per se. Indigenous implants like endoprosthesis have high complication rates like breakage and metallosis (Fig. 25.2).

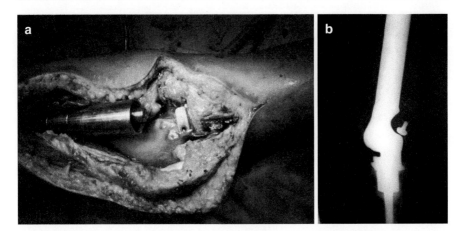

Fig. 25.2 (**a**) Clinical picture of a patient with severe metallosis following implantation of an indigenous endoprosthesis for osteosarcoma. (**b**) Loosening of the axle nut 2 years after surgery in an indigenous endoprosthesis done for an osteosarcoma of the distal femur

4. *Lack of trained personnel*: In resource-challenged environments, there is not only paucity of financial resources but of trained personnel as well. In a country like India, there is a massive shortage of specialist surgeons performing musculoskeletal oncology. Lack of trained para-clinical staff in various aspects of limb salvage makes the surgery not only difficult but outright dangerous for the patient. Concepts of community oncology nurses, community phlebotomists, are totally lacking in countries striving to achieve basic health care for its people. Even the general orthopedic surgeons, who are the primary nodal point of contact for the patient, have a limited exposure to limb salvage procedures during their residency. Thus, in countries like India, the so-called multidisciplinary team (MDT) responsible for care of sarcoma patients is only available at a select few centers.
5. *Poor follow-up*: A good follow-up is essential for the success of any limb salvage procedure. Poor follow-up delays the detection of recurrences thereby jeopardizing the results of good surgery. In countries like India, ensuring regular follow-up is a herculean task. In the presence of poorly functioning community health-care services, follow-up is not ensured thereby leading to high attrition rates and poor final outcome.

25.3 Diagnostic Strategy in Bone Tumors

The diagnosis of malignant bone tumors is the result of sequential, planned array of investigations combined with classical clinical presentations. Besides establishing a diagnosis, it is also essential to stage the disease. Unfortunately, the diagnosis of bone sarcomas is difficult particularly when the tumor is located at an atypical site within the bone or when the clinical picture is distorted with superadded infection, unplanned surgical intervention (like an unplanned biopsy), or attempted surgical excision by an untrained physician. The latter three are common occurrences

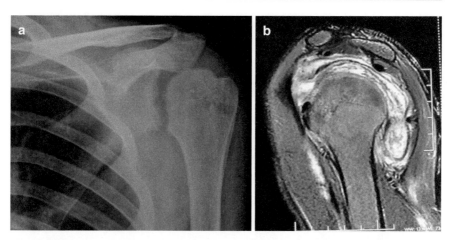

Fig. 25.3 (**a**) Plain radiograph of the left shoulder in a 66-year-old man showing a lytic destruction of the inferior part of the humeral head. (**b**) T2-weighted image MR sequence shows the intense inflammatory exudate surrounding the humeral head. Diagnosis: *TB of the shoulder joint*

in developing countries like India. It is vital to realize the importance of locally endemic diseases when dealing with the radiological picture of a suspected bone tumor. In countries like India, musculoskeletal tuberculosis is a common masquerader of bone tumors and vice versa (Fig. 25.3). An amateur surgeon can mistake a PNET for tubercular osteomyelitis especially in the pediatric age group. Hydatid cyst of bone can resemble an aneurysmal bone cyst.

1. *Plain radiograph*: Still forms the first investigation of choice in a suspected bony lesion. The plain x ray can qualify the lesion and give an immediate working diagnosis. Important parameters which need to be evaluated on a radiograph of a bone tumor are:
   - Site of the lesion: Epiphyseal, metaphyseal (commonest), or diaphyseal. In the Indian context, it is important to remember that diaphyseal lesions like Ewing sarcoma can commonly mimic acute or chronic osteomyelitis, which are a common occurrence in this part of the world (Fig. 25.4).
   - Lytic or sclerotic lesion: It is important to assess whether the lesion is sclerotic or lytic. Lytic destruction in a primary bone tumor indicates aggressiveness of the lesion. In developing countries like India, sclerotic bone lesions may not necessarily be bone-forming tumors. Lytic lesions in the epiphysis can mimic infections, mainly subacute epiphyseal osteomyelitis (Fig. 25.5).
   - Matrix: Of the lesion denotes the underlying tissue. Chondroid lesions show speckled calcification in the matrix. Popcorn calcification in chondrosarcomas is well known (Fig. 25.6).
   - Periosteal reaction: The type of periosteal reaction on a plain radiograph reveals the nature of the underlying disease process. It is important to differentiate the periosteal reaction of an osteosarcoma with that occurring due to atypical pathologies like tuberculosis, the latter being a far more common occurrence in the third world (Fig. 25.7).

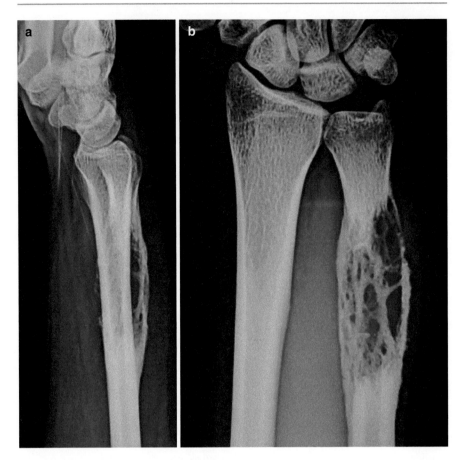

Fig. 25.4 Plain radiograph of the distal forearm in a 22-year-old male. There is a moth-eaten destruction of the ulnar diaphysis with periosteal reaction. Initially treated as osteomyelitis, this turned out to be Ewing sarcoma of the ulna

2. *Magnetic resonance imaging (MRI)*

MRI is used in the staging of bone sarcomas. MRI with specific adapted bone tumor sequences allows an exact local staging of bone sarcomas [7]. MRI is also helpful in the detection of skip lesions and in metachronous osteosarcomas, which are not an uncommon occurrence in cases with late presenting sarcomas as seen in countries like India [8]. Common MRI parameters, which need to be evaluated, include nature of the lesion, its extent, status of neurovascular bundle, presence of other lesions, and involvement of adjacent joints/growth plate [9]. Dynamic MRI studies in osteosarcoma are a useful surrogate to see the amount of angiogenesis in the tumor substance. We were among the first few authors to report the use of dynamic contrast-enhanced MRI as an essential tool in determining tumor angiogenesis in osteosarcomas and hence have an idea about prognosis [10]. However, these studies are available only in few advanced centers of the country.

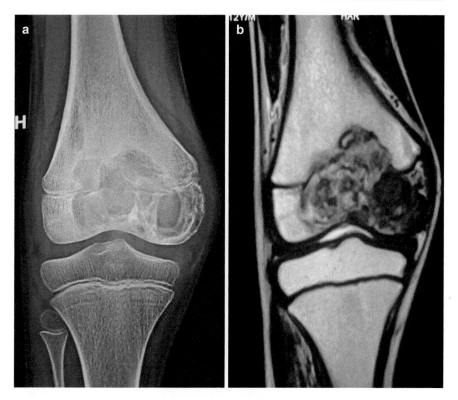

Fig. 25.5 (a) Plain radiograph of the knee in a 12-year-old showing a lytic lesion in the epiphysis. (b) T1-weighted MR scan showing a solid component of the lesion. The child was initially diagnosed as an infective pathology. Final diagnosis: *chondroblastoma*

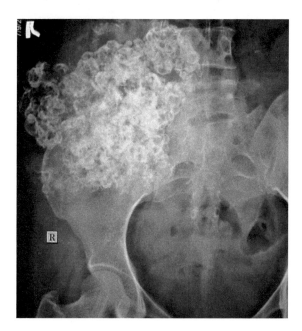

Fig. 25.6 Plain radiograph of the pelvis in a 30-year-old lady with a chondroid lesion of the right iliac wing (note the "popcorn calcification" pattern). Diagnosis: *low-grade chondrosarcoma*

Fig. 25.7 Plain radiograph of the left femur in a 16-year-old boy with tubercular osteomyelitis. Note the presence of a heavy periosteal reaction in the diaphysis. Endosteal sequestrae are also visible

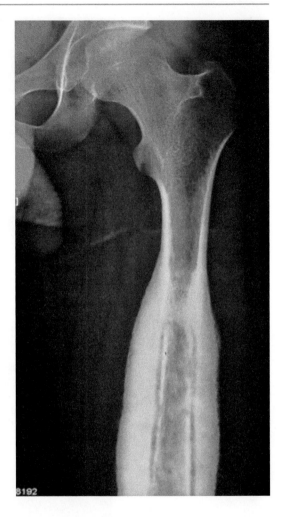

3. *Other imaging modalities*

   In bone sarcomas, it is essential to stage the disease through a three-phase bone scan and a noncontrast CT chest. These investigations should be completed in all patients after the final diagnosis is established through a bone biopsy. Although advanced centers of MSK oncology also use the positron emission tomography CT scan for local and systemic aggressiveness of the lesion, this investigation is sparingly available in developing countries and is only used in specialized centers. We have evaluated the role of PET-CT in the post-chemotherapy assessment of chemotherapy with significant results [11]. We also saw a high degree of accuracy of PET scan in detecting recurrences in patients with recurrent Ewing sarcomas [12].

4. *Biopsy*

   Biopsy is an invasive diagnostic procedure performed with the aim of obtaining a sample of representative abnormal tissue, for histopathological or microbiological analysis. The importance of biopsy in the diagnosis of bone and soft tissue tumors cannot be overemphasized. Biopsy is usually performed as an elective procedure under aseptic precautions preferably in an operating room. Being an invasive procedure, biopsy should be performed only after completing the necessary noninvasive (imaging) examinations such as radiographs and magnetic resonance imaging (MRI).

25.3.1 Biopsy in the Indian Scenario

In resource-challenged environments like ours, there is a lack of trained musculo-skeletal oncologists, which puts the onus of performing a musculoskeletal biopsy on the general orthopedic surgeon. Lack of training in performing a biopsy for a bone and soft tissue tumor leads to an incorrect biopsy procedure and subsequent issues with limb salvage or amputation. Incorrectly done biopsy not only misses the diagnosis but also jeopardizes the anatomy for subsequent surgical intervention.

This is particularly true when the biopsy done is an incisional or an excisional biopsy, with ill-placed surgical scars and oncological pollution of more than one surgical or anatomical plane (Fig. 25.8). In our experience, the chances of recurrences are increased when biopsies are ill placed or performed without care for the soft tissue compartments in malignant bone or soft tissue tumors. Besides oncological contamination, a poorly done biopsy scar also leads to scarring and fibrosis

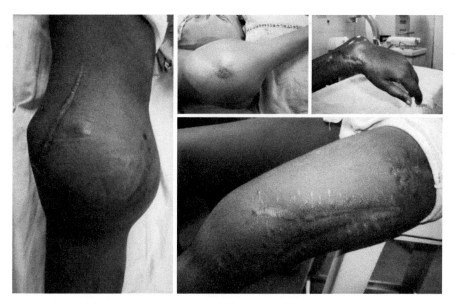

Fig. 25.8 A series of clinical pictures of different patients with poorly done biopsies. This is common in resource-challenged environments where untrained surgeons attempt incisional or excisional biopsies

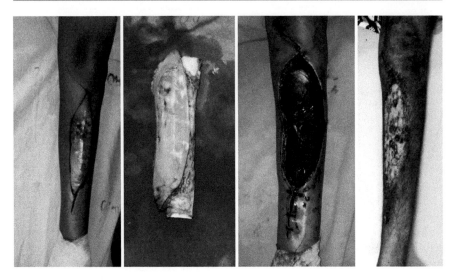

Fig. 25.9 A poorly done biopsy for a tibial osteosarcoma. Reconstruction done using a gastrocnemius flap with excision of the biopsy scar

making soft tissue reconstruction procedures demanding (Fig. 25.9). It is therefore essential that general orthopedic surgeons be adequately trained in performing a biopsy in bone and soft tissue tumors. Biopsy is a complex cognitive skill, which should be performed with adequate care and knowledge.

25.3.2 Types of Biopsy

Based upon the technique utilized, biopsy procedures can be of the following types:

1. Fine needle aspiration cytology/biopsy (FNAC/FNAB)
2. Core needle biopsy
3. Incisional (open) biopsy
4. Excisional biopsy

FNAC is extremely useful in diagnosing carcinomas (malignant neoplasms of epithelial origin), but has little utility in primary diagnosis of bone sarcomas because examining the tissue architecture and matrix formation is important in the diagnosis of sarcomas. Further, fine needle biopsy would provide very little tissue that might preclude further pathological examination such as immunohistochemistry (IHC). However, with advancements in cytological techniques, certain centers in India are favoring FNAC in the diagnosis of soft tissue sarcomas and soft tissue recurrence of bone sarcomas [13, 14].

Core biopsy using a specially designed wide bore needle is the most common biopsy technique utilized in leading cancer centers for diagnosing sarcomas. For primary bony lesions, we prefer the Jamshidi needle (named after its inventor Khosrow Jamshidi), which is a cylindrical trephine needle with a tapered cutting

Fig. 25.10 A Jamshidi needle

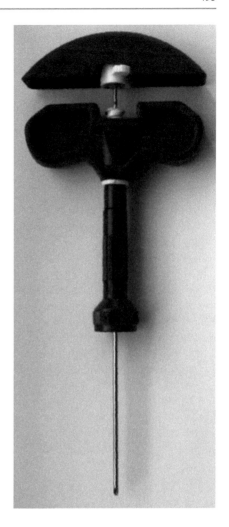

tip (Fig. 25.10). The tip is tapered to retain the core of tissue. Primary soft tissue neoplasms are biopsied using a spring loaded, semiautomated Tru-cut needle. Most biopsies in adults are performed under local anesthesia with or without sedation with general anesthesia being reserved for children and painful conditions.

Incisional (open) biopsy is still the gold standard for biopsy of musculoskeletal lesions. The pathological tissue can be examined visually to locate the ideal site for biopsy. Good quantity of pathological tissue can be obtained thus avoiding inconclusive (repeated) biopsies due to inadequate sample. However, the need for general anesthesia, bigger scar size, and higher chance of contaminating normal tissue has made incisional biopsy less favorable compared to core biopsy. Skrzynski et al. reported 84% success rate of closed needle biopsy when compared to open biopsy which had a success rate of 96% [15].

Excisional biopsy has very little role, if any, in the primary diagnosis of suspected malignant musculoskeletal neoplasms. Excisional biopsy is preferred in certain benign lesions such as osteochondromas and at certain problematic locations like the head of fibula. Excisional biopsy is therapeutic for benign lesions. It is also useful in superficial, soft tissue lesions less than 5 cm with radiological picture suggesting benign etiology. However, if the lesion is beneath the deep fascia or if there is a suspicion of malignancy, we favor Tru-cut biopsy before proceeding with definitive management.

25.3.3 Image-Guided Biopsy

The exact site of biopsy can be located with the help of advanced imaging techniques. Certain locations such as vertebral body and sacrum would require CT-guided biopsy for targeting the lesion accurately. Deeply placed osseous lesions are best biopsied by an interventional radiologist using a CT scan. In our center, due to resource constraints, we prefer CT-guided biopsy only for lesions in the spine, sacrum, or pelvis and in those lesions that are difficult to localize on radiograph (Fig. 25.11). On the other hand, we commonly utilize image intensifier guidance for sampling bone lesions. Certain expansile lesions like an aneurysmal bone cyst should be injected with a radiopaque dye (like Omnipaque) before being biopsied. It helps to identify the loculations and is helpful if the cyst is being injected in the same sitting. Most soft tissue lesions are biopsied under ultrasound guidance except in superficial, palpable lesions.

With recent advancements in imaging techniques, PET-CT-guided biopsies are also being performed. These are mainly reserved for soft tissue lesions like enlarged lymph nodes. Their use in bone tumors is limited.

Even after a satisfactory biopsy, a pathologist may find only dead and necrotic tissue in the biopsy specimen. This is because the biopsy sample could be from the central area of a rapidly growing neoplasm that undergoes necrosis due to inadequate blood supply. To avoid such inconclusive reports, we routinely take biopsy tissue

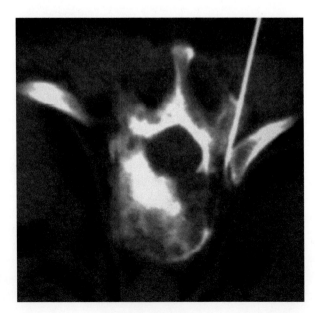

Fig. 25.11 A CT-guided biopsy from the dorsal spine in a patient with metastatic deposit

from the edge of a neoplasm along with a part of normal tissue to aid differentiation. Frozen section or touch smear examination from the biopsy specimen is performed wherever facilities are available, to confirm the presence of representative tumor tissue in the biopsy sample. If a definitive diagnosis cannot be established with the first biopsy, the particular case is discussed at the multidisciplinary team (MDT) meeting to understand the concerns of the pathologist and a re-biopsy is planned accordingly. If two successive core biopsies turn inconclusive, incisional biopsy is preferred. We presume that our re-biopsy rates are higher than developed countries where CT guidance is more commonly employed although we do not have adequate to support our claim. The biopsy scar is excised along with the tumor with wide margins during definitive surgery (Figs. 25.12 and 25.13).

Treating bone sarcomas without biopsies: A large number of patients are referred to our tertiary center with surgery done for the suspected bone sarcoma in the absence of a histopathological diagnosis. The most common error encountered in these referrals is that an unplanned curettage of a lesion was done without a diagnosis and that the curettings were found to be positive for malignancy only during the postoperative period. It is important to stress the fact that despite considerable advances in imaging modalities, these studies are not a substitute for histopathological examination. They only supplement the diagnosis. Any bony lesion suspicious of neoplastic etiology should be biopsied unless it is a "no touch lesion." (Fig. 25.14).

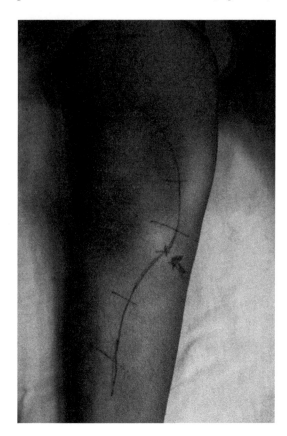

Fig. 25.12 Osteosarcoma of the proximal tibia with (future) surgical incision marked. The *arrow* is the point from where the biopsy will be taken

Fig. 25.13 Biopsy scar
excised along with an
osteosarcoma of the
proximal tibia

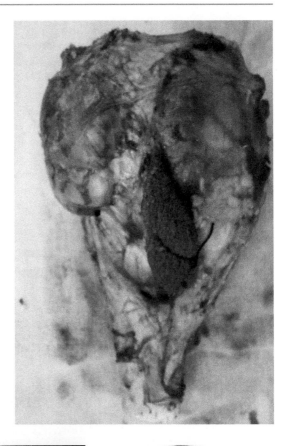

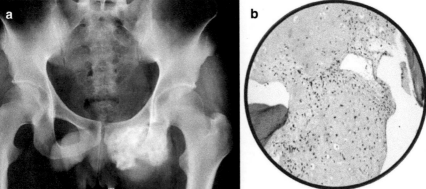

Fig. 25.14 (**a**) Plain radiograph of the pelvis of a 32-year-old man with a sclerotic lesion on the
left inferior pubic ramus. This was excised outside our hospital without any advanced imaging or
biopsy. (**b**) Review of histopathology specimens showed features consistent with a chondrosarcoma

25.4 Chemotherapy Strategies

Once a diagnosis of a bone sarcoma is established, the treatment warrants chemotherapy before limb salvage can be attempted. As in the western world, neo-adjuvant chemotherapy is the gold standard in the treatment of osteosarcoma and Ewing's sarcoma in India. In the absence of standardized protocol and regimen of chemotherapy in bone sarcomas in India, regimens vary at different centers depending upon the local experience. In most tertiary centers, chemotherapy is provided by dedicated medical oncologists specialized in musculoskeletal neoplasms. Tumor board meetings are in place to decide on management of difficult cases that do not fit into the routine protocol. Most centers follow cisplatin- and doxorubicin-based regimens for osteosarcoma [16, 17]. Three cycles of preoperative chemotherapy are followed by surgical excision and three cycles of postoperative chemotherapy. Tumor necrosis rate is determined in the excised specimen to assess response to chemotherapy. If the necrosis rate is more than 90%, then the preoperative regimen is continued. However, if the necrosis rate is less than 90%, it is considered to be a poor prognostic factor. High-dose methotrexate can be added to the chemotherapy regimen as evidence is increasing to support its use. Chemotherapy has increased the disease-free survival of osteosarcoma from less than 20% to 55–75%. Resistance to existing chemotherapeutic drugs is another obstacle to limb salvage surgery. If a tumor progresses rapidly while on neo-adjuvant chemotherapy, upfront ablative surgery is recommended. In our study, we found that chemotherapy response in osteosarcoma can be predicted with dynamic MRI and it correlates well with post chemo necrosis [18]. Newer drugs currently being investigated include gemcitabine, docetaxel, and liposomal formulation of doxorubicin. The regimen for PNET/Ewing's sarcoma group of tumors includes several drugs such as vincristine, doxorubicin, cyclophosphamide, ifosfamide, and etoposide. The first three drugs can be given together alternating with the last two. After the first five cycles, local disease needs to be addressed with surgery or definitive radiotherapy. Definitive radiotherapy is reserved for sites, which are difficult to access such as the centro-axial skeleton. The incidence of second malignancy after radiotherapy is about 2–10%. It may be mentioned that in the absence of skilled musculoskeletal oncologic surgeons in countries like India, relatively more patients receive radiotherapy than those who have surgery for their disease. Postoperative adjuvant radiotherapy can be added if the surgical margins turn out to be positive. Usually postoperative radiotherapy is given within 6–8 weeks following surgery. The risk of infection increases following postoperative radiotherapy in massive endoprosthetic reconstructions. Hence, the risks and benefits need to be assessed at a multidisciplinary clinic before arriving at a decision. Challenges to adjuvant therapy include high cost of chemotherapeutic drugs and lack of infrastructure. Generic drugs are currently being promoted to cut down cost of chemotherapy. Nongovernmental organizations extend support to cancer patients from weaker sections of the society.

25.5   Limb Salvage Surgery

Following wide excision of bone sarcomas, different methods of surgical reconstruction are available. Reconstruction methods following tumor excision can be classified as:

1. Nonbiological methods (mainly includes endoprostheses)
2. Biological methods (autograft, allograft, vascularized grafts, etc.)

However, this division does not include certain other methods of reconstruction such as the nail-cement spacer, a common technique used in developing countries like India.

1. *Nonbiological methods*
   Endoprostheses can be either modular or custom made [19]. In general, the use of endoprosthesis in countries like India is limited by pricing and procuring issues. The main advantage of endoprosthetic reconstruction is that it can restore joint mobility and function apart from restoring limb length. Sufficient muscle should be available to generate power for moving the endoprosthetic joint. As already mentioned, most standard endoprostheses are unaffordable for majority of Indian population. This has forced the development of low cost, indigenous endoprostheses that are widely popular throughout the country (Fig. 25.15). However, loosening and metallosis is a problem with these implants and most bone sarcoma patients require revision within 10 years of the index procedure. The use of prosthesis is also limited by the imminent danger of infection which is common in resource-challenged environments like India.

Biological options for reconstruction in defects following bone sarcoma excision are many. The important options include:

1. Intercalary resection and fibular grafting: This is one of the most common methods of reconstruction for diaphyseal defect. It is also used for metaphyseal sarcomas with reasonable success particularly in achieving arthrodesis of the joint. We have significant experience with resection arthrodesis in distal femoral osteosarcomas using the nonvascularized fibular graft (Figs. 25.16 and 25.17). In our experience, defects less than 12 cm heal well when stabilized by a nonvascularized fibular graft. For larger defects, there is high incidence of nonunion.
2. Reconstruction using irradiated host bone: Irradiating the tumor bone itself with a high single dose of radiotherapy has shown good results for reconstructing bone defects after bone sarcoma excision. Its availability in an institute setup prevents widespread application in the developing world. We have seen good results with the technique, but it can only be used when the joint is uninvolved by the tumor [20]. The resected tumor specimen is denuded of its soft tissue components, and soft tissue component is sent for histopathological examination. The rest of the specimen is packed in a sterile container and irradiated with

Fig. 25.15 Endogenous prostheses used in low-income, resource-challenged situations for limb salvage

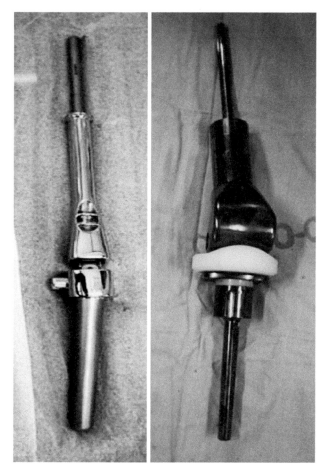

high-dose radiation so as to kill all viable cells. The specimen is then prepared, reimplanted, and fixed using a plate. We prefer a locking plate to achieve higher stability (Fig. 25.18). The medullary canal of the specimen can be either grafted with autologous fibula/iliac crest graft or packed with demineralized bone matrix. The irradiated bone will act as a scaffold over which osteoblasts from adjacent native bone invade by creeping substitution.

3. Vascularized fibular grafting: It is an ideal technique to use in intercalary defects, particularly if the defect length is more than 12 cm. Unfortunately, the procedure needs specialized training and a microvascular team. In the absence of such facilities in the developing world, vascularized fibular graft is used less.

4. Allograft reconstruction: With increase in hip arthroplasty even in countries like India, the availability of allograft has increased. On the contrary, the availability of strut allograft is still low. We use morselized allograft (with or with nonvascularized fibula) in intercalary reconstructions and in achieving joint arthrodesis following excision of bone sarcomas. The use of a resorbable mesh to hold the

Fig. 25.16 Three-year postoperative radiograph of a 15-year-old with osteosarcoma of the distal femur, showing good arthrodesis of the knee using a nonvascularized fibular graft

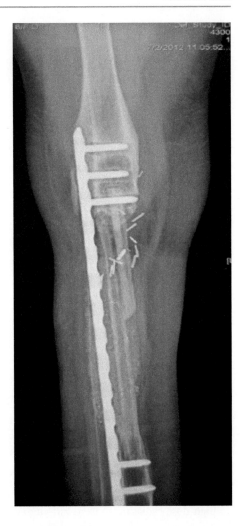

allograft is a useful cost-effective technique (Fig. 25.19). The fibular struts are usually held by locking plates. In fact the advent of angular stable locking plates has encouraged surgeons to go for very close resections [21].

5. Turnoplasty: In huge lesions involving large segments of distal femur or proximal tibia, there is a paucity of available graft. Nonvascularized fibula is usually insufficient. In such patients, coronal half of the femur (for proximal tibial lesions) or coronal half of the tibia (for distal femoral lesions) is used as a sliding autograft to arthrodese the knee. It provides a broad surface of contact with good healing (Fig. 25.20). The procedure is called turnoplasty and is popular in countries with poor facilities to store allografts. [Editor's note: this was described by Enneking and is known as a resection/arthrosis in the USA.]

6. Von Nes rotationplasty: It is another biological option of tumor reconstruction. In this procedure, the tumor is excised along with its soft tissue cover leaving

Fig. 25.17 Four-year postoperative radiograph of
the thigh in a 24-year-old (with Ewing's sarcoma
of the femur) showing a well-incorporated
nonvascularized fibular graft

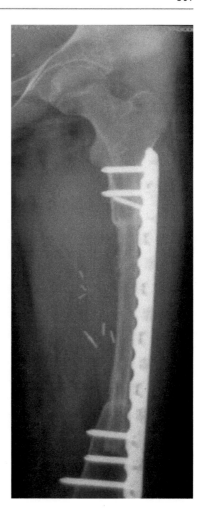

only the neurovascular bundle, and the distal part of the limb is rotated and
reimplanted to the proximal segment and plated. This procedure is useful in salvaging limbs which would otherwise undergo amputation. In the salvaged limb,
the ankle joint will function like a knee joint, and hence the above-knee amputation is converted into a below-knee amputation. The advantage is that the energy
consumption is less and the functional ability is more in the salvaged limb. The
main disadvantage of this procedure is that it is cosmetically disfiguring and
socially unacceptable to some sections of our population [22].

7. Spacers: They are a common method to fill defects created by resection of
   malignant bone tumors. They play an important role as a large number of
   resected tumors are high volume and carry a significant risk of recurrence.
   Hence, spacers can provide as a means of temporary fillers till definitive surgery is planned if the tumor doesn't recur. There are many types of spacers

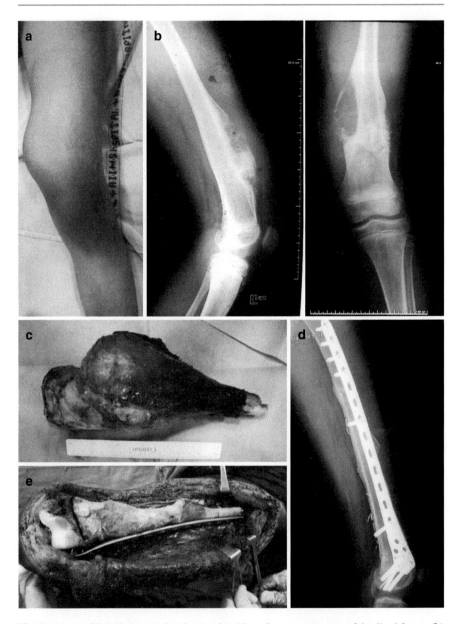

Fig. 25.18 (**a**) Clinical picture of a 12-year-old with surface osteosarcoma of the distal femur. (**b**) Plain radiographs (AP and lateral views) showing the lesion. (**c**) The excised specimen (note the step cut osteotomy proximally). (**d**) Per operative picture of the irradiated tumor bone fixed using a locking compression plate (**e**). Nine months post-op radiograph of the patient showing union in progress both proximally and distally

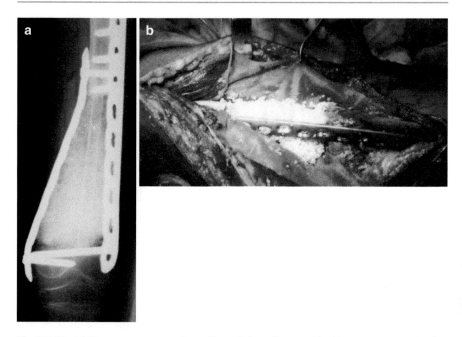

Fig. 25.19 (**a**) Four-year postoperative radiograph in a 13-year-old with osteosarcoma showing good incorporation of morselized allograft and fibular strut using two locking plates. (**b**) Per operative picture showing the placement of morselized allograft over an absorbable mesh (in another patient). The mesh keeps the allograft in place and induces fibrosis

Fig. 25.20 (**a**) Clinical picture of a huge osteosarcoma of the proximal tibia in a 19-year-old boy. (**b**) AP radiograph of the same patient showing the lesion in proximal tibia. (**c**) Intraoperative picture of the patient showing the turnoplasty of distal femur being fixed by a locking plate. (**d**) Two-year postoperative radiograph showing good arthrodesis of the knee with union at the tibiofemoral junction

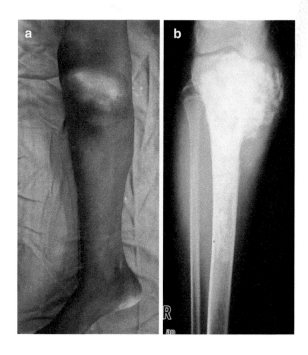

Fig. 25.20 (continued)

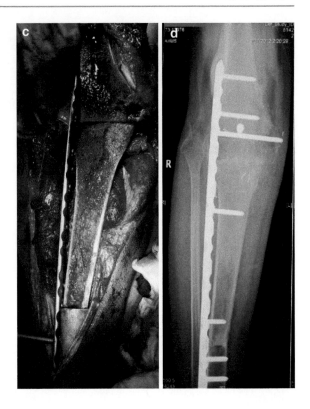

which are used in the developing world. The commonest spacer we use is for proximal humeral tumors where savage of the rotator cuff is not possible and therefore is futile to use an expensive proximal humeral endoprosthesis (Fig. 25.21). Another useful technique of spacers is nail-cement spacer augmented with a plate for rotational stability and is used to achieve arthrodesis (commonly of the knee). One or two stacked K-nails of length approximately 20 cm more than the resection length are used so that they gain purchase of around 10 cm each in the proximal and distal bone. A plate with one-/ two-screw purchase in each bone is added to achieve rotational stability. The advantage of this technique is that it is simple, cheap, and less time consuming and the patient can be mobilized with support. As mentioned earlier, this technique is quite useful in high volume tumors where there is increased chance of wound breakdown. This procedure can be later revised to either arthrodesis or endoprosthetic reconstruction (Fig. 25.22).

Fig. 25.21 Plain radiograph of the left shoulder and arm following excision of a chondrosarcoma of the proximal humerus in a 40-year-old man. The defect is filled with a spacer made of cement and a thick pin. It allows fairly useful movements of the elbow

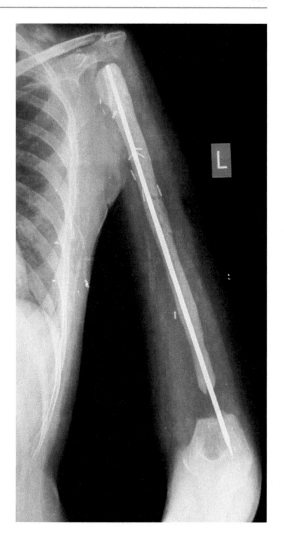

25.5.1 Surgical Choices

In a developing country like India, the patients' demands are low and economic constraints are high. Many patients prefer arthrodesis to amputation/rotationplasty when given an option. This is especially true in the pediatric age group as the parents cannot afford a growing prostheses and children adapt well to an arthrodesed limb. Vascularized fibular graft augmented with autograft/allograft and a plate is the preferred technique of arthrodesis.

Fig. 25.22 Plain radiograph of a nail-plate-cement spacer after resecting an osteosarcoma of the distal femur in a 20-year-old boy

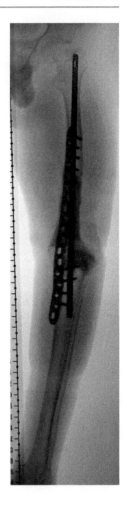

25.6   High Volume Tumors and Salvage

High volume tumors (volume > 500 cm³) are probably more common in India as compared to developed countries. As mentioned earlier, late presentations are common as people waste a lot of useful time with traditional forms of medicine before seeking allopathic treatment. Poverty, illiteracy, and distance of tertiary centers contribute to delay in presentation. Limb salvage surgery becomes difficult in high volume tumors. The duration of surgery as well as the blood loss is increased. Moreover, reconstruction becomes difficult. Contrary to the popular expectation, recurrence rate seems to be unaffected by the volume of tumor if wide surgical margins are achieved [23]. As such, high-volume tumors are not a contraindication for limb salvage surgery if the surgeon is able to achieve wide oncological margins. However, they have a bearing over the method of reconstruction. If a tumor involves most of the compartment, say a distal femoral osteosarcoma involving most muscle of the anterior compartment, it would be wise to go for either rotationplasty or cement spacer application so that definitive reconstruction such as endoprosthesis or arthrodesis can be performed at a later date.

25.7 Amputation for Musculoskeletal Neoplasms

As mentioned in the introduction, amputation probably is the most common surgery performed on bone sarcomas throughout the country. Reasons for considering amputation in a peripheral care center includes lack of training in limb salvage as well as the difficulty in procuring implants for limb salvage at a peripheral center where these procedures are rarely performed. Another important factor to consider is the general misconception that sarcomas do not fare well after limb salvage. In a referral center, amputation is generally considered only if limb salvage is not indicated. Unfortunately, the number of sarcomas requiring amputation is higher than developed nations due to various reasons such as delay in seeking treatment, delay in referral, and unplanned primary procedures. Social factors do play a role in deciding for/against amputation, especially in children. It is well established that the Indian society considers a female child as "less precious" as compared to males as is evident from the high rate of female feticide in India [24]. It is not uncommon to find a parent who would press for limb salvage surgery in a female child who would require amputation because of difficulties in finding a marriage proposal for a girl with amputated limb. Counseling plays a huge role in addressing parental concerns in such cases.

25.8 Follow-Up Strategies and Surveillance

Follow-up of bone sarcoma patients is the most laborious task in the management of sarcoma patients in the developing world. Loss to follow-up is very high and hence recurrences are mostly non-salvageable. Illiteracy, ignorance, poverty, poor healthcare accessibility, and a lack of social support are the main reasons for such high losses. Most patients belong to lower economic class who migrate to cities from villages in search of job opportunities. Once operated, they become economically dependent upon others. We ensure follow-up by educating the patients and their guardians. We also collect the contact numbers of at least three close relatives or friends with whom the patient will be in touch. We routinely follow up our patients once in 3 months in the first 2 years, once in 4 months during the third year, once every 6 months over the fourth and fifth years, and once yearly thereafter. At each follow-up, patient will be assessed for wound condition, joint function, prosthetic complications, local recurrence, and systemic metastasis. Patients who receive adjuvant therapy (chemotherapy/radiotherapy) are followed up more closely depending upon the institute's protocol.

25.9   Rehabilitation

Rehabilitation of sarcoma patients involves a team approach constituted by the musculoskeletal oncologist, medical oncologist, radiation oncologist, counselors/social workers, physiotherapist, and occupational therapist. The role of nongovernmental organizations (NGOs) is pivotal in India. Most oncology centers have dedicated social workers who are actively involved in the rehabilitation process. Procuring a suitable prosthesis/orthoses could be challenging at times due to economic constraints. BMVSS (Bhagwan Mahaveer Viklang Sahayata Samiti) is a nonprofit organization which provides artificial limbs, calipers, and other orthoses free of cost to weaker sections of the society [25]. Several NGOs work closely with oncology centers not only helping the poor with medicines and implants but also rehabilitating them to become useful members of the society [26, 27]. However, rehabilitation of cancer patients gets little attention in peripheral centers lacking rehabilitation experts.

25.10   Soft Tissue Sarcomas

Most of the challenges in treatment of bone sarcomas remain relevant to soft tissue sarcomas as well. This section will deal with those challenges that are specific to soft tissue tumor management. Diagnosis of soft tissue sarcomas largely depends on the experience of the pathologist, and histological peer review is sometimes very essential [28]. Advanced diagnostic tools like immunohistochemistry, FISH (fluorescent in situ hybridization), and PCR (polymerase chain reaction) are not widely available throughout the country due to cost constraints. Hence, erroneous diagnosis is more frequent. Retrieving the slides of primary resection/biopsy for expert review is sometimes not feasible as the onus to get the slides is with the patient and he may decide not to do so because of the distance he needs to travel (say 1000 miles) or other factors. Infrequently, the slides could get lost in transit or the original specimen itself is discarded thus losing valuable data. A vast majority of soft tissue sarcomas are treated by general surgeons who do not have sufficient expertise in treating these tumors. Hence, unplanned excisions are quite common which result in higher risk of recurrence [29]. Most patients are referred to higher centers either after the histopathology of excised specimen confirmed malignancy or after local recurrence of tumor. As expected, tumor bed excision is more frequent in a developing country like India compared to developed nations where guidelines and referral pathways are strictly adhered to. Chandrasekar et al. have reported that 59% of specimens following tumor bed excision had residual tumor [30]. Reconstruction after tumor bed excision is another challenge and many patients would require muscle flaps or skin grafts. It is not uncommon to find a situation when amputation is inevitable. Providing adjuvant therapy can be quite taxing on the resources of the tertiary referral centers as the demand far exceeds the available resources. Certain centers are moving toward alternative options like perioperative interstitial brachytherapy instead of traditional external beam radiotherapy [31]. Chemotherapy protocols also vary between different centers due to

The Beijing JST Hospital has reported 191 cases of excision alcoholization replantation limb salvage treatment with completed follow-up documents from the period of 1965–2003. These cases included 102 male and 89 female patients with an age range of 10–62 years and a median age of 20 years. The postoperative follow-up durations ranged from 1 to 372 months with a median follow-up duration of 32 months. Fifty-two of these cases died. Besides the tumor factors, the total complication incidence rate was 50.3%; local complications included nonunion in 33 cases (17.3%), inactivated bone fractures in 39 cases (20.4%), infection in 39 cases (20.4%), internal fixation fracture in 15 cases (7.9%), and joint instability or subluxation in 5 cases (2.6%). The 5-year survival rate associated with inactivated bone was 55%. The satisfaction rate according to the Mankin function evaluation criterion was 50.3%.

For a long period of time, allograft transplantation has been used as an effective method for bone defect reconstruction. Its advantages include abundant sources, numerous shape and size options, host bone to allograft healing, shaping ability, ligament reattachment and reconstruction, and viable articular surfaces. Since the 1950s, the Beijing JST Hospital has used large bone allograft to reconstruct bone defects resulting from bone tumor resection. For historical reasons, the documents from some early cases were lost and were therefore not included in the statistical analysis (Fig. 26.14). The allogeneic bones were initially preserved by the addition of chemical agents, but since the end of 1991, cryopreservation has been used for bone preservation.

The Beijing JST Hospital has reported 149 well-documented cases with more than 1 year of follow-up that involved the application of cryopreserved allogeneic bones (fresh frozen) for the treatment of bone defects resulting from bone tumor resections [11–13]. These cases included 82 male and 67 female patients. Their ages

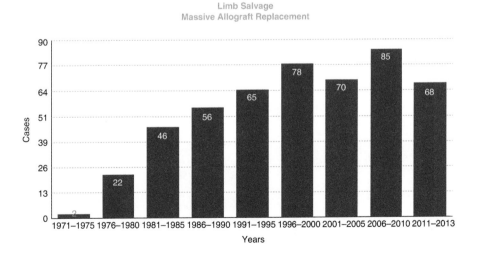

Fig. 26.14 The numbers of cases treated via the bone allograft method in previous years

ranged from 12 to 65 years with an average age of 22.3 years. The reconstruction methods included 91 cases of one-half joint transplantation, 13 cases of one-quarter joint transplantation, 11 cases of allograft prosthetic composite, 19 cases of large bone allograft transplantation, 12 cases of diaphyseal allograft transplantation, and 3 cases of pelvic allograft transplantation. The average follow-up duration was 33.6 months with a satisfaction rate of 74.5%, a recurrence rate of 11.4%, a mortality rate of 5.3%, and a final limb salvage rate of 93.3%. The complication incidence rate was 46.3%; including infection (11.4%), nonunion (24.2%), internal fixation fracture (6%), instable joint (8.7%), and bone fracture (7.4%). According to our experiences, the en bloc bone allograft transplantation reconstruction method is associated with a high complication rate. The complication rate decreases as the bone allograft size decreases, leading to better limb function. Infection and nonunion are the major complications. Following en bloc allograft reconstruction, the limb requires brace protection and non-weight-bearing while walking for a period of time. The early-stage limb function is poor and therefore cannot provide a high quality of life. If an oncological issue such as distant metastasis or local recurrence occurs, the patient will not have the benefit of limb salvage. For long-term survival patients, late-stage complications (e.g., fracture and infection) are more crucial issues that threaten the patients' quality of life (Figs. 26.15, 26.16, and 26.17).

With the evolution of limb salvage techniques and rapid growth in endoprosthesis manufacturing technology, the application of endoprosthesis for bone defect reconstruction following malignant bone tumor resection is becoming the preferred choice. Since the 1970s, the Beijing JST Hospital has incorporated an endoprosthesis reconstruction method (Fig. 26.18). However, endoprosthetic replacements were not used extensively during the years immediately following their introduction because of the limited economic development and consequent high cost. To date, although surgeons can select either imported (Western countries) or domestic endoprosthesis, this method remains an expensive choice for some patients because of the economic imbalances and imperfect health insurance system in China (Figs. 26.19, 26.20, and 26.21).

The Beijing JST Hospital reported 84 cases of primary endoprosthetic replacement reconstruction around the knee area, including 65 cases of distal femur and 19 cases of proximal tibia. These cases included 47 male and 37 female patients. The average patient age was 27 years (range: 10–75 years). There were 60 cases of osteosarcoma, with an average follow-up period of 22 months (range: 3–43 months).

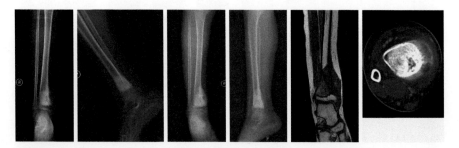

Fig. 26.15 An 11-year-old male who underwent treatment for a right distal tibia osteosarcoma. *Left* to *right*: X-ray images before and after chemotherapy, CT, and MRI images

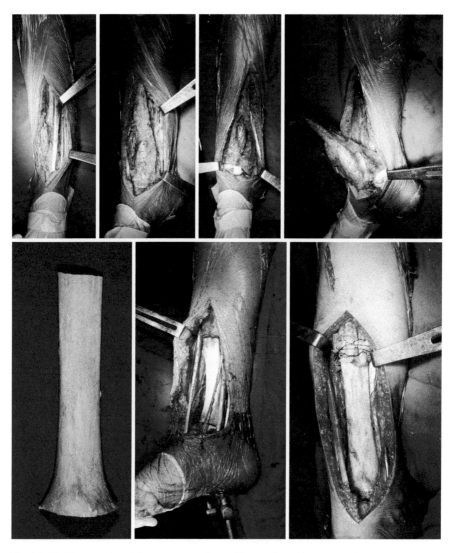

Fig. 26.16   Photographs of the tumor resection and bone allograft reconstruction surgery

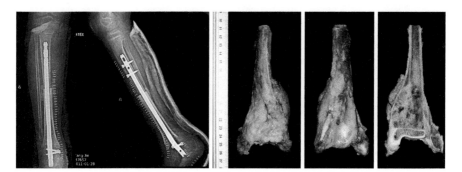

Fig. 26.17   Postoperative X-ray and specimen images

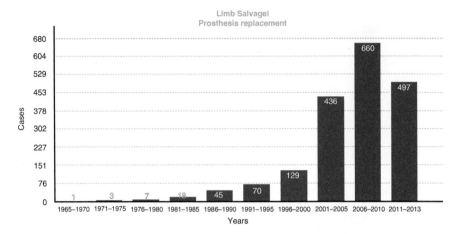

Fig. 26.18 The numbers of cases treated via the artificial joint method in previous years

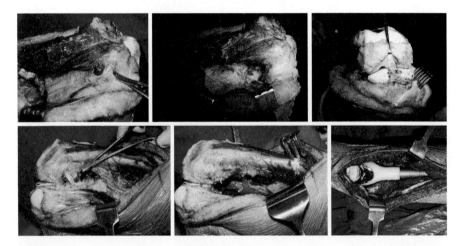

Fig. 26.19 A 17-year-old female with a right distal femur osteosarcoma. X-ray images before and after chemotherapy, computed tomography images, magnetic resonance images, and a preoperative plan for resection with wide margins

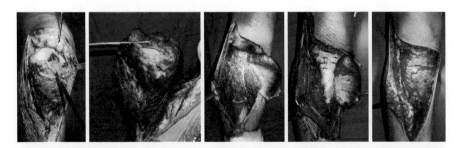

Fig. 26.20 Intraoperative photographs

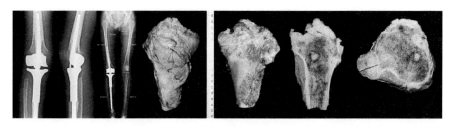

Fig. 26.21 Postoperative X-ray images and specimens

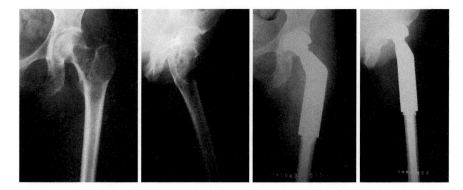

Fig. 26.22 A 40-year-old female with bone giant cell tumor of left proximal femur and performed mega prosthesis reconstruction

Eight of these cases (9.5%) developed wound complications. Three cases (3.6%) experienced wound nonunion, which were cured after local debridement. Five cases developed deep wound infections (5.9%): two of these cases were cured following several debridements, two developed recurrent infection after debridement and finally underwent amputation, and one underwent prosthesis removal after debridement followed by surgery for antibiotic bone cement temporary spacer implantation. This latter patient was cured after a staged endoprosthesis replantation.

Regarding the cases involving aseptic loosening or fracture of a prosthesis, we attempted to apply an intramedullary fixed short-stemmed cemented prosthesis, the bottom of which features biological coatings that can be fixed in an extramedullary fashion to the distal end of the remaining host bone. Short-term effects showed to be good, but further follow-ups are needed (Figs. 26.22, 26.23, 26.24, and 26.25).

Allograft prosthetic composite comprises a prosthesis that is surrounded and fixed by a large bone allograft. This method can be used for large-scale bone defect reconstruction around the knee joint, proximal humerus, and proximal femur. Theoretically, the combination of a bone allograft and endoprosthesis should be more effective than a single prosthesis considering soft tissue reattachment reconstruction. This method can prevent joint dislocation with best function. The fusion of allograft and host bone can reduce stress on the host bone and avoid bone absorption. However, this strategy leads to the superimposition

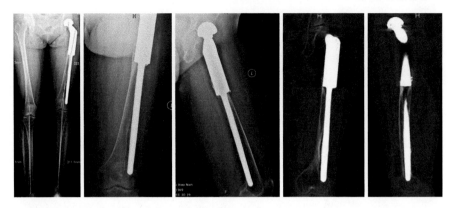

Fig. 26.23 Mega prosthesis loosing after 16 years later

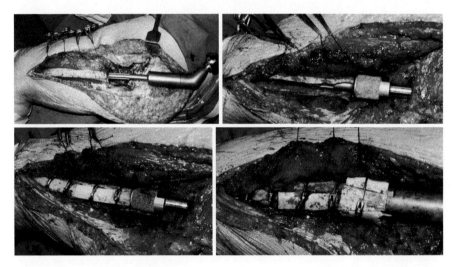

Fig. 26.24 Intraoperative photographs of revision with short-stemmed cemented prosthesis and extra medullary biological fixation

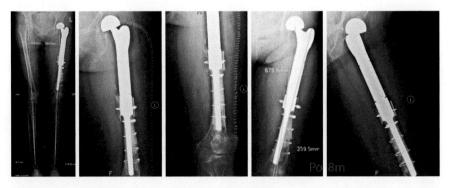

Fig. 26.25 X-ray of postoperation and follow-up 8 months later

of the complication rates associated with both methods. Therefore, we hold a prudent attitude when selecting an allograft prosthetic composite.

26.6 Computer Navigation System in Limb Sarcoma Resection and Reconstruction

The surgical treatment of bone tumors should fulfill the requirements of both oncology and orthopedics, i.e., complete resection of tumors with safe surgical margins to avoid oncological treatment failure and orthopedic reconstruction necessary for postoperative function. Currently, in the division, tumor imaging in preoperative bone tumor surgical planning is mainly based on the experience of surgeons, followed by designs of tumor prostheses without incorporating current digital technological advantages. Digital images could be fully utilized to achieve accurate tumor resection and functional reconstruction, such as computer-aided navigation. The navigation could provide: (1) a precise design based on the preoperative computed tomography (CT) and magnetic resonance (MR) image-based detection and determination of the tumor resection area, (2) simulations and reconstruction designs of the bone defects resulting from tumor resection via "mimics" and other design software, and (3) the registration of operative images and their fusion with preoperative images to achieve navigated and precise tumor resection and reconstruction.

At present, computer navigation can be applied to the entire diagnostic and treatment process associated with bone tumor surgery, from biopsy, preoperative planning, surgery, to postoperative evaluation, including the resection of pelvic tumors, surgical margin determination during extremity tumor curettage surgery, the precise localization of bone tumors with complicated anatomical locations, minimally invasive surgery (Figs. 26.26, 26.27, and 26.28), and the preoperative planning and operative implementation of tumor mega prostheses (Figs. 26.29, 26.30, 26.31, 26.32, 26.33, and 26.34). Evidence-based studies have demonstrated that the two most crucial reasons for pelvic tumor surgical failure are recurrence and complications. The navigation technology can precisely illustrate the three-dimensional configurations of tumors, thus helping to minimize the post-resection recurrence rate. This technology has an incomparable advantage in terms of surgery within the pelvic region (details are discussed in the pelvic tumor part). Extremity tumor curettage surgery is primarily used in benign and intermediate tumors or occasionally low-grade limb chondrosarcoma, such as the extended curettage treatment of giant bone cell tumors. Other than surgeon's experience, with assistance from computer navigation, surgeons could clearly determine the curettage regions, or any remaining areas of tumor during surgery, and preserve as much normal bone as possible. Osteoid osteomas usually occur on the diaphysis of long bones. Repeated scans are common during surgery because of the lack of anatomical landmarks. CT-guided radiofrequency ablation is also constrained by the non-sterile conditions of the CT room and cooperation with the anesthesiology team. The use of navigation

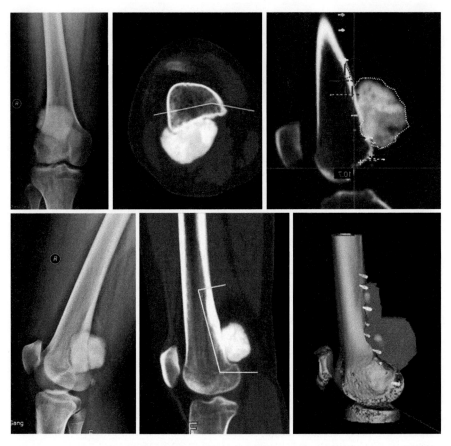

Fig. 26.26 A 35-year-old male with a right distal femur parosteal osteosarcoma; preoperative X-ray, computed tomography (CT) images, and navigated preoperative resection design

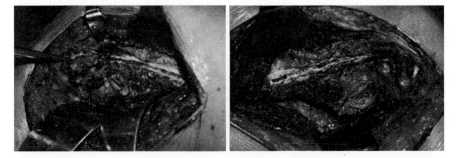

Fig. 26.27 Surgical margins of the tumor under operative navigation, bone allograft preparation under navigation, bone allograft transplantation, and specimen resection

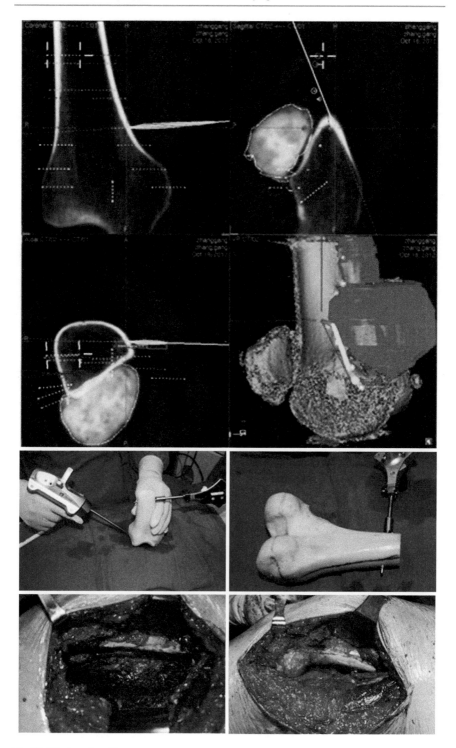

Fig. 26.27   (continued)

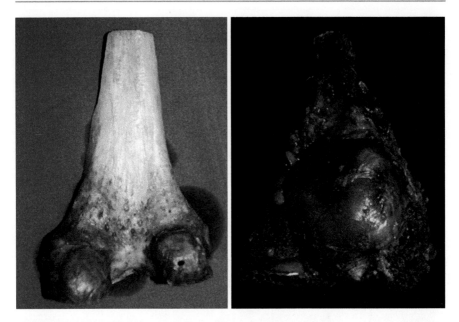

Fig. 26.27 (continued)

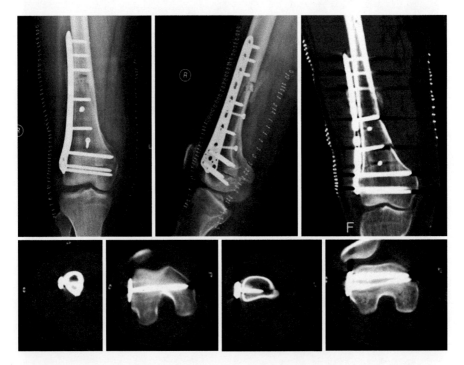

Fig. 26.28 Postoperative X-ray and CT images

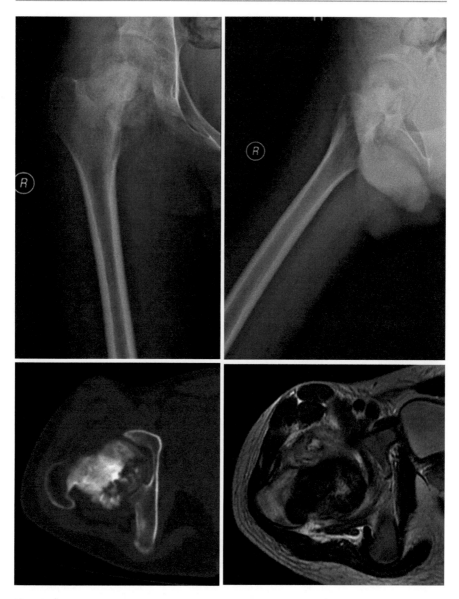

Fig. 26.29 A 16-year-old male with a right proximal femur osteosarcoma; preoperative X-ray, computed tomography, and magnetic resonance images

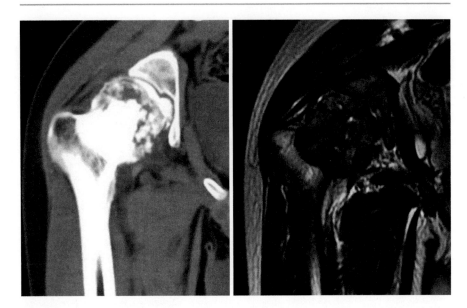

Fig. 26.29 (continued)

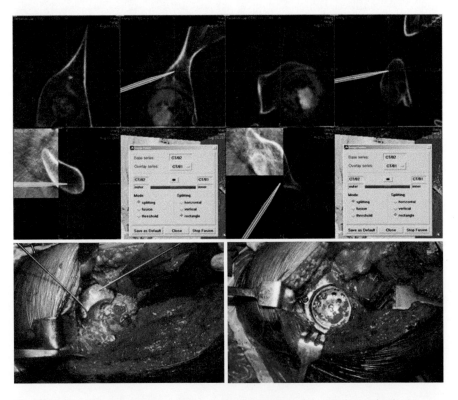

Fig. 26.30 Tumor resection and total hip joint reconstruction under operative navigation

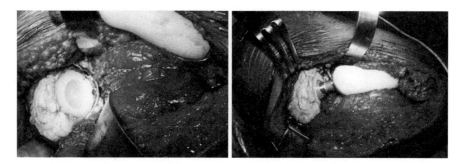

Fig. 26.30   (continued)

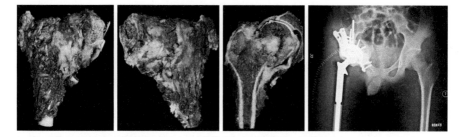

Fig. 26.31   The postoperative specimen and a postoperative X-ray image

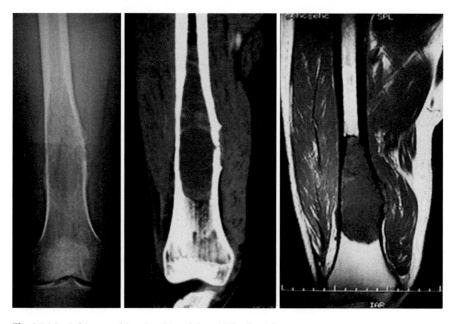

Fig. 26.32   A 31-year-old male with a right middle-distal femur osteosarcoma

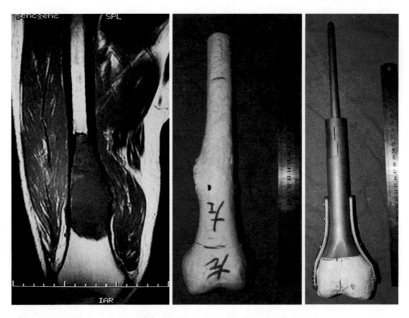

Fig. 26.33 Preoperative three-dimensional osteotomy and special prosthesis design

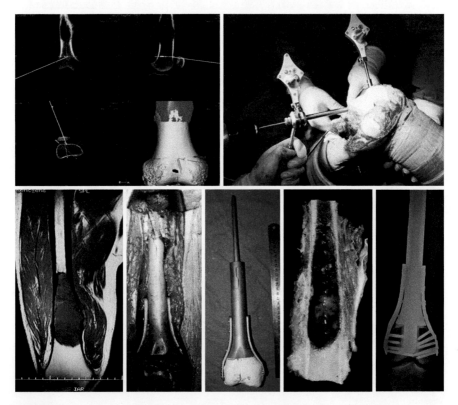

Fig. 26.34 Operative navigation, preoperative magnetic resonance image, preoperative planning, postoperative specimen, and X-ray image comparison

solves not only the above-described issues but also provides confidence to the surgeon regarding precise tumor resection. The patient can undergo simultaneous minimally invasive radiofrequency ablation under navigation.

In situations where special tumor prostheses require a high degree of matching, the use of navigation covers the entire process of preoperative tumor surgical margin determination, prosthesis design, surgical simulation, and the actual surgery.

26.7   Treatment Strategy for Malignant Pelvic Tumors

Although the incidence of malignant pelvic tumors is not very high, the prognosis of these tumors is much worse than those in the extremities. These tumors remain a considerable challenge for orthopedic oncologists. The Beijing JST Hospital has reported 366 well-documented cases of primary malignant pelvic tumors from March 1958 to October 2011 [14]. Among these, 221 were male and 145 were female patients, with a male to female ratio of 1.52:1. The age of onset ranged from 8 to 73 years, with median and average ages of 39.0 and 38.3 years, respectively. Additionally, 215 of the cases were chondrosarcoma, 69 were osteosarcoma, and 31 were Ewing's sarcoma. Region I was the tumor predilection site, and 148 cases were observed in this region. Among these cases, chondrosarcoma was the most common type (73 cases), followed by osteosarcoma (33 cases). Fifty-five cases occurred in region II; these were primarily chondrosarcoma (31 cases), osteosarcoma (17 cases), and malignant fibrous histiocytoma (6 cases). Fifty-two cases occurred in region III, including 39 cases of chondrosarcoma and 5 cases of osteosarcoma. We have listed the numbers of pelvic tumor cases throughout the years as listed in the digital musculoskeletal tumor database in Fig. 26.35.

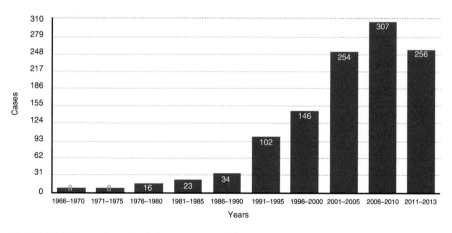

Fig. 26.35 The numbers of pelvic tumors treated in our institution

The staging system for bone and soft tissue tumors was firstly developed by Enneking in the 1980s and has been globally accepted as a bone tumor treatment guideline. The most brilliant part of this system involves surgical margin determination. If surgical treatment achieves certain margins, the local tumor control rate will be effectively increased. However, Enneking had considered the complexities of pelvis tumors as early as the period during which he developed his staging system. He did not believe that a surgical staging system intended for extremity tumor staging could be applied to the spine and pelvis. Therefore, the evaluation of the safe pelvic tumor resection regions remains an unresolved question. Not all malignant pelvic tumor resections require subsequent functional reconstruction. However, as the pelvis performs the function of lower limb weight transmission and is an important structure in the maintenance of normal working abilities, in many cases reconstruction can provide potential limb functional recovery. Given the complex stress distribution in the pelvic region, each different type of current reconstruction methods addresses certain issues, and there is no currently well-accepted reconstruction method.

The Beijing JST Hospital has reported a retrospective study of 79 well-documented patients with primary malignant pelvic bone tumors who were treated from October 1992 to July 2007. Of these, 23 had stage IB disease and 56 had stage IIB disease. For these patients, the follow-up duration ranged from 0 to 183 months with an average of 28.6 months. The minimum follow-up duration for surviving patients was 4 months. Of the 70 limb salvage cases, 28 and 42 patients did and did not undergo reconstruction, respectively. Additionally, there were nine amputation cases. The postoperative Musculoskeletal Tumor Society (MSTS) functional scores of the non-reconstruction patients ranged from 2 to 30 points with an average of 15 points. The postoperative MSTS functional scores of reconstruction patients ranged from 5 to 29 points with an average of 15 points. Twenty-five cases developed local recurrence (31.6%), of which 3 had stage IB disease (13.0%) and 22 had stage IIB disease (39.3%, $P = 0.023$). Twenty-one limb salvage patients (30.0%) and four amputation patients (44.4%) developed recurrences. Patients with inadequate intralesional resection or marginal resection margins had a local recurrence rate of 38.1%. However, patients with wide adequate resection margins had a local recurrence rate of 6.3% ($P = 0.014$).

Generally, for region I tumors, functional reconstruction is unnecessary if the integrity of the pelvic ring still exists. Patients with tumor in this region usually have good postoperative function (Figs. 26.36, 26.37, 26.38, and 26.39). Not many malignant tumor cases involve region III alone, but if a safe resection can be achieved via region III resection alone, postoperative reconstruction is unnecessary and the patient can obtain good postoperative functioning (Figs. 26.40 and 26.41). However, some patients with this tumor type may still experience back

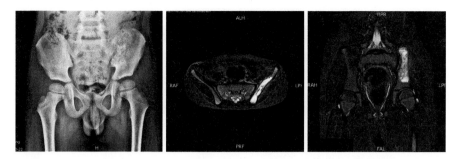

Fig. 26.36 An 8-year-old male with left iliac Ewing's sarcoma; post-chemotherapy X-ray and magnetic resonance images that illustrate a clear tumor region

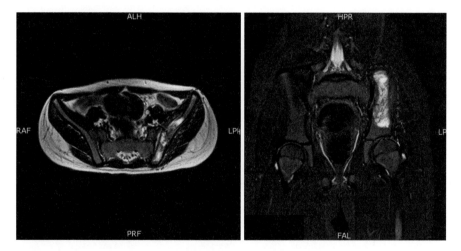

Fig. 26.37 The extensive resection region during preoperative planning

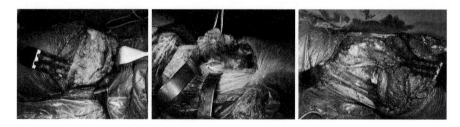

Fig. 26.38 Intraoperative photographs of the lateral and medial sides of the ilium and the sacral osteotomy plane after tumor resection

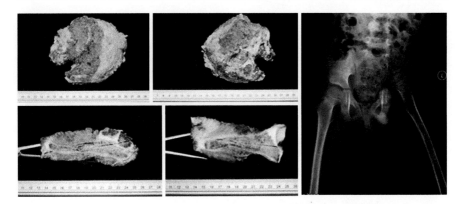

Fig. 26.39 Photographs of the lateral side of the specimen, including the sacroiliac joints and the specimen cross section along the axis of the acetabulum. Postoperative X-ray image

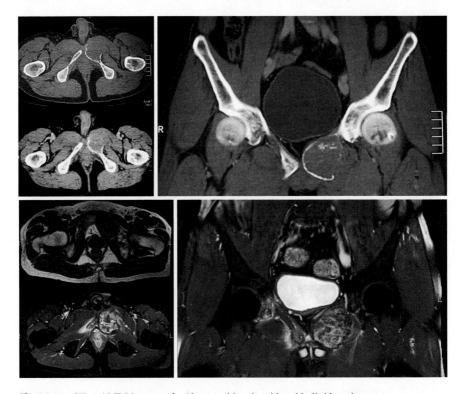

Fig. 26.40 CT and MRI images of a 40-year-old male with epithelioid angiosarcoma

discomfort due to the concentration of stress on the sacroiliac joint. The challenge of functional reconstruction after malignant pelvic tumor resection is primarily associated with region II lesions. Following region II lesion resection, the hip joint exhibits structural damage and lower limb function is severely affected. The

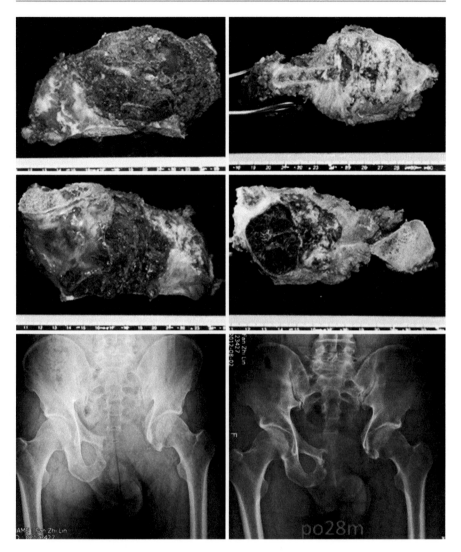

Fig. 26.41 Resection of pelvic region III without reconstruction. Photographs of specimen and X-ray of postoperation and follow-up 28 months later

reconstruction method for region II + III defects is similar to that for single region II defects. In recent years, we have incorporated computer-aided navigation technology into the preoperative surgical margin design, precise intraoperative resection, and post-resection reconstruction of many complex malignant pelvic tumor surgeries. We can design precise surgical margins based on preoperative imaging data and surgical margin rules. We are subsequently able to match these preoperatively designed borders with the exposed surgical field to identify the suitable surgical margins. Using this strategy, we can achieve the required surgical margins and fulfill the tumor resection requirements. Furthermore, we can retain larger amounts of normal tissues to allow better and simpler reconstructions and maintain more function. When treating region II malignant pelvic tumors, for which a portion of the acetabular region can be retained after the resection, computer-navigated resection is applied, followed by total hip joint replacement and reconstruction (Figs. 26.42, 26.43, and 26.44). For the reconstruction of combined region II + III defects, we have applied iliofemoral fusion and iliac arthroplasty (Figs. 26.45 and 26.46), which can lead to fewer postoperative complications but may cause limb length inequality. Recently, we have attempted to treat pelvic region II + III defects using reconstruction methods that involve the femur upward rotation and fusion with remain ilium or sacrum and bone allograft via internal fixation. With this strategy, we can address both the issue of limb shortening and the nonuniform load transfer between the femoral head and sacroiliac joint. Furthermore, the area of contact between the autologous and bone allograft will increase, thus promoting the healing process (Figs. 26.47, 26.48, and 26.49).

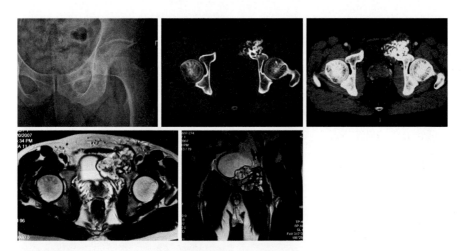

Fig. 26.42 A 33-year-old male with a chondrosarcoma in the left pelvic region II; preoperative X-ray, computed tomography (CT), and magnetic resonance images

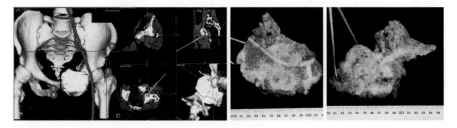

Fig. 26.43 Operative navigation images and postoperative specimen cross sections

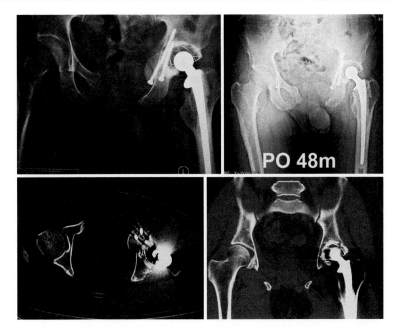

Fig. 26.44 Postoperative X-ray images immediately after surgery and at 48 months after surgery; postoperative CT image

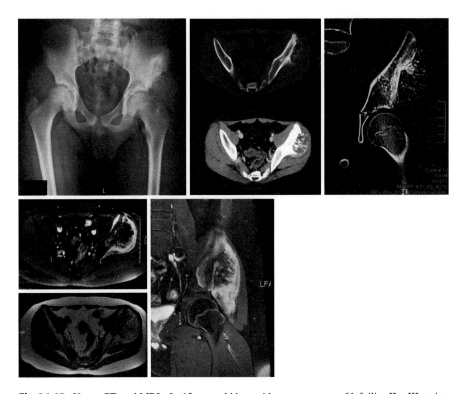

Fig. 26.45 X-ray, CT, and MRI of a 13-year-old boy with osteosarcoma of left iliac II + III regions

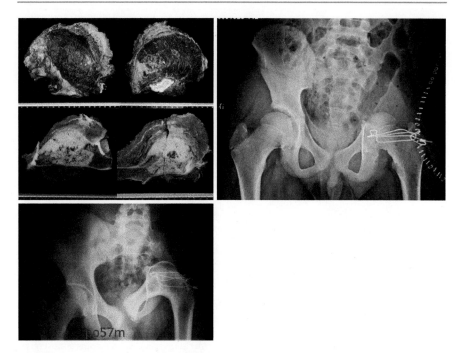

Fig. 26.46 Resection of pelvic II + III regions with hip joint fusion. Photographs of specimen and X-ray of postoperation and follow-up 57 months later

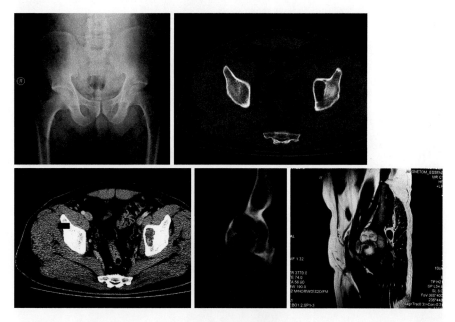

Fig. 26.47 A 43-year-old male with a top left acetabular chondrosarcoma; preoperative X-ray, computed tomography (CT), and magnetic resonance images

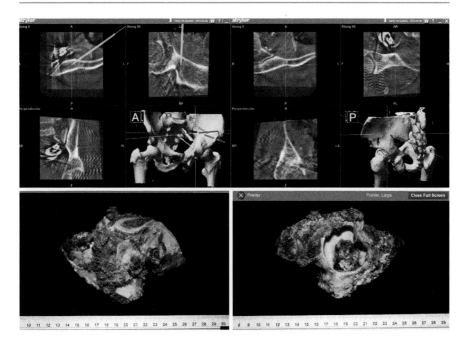

Fig. 26.48 Operative navigation images and photographs of the postoperative specimen and its cross sections

In particular, we should indicate that overemphasizing bone defect reconstruction following malignant pelvic tumor resection may lead to two undesirable tendencies: first, an emphasis on reconstruction while discounting resection margin and an emphasis on short-term functioning while discounting long-term follow-up will result in oncological treatment failure; second, despite successful tumor resection, excess reconstruction will increase the risk of complications and place the entire surgical treatment process at risk. Following pelvic tumor resection, reconstruction methods mainly include biological and mechanical reconstruction. Biological reconstruction refers to the use of autogenous and allogeneic bone grafts, excision alcoholization replantation, or a direct end–end fusion method for post-tumor resection bone defect reconstruction. The objective of biological reconstruction is to achieve bone healing and a durable long-term reconstruction. Although bone allograft and excision alcoholization replantation are the best morphological reconstruction methods, the associated complication rates are very significant. These complications mainly include infection, resorption, nonunion, allograft reaction, and fracture. The good functioning associated with these methods is predicated on uncomplicated bone healing, which cannot be achieved by most patients. Furthermore, new complications will continuously emerge over time. Recently, we have less frequently used bone allograft and excision alcoholization replantation. Prosthetic reconstruction refers to the use of metal prostheses for post-tumor resection bone defect reconstruction. Although computer simulation-designed prostheses

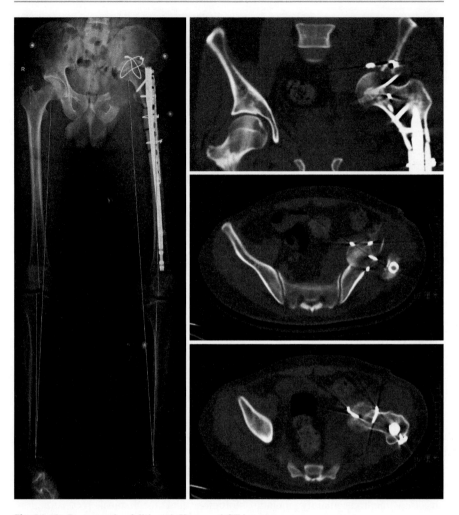

Fig. 26.49 Postoperative full-length X-ray and CT images

have potential advantages because of their simple components and reasonable fixations (e.g., vertical compressive stress, bone ingrowth into coatings, inner cylindrical bone fixation), the persistence and frequency of surgical complications continue to raise concerns. To date, there have been no reports of satisfactory long-term follow-ups resulting from this procedure. Given the above reasons, we prefer to conduct more simple and effective biological reconstructions under the premise of guaranteeing adequate tumor resection margins.

For patients with large tumors that have invaded major blood vessels and for which safe surgical resection margins cannot be achieved, external hemipelvectomy remains the most preferred treatment plan. However, for some patients with

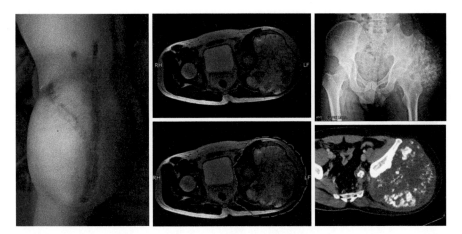

Fig. 26.50 A 30-year-old male with a recurrent left pelvis chondrosarcoma following a second operation. Positional photograph before the third operation; preoperative magnetic resonance image and surgical margin design; preoperative X-ray and computed tomography (CT) image

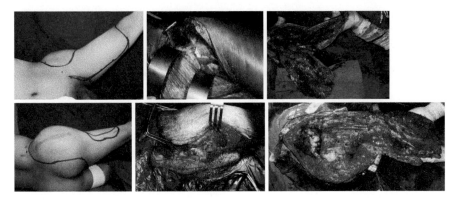

Fig. 26.51 The anterior and posterior incision photographs during the anterior flap external hemipelvectomy and the related anterior and posterior surgical photographs

contamination in the posterior flap area, anterior flap external hemipelvectomy remains the preferred method (Figs. 26.50, 26.51, and 26.52). Resection and reconstruction remain the basic stages of pelvic tumor treatment. Resection aims to remove tumors based on safe surgical margins in order to prevent tumor spread and reduce mortality, whereas functional reconstruction aims to improve the patient's quality of life.

In conclusion, the surgical treatment of malignant pelvic tumors is still quite challenging. This procedure is not only associated with high local recurrence and complication rates but also with a high perioperative mortality rate and low long-term survival rate.

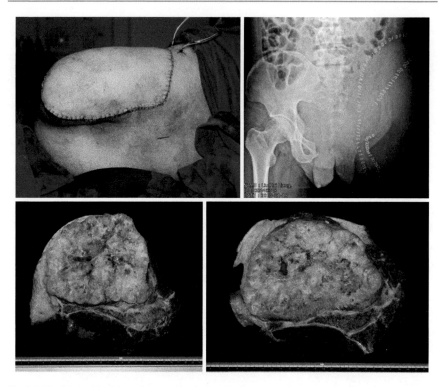

Fig. 26.52 Sutured incision photographs during the operation; postoperative X-ray image; specimen cross section photographs

26.8   The Treatment Strategy for Malignant Sacral Tumors

The incidence of primary malignant sacral tumors is low. Beginning in the 1970s, Beijing JST Hospital initiated surgical treatment for the sacral tumors in China, thus breaking the former convention that a sacral tumor represented a surgical contraindication. With the tumor database, we identified data from sacral tumor cases throughout the years (Fig. 26.53). There were 165 cases of chordoma, 154 of which occurred at the sacrum (93.33% of the total number). Chordoma is the most common primary malignant sacral bone tumor. As such, the following discussion uses chordoma as an example. The Beijing JST Hospital reported 68 cases of sacral chordoma from October 1978 to October 2000, involving 60 male and 8 female patients. The patients' age ranged from 25 to 74 years with a median age of 55.5 years. There were 104 related surgeries. There were 48 primary cases were initially treated in our department and 20 secondary recurrent cases. In terms of the tumor surgical margins, there were 4 cases of wide resection (8.3%), 21 cases of marginal resection (43.7%), and 23 cases of intralesional resection (48.0%). The follow-up period ranged from 1 to 365 months with an average of 81.84 months. Overall, 53

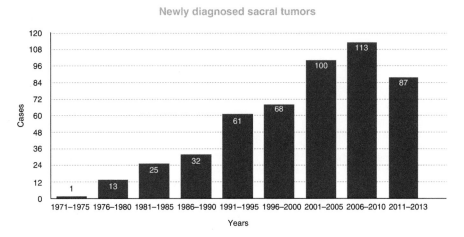

Fig. 26.53   The distribution of sacral tumor cases per year

cases survived (77.9%) and 15 cases died (22.1%). Seven of the deceased patients died during the perioperative period; these represented 46.7% of all deceased cases. The 5-year and 10-year overall survival rates were 87.3% and 73.3%, respectively. The median survival duration was 282.0 ± 88.7 months. Additionally, 34 intralesional resection cases (81.0%) and 8 marginal resection cases (36.4%) developed recurrences ($P = 0.000$).

Chordoma is a primary low-grade malignant sarcoma that is insensitive to radiotherapy and chemotherapy. As such, the primary treatment is surgery. Therefore, the crucial part of chordoma treatment is precise tumor resection according to perfect resection margins. However, chordoma usually occurs on the sacrum. An additional focus of attention is the maintenance of the normal uninvaded sacral nerve function while achieving satisfactory surgical margins. In recent years, to address these conflicting issues, we have applied computer navigation technology during the preoperative planning and intraoperative resection stages of sacral chordoma resection surgery and have achieved excellent results. The improvements in imaging technologies allow the implementation of preoperative three-dimensional reconstruction, computed tomography (CT) and magnetic resonance (MR) image fusion, and precise tumor region evaluation. Intraoperative navigation technology allows visualization of the precise tumor resection plan and assists the surgeon in achieving the preoperatively designed orthopedic tumor resection margins; in some cases, this allows the achievement of a marginal or wide resection and thus reduces the risk of recurrence.

Each computer-navigated sacral tumor resection surgery requires an initial preoperative plan, for which X-ray, CT, and MR image analyses are needed to determine the location and size of the tumor and its structural relationships with the surrounding tissues. This preoperative plan can also be designed so that the surgical tumor

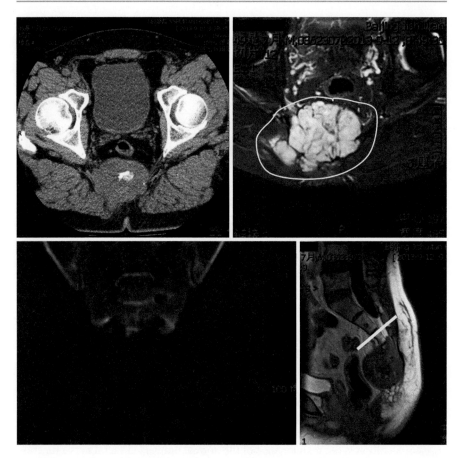

Fig. 26.54 A 49-year-old male; preoperative computed tomography and magnetic resonance images of a sacral chordoma; simulated bone and soft tissue surgical margins for wide resection

resection margins include the normal soft tissue intended for removal and the osteotomy plane design. Together with the preoperative plan, real-time navigation can be used during surgery to complete the tumor resection. After surgery, the resected tumor specimen should be compared with the preoperative plan and subjected to a strict evaluation of how accurately the preoperatively plan was adhered to. The detailed procedure is as follows: (1) collection of the original CT and MR data/images of the sacral tumor (Fig. 26.54). (2) Uploading DICOM-formatted original CT and MR data into a dedicated computer navigation system workstation and fusion of these data. As CT is superior with respect to bony tumor margin determinations (i.e., extent of bony destruction) and MR is superior with respect to soft tissue tumor margin determination, a combination of both imaging techniques can provide good illustrations of both bony and soft tissue tumor margins (Fig. 26.55). (3) Based on the precisely imaged tumor margins obtained from the CT-MR fusion, we can mark the bony and soft tissue tumor regions on the CT images. Meanwhile, we can construct

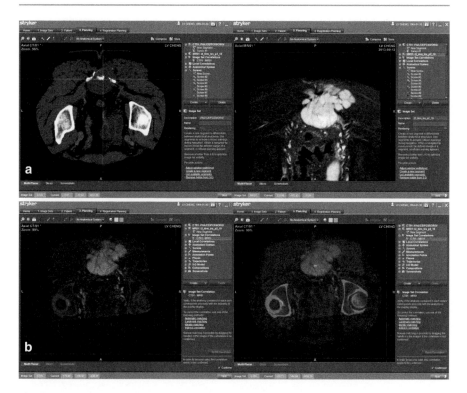

Fig. 26.55 (**a**) CT and MR images and (**b**) their fusion

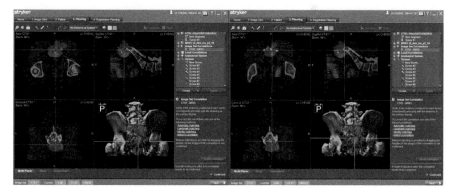

Fig. 26.56 The three-dimensional tumor model after marking the tumor borders

a three-dimensional tumor model from the CT DICOM data in order to better appreciate the real tumor configuration (Fig. 26.56). (4) Using the three-dimensional positioning of navigation symbols (screw tools), we can ensure and mark the closest bone and soft tissue tumor resection margins. The preoperative plan is shown in Figs. 26.57 and 26.58. (5) The navigation system is activated during surgery and introduces the

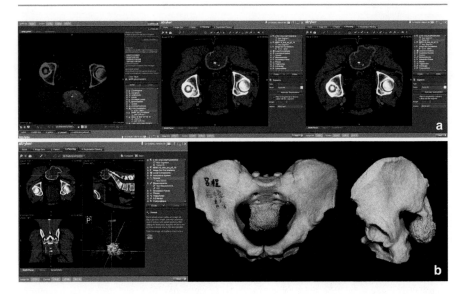

Fig. 26.57 (**a**, **b**) Layer by layer completion of the soft tissue tumor borders; positions of the screws were marked

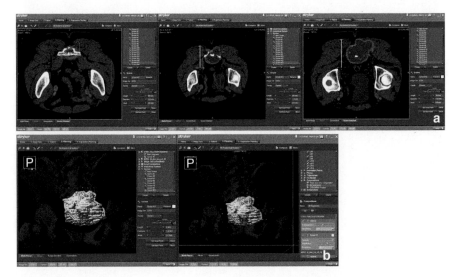

Fig. 26.58 (**a**) Fifteen millimeter from the highest intra-bone point of the tumor; marked screws were horizontally placed on the sacrum. (**b**) The smallest intra-bone and soft tissue resection margins were completed

completed preoperative plan from the navigation workstation into the intraoperative navigation system. CT is used to localize and scan the tumor region during surgery. The intraoperative CT images are fused with the preoperative CT images to complete a unified composite representation of the navigated preoperative design and

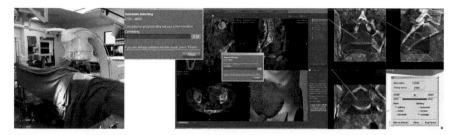

Fig. 26.59 Activation of the navigation system during surgery; computed tomography (CT) localization and scan of the tumor region; the fusion process of intraoperative and preoperative CT images

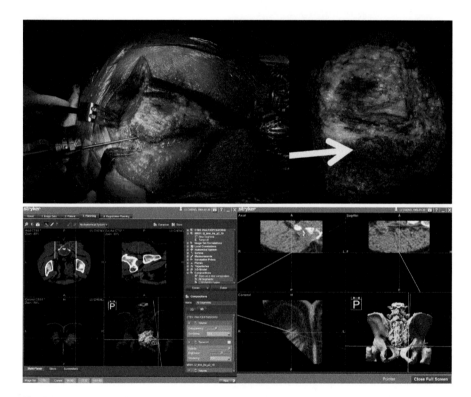

Fig. 26.60 Intraoperative real-time navigation of the soft tissue tumor resection margin determination; a comparison with the postoperative specimen

intraoperative real-time navigation data (Fig. 26.59). (6) Intraoperative real-time navigation can complete the determination of the sacral tumor and soft tissue margins and facilitate surgery completion (Figs. 26.60, 26.61, and 26.62). (7) Finally, a comparison of the postoperative specimen and CT images with the preoperative design and completion of the specimen surgical border evaluation will confirm adherence to the preoperative plan (Fig. 26.63).

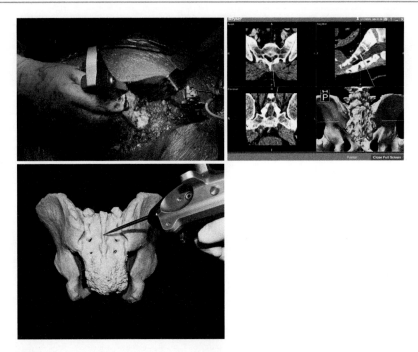

Fig. 26.61 Determination of the sacral osteotomy level and comparison with the three-dimensional tumor images

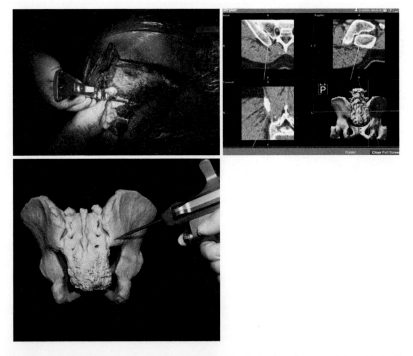

Fig. 26.62 Determination of the sacroiliac joint osteotomy level and comparison with the three-dimensional tumor images

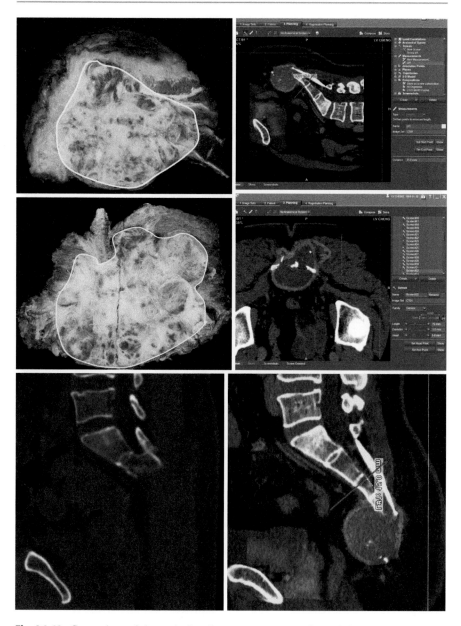

Fig. 26.63 Comparison of the sagittal and transverse cross sections of the specimen with the preoperative design; comparison of the postoperative computed tomography image with the preoperative design

References

1. Feng C, Yu D, Lin J. Orthopaedics in China: its past and present. Chin Med J. 1996;109(6):419.
2. Song XW. Excision-alcohol-replantation (EAR) method for bone grafting after tumor resection. Chin Med J. 1986;99(2):97.
3. Sung HW, Wang HM, Kuo DP, Hsu WP, Tsai YB. EAR method: an alternative method of bone grafting following bone tumor resection (a preliminary report). Semin Surg Oncol. 1986;2(2):90–8.
4. Xian-wen S. Excision alcohol replantation (EAR) method for bone grafting after tumor resection. Plast Reconstr Surg. 1987;79(5):855.
5. Van Doorslaer E, O'Donnell O, Rannan-Eliya RP, Somanathan A, Adhikari SR, Garg CC, et al. Effect of payments for health care on poverty estimates in 11 countries in Asia: an analysis of household survey data. Lancet. 2006;368(9544):1357–64.
6. DeVita VT, Lawrence TS, Rosenberg SA. DeVita, Hellman, and Rosenberg's cancer: principles & practice of oncology. Philadelphia: Wolters Kluwer Health/Lippincott Williams & Wilkins; 2011.
7. Niu X, Wang J. The professional consensus of classical osteosarcoma clinical treatments. Clin Oncol. 2012;17(10).
8. Enneking WF, Spanier SS, Goodman MA. A system for the surgical staging of musculoskeletal sarcoma. Clin Orthop Relat Res. 1980;153:106–20.
9. Kawaguchi N, Ahmed AR, Matsumoto S, Manabe J, Matsushita Y. The concept of curative margin in surgery for bone and soft tissue sarcoma. Clin Orthop Relat Res. 2004;419:165–72.
10. Matsumoto S, Kawaguchi N, Manabe J, Tanizawa T, Koyama S, Ae K, et al. Surgical treatment for bone and soft tissue sarcoma. Gan To Kagaku Ryoho. 2004;31(9):1314.
11. Niu XH, Cai YB, Hao L, Zhang Q, Ding Y, Liu WS, et al. Allograft replacement in management of giant cell tumor of bone: a report of 77 cases. Zhonghua Wai Ke Za Zhi. 2005;43(16):1058.
12. Niu X, Zhang Q, Hao L. Complications after allograft implantation. Chin J Bone Tumor Bone Dis. 2006;5(1):7–11.
13. Niu XH, Hao L, Zhang Q, Ding Y. Massive allograft replacement in management of bone tumors. Zhonghua Wai Ke Za Zhi. 2007;45(10):677.
14. Ding Y, Niu XH, Zhang Q, Ma K, Liu WF. The surgical treatment of primary malignant bone tumors of pelvis. Zhonghua Wai Ke Za Zhi. 2008;46(12):886.

Is It Reasonable for Orthopedic Surgeons to Do Chemotherapy for Patients with High-Grade Bone Sarcoma? A Paradigm for Treatment Individualization

27

Wei Guo, Lu Xie, and Jie Xu

27.1 Introduction

Malignant mesenchymal tumors arising from the bone and soft tissue, also known as sarcoma, are relatively rare forms of cancer and often require treatment with surgery, chemotherapy, radiation therapy, and other adjuvant treatments. Sarcomas are heterogenous groups of diseases, thus their treatments and patients outcomes are different. Doctors make their decisions for those particular patients according to the pathological diagnosis, stages, and general conditions. Musculoskeletal tumors are rare diseases. Let's take the most common disease for example: osteosarcoma. Osteosarcoma is classified as an orphan disease, with an overall incidence of 0.2–3/100,000 per year (0.8–11/100,000 per year in the age group 15–19 years) in the EU [1]. From the perspectives of pathologists, correct diagnosis requires abundant experience with pathological microscopic findings combined with clinical and radiographic features. Osteosarcoma is defined as a primary malignant tumor of the bone in which proliferating neoplastic cells produce osteoid and/or bone, if only in small amounts. This histological principle defines a tumor that usually affects young males more frequently than females and disproportionately involves the long bones of the appendicular skeleton. However, osteosarcoma is not a single disease but a family of neoplasms, sharing the single histological finding of osseous matrix production in association with malignant cells [2]. The majority (i.e., 75%) of cases are relatively stereotypical from the demographic, clinical, radiographic, and histological points of view. These tumors generally occur in the metaphyseal portion of the medullary cavity of the long bone and are referred to as conventional osteosarcoma. This group is subclassified by the form of the dominant matrix present within the tumor, which may be the bone, cartilage, or fibrous tissue, correspondingly referred

W. Guo, M.D., Ph.D. (✉) • L. Xie, M.D. • J. Xu, M.D.
Musculoskeletal Tumor Center, Peking University People's Hospital, Beijing, China
e-mail: bonetumor@163.com

© Springer International Publishing Switzerland 2017
R.M. Henshaw (ed.), *Sarcoma*, DOI 10.1007/978-3-319-43121-5_27

to as osteoblastic, chondroblastic, and fibroblastic osteosarcoma. The remaining 25% of cases have unique parameters that allow reproducible identification of tumors biologically different from conventional osteosarcoma and are referred to as variants. The parameters identifying variants fall into one of three major groups: (1) clinical factors, (2) histological findings, and (3) location of origin (e.g., within or on the cortex). Because of their inherent biological difference from conventional osteosarcoma, the variants identify cases which must be excluded from the analysis of data pertaining to the treatment of the majority of cases. Sometimes it is really difficult for even senior pathologists to give a correct or accurate diagnosis. In China, it is quite common for clinicians to confirm or even correct errors in diagnosis based on their clinical experience.

Moreover, current management for osteosarcoma comprises preoperative (neoadjuvant) chemotherapy followed by surgical removal of all detectable disease (including metastases) and postoperative (adjuvant) chemotherapy, preferably within the setting of clinical trials [3]. Preoperative chemotherapy is generally administered for a period of about 8–10 weeks prior to surgery. Following surgical resection and a brief lapse to allow for wound healing, postoperative adjuvant chemotherapy is continued for a period of another 12–29 weeks [4]. However, for neoadjuvant chemotherapy, 8–10 weeks is an obscure concept. When should we stop delivering the chemotherapy and prepare to do the operation is a question which needs to be discussed. Different patients and different subtypes of the osteosarcoma have different sensibilities to chemotherapy. Should each tumor center use a single preoperative chemotherapy strategy to treat those different people? During neoadjuvant chemotherapy, there are some situations that require clinicians to actively intervene, such as when tumor progression occurs during treatment.

Recently, most chemotherapy regimens used for osteosarcoma have been based around four drugs: high-dose methotrexate (HDMTX) with leucovorin rescue, doxorubicin (Adriamycin), cisplatin, and ifosfamide [5]. These agents were integrated into various chemotherapy protocols. Most current protocols include a period of preoperative (neoadjuvant) chemotherapy, even though this has not been shown to add a survival benefit over postoperative (adjuvant) chemotherapy alone [6]. The extent of histological response to preoperative chemotherapy, however, offers important prognostic information. Nowadays, from the perspective of pathological evaluation, during neoadjuvant chemotherapy, the tumor cell necrosis rate>90% for osteosarcoma can be seen in only 50–70% according to literature [1, 4, 7], which means there are around 30–50% patients who don't respond well to preoperative chemotherapy. For those patients, how can we identify them in a timely fashion and operate or intervene earlier? Clinicians who are also orthopedic surgeons may have advantages in doing this.

Osteosarcoma combined with pathologic fracture is also a difficult condition which needs to be handled properly. Different situations often imply a completely different prognosis [8]. For example, osteosarcoma of extremities with pathologic fracture due to minor trauma prior to treatment, in which the fracture heals during neoadjuvant chemotherapy, might benefit from preoperative chemotherapy and could acquire a more favorable prognosis. Those patients needed to be immobilized appropriately and started on preoperative chemotherapy with close observation in case of displacement or other orthopedic situations happened. When pathologic fractures happened during neoadjuvant chemotherapy without obvious trauma, this may indicate the tumor is responding poorly to chemotherapy and might need surgical intervention immediately. The right time and appropriate intervention measure might be handled better under the direct care of orthopedists specialized in musculoskeletal tumor.

27.2 Bone and Soft Tissue Sarcomas Need Individualized Therapy and Multidisciplinary Cooperation

Chemosensitivity varies in different kinds of sarcoma, according to their histological type. For some bone and soft tissue sarcomas, their histological features make them insensible to chemotherapy, for example, classical chondrosarcoma and some types of soft tissue sarcoma. There is no need to force these patients to go through chemotherapy. As noted for osteosarcoma, which is one of the most common types of bone cancer in children and adolescent, neoadjuvant chemotherapy followed by appropriate surgery and adjuvant chemotherapy has become the standard treatment in recent decades. For other kinds of sarcoma consisting of small round cells, such as Ewing sarcoma family of tumors and alveolar rhabdomyosarcoma, systematic chemotherapy may be more important than in other sarcomas. Soft tissue sarcoma (STS) is more complicated compared with bone sarcoma. The role of chemotherapy is controversial in STS. The decision of whether chemotherapy should be given is made according to the histology, clinical stages, tumor surgical margins, and the patients' general conditions. Broadly speaking, therapy should be individualized.

The department of surgical oncology in China is an offshoot of the general surgery department. Most medical oncology departments have been set up over the last 40 years, but the number of doctors remain particularly small because of low interest. In some remote provinces, there are even less than ten doctors with experience in musculoskeletal tumor. An appropriate medical team for sarcoma requires the engagement of surgeons, oncologists, radiologists, pathologists, and radiotherapists. In many hospitals, there are not enough doctors who majored in this area; thus surgeons, as the leading members in the whole medical team, are required to give chemotherapy. These surgeons became the precursor to chemosurgeons.

27.3 Classification of Chemosurgeons in China

There are two patterns of chemosurgeons in China. The first type is seen in the community or relatively small hospitals. Medical resources in China are concentrated in large hospitals, which have resulted in the serious lack of health-care resources for small communities. There are merely one or two professional surgeons in an entire province, let alone medical oncologists in these basic hospitals. Under this condition, these surgeons collaborate with oncologists specialized in other tumors, such as gastric cancer or lung cancer, developing and providing care as best they can. This kind of chemosurgeon is both a surgeon and chemotherapist. Most of the time, they work as surgeons, but they also administer chemotherapy when necessary.

The second type of chemosurgeon refers to surgeons receiving years of training in medical oncology in addition to surgery and is more common. Larger hospitals are richer in various kinds of medical resources and have more trained and experienced surgeons. As a result, they become more attractive to patients. For example, the incidence of osteosarcoma is merely three per million people, but in Peking University People's Hospital's Musculoskeletal Tumor Center, we perform more than 200 osteosarcoma operations per year. On the basis of a large number of patients, doctors in such a tumor center are expected to be more experienced and professional. Given its low incidence, neither surgeons nor medical oncologists who graduated from medical college with a doctor's degree are familiar enough with this kind of disease. Sarcoma itself is complex and calls for years of special training. Residents with surgical degrees working in this tumor center are provided the opportunity to manage patients with these kinds of rare diseases and understand those diseases better than those residents with an ordinary oncological degree or internal medical degree. At Peking University People's Hospital, for example, there are two wards in our institute, namely, the operation ward and the chemotherapy ward. Every doctor specializing in tumor surgery is trained in the operation ward for at least 3 years. After that, those who choose to be surgeons will be sent to the chemotherapy ward and receive medical oncology training for at least 3 months and then return to the surgical ward. Those who choose chemotherapy as their career will receive medical oncology training for a longer time and remain in the chemo ward for their career. The latter are referred to as chemosurgeons. Both the surgeons and the chemosurgeons work in the same tumor center and hold morning rounds together to discuss the patient treatment plans weekly.

27.4   Diagnosis and Treatment Procedures for Bone and Soft Tissue Sarcoma in China

Once bone or soft tissue sarcoma is suspected based on clinical and imaging features, patients diagnosed in community hospitals are advised to go to a professional multidisciplinary tumor center for further treatment, where doctors in multidisciplinary teams work together to make the patient's overall treatment plan. Biopsy, which is a complex cognitive skill for the surgeon, often comes as the first step in the whole procedure. After the tumor is confirmed by pathology, treatment options and recommendations are made depending on several factors, including the type and stage of tumor, possible side effects, and the patient's preferences and ECOG scores [9]. For this purpose, CT scan of the chest, whole-body bone SPECT, and sometimes PET-CT are indispensable. If the tumor is sensitive to some certain kind of drugs, and patient's ECOG Performance Status is less than two, neoadjuvant chemotherapy before surgery is recommended to reduce the size of tumor or relieve pain and other symptoms. This part of therapy will be done in the chemo ward where chemosurgeons are responsible for patient care. Chemosurgeons evaluate the benefits and the risks of drugs according to clinical manifestation, drug concentration, side effect, parameters in the lab, and changes in medical images and choose the best time to perform surgery.

When the patient recovers from chemotherapy, surgeons in the operation ward take over and select proper surgical methods balancing adequacy of oncologic resection, skeletal reconstruction, and functional outcome. For a tumor that can be surgically removed, clear oncological margin usually comes first. As soon as the patients recover from surgery, often 2 weeks later, they return to the same chemosurgeons to get adjuvant chemotherapy. This treatment regimen will be carefully selected considering their response to neoadjuvant therapy, necrosis rate, and tumor margin. Functional training after surgery will continue throughout the whole period of adjuvant chemotherapy, where chemosurgeons have a distinct advantage over ordinary medical oncologists. If necessary, chemosurgeons will discuss some patients' cases together with surgeons about whether the patient may need to do local radiotherapy and when to do it. Then during or after adjuvant chemotherapy, the patients may be transferred to radiotherapy ward to receive further treatment.

During the whole course of treatment, patients stay in the same tumor center, although they are transferred between different wards. Surgeons and chemosurgeons work together to observe and record the whole treatment course, thus facilitating them to formulate individualized strategy.

27.5   The Advantages of Orthopedists Doing Chemotherapy in China from the Perspective of Multidisciplinary Collaboration

1. It allows the orthopedists to monitor the whole course of the treatment of sarcoma, which will be beneficial for patients as their doctor to have an integrated and profound understanding of these diseases.

   Following the implementation of chemotherapy in the 1960s, the treatment of high-grade osteosarcoma (OS) has made important progress [10]. However, survival rates continue to be unsatisfactory in the metastatic and recurrent setting. Long-term outcome for patients with high-grade osteosarcoma has improved with the addition of systemic chemotherapy. Modern, multiagent, dose-intensive chemotherapy in conjunction with surgery achieves a 5-year event-free survival of 60–70% in extremity localized, nonmetastatic disease [7]. According to Zhang et al. [11], the mean 2-year overall survival of osteosarcoma was 64% in China (ranging from 37.5 to 77.6%); limb-salvage rate was 79%; relapse rate was 9.1% (ranging from 0.8 to 22.0%). Due to the different kinds of medical education available in different districts of China and the complicated development of musculoskeletal tumor centers, orthopedists provided chemotherapy for their patients in most hospitals.

As professional orthopedists specializing in musculoskeletal tumor, it is valuable to observe patients throughout their whole treatment course for sarcoma. This would especially benefit those junior residents who wish to specialize in musculoskeletal tumors, for they would have an integrated and profound understanding of these diseases. Young surgeons can learn to perform safe and effective biopsy techniques, learn to deliver neoadjuvant chemotherapy, evaluate the clinical chemotherapy effect on these tumors, and then assist with the surgical resection. They can learn how preoperative chemotherapy or the biopsy should be done to minimize problems with obtaining wide surgical margins and to facilitate limb-sparing surgery. After surgery, they could choose appropriate therapy for those patients, such as adjuvant chemotherapy and/or radiotherapy. Through involvement with those surgeries, they know what kind of therapy might be more useful. The rationale for a multidisciplinary treatment approach requires collaboration and teamwork. This experience for residents specializing in orthopedic tumors in their early years under the supervision of senior doctors helps them to collaborate better in their entire medical career.

2. It is more convenient for orthopedists to observe patients' postoperative recovery in progress, guide the postoperative rehabilitation training, and notice local recurrence as early as possible.

After surgery, most patients are transferred to the chemotherapy ward to receive further treatment. There are lots of conditions which need to be managed by orthopedists. For example, observing the wound healing progress so as to choose most appropriate timing to deliver postoperative chemotherapy needs to be dealt with immediately after surgery and is managed better by professional orthopedists. If too early, the chemotherapy might interfere with wound healing, causing increased wound effusion (especially for patients with arthroplasty), while if too late, it would delay the systemic treatment.

During the first half year after surgery, patients usually stay in the chemotherapy ward or frequently visit oncologists. If those doctors have orthopedic knowledge, they could supervise those patients for postoperative rehabilitation. Even more, they could adjust the training program according to the patients' chemotherapy course individually, which benefits patients more.

A total of 30–40% of patients with localized osteosarcoma will develop a local recurrence or distant metastasis [12]. Approximately 90% of relapses are lung metastasis, which usually occur in the first 2–3 years [13]. Osteosarcoma recurrences are associated with a rather poor prognosis [14]. Five-year overall survival (OAS) for recurrent osteosarcoma has been reported to be 23–29% (pulmonary metastases only 28–33%) [15]. The outlook is considered to be extremely poor for patients who present with synchronous regional bone metastasis (skip metastasis), either in the primary bone site or transarticular [15]. During the first year after operation, patients are usually monitored with routine radiological reexamination in the chemotherapy ward. Orthopedists who do double as oncologists are better suited to discover early local recurrences or bone metastasis and to perform surgical interventions early for the purpose of improving prognosis.

3. Orthopedists could make more precise clinical and radiologic evaluations for patients who receive chemotherapy.

Up to now, standardized clinical evaluation for bone tumors' response to chemotherapy has remained unclear. Some centers have used RECIST, which stands for Response Evaluation Criteria in Solid Tumor, to evaluate the effect of chemotherapy [16]. In the early 2009, RECIST 1.1 [17] was introduced and made some updates based on "the old RECIST," which included changes in evaluation for the number of lesions, pathological evaluation of lymph nodes, further refining of curative effect, and so on. However, "RECIST 1.1" continues to have its limitation for bone sarcoma. Because most sarcomas are originated from the bone or involve the bone, the maximum diameter to measure may not be obvious. This is because osseous lesions won't shrink as typically seen in soft tissue. Plus, sarcoma usually spreads by hematogenous seeding; lymph nodes are not as important as they are for other solid tumors. At the same time, there are many other osseous manifestations which were not included in the RECIST 1.1, for example, increase of ossification, bony shell formation of the tumor, emerging of sequestrum, and so on. Those imaging manifestations may easily be observed by professional orthopedists, and those orthopedic surgeons specialized in musculoskeletal tumor could make more precise clinical evaluation of neoadjuvant chemotherapy for patients with bone tumors.

4. It may be more convenient for orthopedists to carry out other kinds of adjuvant therapy, such as arterial infusion chemotherapy.

The neoadjuvant treatment of osteosarcoma using intravenous agents has resulted in survival rates of 55–77% [18]. Most treatment plans used multiagent drugs with cumulative side effects that effectively limited the dose and duration of any one drug in the regimen. At the same time, there were no concentration of chemotherapy at the site of the primary tumor, and normal healthy tissues received chemotherapeutic doses equal to that of the diseased tissues. Based on these observations, dose-intensified intra-arterial (IA) cisplatin was administered in some tumor centers in China. This response-based regimen used arteriography to serially assess tumor neovascularity and treatment response. It required doctors' acquaintance with anatomy, limb ischemic preconditioning, and post-conditioning knowledge. Thus, IA administration may be more appropriate for orthopedists specialized in oncology to carry out these clinical trials than conventional oncologists.

27.6 The Disadvantages of Chemosurgeons Administering Chemotherapy

Like any other new endeavor, this training system and treatment pattern in China has its shortcomings. We must face these difficulties, bear the risks, and explore various means of solving these problems.

1. Chemosurgeons have some difficulties in dealing with combined treatment and adverse effects, for they lack long-term practice and experience working as physicians.

   Chemosurgeons, who were trained in surgery while obtaining their MD, stay in the operation ward during their early residency, which means they lack long-term education, practice, and experience working as physicians. Even in the same institute, the chemotherapy ward is always separated from the operation ward, with totally different medical environments. Chemotherapy, tracing its root, developed from internal medicine. The whole therapeutic procedure of chemotherapy is long, precise, and individualized. Each chemotherapeutic drug has its unique characteristics, including pharmacokinetic pattern, dosage, administration, adverse reaction, and so on. Patients should be carefully monitored for toxicity. Severe adverse reaction, such as myelosuppression, can be lethal. It is extremely dangerous for untrained doctors to deliver chemotherapy. Acute infusion-related reactions in some new drugs are very common. It has been reported that patients with osteosarcoma get more benefit using pegylated liposomal doxorubicin than classic doxorubicin [19]. However, acute infusion-related reactions of this new form of doxorubicin include flushing, shortness of breath, facial swelling, headache, chills, back pain, tightness in the chest or throat, and/or hypotension in up to 10% of patients [20]. Medications/emergency equipment to treat such reactions should be available for immediate use. And most important of all, the doctors should be familiar with those medications and equipment to make good use of them.

   Adverse reactions, such as hand-foot syndrome, hepatic and renal function damage, hematologic toxicities, and stomatitis should be managed by dose delay and adjustments. Chemosurgeons, the so-called "midcareer" chemotherapists, are not familiar with these drugs so much as physicians, as a result of different priorities in the training system of surgeons and physicians. They lack experience in the use of chemo drugs, let alone in combined or compounded protocols, and sometimes are unprepared for various complications, especially for newcomers.

2. Chemosurgeons are focused only on sarcoma, which may impair their ability to use new drugs or promising clinical trials.

   The second question, which arises from the background of surgeons and the departments they belong to, is that chemosurgeons are unfamiliar with new drugs and treatments. Classically trained medical oncologists undergo a long term of training in different kinds of tumors, ensuring them a broad, general knowledge of cancer and antineoplastic drugs. Due to its low incidence, few pharmacological companies are motivated to design new agents for sarcoma, which means the systematic treatment of sarcoma often must borrow treatments introduced for other types of cancer, such as lymphoma, leukemia, and lung cancer. Chemosurgeons specialized in sarcoma do not have training experience in other cancer, and consequently, the opportunities are limited to learn about new drugs and other treatment methods. Thus chemosurgeons get fewer chances to take part in the development of new drugs, and what's more, they become less competitive in clinical trials and basic research.

For example, imatinib, the first tyrosine kinase inhibitor developed initially for CML and then for metastatic GIST, was first introduced in the treatment of musculoskeletal tumors in 2008 by Blay et al., who described the role of imatinib in diffuse type tenosynovial giant cell tumor (TGCT), also known as pigmented villonodular synovitis (PVNS) [21]. Another promising drug, trabectedin, an alkylating agent that binds to the DNA minor groove, originally isolated from the Caribbean sea squirt *Ecteinascidia turbinata,* has demonstrated its efficacy in the treatment of liposarcoma and leiomyosarcoma, as well as synovial sarcoma, beginning in 2009 [22, 23]. Chemosurgeons have had little experience with these drugs, impairing their ability to participate in promising clinical trials.

27.7 Methods to Solve These Problems

To solve these problems, we should reevaluate chemosurgeons' training procedures or working mode as the first step. Given the two kinds of chemosurgeons in China as described above, those who choose chemotherapy as their career after years of training in the operation ward appear to be on a better pathway for chemosurgeons.

Better knowledge of operation methods and adequate training of surgical skills facilitate chemosurgeons to perform their own biopsies, give reasonable advice in the postoperative rehabilitation, and notice local recurrence as soon as possible. However, once they have finished the training in the operation ward, they are sent to the chemo ward in the same department, where they are unfamiliar with some basic medical oncological knowledge and techniques, including adjustment of dosage, combination of drugs, and the ability to deal with adverse effect. What's more, an early insulation from other kinds of cancer with much higher incidence unfortunately impairs their familiarity with new or existing medications used in other fields. To overcome this difficulty, those who choose chemotherapy as their future career should be sent to a more comprehensive tumor center to receive general medical oncology training in all kinds of tumor for several years and then go back to their own battlefield. On the other hand, chemosurgeons majored in sarcoma are expected to take a more active part in medical oncology associations and conferences in the future, to collaborate and communicate further with experts in other fields, through which they can get a better sense of new promising drugs and treatment methods.

Furthermore, closer cooperation between orthopedists and chemosurgeons is required. Both the orthopedists and the chemosurgeons should work in the same tumor center and hold morning meetings at least once a week to discuss the treatment plan together. This close collaboration allows the orthopedists to monitor the whole course of the treatment of sarcoma and provides the chemosurgeons with important surgical information, such as neoplastic gross manifestation, surgical margins, and so on. It will be beneficial to have a better understanding of the therapeutic strategy of patients, opening the windows to the meaningful individualized multidisciplinary treatment. Finally we all think that "chemosurgeons" are just a temporary phenomenon here in China in the long-time development of Chinese medical teams specialized in sarcoma. It is apparent that close team work is essential for sarcoma treatment. And we also think that with more years' experience on clinical work, we will have more surgeons, oncologists as well as radiology doctors specially trained for sarcoma.

References

1. Bielack S, Carrle D, Casali PG, Group EGW. Osteosarcoma: ESMO clinical recommendations for diagnosis, treatment and follow-up. Ann Oncol. 2009;20(Suppl 4):137–9.
2. Raymond AK, Jaffe N. Osteosarcoma multidisciplinary approach to the management from the pathologist's perspective. Cancer Treat Res. 2009;152:63–84.
3. Chou AJ, Geller DS, Gorlick R. Therapy for osteosarcoma: where do we go from here? Paediatr Drugs. 2008;10:315–27.
4. Geller DS, Gorlick R. Osteosarcoma: a review of diagnosis, management, and treatment strategies. Clin Adv Hematol Oncol. 2010;8(10):705–18.
5. Ta HT, Dass CR, Choong PF, Dunstan DE. Osteosarcoma treatment: state of the art. Cancer Metastasis Rev. 2009;28(1–2):247–63.
6. Goorin AM, Schwartzentruber DJ, Devidas M, Gebhardt MC, Ayala AG, Harris MB, Helman LJ, Grier HE, Link MP, Pediatric OG. Presurgical chemotherapy compared with immediate surgery and adjuvant chemotherapy for nonmetastatic osteosarcoma: Pediatric Oncology Group Study POG-8651. J Clin Oncol. 2003;21-8:1574–80.
7. Luetke A, Meyers PA, Lewis I, Juergens H. Osteosarcoma treatment—Where do we stand? a state of the art review. Cancer Treat Rev. 2014;40(4):523–32.
8. Xie LGW, Li Y, Ji T, Sun X. Pathologic fracture does not influence local recurrence and survival in high-grade extremity osteosarcoma with adequate surgical margins. J Surg Oncol. 2012;106-7:820–5.
9. Oken MM, Creech RH, Tormey DC, Horton J, Davis TE, McFadden ET, Carbone PP. Toxicity and response criteria of the Eastern Cooperative Oncology Group. Am J Clin Oncol. 1982; 5(6):649–55.
10. Osteosarcoma: advances in treatment or changing natural history? Lancet. 1978;2(8080): 82–3.
11. Zhang Qing XW, Guo W. The current status of the treatment for osteosarcoma in China. Chin J Bone Tumor Bone Dis. 2009;8(3):129–32.
12. Kempf-Bielack B, Bielack SS, Jurgens H, Branscheid D, Berdel WE, Exner GU, Gobel U, Helmke K, Jundt G, Kabisch H, Kevric M, Klingebiel T, Kotz R, Maas R, Schwarz R, Semik M, Treuner J, Zoubek A, Winkler K. Osteosarcoma relapse after combined modality therapy: an analysis of unselected patients in the Cooperative Osteosarcoma Study Group (COSS). J Clin Oncol. 2005;23(3):559–68.
13. Ferrari S, Briccoli A, Mercuri M, Bertoni F, Picci P, Tienghi A, Del Prever AB, Fagioli F, Comandone A, Bacci G. Postrelapse survival in osteosarcoma of the extremities: prognostic factors for long-term survival. J Clin Oncol. 2003;21(4):710–5.
14. Franke M, Hardes J, Helmke K, et al. Solitary skeletal osteosarcoma recurrence. Findings from the Cooperative Osteosarcoma Study Group. Pediatr Blood Cancer. 2011;56:771–6.
15. Carrle D, Bielack S. Osteosarcoma lung metastases detection and principles of multimodal therapy. Cancer Treat Res. 2009;152:165–84.

16. Therasse P, Arbuck SG, Eisenhauer EA, Wanders J, Kaplan RS, Rubinstein L, Verweij J, Van Glabbeke M, van Oosterom AT, Christian MC, Gwyther SG. New guidelines to evaluate the response to treatment in solid tumors. European Organization for Research and Treatment of Cancer, National Cancer Institute of the United States, National Cancer Institute of Canada. J Natl Cancer Inst. 2000;92(3):205–16.

17. Duffaud F, Therasse P. New guidelines to evaluate the response to treatment in solid tumors. Bull Cancer. 2000;87(12):881–6.

18. Bacci G, Ferrari S, Longhi A, Forni C, Bertoni F, Fabbri N, Zavatta M, Versari M. Neoadjuvant chemotherapy for high grade osteosarcoma of the extremities: long-term results for patients treated according to the Rizzoli IOR/OS-3b protocol. J Chemother. 2001;13(1):93–9.

19. Gabizon AA. Pegylated liposomal doxorubicin: metamorphosis of an old drug into a new form of chemotherapy. Cancer Invest. 2001;19(4):424–36.

20. Gibbs DD, Pyle L, Allen M, Vaughan M, Webb A, Johnston SR, Gore ME. A phase I dose-finding study of a combination of pegylated liposomal doxorubicin (Doxil), carboplatin and paclitaxel in ovarian cancer. Br J Cancer. 2002;86(9):1379–84.

21. Blay JY, El Sayadi H, Thiesse P, Garret J, Ray-Coquard I. Complete response to imatinib in relapsing pigmented villonodular synovitis/tenosynovial giant cell tumor (PVNS/TGCT). Ann Oncol. 2008;19(4):821–2.

22. Gronchi A, Bui BN, Bonvalot S, Pilotti S, Ferrari S, Hohenberger P, Hohl RJ, Demetri GD, Le Cesne A, Lardelli P, Perez I, Nieto A, Tercero JC, Alfaro V, Tamborini E, Blay JY. Phase II clinical trial of neoadjuvant trabectedin in patients with advanced localized myxoid liposarcoma. Ann Oncol. 2012;23(3):771–6.

23. Grosso F, Sanfilippo R, Virdis E, et al. Trabectedin in myxoid liposarcoma (MLS): a long-term analysis of a single-institution series. Ann Oncol. 2009;20:1439–44.

The Current Situation and Experience of Multidisciplinary Treatment of Soft Tissue Sarcoma in China

28

Chunlin Zhang, Zhongsheng Zhu, and Kun Peng Zhu

28.1 Introduction

STS are a heterogeneous group of rare tumors that arise predominantly from the embryonic mesoderm. STS has more than 50 distinct histological subtypes and occur in various anatomic locations in addition to the extremities, including the chest wall, retroperitoneum, and head/neck. Extremity soft tissue sarcomas exhibit numerous histological subtypes, with undifferentiated pleomorphic sarcoma, liposarcoma, leiomyosarcoma, synovial sarcoma, epithelioid sarcoma, and malignant peripheral nerve sheath tumor being among the most common subtypes in adults. They may be low or high grade and subcutaneous or deep in location. The vast majority metastasize hematogenously, though select subtypes can also spread through the lymphatic system [1]. Although they are rare, accounting for less 1% of all malignant tumors, half of patients diagnosed will die from the sarcoma [2]. Patients typically demonstrate a median survival ranging from 11 to 18 months from the time of diagnosis with advanced disease [3].

Optimal management of soft tissue sarcoma relies upon an appropriately performed biopsy, accurate diagnosis and staging, an effective surgical plan and execution, rational utilization of adjuvant therapies, and close surveillance following resection. This is best carried out at a tertiary care center with an experienced multidisciplinary team specializing in the care of sarcoma patients. The cancer multidisciplinary team (MDT) represents a new clinical model, capable of breaking the barriers between disciplines, exploring new ideas, and brainstorming with

C. Zhang, M.D. (✉) • K.P. Zhu, M.D.
Department of Orthopaedic Surgery, Shanghai Tenth People's Hospital, Tongji University, Shanghai, China
e-mail: shzhangchunlin@163.com

Z. Zhu, M.D.
Department of Orthopaedic Surgery, Central Hospital of Fengxian District, Shanghai Sixth People's Hospital, Shanghai Jiao Tong University, Shanghai, China

© Springer International Publishing Switzerland 2017
R.M. Henshaw (ed.), *Sarcoma*, DOI 10.1007/978-3-319-43121-5_28

colleagues from different specialties. Radiotherapy, chemotherapy, and surgery are the main methods of treatment of soft tissue sarcoma in China. Among these three treatments, whether used alone or combined, surgery remains the main method. For some highly selected cases, a small scale of resection of soft tissue sarcoma, with postoperative inside or outside irradiation, can reduce damage to important structures, preserving more function, without an increase in the local recurrence rate.

28.2   Clinical Presentation

The typical presenting complaint of a patient diagnosed with soft tissue sarcoma is that of a painless enlarging mass. Characteristics such as size greater than 5 cm, location deep to fascia, and rapid tumor growth are worrisome and should raise suspicion of a sarcoma. Appropriate workup of a suspected sarcoma should begin with a careful history and physical examination. Important elements of the history are duration of mass, rate of growth, pain, weakness or numbness, history of trauma, exposure to radiation or other carcinogenic toxins, personal or family history of cancer, and smoking history. Clinical symptoms and signs of sarcoma, apart from a mass effect, may include joint activity limitation and neurovascular compression. The examination should note the characteristics of the size, margins and consistency of the mass, transillumination to rule out cyst, presence of pain with palpation, its anatomic compartment and location relative to the fascia and neurovascular structures, regional lymph node examination, and neurovascular examination of the affected extremity.

28.3   Imaging

Any patient in China with a suspected STS should be referred to a diagnostic center for triple assessment with clinical history, imaging, and biopsy. Radiographs of the affected extremity should be obtained and scrutinized for the presence and size of a soft tissue shadow, bony destruction, and intratumoral calcifications. Magnetic resonance imaging (MRI) is the necessary examination for evaluation of a potential soft tissue sarcoma, both for diagnostic characterization and staging purposes to plan effective management. A soft tissue sarcoma will typically exhibit heterogeneous high signal intensity on T2-weighted images. There may also be substantial peritumoral edema. T1-weighted images best demonstrate normal anatomy and its relation to the tumor and typically are relied upon for preoperative planning and surgery border. While the preferred method of imaging is MRI, other options including computerized tomography (CT) or ultrasound may be appropriate depending on local expertise. Patients with a confirmed STS should be staged with a high-resolution CT chest to exclude pulmonary metastases and abdominal ultrasound to observe abdominal situation prior to definitive treatment [4]. Isotope bone scan is not recommended as routine examination in China, as the incidence of bone metastasis is extremely low. CT abdomen and pelvis are included for myxoid liposarcomas and other sarcomas that can go to lymph nodes. There are several roles for FDG-PET in soft tissue sarcoma including: grading of tumors, initial staging, assessing response to neo-adjuvant therapy, determining prognosis, and investigating potential local recurrence [5]. However, PET imaging cannot be recommended as a routine staging investigation in patients with STS because of its expense for most patients as it is not covered by medical insurance in China, although it is used in patients who can afford the cost.

28.4 Biopsy

A histological diagnosis is needed to guide treatment planning. The standard approach to diagnosis of a suspicious mass is core needle biopsy: it is quicker than open biopsy and cheaper, and morbidity is lower, while open incision biopsy has a high complication rate (12–17%) [6]. However, an incisional biopsy may be necessary on occasion, and excisional biopsy may be the most practical option for superficial lesions <5 cm diameter. The biopsy should be planned in such a way that the biopsy tract can be safely removed at the time of definitive surgery to reduce the risk of seeding and should be performed either at a diagnostic clinic or by a sarcoma surgeon or radiologist following discussion with the surgeon. In China, most biopsies are completed by the orthopedic surgeon, who will choose a core needle biopsy or open biopsy based on the location of the lesion and the surgeon's preferences. X-ray or CT-guided biopsy can increase the accuracy of needle biopsy. In large tumor centers, needle biopsy has increasingly replaced open incision biopsy. We usually use 9G–11G needles for this purpose.

28.5 Staging

Information on tumor stage can help estimate prognosis and survival and plan management. Several systems are used to stage soft tissue sarcoma in the world. The most widely accepted STS classification system is the TMN system produced jointly by the American Joint Committee on Cancer (AJCC) (Table 28.1) [7], which includes information on both the grade and stage of the tumor. Although compartmental extent has not been shown to definitively affect prognosis, it is widely accepted as an important surgical consideration and is represented in the system described by Enneking and adopted by the Musculoskeletal Tumor Society (MSTS) (Table 28.2) [8]. We use the MSTS tumor grading system in our center. In China, medical oncologists like to use AJCC staging system, while surgeons prefer to use MSTS staging system. This is likely due to physicians being concerned about the patients' systemic situation, while the surgeon mainly focuses on the scope and modalities of operation.

Table 28.1 American Joint Committee on Cancer grading system (AJCC)

Tumor size				
T1		5 cm or less		
T2		>5 cm		
Location				
a		Superficial		
b		Deep		
Lymph nodes				
N0		No nodal metastases		
N1		Nodal metastasis present		
Distant metastases				
M0		No distant metastases		
M1		Distant metastases present		
Histologic grade				
G1		Low		
G2		Intermediate		
G3		High		
Group/stage	T	N	M	Histologic grade
IA	T1a/b	N0	M0	G1
IB	T2a/b	N0	M0	G1
IIA	T1a/b	N0	M0	G2,G3
IIB	T2a/b	N0	M0	G2,G3
III	T2a/b	N0	M0	G3
IV	Any T	N1	M1	Any G

Table 28.2 Musculoskeletal Tumour Society staging system/Enneking

Stage	Grade	Site
IA	Low	Intracompartmental
IB	Low	Extracompartmental
IIA	High	Intracompartmental
IIB	High	Extracompartmental
III	Any	Regional or distant metastases (or both)

28.6 Management Options

Limb salvage indications: (1) limb salvage surgery can obtain a satisfactory surgical border (margin), (2) important neurovascular bundle remains uninvolved, (3) soft tissue coverage is obtainable, (4) preserved limb function is better than expected artificial limb (prosthesis), and (5) distant metastasis is not a contraindication for limb salvage.

Table 28.3 Classification of surgical margins in soft tissue sarcoma [9]

Type	Surgical dissection	Outcome
Intralesional	Margin runs through the tumor	Microscopic disease remains
Marginal	Surgical margin runs through pseudocapsule or reactive zone	Tumor satellites remain in the reactive tissue—high local recurrence rate
Wide	En bloc resection within the same compartment as the tumor with a cuff of normal tissue	May leave skip lesions—low recurrence rate
Radical	En bloc resection of the entire compartment	No residual—minimal risk of local recurrence

Amputation indications: (1) patient request or consent to amputation, (2) important neurovascular bundle involved, (3) lack of reconstruction options for bone or soft tissue defects after limb salvage, (4) artificial limb function better than expected salvage limb, and (5) regional or distant metastasis not a contraindication for surgical amputation.

The major therapeutic goals are long-term survival, avoidance of local recurrence, maximizing function, and minimizing morbidity. Surgery is the standard treatment for all patients with adult-type, localized soft tissue sarcomas. It aims to excise the soft tissue sarcoma completely, along with a biological barrier of normal tissue, commonly accepted as 3–5 cm soft tissue. However, a tumor's proximity to important anatomical structures such as nerves and blood vessels can make it difficult to achieve an acceptable tumor-free margin. In this situation, we must evaluate the resectability of a tumor by the surgeon in consultation with the MDT and decide the upon the surgical plan (Table 28.3) accord to the tumor stage, patient's physical condition, risks of recurrence, morbidity of more radical surgery, and patient's demands. For patients who have undergone surgery and/or have an unplanned positive margin, re-excision should be undertaken if adequate margins can be achieved. Advances in reconstructive techniques have enabled limb preservation in complex cases by use of pedicle flaps and free tissue transfers.

In some situations, amputation may be the most appropriate surgical option to obtain local control and offer the best chance of cure. The main indications for amputation are related to tumor size and extent, NV involvement, difficult soft and bone tissue reconstruction, unresectable recurrence, uncontrolled infection, and presence of fungating mass. Typically in patients with high grade, large, or recurrent disease, the tumors often affect anatomically important sites. They are likely to have poor long-term survival, and the need to relieve local symptoms such as pain or fungation may outweigh negative factors associated with amputation.

The benefit of adjuvant radiation therapy has been clearly demonstrated in the treatment of soft tissue sarcomas. Most intermediate- or high-grade soft tissue sarcomas, large deep low-grade sarcomas, and incompletely resectable tumors that are close to important structures (such as nerves and blood vessels) are candidates for radiotherapy [10]. The effect of radiation is believed to be exerted by sterilization of the tumor capsule, i.e., killing the microscopic extensions of the tumor. This both decreases the intrinsic risks of local recurrence and also permits the sparing of critical normal tissue structures with focal marginal resection planes. In general, a standard dose of preoperative radiation involves 50Gy delivered over a 5-week period. Surgery then follows after a 3–4-week "rest" period to allow the overlying soft tissues to heal. Postoperative radiation doses are higher, approximately 65Gy delivered over 6–7 weeks, and are usually delivered after the wound has been determined to heal (usually at 3–6 weeks postoperatively).

The optimum timing of radiotherapy relative to surgery for soft tissue sarcoma of the extremities has been controversial since the 1980s. The difference in the rate of tumor recurrence and overall survival between preoperative radiotherapy and postoperative radiotherapy are inconsistent from various reports, and both alternatives have benefits and drawbacks. Preoperative radiotherapy has the potential advantage of producing a better functional outcome than postoperative radiotherapy, due to smaller treatment volumes and lower doses, but the main disadvantage of preoperative radiation is a higher risk of acute wound healing complications. The complications associated with postoperative radiotherapy include joint stiffness, edema, and pathological fractures; on balance we prefer postoperative radiotherapy.

The role of adjuvant chemotherapy in the management of soft tissue sarcoma of the extremities is controversial, particularly when comparing adjuvant chemotherapy versus neoadjuvant chemotherapy, as the evidence for its use is conflicting. In general, these regimens are highly toxic and have failed to show long-term survival benefits. Different histological subtypes vary greatly to chemosensitivity so the decision of whether chemotherapy should be given is made according to the histology, clinical stages, tumor surgical margins, and the patients' general conditions. Broadly speaking, therapy should be individualized. Evidence showed that there are effective chemotherapy drugs for rhabdomyosarcoma, angiosarcoma, synovial sarcoma, and liposarcoma [11], but there is a lack of large case reports or prospective clinical studies. Due to unbalanced development of musculoskeletal tumor centers in China and the complexity of soft tissue sarcoma chemotherapy, chemotherapy of soft tissue sarcoma may be administered by oncology physicians, although there are a few musculoskeletal tumor centers where surgeons administer chemotherapy themselves.

Currently, the first-line chemotherapy program in soft tissue sarcoma mainly includes 2–4 cycles preoperation: (1) MAID program:Mesna + ADM + IFO + DTIC; (2) AIM program:ADM + IFO + Mesna; and (3) AC + IE program, (ADM + CTX) + (IFO + VP16) alternately. Second-line chemotherapy included: (1) GT program:GEM + TXT and (2) IEP program:IFO + VP16 + DDP.

Indications for neoadjuvant chemotherapy include: (1) chemosensitive soft tissue sarcoma, (2) expected poor limb function, (3) waiting period before palliative surgery, and (4) isolated limb perfusion chemotherapy. Indications for adjuvant chemotherapy include: (1) high-risk patients, (2) highly malignant tumor (G3), and (3) marginal resection of highly malignant tumor (including intraoperative tumor contamination).

If neoadjuvant chemo tumor necrosis is less than 90%, we prefer to change to another chemo protocol. Isolated limb perfusion is used to treat melanoma. This treatment can be used to reduce tumor size to enable limb salvage procedures or for palliative treatment. It is widely used in Europe to treat soft tissue sarcoma of the extremities, but it is rarely used in China.

Following definitive treatment of a soft tissue sarcoma, it is very important that patients be followed closely for potential development of local recurrence or metastatic disease in order to permit early detection and treatment. This reinforces the need for close surveillance, including regular history and clinical examination to look for local recurrence, with ultrasound or magnetic resonance imaging as needed. As most metastases are likely to occur within the lung, CT scanning of the chest at routine intervals for surveillance is indicated. In China, we recommend a CT scan of the chest every 3 months for the first 2 years postoperatively, every 6 months for the third year, and after once a year thereafter.

28.7   Multidisciplinary Approach in China

Management of soft tissue sarcomas requires a multidisciplinary approach which is also performed in China. Decisions about surgery, chemotherapy, radiotherapy, and the timing of all these modalities should be made by the sarcoma MDT. The sarcoma MDT members consist of orthopedics, medical oncology, general surgery, radiology, pathology, interventional radiology, and other relevant departments to jointly establish a treatment group. MDTs are supported financially by the hospital's leadership. In addition, we have set up a sarcoma MDT clinic to see patients as a team. The MDT holds regular meetings, usually once a month or when special, and emergent cases need to be discussed. The content of MDT meeting includes:

(1) Case presentations to confirm the treatment protocol for patients newly diagnosed, to review postoperative cases and recurrent cases, discuss patients not suitable for standard treatment, review difficult and complicated cases, and consider efficacy assessments

(2) Development of clinical practice guidelines for soft tissue sarcoma, updated yearly

(3) Education through the introduction of the latest developments in respective professional disciplines within the MDT project team members, in order to exchange information and share resource.

At our facility, the orthopedists (orthopedic oncologists) monitor the whole course of the treatment of soft tissue sarcoma. The team will take into account the tumor's site, stage, the patient's comorbidities, and treatment preferences. Limb salvage surgery combined with postoperative radiotherapy is standard treatment of limb and truncal tumors in China and achieves high rates of local control while maintaining optimal function. Our current protocols for the diagnosis and treatment of soft tissue sarcoma are summarized as flow charts. (Figs. 28.1–28.4).

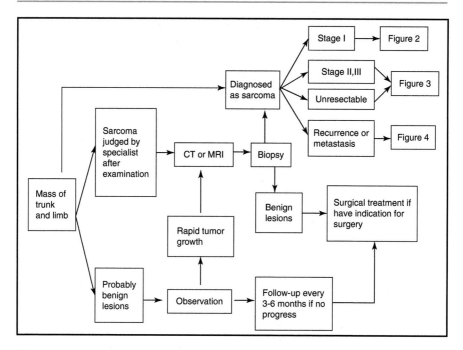

Fig. 28.1 Procedures of diagnosis and treatment of soft tissue tumor

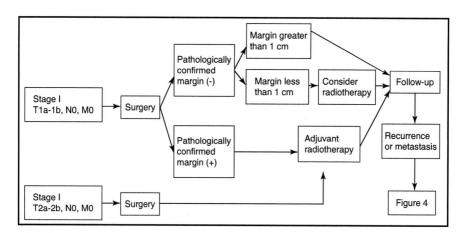

Fig. 28.2 Procedures of diagnosis and treatment for stage I soft tissue sarcoma

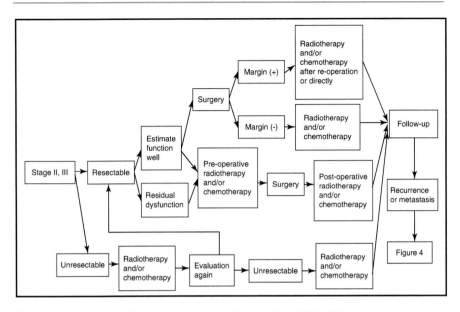

Fig. 28.3   Procedures of diagnosis and treatment for stage II and III soft tissue sarcoma

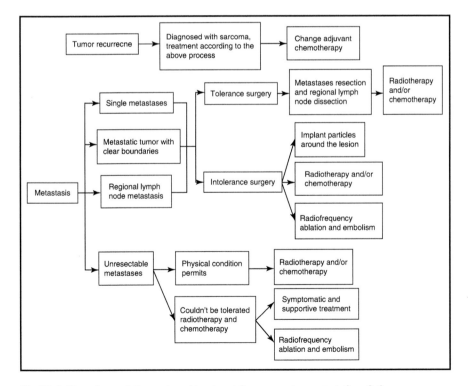

Fig. 28.4   Procedures of diagnosis and treatment for recurrent or metastatic soft tissue sarcoma

28.8 Conclusion

1. The use of limb perfusion in China is much less than that in Europe.
2. Postoperative radiotherapy is performed more frequently than preoperative radiotherapy, different from Australia.
3. Conventional chemotherapy is applied before and after surgery.
4. Open biopsy used more frequently than needle biopsy.
5. En bloc resection remains the goal of surgical treatment.
6. Follow-up in accordance with international conventions is encouraged.

28.9 Case Example

28.9.1 Patient Data

One male patient, aged 52 years, had an enlarging soft tissue mass involving the right thigh for more than 2 months and was admitted to the hospital. This patient had no history of trauma or local radiation exposure. The mass had been growing rapidly and painlessly.

Physical examination: Examination revealed a 8 × 12 cm palpable mass that was observed and palpated on the anteromedial of the right proximal thigh, with hard texture, border clearance, fixed position, no tenderness, no local skin warmth, no venous engorgement, and no enlarged lymph nodes in the groin area.

28.9.2 Imaging

Ultrasound examination: there was a cystic mass and scattered blood flow signal within the muscle of right thigh. X-ray: soft tissue mass with punctate calcification in right proximal thigh and no bone destruction and periosteal reaction in the right femur (Fig. 28.5). MRI: a 12 × 8 × 5 cm oval mass was in the quadriceps gap of the right thigh. There was equal and patchy low signal on T1-weighted image, while high signal was apparent in the center of the mass on T2-weighted images surrounded by a peripheral portion that was significantly intensified after administration of contrast. Small punctate low-signal image observed in the tumor mass with T2-weighted images was considered to represent calcification. There was no involvement of the femur. MRA was performed: the tumor was supplied by the lateral femoral circumflex artery (Fig. 28.6). Isotope bone scan: radiation uptake was displayed in right proximal thigh. CT chest showed no metastasis.

Fig. 28.5 X-ray
demonstrated a soft tissue
shadow and intratumoral
calcifications with no bony
destruction in proximal
thigh

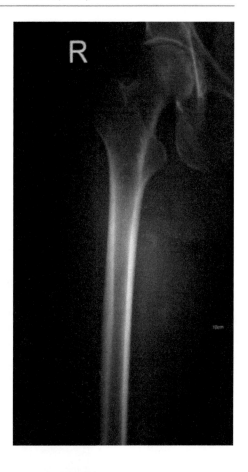

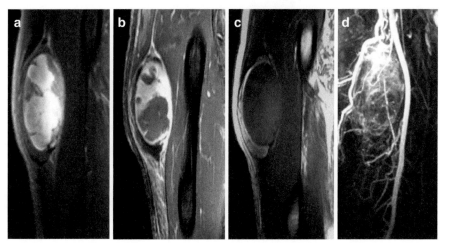

Fig. 28.6 MRI (**a–c**) and MRA (**d**) showed myxoid mass T1 low signal, T2 high signal, the
borders of the tumor, and the relationship with the surrounding neurovascular clearly

28.9.3 Biopsy

The tumor biopsy was performed with a core needle biopsy; microscopic examination revealed tumor cells demonstrating spindle-shaped cells organized as small polygons with osteoid formation, with mitotic figures. Ki-67 was expressed about 25% positive by immunohistochemistry. Preoperative clinical diagnosis: malignant soft tissue tumor in upper right thigh, extraskeletal osteosarcoma, Enneking stage system IIB.

28.9.4 Treatment

This patient received two cycles of neoadjuvant chemotherapy (AP + MTX + IFO). After two cycles, assessment showed no change of symptoms, physical signs or change in pre- and post-contrast MRI images. En bloc surgery with limb salvage was decided by the multidisciplinary team, and surgery was performed by orthopedic surgeons (orthopedic oncologists). Tumor was found mainly located between the vastus intermedius and vastus medialis with involvement of part of the rectus femoris, but did not invade the femur or periosteum. The surgical goal was wide resection of the tumor, requiring removal of the vastus intermedius, vastus medialis, and most of the rectus femoris. Resection of the primary biopsy tract and skin and ligation of the tumor blood vessels were also performed. Tumor specimen (Fig. 28.7) was sent for pathological examination after excision. Pathological diagnosis was well-differentiated extraskeletal osteosarcoma, with many mitotic figures and a lot of cartilage-like matrix. Immunohistochemical staining of tumor tissue showed the

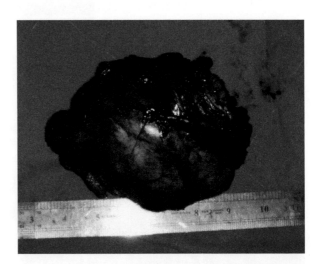

Fig. 28.7 Soft tissue sarcoma specimen

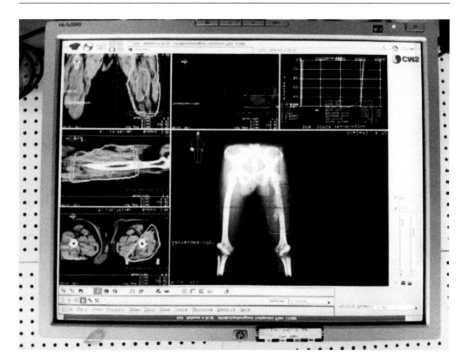

Fig. 28.8 Plan of radiation therapy; the *green* part represented the original tumor bed, and *purple* part was the radiation field

following: SMA (+), S-100 (+), HMB45 (−), and DES (−) CK (−). After recovery from surgery, the patient received four cycles of chemotherapy (AP + MTX + IFO), starting 3 weeks postoperatively.

The tumor bed was treated with external irradiation over a 6-week period starting 4 weeks postoperatively in the department of radiation oncology (Fig. 28.8). The target volume was the original tumor bed with a 5 cm margin in all planes. The treatment plan was optimized by using TPS (treatment plan system) with 6MVX line with the same center of daily irradiation, first giving DT 50Gy/25Fx/5w, with a shrinking field for the local tumor bed at the sixth week boosting the total dose to the tumor bed, DT 60Gy/30Fx/6w.

28.9.5 Follow-Up

The patient was able to be followed according to our soft tissue tumor surveillance schedule and had a good outcome with no recurrence or metastasis during 5 years of follow-up.

Conclusion

Overall, multidisciplinary collaboration plays a vital role in the diagnosis and treatment of soft tissue sarcoma. Soft tissue sarcoma patients in China have benefited from the MDT treatment.

References

1. Cormier JN, Pollock RE. Soft tissue sarcomas. CA Cancer J Clin. 2004;54:94–109.
2. Rydholm A. Improving the management of soft tissue sarcoma. Diagnosis and treatment should be given in specialist centres. BMJ. 1998;317:93–4.
3. Italiano A, Mathoulin-Pelissier S, Cesne AL, Terrier P, Bonvalot S, et al. Trends in survival for patients with metastatic soft-tissue sarcoma. Cancer. 2011;117:1049–54.
4. Christie-Large M, James SL, Tiessen L, Davies AM, Grimer RJ. Imaging strategy for detecting lung metastases at presentation in patients with soft tissue sarcomas. Eur J Cancer. 2008;44: 1841–5.
5. Conrad 3rd EU, Morgan HD, Vernon C, Schuetze SM, Eary JF. Fluorodeoxyglucose positron emission tomography scanning: basic principles and imaging of adult soft-tissue sarcomas. J Bone Joint Surg Am. 2004;86-A(Suppl 2):98–104.
6. Strauss DC, Qureshi YA, Hayes AJ, Thway K, Fisher C, et al. The role of core needle biopsy in the diagnosis of suspected soft tissue tumours. J Surg Oncol. 2010;102:523–9.
7. AJCC cancer staging manual, 7th edn, New York: Springer; 2009.
8. Enneking WF, Spanier SS, Goodman MA. A system for the surgical staging of musculoskeletal sarcoma. Clin Orthop Relat Res. 1980;153:106–20.
9. Enneking WF, Spanier SS, Goodman MA. A system for the surgical staging of musculoskeletal sarcoma. 1980. Clin Orthop Relat Res. 2003;415:4–18.
10. O'Sullivan B, Davis AM, Turcotte R, Bell R, Catton C, et al. Preoperative versus postoperative radiotherapy in soft-tissue sarcoma of the limbs: a randomised trial. Lancet. 2002;359: 2235–41.
11. Gortzak E, Azzarelli A, Buesa J, Bramwell VH, van Coevorden F, et al. A randomised phase II study on neo-adjuvant chemotherapy for 'high-risk' adult soft-tissue sarcoma. Eur J Cancer. 2001;37:1096–103.